# Advances in Drug Development Research

# Advances in Drug Development Research

Edited by **Ned Burnett**

SYRAWOOD
PUBLISHING HOUSE

New York

Published by Syrawood Publishing House,
750 Third Avenue, 9th Floor,
New York, NY 10017, USA
www.syrawoodpublishinghouse.com

**Advances in Drug Development Research**
Edited by Ned Burnett

International Standard Book Number: 978-1-68286-192-9 (Hardback)

Printed in the United States of America.

# Contents

# Preface

Drug development is extremely necessary to cure the critical diseases and also to enhance the therapeutic effect of existing drugs. This book consists of contributions made by international experts of pharmaceutical sciences. Various aspects of chemically defined therapeutic and toxic agents, experimental pharmacology, clinical trials, etc. have been elucidated in this book. Also included are significant researches that will provide a thorough understanding of the current status of this scientific discipline. As a reference material, this book will be highly beneficial for post graduate students and research scholars pursuing pharmaceutical sciences.

After months of intensive research and writing, this book is the end result of all who devoted their time and efforts in the initiation and progress of this book. It will surely be a source of reference in enhancing the required knowledge of the new developments in the area. During the course of developing this book, certain measures such as accuracy, authenticity and research focused analytical studies were given preference in order to produce a comprehensive book in the area of study.

This book would not have been possible without the efforts of the authors and the publisher. I extend my sincere thanks to them. Secondly, I express my gratitude to my family and well-wishers. And most importantly, I thank my students for constantly expressing their willingness and curiosity in enhancing their knowledge in the field, which encourages me to take up further research projects for the advancement of the area.

**Editor**

# Pharmacokinetics and tolerability of zibotentan (ZD4054) in subjects with hepatic or renal impairment: two open-label comparative studies

Helen Tomkinson*, John Kemp, Stuart Oliver, Helen Swaisland, Maria Taboada, Thomas Morris

## Abstract

**Background:** Zibotentan (ZD4054) is a specific endothelin A ($ET_A$) receptor antagonist being investigated for the treatment of prostate cancer. As zibotentan is eliminated by renal and metabolic routes, clearance may be reduced in patients with hepatic or renal impairment, leading to greater drug exposure.

**Methods:** Open-label studies investigated the PK and tolerability of zibotentan in subjects with hepatic or renal impairment, compared with those with normal organ function. In the hepatic and renal studies, respectively, subjects were divided into categories using Child-Pugh classification or 24-hour urine creatinine clearance (mild, moderate, or severe impairment and normal function). Each subject received a single oral dose of zibotentan 10 mg and PK sampling was undertaken. Within the hepatic study, AUC and $C_{max}$ were expressed as the ratio of geometric means and 90% CI for each impairment group compared with the normal function group. The possibility that hepatic impairment had a clinically relevant effect on exposure was considered if the upper 90% CI for the ratio exceeded 2. In the renal study, AUC, $C_{max}$ and $t_{1/2}$ were analyzed using linear regression fitting effects for creatinine clearance and age.

**Results:** In the hepatic and renal studies respectively, 32 subjects (eight per group) and 48 subjects received treatment (n = 18 normal, n = 12 mild, n = 9 moderate, n = 9 severe). Zibotentan $C_{max}$ was not significantly affected by hepatic or renal impairment. Compared with the normal function group, zibotentan AUC was 40% (1.40; 90% CI 0.91-2.17), 45% (1.45; 90% CI 0.94-2.24) and 190% (2.90; 90% CI 1.88-4.49) higher in subjects with mild, moderate and severe hepatic impairment, respectively, and 66% (1.66; 90% CI 1.38-1.99), 89% (1.89; 90% CI 1.50-2.39) and 117% (2.17; 90% CI 1.64-2.86) higher in subjects with mild, moderate and severe renal impairment, respectively. In both studies mean $t_{1/2}$ increased and zibotentan clearance decreased with the degree of impairment. Headache was the most common AE in all groups.

**Conclusions:** Zibotentan absorption was unchanged, however, exposure was higher in subjects with hepatic or renal impairment due to slower clearance. This increased exposure did not result in differences in the range or severity of AEs observed.

**Trial Registration:** ClinicalTrials.gov: NCT00672581 and AstraZeneca study number D4320C00016 (renal trial; conducted in Germany).

## Background

Prostate cancer is a leading cause of death in men in the Western world, accounting for an estimated 28% of new cancer cases in men in the US in 2010 [1]. Patients with advanced prostate cancer are initially treated with androgen deprivation therapy; however, disease progression will eventually occur in many men despite castrate serum androgen levels. This stage of disease is defined as castration-resistant prostate cancer (CRPC) for which treatment is currently limited to further hormonal manipulation or cytotoxic chemotherapy [2].

The endothelin (ET) axis has been implicated in several mechanisms that promote cancer progression. Endothelin-1 (ET-1) acting through the endothelin A ($ET_A$)

* Correspondence: helen.tomkinson@astrazeneca.com
AstraZeneca, Alderley Park, Macclesfield, UK

receptor is believed to promote tumour proliferation, angiogenesis, migration and invasion, as well as inhibiting apoptosis [3]. Conversely, activation of the $ET_B$ receptor by ET-1 promotes apoptosis and inhibits ET-1 production [4,5]. In prostate cancer, increased expression of the $ET_A$ receptor correlates significantly with increased tumour stage and aggressiveness whilst $ET_B$ receptor expression appears to be reduced or absent in CRPC [6]. Furthermore, activation of the $ET_A$ receptor by ET-1 is thought to be a key factor driving bone metastasis, which is a marked feature of CRPC [7,8]. In addition to its prominent role in CRPC, the ET axis has recently been implicated in a number of female malignancies including gynecological and breast cancers [9].

Zibotentan (ZD4054) is an oral specific $ET_A$ receptor antagonist in clinical development for the treatment of CRPC. A Phase II study of zibotentan monotherapy demonstrated a good tolerability profile and a promising overall survival signal in patients with metastatic CRPC who were pain free or mildly symptomatic for pain [10]. Zibotentan is being further assessed in a large Phase III clinical trial programme in this disease setting [11,12]. Preclinical investigations of zibotentan in other tumour types, including ovarian cancer, are ongoing [13,14].

Zibotentan exposure exhibited a dose-linear increase between 5 and 15 mg doses in Caucasian patients with CRPC. Following repeated dosing of zibotentan, there was minimal accumulation and no temporal change in the pharmacokinetics of zibotentan [15]. A pharmacokinetic (PK), metabolism and disposition study using [$^{14}$C]-zibotentan has demonstrated that both renal excretion and metabolism are important clearance mechanisms for zibotentan [16]. The drug and its metabolites are predominantly eliminated in urine with ~58% of parent compound being eliminated by renal clearance. Metabolism of zibotentan is known to be mediated by the CYP3A4 isozyme [16,17]. When zibotentan was administered in combination with the potent inhibitor of CYP3A4, itraconazole, exposure evaluated by the area under the plasma concentration time curve from time zero to infinity (AUC) was increased by 28% [17]. Therefore, patients with hepatic or renal impairment may have reduced drug clearance which could potentially lead to a greater exposure to zibotentan than in patients with normal organ function.

Many patients with CRPC have acute renal failure due to obstruction of the urinary outflow tracts by the prostate tumour [18]. Furthermore, chemotherapy and some bisphosphonates, such as zoledronic acid, which are used widely in this disease setting, have also been associated with the development and progression of renal failure [19,20]. As zibotentan may be given to patients with CRPC prior to, or in conjunction with, chemotherapy and/or bisphosphonates it is important to establish whether the presence of hepatic or renal impairment has any impact on its exposure.

The aim of the two studies presented here was to determine whether hepatic or renal impairment (in subjects without CRPC) has any clinically relevant effect on exposure to zibotentan by assessment of PK, safety and tolerability parameters.

## Methods
### Study design and participants
#### Hepatic impairment study
This was an open-label, two-centre, single-dose, parallel-group study which assessed the effect of mild, moderate and severe hepatic impairment on the PK, safety and tolerability profile of zibotentan 10 mg. Subjects were divided into four groups (n = 8 per group [n ≥ 2 subjects of each sex per group]) using the Child-Pugh classification of hepatic impairment [21] based on scores for encephalopathy, ascites, serum bilirubin, serum albumin and prothrombin time (Table 1): normal hepatic function, matched to the hepatically impaired subjects with respect to age, gender and weight (control); mild hepatic impairment (Child-Pugh A); moderate hepatic impairment (Child-Pugh B); severe hepatic impairment (Child-Pugh C).

Male and female subjects aged 18-75 years with a BMI of 18-34 kg/m$^2$ were included in the study. Subjects with normal hepatic function were required to be hepatitis B and C negative and have normal values for clinical laboratory tests and a normal medical history and examination. Females were to be surgically sterile or postmenopausal. Hepatically impaired subjects were required to have stable liver cirrhosis and hepatic impairment for at least 3 months prior to screening. Subjects were excluded if they had taken drugs with known significant cytochrome P450 (CYP) inducer/inhibitory effects within 30 days prior to zibotentan dosing; had abnormal resting

**Table 1 Child-Pugh classification of hepatic impairment**

|  | Points scored for observed findings | | |
|---|---|---|---|
|  | 1 point | 2 points | 3 points |
| Encephalopathy grade* | Absent | 1 or 2 | 3 or 4 |
| Ascites | Absent | Slight | Moderate |
| Serum bilirubin (µmol/L) | <34.2 | 34.2-51.3 | >51.3 |
| Serum albumin (g/L) | >35 | 28-35 | <28 |
| Prothrombin time (INR) | <1.16 | 1.16-1.56 | >1.56 |
|  | **Classification** | | |
| Child-Pugh grade | Child-Pugh A | Child-Pugh B | Child-Pugh C |
| Points required | 5-6 | 7-9 | 10-15 |

INR, international normalized ratio. *Encephalopathy: Grade 0: normal consciousness, personality, neurological examination, electroencephalogram. Grade 1: restless, sleep disturbed, irritable/agitated, tremor, impaired handwriting, 5 cps waves. Grade 2: lethargic, time disorientated, inappropriate, asterixis, ataxia, slow triphasic waves. Grade 3: somnolent, stuporous, place disorientated, hyperactive reflexes, rigidity, slower waves. Grade 4: unrousable coma, no personality/behaviour, decerebrate, slow 2-3 cps delta activity.

vital signs of supine blood pressure >160 mmHg or <90 mmHg systolic or >95 mmHg or <50 mmHg diastolic or supine pulse ≥100 beats per minute (bpm) or ≤40 bpm; had a history or presence of gastrointestinal or renal disease or other condition known to interfere with the PK profile of drugs. Subjects were excluded from the control group if they had a history or presence of hepatic disease. Exclusion criteria from the hepatically impaired groups included: fluctuating or rapidly deteriorating hepatic function or presence of a hepatocellular carcinoma or an acute liver disease caused by drug toxicity or by an infection, significant renal dysfunction (creatinine clearance below 50 mL/min), severe portal hypertension (with exception of subjects in Child-Pugh C class) or surgical porto-systemic shunts, presence of severe hepatic encephalopathy, refractory ascites, or a platelet count below $40 \times 10^9$/L and/or neutrophil count <1.5 × $10^9$/L and/or hemoglobin <90 g/L.

### Renal impairment study

This was an open-label, single-centre, single-dose study which evaluated the effect of varying degrees of renal impairment on the PK, safety and tolerability profile of zibotentan 10 mg. Subjects were divided into four groups at screening (n = 12 per group [n ≥ 2 subjects of each sex per group, 50% of each group were to be >50 years]) using estimated creatinine clearance ($CL_{CR}$) values (estimated using the Cockcroft-Gault equation) [22]; normal renal function (>80 mL/min); mild renal impairment (≥50 to ≤80 mL/min); moderate renal impairment (≥30 to <50 mL/min); severe renal impairment (<30 mL/min). Prior to analyzing the data, subjects were re-classified into their appropriate renal impairment groups based upon their measured creatinine clearance value determined using 24-hour urine collections on day -1 and serum creatinine levels obtained pre-dose on day 1.

Male and female subjects aged 25-75 years with a BMI of 18-32 kg/m$^2$ were included in the study. All subjects were required to be hepatitis B and C negative and all females were required to be surgically sterile or postmenopausal. Subjects with normal renal function were required to have normal values for clinical laboratory tests and a normal medical history and examination. Renally impaired subjects were to have had stable renal impairment for at least 2 months prior to zibotentan dosing. Subjects were excluded if they had taken drugs with known significant CYP inducer/inhibitory effects within 30 days prior to zibotentan dosing, had a history or presence of gastrointestinal or hepatic disease or other condition known to interfere with the PK of drugs. Subjects were excluded from the control group if they had a history or presence of renal disease, had abnormal resting vital signs of supine blood pressure >160 mmHg systolic or >100 mmHg diastolic or supine heart rate ≥90 bpm or ≤50 bpm. Exclusion criteria for renally impaired subjects included: renal

transplant and end stage renal disease patients, use of drugs that affect creatinine clearance (such as cephalosporin antibiotics, ascorbic acid, trimethoprim, cimetidine and quinine) within 8 days of dosing and abnormal resting vital signs of supine blood pressure >180 mmHg or <110 mmHg systolic or >110 mmHg or <65 mmHg diastolic or supine heart rate ≥90 bpm or ≤50 bpm.

In both studies, all subjects received a single oral dose of zibotentan 10 mg and remained resident at the study unit from the night before the zibotentan dose was administered until 48 hours post dose.

The design of both trials followed the Food and Drug Administration (FDA) [23,24] and the European regulations [25,26] on the design and conduct of *in vivo* hepatic or renal impairment studies. These studies were performed in accordance with the Declaration of Helsinki [27], consistent with the ethical principles of the International Conference on Harmonization/Good Clinical Practice [28]. The hepatic study was approved by the Ethics Committee of the Institute for Clinical and Experimental Medicine and Faculty Thomayer Hospital, Prague, Czech Republic and the renal study was approved by the Bavarian Physicians Board, Ethics Committee, Munich, Germany. All subjects provided written informed consent prior to enrolment in the study and subsequent screening.

### Study objectives

The primary objective of these studies was to investigate the PK of a single oral dose of zibotentan 10 mg in subjects with hepatic or renal impairment compared with healthy subjects. The secondary objectives were to assess the safety and tolerability of a single oral dose of zibotentan 10 mg in these subjects.

### Procedures

Blood samples were collected for the determination of plasma concentrations of zibotentan pre dosing and at pre-defined intervals up to 96 and 120 hours, following receipt of a single oral dose of zibotentan 10 mg for subjects in the renal and hepatic impairment studies, respectively. Blood samples were centrifuged at 4°C for 10 minutes at 1500*g* to provide plasma. An additional blood sample was taken at 3 hours post dose for the determination of protein binding of zibotentan and was centrifuged at 37°C for 10 min at 1500*g* to provide plasma. Plasma samples were transferred into Amicon Centrifree cartridges (30,000 molecular cut off; Millipore, Watford). The cartridges were centrifuged in a fixed angle rotor at 1000-2000*g* at 37°C for 30 minutes to produce plasma ultrafiltrate. The collection cup was removed and stored at -20°C. In the renal impairment study, urine samples were collected from 0-6, 6-12, 12-24, 24-36 and 36-48 hours post dosing for the determination of zibotentan concentrations. The volume of each urine collection was recorded.

Plasma, plasma ultrafiltrate and urine samples for zibotentan analysis were stored at -20°C and transported to York Bioanalytical Solutions Ltd (York, UK). Zibotentan plasma and plasma ultrafiltrate concentrations were determined as described previously [17]. An additional calibration curve ranging from 5 to 5000 ng/mL which used an internal standard concentration of 10,000 ng/mL in water (rather than the 100 ng/mL solution previously reported for the 0.5 to 500 ng/mL calibration range) was used for plasma samples in the renal study and for plasma ultrafiltrate samples. The performance of the assay was monitored during each run using quality control samples at concentrations of 1.5, 200, 400 and 800 ng/mL where sample dilution was required (for the 0.5 to 500 ng/mL range) and 15, 2000 and 4000 ng/mL (for the 5 to 5000 ng/mL range) spiked into control human plasma samples or into control human plasma ultrafiltrate samples for the ultrafiltrate analysis. These were prepared prior to commencement of the analysis of study samples and stored at -20°C until required. In the hepatic study the CV of the assay was ≤12% at all concentrations and accuracy was typically between 98 and 103%. In the renal study the CV of the assay was ≤9.3% and the accuracy was typically 96 and 103%. Following analysis of the plasma ultrafiltrate samples, the CV of the assay was ≤8.4% in the hepatic study and ≤7% in the renal study and accuracy ranged from 101 to 106% and 97.8 to 107% for the hepatic and renal studies, respectively. Zibotentan urine sample concentrations were determined by dilution followed by HPLC with mass spectrometric detection (HPLC-MS-MS). Urine samples were aliquoted (100 μL) into polypropylene tubes with acetonitrile (100 μL). Samples were vortex mixed and sonicated at 40°C for 30 minutes. A 25 μL portion of each sample was aliquoted into a 2 mL square well plate and internal standard (900 μL, 1400 ng/mL) was added to each sample, except appropriate blanks, to which mobile phase (900 μL) was added. The plate was vortex mixed and centrifuged (3 minutes, 2500 rpm, 20°C), prior to being submitted for HPLC-MS-MS analysis as previously described [17]. The CV of the assay was ≤7.2% and the accuracy typically ranged from 101 to 107%.

Zibotentan PK parameters determined included maximum plasma concentration ($C_{max}$), time to $C_{max}$ ($t_{max}$), area under the concentration-time curve from zero to infinity (AUC), area under the concentration-time curve from zero until the last measurable concentration ($AUC_{0-t}$), terminal half-life ($t_{1/2}$), total apparent plasma clearance (CL/F), apparent volume of distribution at steady state ($V_{ss}/F$), ratio of unbound drug in plasma (Fu), free $C_{max}$, free AUC, and unbound CL/F. Renal clearance ($CL_R$) and the fraction of dose excreted

unchanged (Fe) were evaluated in the renal study only. Non-compartmental methods were used for the evaluation of the plasma concentration-time data and $C_{max}$ and $t_{max}$ were determined by inspection of the concentration-time profiles. Where possible, the terminal elimination rate constant ($\lambda_z$) was calculated by log-linear regression of the terminal portion of the concentration-time profiles, and $t_{1/2}$ was calculated as $Ln2/\lambda_z$. $AUC_{0-t}$ was determined using the linear trapezoidal rule, and where appropriate, the $AUC_{0-t}$ was extrapolated to infinity using $\lambda$ to obtain AUC. CL/F was calculated from the ratio of dose/AUC and Vss/F was determined from the mean residence time (MRT) × CL/F. The percentage of free zibotentan was determined by comparison of the free and total zibotentan concentrations at 3 hours post dose; free $C_{max}$ and free AUC were calculated using $C_{max}$ or AUC x percentage free zibotentan, respectively, and unbound CL/F was determined by CL/F/percentage free zibotentan. The amount of zibotentan excreted in the urine was determined from the concentration of zibotentan in each collection and the volume of urine collected. $CL_R$ of zibotentan was calculated from the total amount of zibotentan excreted/plasma AUC and the Fe of zibotentan was calculated as the total drug excreted unchanged/dose. The methods for the PK parameter assessments and calculations reported in this study have been described previously [29]. AUC, free AUC, $AUC_{0-t}$, $C_{max}$, and free $C_{max}$ were presented as geometric mean (CV) for each hepatic or renal study group. CL/F, unbound CL/F, $t_{1/2}$, Vss/F, $CL_R$, Fe and Fu were presented as arithmetic mean (± standard error [SE]).

Safety and tolerability was evaluated by recording the incidence of adverse events (AEs) according to Medical Dictionary for Regulatory Activities (MedDRA) vocabulary and the Common Terminology Criteria for Adverse Events (CTCAE) Version 3, laboratory tests (hematology, urinalysis and clinical chemistry), physical examination, and measurement of vital signs.

## Statistical methods

In the hepatic impairment study AUC and $C_{max}$ were logarithmically transformed using natural logarithms (back-transformed results were reported). These parameters were analyzed using an analysis of variance model (ANOVA) with a factor fitting for hepatic impairment status (mild/moderate/severe or normal). Ratios of geometric means of each hepatically impaired group compared to the normal function group (mild/moderate/severe: control) and 90% confidence intervals (CIs) were reported. An effect of hepatic impairment was predefined to have occurred if the upper 90% CI for the ratio did not lie below 2. This was chosen as zibotentan 15 mg has previously been tolerated in patients with CRPC; however, zibotentan 22.5 mg was not tolerated, therefore

**Table 2 Demographic and baseline characteristics for subjects in the hepatic and renal impairment studies**

| | | Degree of hepatic impairment | | | | Degree of renal impairment | | |
|---|---|---|---|---|---|---|---|---|
| | Normal hepatic function (n = 8) | Mild (n = 8) | Moderate (n = 8) | Severe (n = 8) | Normal renal function (n = 18) | Mild (n = 12) | Moderate (n = 9) | Severe (n = 9) |
| Male, n (%) | 5 (63) | 6 (75) | 5 (63) | 5 (63) | 13 (72) | 9 (75) | 7 (78) | 7 (78) |
| Female, n (%) | 3 (38) | 2 (25) | 3 (38) | 3 (38) | 5 (28) | 3 (25) | 2 (22) | 2 (22) |
| Mean age, years (range) | 58.4 (55-62) | 56 (45-63) | 59.3 (49-68) | 52 (37-67) | 60 (47-71) | 58 (38-71) | 60 (48-69) | 57 (32-69) |

doubling of the zibotentan dose was to be eliminated [30].

For the renal impairment study, statistical analysis of AUC, $C_{max}$ (using natural logarithm transformed data) and $t_{1/2}$ (using untransformed data) was performed using linear regression fitting effects for creatinine clearance and age as explanatory variables. The slope parameter and corresponding SE were used to provide point estimates and 90% confidence intervals (CIs) for the ratio (or difference for $t_{1/2}$) of zibotentan exposures in subjects with severe, moderate and mild renal impairment compared to subjects with normal renal function.

## Results

### Patient demographics

Thirty-seven subjects were enrolled in the hepatic impairment study, 32 of whom received zibotentan and completed the study. In the renal impairment study, 52 subjects were enrolled and 48 subjects received zibotentan and completed the study. Twenty-four hour urine collections could not be taken until subjects had given consent and were admitted to the investigational site, therefore

estimated creatinine clearance values using the Cockcroft-Gault equation were used at screening to classify subjects with varying degrees of renal impairment, to achieve 12 subjects per group. Subjects were subsequently re-classified within the renal impairment categories according to their actual serum creatinine clearance values obtained on day 1, resulting in a disproportionate number of subjects within each category. In both studies, all subjects were Caucasian, cohorts were balanced with respect to age and there were more males than females (Table 2).

### Pharmacokinetics

#### Hepatic impairment study

The PK parameters and plasma concentrations of zibotentan 10 mg in subjects with varying degrees of hepatic impairment are presented in Table 3 and Figure 1a, respectively. The results of the statistical analysis are presented in Table 4 and Figure 2. Following a single oral dose of zibotentan 10 mg, $C_{max}$ was unchanged in subjects with mild, moderate and severe hepatic impairment compared with those with normal hepatic function (Table 4). Exposure in terms of AUC was significantly

**Table 3 Pharmacokinetic parameters of zibotentan in subjects with normal renal function and varying degrees of renal impairment, normal hepatic function and varying degrees of hepatic impairment**

| PK parameter | | Degree of hepatic impairment | | | | Degree of renal impairment | | |
|---|---|---|---|---|---|---|---|---|
| | Normal hepatic function (n = 8) | Mild (n = 8) | Moderate (n = 8) | Severe (n = 8) | Normal renal function (n = 18) | Mild (n = 12) | Moderate (n = 9) | Severe (n = 9) |
| $AUC_{(0-t)}$ (ng·h/mL)* | 5460 (46.2) | 7560 (65.1) | 7850 (50.3) | 15100 (49.8) | 5560 (36.9) | 6910 (57.5) | 9090 (35.2) | 9640 (37.7) |
| AUC (ng·h/mL)* | 5480 (46.0) | 7680 (68.8) | 7940 (50.7) | 15900 (52.9) | 5490 (39.0)$^{\$}$ | 6950 (58.3) | 8710 (3.8)$^{£}$ | 9750 (38.8) |
| $C_{max}$ (ng/mL)* | 566 (25.6) | 526 (22.3) | 505 (23.0) | 536 (30.2) | 545 (22.7) | 531 (28.8) | 550 (9.9) | 619 (20.6) |
| $t_{max}$ (h)$^{†}$ | 2 (1-2) | 2 (1-4) | 2 (1-6) | 2 (1-4) | 1 (1-3) | 1 (1-4) | 2 (1-8) | 1 (1-3) |
| $t_{1/2}$ (h)$^{‡}$ | 9.3 (3.6) | 13.0 (9.4) | 14.6 (6.5) | 24.8 (10.9) | 10.8 (2.7)$^{\$}$ | 11.3 (4.0) | 13.5 (4.3)$^{£}$ | 13.2 (4.7) |
| CL/F (mL/min)$^{‡}$ | 33.2 (15.6) | 25.0 (12.1) | 23.6 (14.2) | 11.9 (7.3) | 32.7 (14.2)$^{\$}$ | 27.9 (18.9) | 20.1 (6.5)$^{£}$ | 18.2 (6.5) |
| $V_{ss}/F$ (L)$^{‡}$ | 19.0 (6.1) | 19.8 (3.1) | 21.2 (7.2) | 21.9 (7.1) | 22.6 (7.0)$^{\$}$ | 20.8 (5.8) | 19.3 (2.0)$^{£}$ | 17.8 (3.4) |
| Fu (%)$^{‡}$ | 22.5 (7.5) | 23.4 (4.0) | 20.2 (4.8) | 29.2 (9.4) | 22.8 (6.2) | 25.4 (6.7) | 26.6 (2.9) | 27.9 (5.3) |
| $CL_R$ (mL/min)$^{‡}$ | - | - | - | - | 17.4 (13.9)$^{\$}$ | 10.3 (16.8) | 3.2 (5.6)$^{£}$ | 2.3 (2.7)$^{£}$ |
| Fe (%)$^{‡}$ | - | - | - | - | 47.2 (18.0) | 27.1 (19.5) | 12.7 (16.9) | 10.5 (9.0)$^{£}$ |
| Free $C_{max}$ (ng/mL)* | 121 (58.7) | 123 (21.9) | 97.3 (32.4) | 149.2 (52.6) | 121 (32.3) | 131 (22.9) | 145 (13.4) | 170 (18.2) |
| Free AUC (ng·h/mL)* | 1170 (69.3) | 1800 (54.7) | 1460 (56.5) | 4430 (40.0) | 1230 (39.1)$^{\$}$ | 1720 (60.6) | 2260 (34.5)$^{£}$ | 2680 (38.9) |
| Unbound CL/F (mL/min)$^{‡}$ | 167 (98.4) | 103 (46.8) | 129 (69.8) | 40 (14.7) | 146 (67.3)$^{\$}$ | 115 (83.8) | 77.4 (24.1)$^{£}$ | 65.8 (22.3) |

*Geometric mean (coefficient of variation, %), $^{†}$median (range), $^{‡}$arithmetic mean (standard deviation), $^{\$}$n = 16, $^{£}$n = 8. $AUC_{(0-t)}$, area under the plasma concentration-time curve from 0 to the time of the last quantifiable concentration; AUC, area under the plasma concentration-time curve from 0 to infinity; CL/F, total apparent drug clearance; $CL_R$, renal clearance; $C_{max}$, maximum plasma concentration; Fe, fraction of dose excreted unchanged; Fu, ratio of unbound drug in plasma; $t_{max}$, time to reach $C_{max}$; $t_{1/2}$, terminal half-life; Vss/F, volume of distribution at steady state.

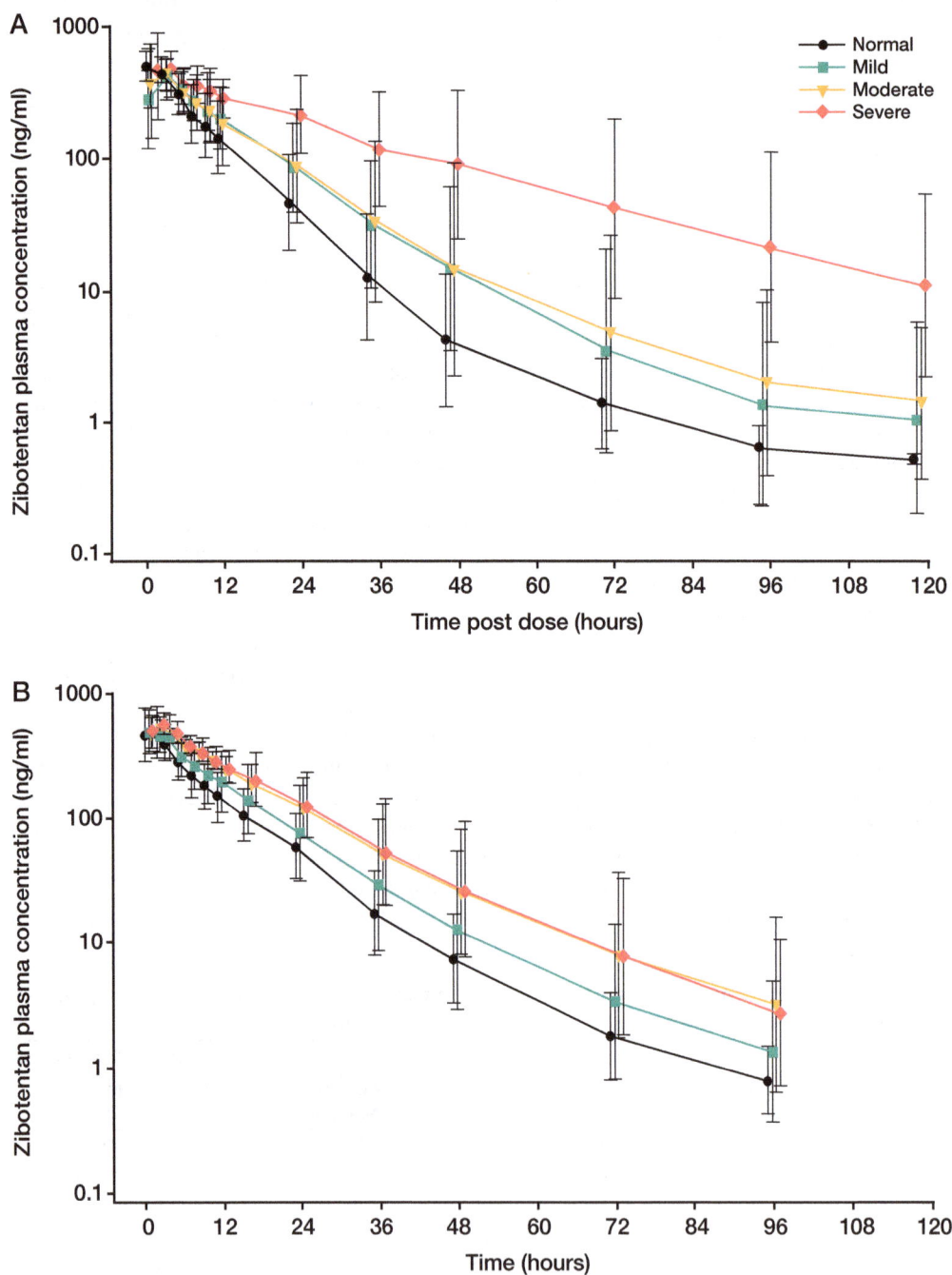

*Values are presented as geometric mean (± standard deviation)*

**Figure 1 Zibotentan plasma concentration-time curves**. Zibotentan plasma concentration-time curves for (a) subjects with normal hepatic function and varying degrees of hepatic impairment and (b) subjects with normal renal function and varying degrees of renal impairment.

increased in subjects with hepatic impairment (Table 4; Figure 2). Zibotentan clearance (CL/F) was decreased in subjects with hepatic impairment with the magnitude of decrease being related to the degree of hepatic impairment (Figure 3). There was no statistical analysis of $t_{1/2}$ values but the data demonstrated an increase in $t_{1/2}$ in

subjects with hepatic impairment compared with subjects with normal hepatic function (Table 3). The magnitude of the increase in this parameter was related to the degree of hepatic impairment. There was little difference in plasma protein binding between subjects with normal and impaired hepatic function, thus changes in

**Table 4 Ratios of pharmacokinetic parameters of zibotentan in subjects with varying degrees of renal impairment compared with subjects with normal renal function, and in subjects with varying degrees of hepatic impairment compared with subjects with normal hepatic function**

| PK parameter | Degree of hepatic impairment* | | | Degree of renal impairment[†] | | |
|---|---|---|---|---|---|---|
| | Mild | Moderate | Severe | Mild | Moderate | Severe |
| $C_{max}$ ratio (90% CI) | 0.93 (0.75-1.15) | 0.89 (0.72-1.10) | 0.95 (0.77-1.17) | 1.07 (0.97-1.19) | 1.09 (0.96-1.24) | 1.12 (0.96-1.30) |
| AUC ratio (90% CI) | 1.40 (0.91-2.17) | 1.45 (0.94-2.24) | 2.90 (1.88-4.49) | 1.66 (1.38-1.99) | 1.89 (1.50-2.39) | 2.17 (1.64-2.86) |
| $t_{1/2}$ difference, h (90% CI) | - | - | - | 1.87 (0.06-3.68)** | 2.37 (0.08-4.66)** | 2.87 (0.1-5.64)** |

*Point estimate of geometric mean ratio in relation to control; [†]Point estimate of geometric least squares ratio in relation to control; **Least squares mean difference in relation to control; AUC, area under the plasma concentration-time curve from zero to infinity; $C_{max}$, maximum plasma concentration; $t_{1/2}$, terminal half-life; CI = confidence interval.

free $C_{max}$, free AUC and unbound CL/F across the groups were similar to changes in $C_{max}$, AUC and CL/F (Table 3).

### Renal impairment study

The PK parameters and plasma concentrations of zibotentan 10 mg in subjects with varying degrees of renal impairment are presented in Table 3 and Figure 1b, respectively. The results of the statistical analysis are presented in Table 4 and Figure 2. Following a single oral dose of zibotentan 10 mg, $C_{max}$ was unchanged in subjects with mild, moderate and severe renal impairment compared with subjects with normal renal function (Table 4). Exposure, in terms of AUC, was significantly increased in subjects with renal impairment and the magnitude of this increase was related to the degree of renal impairment; AUC was 66%, 89%, and 117% higher, respectively, in subjects with mild, moderate or severe renal impairment compared with subjects with normal renal function (Table 4; Figure 2). Zibotentan clearance (CL/F) decreased as the severity of renal impairment increased, with mean CL/F being 39% and 44% lower in the moderate and severe renal impairment groups, respectively, compared with subjects with normal renal function (Figure 4). Analysis of $t_{1/2}$ indicated a difference with degree of renal impairment, with longer $t_{1/2}$ values being observed as the severity of renal impairment increased (Table 3). There was little difference in plasma protein binding between subjects with normal and impaired renal function, thus changes in free $C_{max}$, free AUC and unbound CL/F across the groups were similar to those observed for $C_{max}$, AUC and CL/F (Table 3).

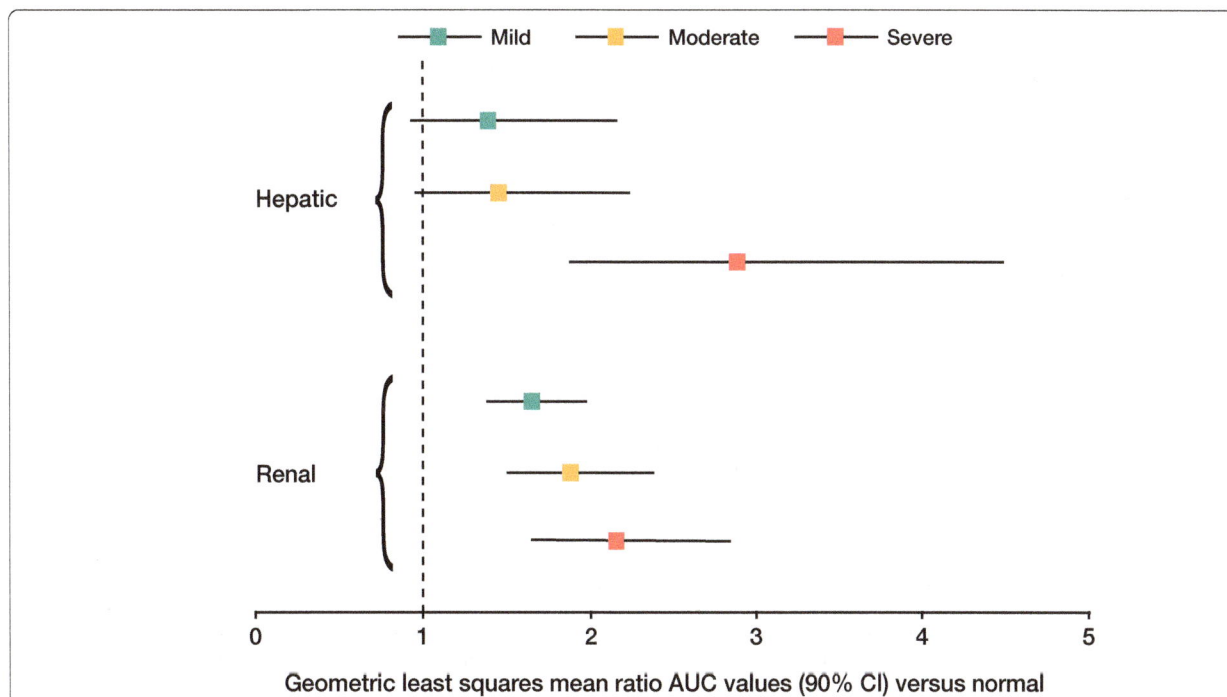

**Figure 2 Forest plot of the ratios of zibotentan exposure.** Forest plot of the ratios of zibotentan exposure (AUC) in subjects with varying degrees of renal impairment compared with subjects with normal renal function, and in subjects with varying degrees of hepatic impairment compared with subjects with normal hepatic function.

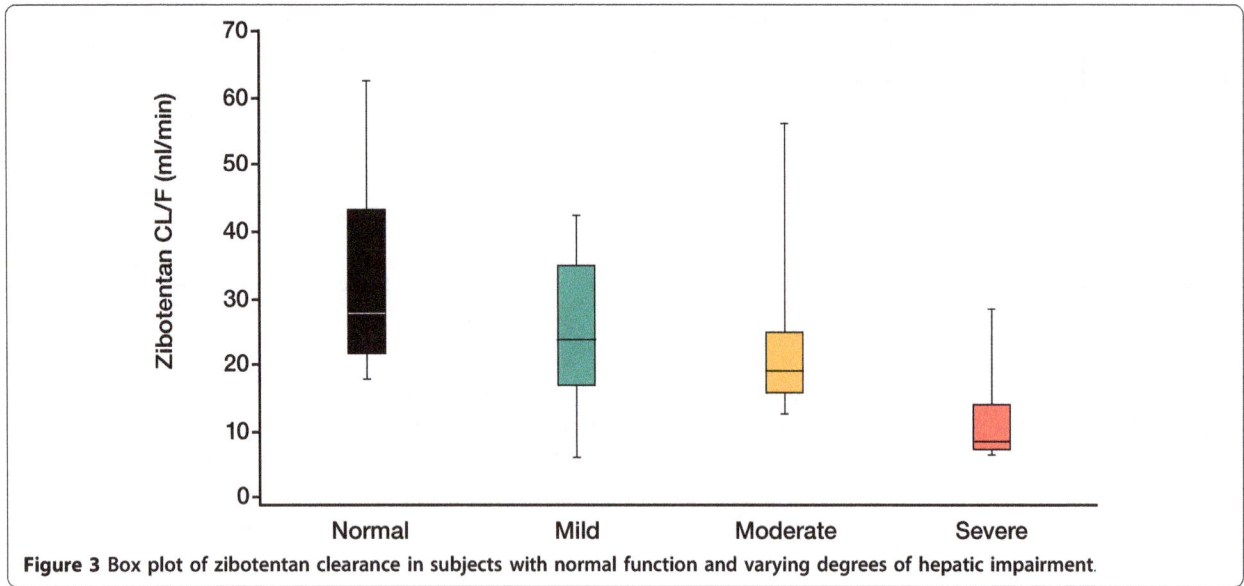

**Figure 3** Box plot of zibotentan clearance in subjects with normal function and varying degrees of hepatic impairment.

## Safety profile

Zibotentan was well tolerated in both studies and all AEs were CTCAE Grade 1 or 2. Headache (seven subjects [22%]) was the most common AE in the hepatic study which was reported in at least one subject in all groups, with the frequency increasing with the severity of hepatic impairment (Table 5). Vomiting was the second most common AE in the hepatic study, which was reported in two (6%) subjects. One subject with moderate hepatic impairment experienced a QT prolongation

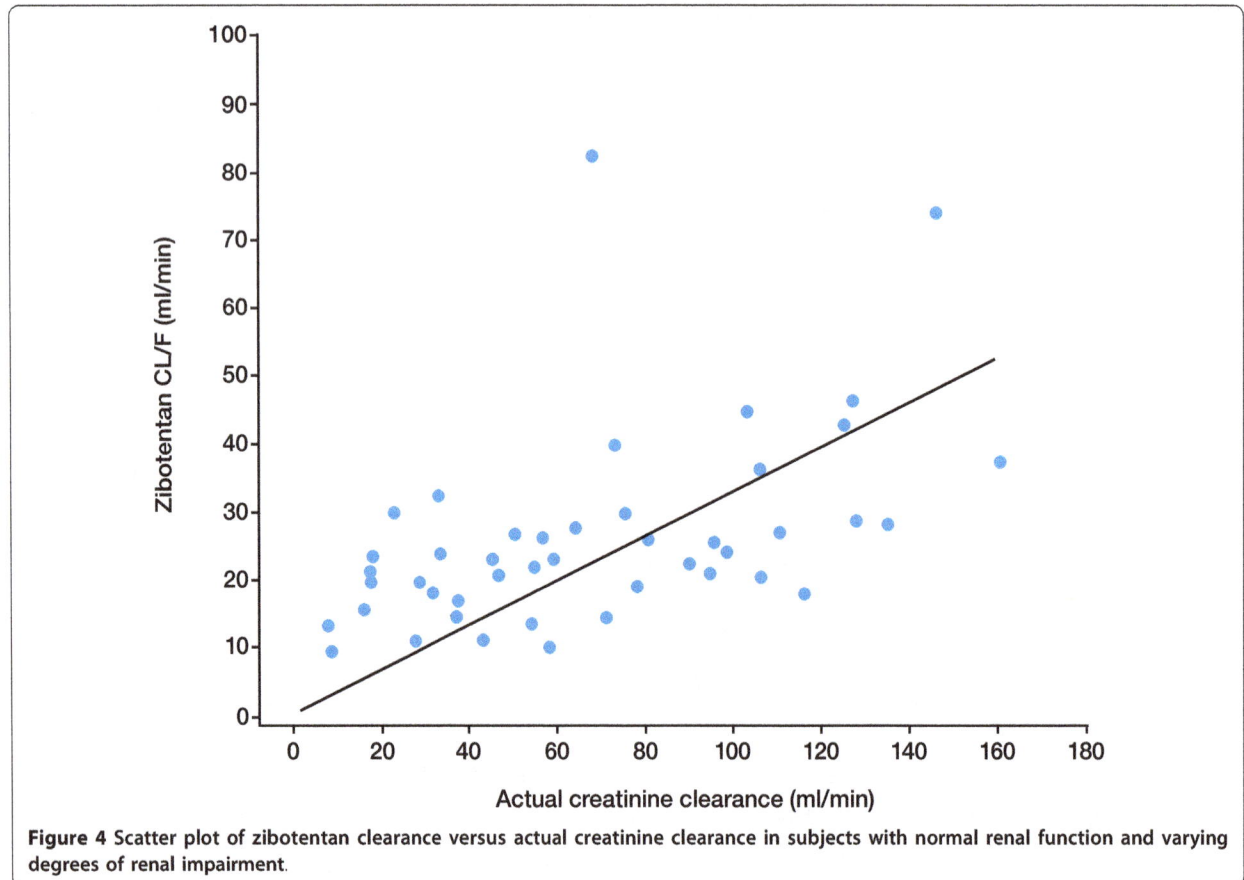

**Figure 4** Scatter plot of zibotentan clearance versus actual creatinine clearance in subjects with normal renal function and varying degrees of renal impairment.

**Table 5 AEs reported in >1 subject with normal hepatic function and varying degrees of hepatic impairment**

| Adverse event, n (%) | Normal hepatic function (n = 8) | Degree of hepatic impairment | | |
| --- | --- | --- | --- | --- |
| | | Mild (n = 8) | Moderate (n = 8) | Severe (n = 8) |
| Any AE | 1 (13) | 1 (13) | 3 (38) | 4 (50) |
| Headache | 1 (13) | 1 (13) | 2 (25) | 3 (38) |
| Vomiting | 1 (13) | 0 | 0 | 1 (13) |

from 422 ms pre dose to 455 ms 4 hours post dose; however, this event was not considered to be related to zibotentan treatment and likely reflects normal variability in this parameter.

Headache was also the most commonly reported AE in the renal impairment study; however, the incidence of headache did not appear to correlate with the severity of renal impairment (Table 6). Other AEs reported in more than two subjects included nasopharyngitis (n = 4), fatigue (n = 4), somnolence (n = 3) and nausea (n = 3).

In both studies, AEs of headache were assessed by the investigator as being causally related to zibotentan treatment and either resolved without medication or were managed with paracetamol. Minor reductions in systolic and diastolic blood pressure were noted following zibotentan dosing in most subjects in both studies; however, these changes were not associated with any symptoms and were not considered to be clinically relevant. There were no deaths, serious AEs, discontinuations due to AEs, or other significant AEs in either study.

## Discussion

A previous PK, metabolism and disposition study has indicated that zibotentan and its metabolites are predominately eliminated in urine. Between 71 and 94% of dosed drug is eliminated in the urine with 58% of an administered dose renally cleared as parent compound [16]. *In vitro* investigations have demonstrated that CYP3A4 is responsible for the metabolism of zibotentan [17]. Furthermore, when zibotentan was administered in combination with itraconazole, a potent inhibitor of CYP3A4, AUC increased by 28% [17]. Consequently, patients with hepatic or renal impairment may have reduced clearance of zibotentan, which could potentially lead to a greater exposure to zibotentan. A significant proportion of patients with CRPC are likely to have varying degrees of renal failure due to obstruction of the urinary outflow tracts by the tumour [18] and as a consequence of previous chemotherapy treatment regimens [19]. These observations support an assessment of the effects of hepatic or renal impairment on the PK of zibotentan.

The PK parameters of zibotentan in normal healthy subjects were similar between the two studies and were consistent with the findings of previous PK studies [17]. In subjects with mild, moderate or severe hepatic or renal impairment, there was no significant difference in the $C_{max}$ of zibotentan following a single oral dose of zibotentan 10 mg compared with those subjects with normal organ function, indicating that absorption of the drug was unchanged. Hepatic or renal impairment did, however, significantly increase zibotentan exposure (AUC), as a consequence of slower clearance of zibotentan. Furthermore, exposure increased with degree of hepatic or renal impairment. Of note, in the hepatic impairment study, the PK profile of one subject in the mild impairment group was similar to the PK profile of subjects in the severe impairment group and therefore the data from this subject will have influenced the mean PK values for the mild group and contributed to the wide variability observed (Figure 2). Indeed, when this

**Table 6 AEs reported in >1 subject with normal renal function and varying degrees of renal impairment**

| Adverse event, n (%) | Normal renal function (n = 18) | Degree of renal impairment | | |
| --- | --- | --- | --- | --- |
| | | Mild (n = 12) | Moderate (n = 9) | Severe (n = 9) |
| Any AE | 14 (78) | 7 (58) | 8 (89) | 7 (78) |
| Headache | 14 (78) | 6 (50) | 5 (56) | 4 (44) |
| Nasopharyngitis | 1 (6) | 1 (8) | 2 (22) | 0 |
| Fatigue | 0 | 1 (8) | 1 (11) | 2 (22) |
| Somnolence | 2 (11) | 1 (8) | 0 | 0 |
| Nausea | 1 (6) | 1 (8) | 0 | 1 (11) |
| Neck pain | 0 | 2 (17) | 0 | 0 |
| Back pain | 1 (6) | 1 (8) | 0 | 0 |
| Dizziness | 0 | 0 | 2 (22) | 0 |
| Dyspepsia | 1 (6) | 0 | 0 | 1 (11) |

subject was removed from the analysis, the upper confidence limit of the AUC treatment ratio fell below the predefined limit of 2. In both studies there was an increase in the elimination half-life of zibotentan as the degree of hepatic or renal impairment increased, although this was more evident in subjects with hepatic impairment. Hepatic and renal dysfunction has been shown to cause changes in plasma protein binding, therefore the fraction of unbound zibotentan was calculated at 3 hours post dose to determine free $C_{max}$, free AUC and unbound CL/F. Little change was documented in protein binding across the groups in either study, and consequently changes in free $C_{max}$, free AUC and unbound CL/F across the groups were similar to changes in $C_{max}$, AUC and CL/F.

Data from the hepatic study have demonstrated that although mild and moderate impairment had only a small impact on the average PK profile of zibotentan, the impact of severe hepatic impairment was much greater. Total plasma clearance of zibotentan in individuals with severe hepatic impairment was 64% lower than that in individuals with normal function (Figure 3), resulting in an approximate 190% increase in exposure to zibotentan. Across the three hepatically impaired groups there was a large amount of variability. Although the average increase in exposure was 40 to 45% for the mild and moderately impaired groups, increases of more than 2 could not be ruled out. For the severely impaired group, increases of 4.5 fold could not be ruled out. Data from the renal study have shown that mild renal impairment had only a small impact on the PK profile of zibotentan with average exposure increasing 66% and the upper CI remaining below 2, whereas, in this case, the impact of moderate and severe renal impairment was progressively greater. Total plasma clearance of zibotentan in individuals with a moderate or severe degree of renal impairment was 39% and 44% lower, respectively, than in subjects with normal renal function, resulting in increases in zibotentan exposure of 89% and 117%, respectively.

In a Phase II study of zibotentan in patients with metastatic CRPC and bone metastases, zibotentan 15 mg was well tolerated, with headache being the most commonly reported AE [31]. Patients with mild renal impairment who receive zibotentan 10 mg may have exposures equivalent to those in patients receiving zibotentan 15 mg in the Phase II study, and therefore zibotentan is likely to be well tolerated. In contrast, in a Phase I study of patients with metastatic CRPC, patients taking zibotentan 22.5 mg reported dose-limiting toxicities of Grade 3 peripheral edema and intraventricular hemorrhage [30]. The most common AEs reported in this study were headache, peripheral edema, fatigue, nasal congestion, arthralgia and nausea.

Groups of patients who get more than a doubling in mean drug plasma concentrations compared with normal patients could therefore be exposed to greater risks with zibotentan therapy. As such, caution and careful monitoring may be required if considering using zibotentan 10 mg/day in patients with hepatic insufficiency or moderate or severe renal insufficiency.

A single oral dose of zibotentan 10 mg was generally well tolerated in subjects with normal renal and hepatic function, and in those subjects with mild, moderate or severe hepatic or renal impairment. The most commonly reported AE in both studies was headache, which is consistent with reports from previous studies of zibotentan and other endothelin receptor antagonists [31,32]. The occurrence of headache increased with the degree of hepatic impairment, but not with the degree of renal impairment, where the incidence of headache was highest in subjects with normal renal function. In both studies, headache was reported to resolve without medication or was managed with paracetamol. Overall, there was an increase in the total number of AEs reported as the severity of hepatic impairment increased; 13% and 50% of subjects experienced AEs in the normal and severe hepatic impairment groups, respectively. In contrast, in the renal impairment study, the number of AEs reported was similar across all groups. This finding suggests that the increased exposure to zibotentan in subjects with moderate or severe renal impairment had little effect on the tolerability of zibotentan.

## Conclusions

Following administration of a single oral dose of zibotentan 10 mg to subjects with hepatic or renal impairment, the $C_{max}$ of zibotentan was unchanged, although zibotentan exposure (AUC) was higher in subjects with hepatic or renal impairment as a consequence of slower clearance of zibotentan. The magnitude of the increase in exposure was related to the degree of hepatic or renal impairment. Despite this increased exposure, there were no differences in the type or severity of AEs. Zibotentan 10 mg is currently undergoing further clinical investigation in patients with CRPC in a large Phase III clinical programme [11].

**Acknowledgements**
We thank Angelika Weil, Eva Engelhardt and Karin Schmid from APEX GmbH (Germany) and Blanka Cieslarová from PRA International (Czech Republic) for recruiting volunteers and conducting the studies locally, and Dr Claire Routley from Mudskipper (UK) who provided editorial assistance funded by AstraZeneca. This study was funded by AstraZeneca.

**Authors' contributions**
HT performed the PK analysis of the renal study and drafted the manuscript. JK performed the PK analysis of the hepatic study. SO was the study physician in the renal study. MT performed the statistical analyses of both studies. TM and HS participated in the design and concept of the studies. All authors contributed to and approved the final manuscript.

**Competing interests**
This study was sponsored by AstraZeneca. Helen Tomkinson, John Kemp, Stuart Oliver, Helen Swaisland, Maria Taboada and Thomas Morris are all employees of AstraZeneca.

**References**
1.  Jemal A, Siegel R, Xu J, Ward E: **Cancer Statistics, 2010.** *CA Cancer J Clin* 2010, **60**:277-300.
2.  Di Lorenzo G, Buonerba C, Autorino R, De Placido S, Sternberg CN: **Castration-resistant prostate cancer: current and emerging treatment strategies.** *Drugs* 2010, **70**:983-1000.
3.  Nelson JB: **Endothelin inhibition: novel therapy for prostate cancer.** *J Urol* 2003, **170**:S65-S68.
4.  Okazawa M, Shiraki T, Ninomiya H, Kobayashi S, Masaki T: **Endothelin-induced apoptosis of A375 human melanoma cells.** *J Biol Chem* 1998, **273**:12584-12592.
5.  Fukuroda T, Fujikawa T, Ozaki S, Ishikawa K, Yano M, Nishikibe M: **Clearance of circulating endothelin-1 by ETB receptors in rats.** *Biochem Biophys Res Commun* 1994, **199**:1461-1465.
6.  Nelson JB, Hedican SP, George DJ, Reddi AH, Piantadosi S, Eisenberger MA, Simons JW: **Identification of endothelin-1 in the pathophysiology of metastatic adenocarcinoma of the prostate.** *Nat Med* 1995, **1**:944-949.
7.  Nelson JB: **Endothelin receptors as therapeutic targets in castration-resistant prostate cancer.** *Eur Urol Suppl* 2009, **8**:20-28.
8.  Bagnato A, Natali PG: **Endothelin receptors as novel targets in tumor therapy.** *J Transl Med* 2004, **2**:16.
9.  Smollich M, Wülfing P: **Targeting the endothelin system: novel therapeutic options in gynecological, urological and breast cancers.** *Expert Rev Anticancer Ther* 2008, **8**:1481-1493.
10. James ND, Caty A, Payne H, Borre M, Zonnenberg BA, Beuzeboc P, McIntosh S, Morris T, De Phung H, Dawson NA: **Final safety and efficacy analysis of the specific endothelin A receptor antagonist zibotentan (ZD4054) in patients with metastatic castration-resistant prostate cancer and bone metastases who were pain free or mildly symptomatic for pain: A double-blind, placebo-controlled, randomised Phase II trial.** *BJU Int* 2010, **106**:966-973.
11. Fizazi K, Miller K: **Specific endothelin-A receptor antagonism for the treatment of advanced prostate cancer.** *BJU Int* 2009, **104**:1423-1425.
12. Fizazi K, Sternberg CN, Fitzpatrick JM, Watson RW, Tabesh M: **Role of targeted therapy in the treatment of advanced prostate cancer.** *BJU Int* 2010, **105**:748-767.
13. Rosano L, Di Castro V, Spinella F, Decandia S, Natali PG, Bagnato A: **ZD4054, a potent endothelin receptor A antagonist, inhibits ovarian carcinoma cell proliferation.** *Exp Biol Med (Maywood)* 2006, **231**:1132-1135.
14. Rosanò L, Di Castro V, Spinella F, Nicotra MR, Natali PG, Bagnato A: **ZD4054, a specific antagonist of the endothelin A receptor, inhibits tumor growth and enhances paclitaxel activity in human ovarian carcinoma *in vitro* and *in vivo*.** *Mol Cancer Ther* 2007, **6**:2003-2011.
15. Ranson M, Wilson R, O'Sullivan JM, Maruoka M, Yamaguchi A, Cowan RA, Logue JP, Tomkinson HK, Tominaga N, Swaisland H, Oliver S, Usami M: **Pharmacokinetic and tolerability profile of once-daily zibotentan (ZD4054) in Japanese and Caucasian patients with hormone-resistant prostate cancer.** *Int J Clin Pharm Ther* 2010, **48**:708-717.
16. Clarkson-Jones J, Kenyon A, Kemp J, Lenz E, Oliver S, Phillips P, Sandall D, Swaisland H: **Metabolism of [$^{14}$C]-ZD4054 in healthy volunteers.** *Eur J Cancer Suppl* 2007, **5**:114.
17. Swaisland HC, Oliver SD, Morris T, Jones HK, Bakhtyari A, Mackey A, McCormick AD, Slamon D, Hargreaves JA, Millar A, Taboada MT: **In vitro metabolism of the specific endothelin-A receptor antagonist ZD4054 and clinical drug interactions between ZD4054 and rifampicin or itraconazole in healthy male volunteers.** *Xenobiotica* 2009, **39**:444-456.
18. Thadhani R, Pascual M, Bonventre JV: **Acute renal failure.** *N Engl J Med* 1996, **334**:1448-1460.
19. Oh WK, Proctor K, Nakabayashi M, Evan C, Tormey LK, Daskivich T, Antràs L, Smith M, Neary MP, Duh MS: **The risk of renal impairment in hormone-refractory prostate cancer patients with bone metastases treated with zoledronic acid.** *Cancer* 2007, **109**:1090-1096.
20. Humphreys BD, Soiffer RJ, Magee CC: **Renal failure associated with cancer and its treatment: an update.** *J Am Soc Nephrol* 2005, **16**:151-161.
21. Pugh RN, Murray-Lyon IM, Dawson JL, Pietroni MC, Williams R: **Transection of the oesophagus for bleeding oesophageal varices.** *Br J Surg* 1973, **60**:646-649.
22. Cockcroft DW, Gault MH: **Prediction of creatinine clearance from serum creatinine.** *Nephron* 1976, **16**:31-41.
23. FDA Guidance for industry: **Pharmacokinetics in patients with impaired renal function: Study design, data analysis and impact on dosing and labeling.** 1998 [http://www.fda.gov/downloads/Drugs/ GuidanceComplianceRegulatory%20Information/Guidances/UCM072127.pdf].
24. FDA Guidance for industry: **Pharmacokinetics in patients with impaired hepatic function: Study design, data analysis and impact on dosing and labeling.** 2003 [http://www.fda.gov/downloads/Drugs/ GuidanceComplianceRegulatoryInformation/Guidances/ucm072123.pdf].
25. The European Agency for the evaluation of medicinal products: **Guideline on the evaluation of the pharmacokinetics of medicinal products in patients with impaired renal function.** 2004 [http://www.ema.europa.eu/docs/en_GB/ document_library/Scientific_guideline/2009/09/WC500003123.pdf].
26. The European Agency for the evaluation of medicinal products: **Guideline on the evaluation of the pharmacokinetics of medicinal products in patients with impaired hepatic function.** 2004 [http://www.ema.europa. eu/docs/en_GB/document_library/Scientific_guideline/2009/09/ WC500003122.pdf].
27. World Medical Association (WMA). Declaration of Helsinki: **Ethical principles for medical research involving human subjects.** Adopted by the 18th WMA General Assembly, Helsinki, Finland, June; 1964 [http://www.wma.net/ en/30publications/10policies/b3/index.html].
28. European Medicines Agency: **ICH harmonised tripartite guideline; Guideline for good clinical practice E6(R1).** 2002 [http://www.ema.europa. eu/pdfs/human/ich/013595en.pdf].
29. Rowland M, Tozer TN: **Clinical Pharmacokinetics: Concepts and Applications.** Lippincott, Williams & Wilkins, 3 1995.
30. Schelman WR, Liu G, Wilding G, Morris T, Phung D, Dreicer R: **A phase I study of zibotentan (ZD4054) in patients with metastatic, castrate-resistant prostate cancer.** *Invest New Drugs* 2009, **29**:118-125.
31. James ND, Caty A, Payne H, Borre M, Zonnenberg BA, Beuzeboc P, McIntosh S, Morris T, De Phung H, Dawson NA: **Final safety and efficacy analysis of the specific endothelin A receptor antagonist zibotentan (ZD4054) in patients with metastatic castration-resistant prostate cancer and bone metastases who were pain free or mildly symptomatic for pain: A double-blind, placebo-controlled, randomised Phase II trial.** *BJU Int* 2010, **106**:966-973.
32. Carducci MA, Nelson JB, Bowling MK, Rogers T, Eisenberger MA, Sinibaldi V, Donehower R, Leahy TL, Carr RA, Isaacson JD, Janus TJ, Andre A, Hosmane BS, Padley RJ: **Atrasentan, an endothelin-receptor antagonist for refractory adenocarcinomas: safety and pharmacokinetics.** *J Clin Oncol* 2002, **20**:2171-2180.

# An evaluation of ciprofloxacin pharmacokinetics in critically ill patients undergoing continuous veno-venous haemodiafiltration

Almath M Spooner[1], Catherine Deegan[2], Deirdre M D'Arcy[1], Caitriona M Gowing[3], Maria B Donnelly[2*] and Owen I Corrigan[1]

## Abstract

**Background:** The study aimed to investigate the pharmacokinetics of intravenous ciprofloxacin and the adequacy of 400 mg every 12 hours in critically ill Intensive Care Unit (ICU) patients on continuous veno-venous haemodiafiltration (CVVHDF) with particular reference to the effect of achieved flow rates on drug clearance.

**Methods:** This was an open prospective study conducted in the intensive care unit and research unit of a university teaching hospital. The study population was seven critically ill patients with sepsis requiring CVVHDF. Blood and ultrafiltrate samples were collected and assayed for ciprofloxacin by High Performance Liquid Chromatography (HPLC) to calculate the model independent pharmacokinetic parameters; total body clearance (TBC), half-life ($t_{1/2}$) and volume of distribution (Vd). CVVHDF was performed at prescribed dialysate rates of 1 or 2 L/hr and ultrafiltration rate of 2 L/hr. The blood flow rate was 200 ml/min, achieved using a Gambro blood pump and Hospal AN69HF haemofilter.

**Results:** Seventeen profiles were obtained. CVVHDF resulted in a median ciprofloxacin $t_{1/2}$ of 13.8 (range 5.15-39.4) hr, median TBC of 9.90 (range 3.10-13.2) L/hr, a median $V_{dss}$ of 125 (range 79.5-554) L, a CVVHDF clearance of 2.47 +/-0.29 L/hr and a clearance of creatinine ($Cl_{cr}$) of 2.66+/-0.25 L/hr. Thus CVVHDF, at an average flow rate of ~3.5 L/hr, was responsible for removing 26% of ciprofloxacin cleared. At the dose rate of 400 mg every 12 hr, the median estimated $C_{pmax}$/MIC and $AUC_{0-24}$/MIC ratios were 10.3 and 161 respectively (for a MIC of 0.5 mg/L) and exceed the proposed criteria of >10 for $C_{pmax}$/MIC and > 100 for $AUC_{0-24}$/MIC. There was a suggestion towards increased ciprofloxacin clearance by CVVHDF with increasing effluent flow rate.

**Conclusions:** Given the growing microbial resistance to ciprofloxacin our results suggest that a dose rate of 400 mg every 12 hr, may be necessary to achieve the desired pharmacokinetic - pharmacodynamic (PK-PD) goals in patients on CVVHDF, however an extended interval may be required if there is concomitant hepatic impairment. A correlation between ciprofloxacin clearance due to CVVHDF and creatinine clearance by the filter was observed ($r^2$ = 0.76), providing a useful clinical surrogate marker for ciprofloxacin clearance within the range studied.

**Trial Registration:** Current Controlled Trials ISRCTN52722850

## Background

Severe sepsis is a significant contributor to Intensive Care Unit (ICU) admission and reports vary from 12% to 27% of ICU admissions in different countries [1]. Many more patients develop sepsis following ICU admission. EPIC 2 demonstrated that 51% of ICU inpatients were classified as infected on the day of the point prevalence study. In this study 62% of isolates were identified to be Gram negative, which is worrisome given the dearth of in-development antimicrobials with gram negative coverage [2]. Under dosing of antibiotics has enabled the genesis of resistant strains and this is particularly an issue with fluoroquinolones, aminoglycosides and beta lactams [3,4]. Of particular concern is the ability of fluoroquinolones to engender resistance to other classes of antibiotics [5]. Altered drug

* Correspondence: maria.donnelly@amnch.ie
[2]Intensive Care Medicine, Adelaide and Meath Hospital, Dublin, Incorporating the National Children's Hospital, Tallaght, Dublin 24, Ireland
Full list of author information is available at the end of the article

pharmacokinetics, due to disease, results in variable antimicrobial drug clearance in critically ill patients (antibiotic regimens are often developed on the basis of drug disposition in non-critically ill volunteers) and further complicates the selection of appropriate dosing schedules for these patients. For optimal dosing, it is necessary to consider the kill characteristics of the antibiotic.

Pharmacokinetic-pharmacodynamic (PK-PD) parameters can be used to indicate the potential for bacterial eradication with antimicrobial therapy. Bactericidal activity can be time-dependent or concentration-dependent. Quinolones exhibit concentration-dependent bacterial killing [6-10]. Consequently bactericidal activity becomes more pronounced as serum drug concentrations increase to approximately 10 times the minimum inhibitory concentration (MIC.). The goal of ciprofloxacin therapy is to maximise the 24-hr AUC/MIC and the peak/MIC ratios [10]. There is general concern about the emergence of resistance as a result of inadequate doses of ciprofloxacin [9]. A $C_{pmax}$/MIC ratio, where $C_{pmax}$ is the maximum steady state serum concentration, of >10 and an $AUC_{24}$/MIC ~> 100 have been proposed as predictors of therapeutic efficacy [10-12]. In clinical practice, $C_{pmax}$ is equated with the serum peak level. A number of papers have highlighted the requirement for a re-evaluation of currently recommended antimicrobial dosage regimens for critically ill patients [13,14].

Ciprofloxacin disposition is affected by critical illness, particularly by the presence of organ failure and dosage adjustment is advised in patients with renal failure [15]. In patients with severely impaired renal function, a 50% dosage reduction has been recommended [16]. Some data are extrapolated from non-critical patients with renal failure and others from critically ill patients without renal failure. Doses ranging from 200 mg twice daily to 400 mg three times daily have been used for critically ill patients without renal impairment [17,18].

Renal elimination, including both glomerular filtration and tubular secretion accounts for approximately 66% of ciprofloxacin clearance [19]. In healthy volunteers, the hepatic route accounts for approximately 20% of elimination, with transintestinal excretion also playing a possibly significant role. This is thought to represent a notable compensatory pathway preventing drug accumulation in renal failure. In terms of clearance during continuous renal replacement therapy (CRRT), the method of CRRT used has been presented as an important determinant of the effect of CRRT on clearance, with increased drug clearance via CVVHDF compared to continuous veno-venous haemofiltration (CVVH) [20]. Nonetheless, clearance via CVVH of up to 25% has been reported [21]. It has been recommended therefore that dosing during CVVHDF is focussed on attaining clinically adequate drug concentrations, preferably with concurrent therapeutic drug monitoring.

As a result of the reported variability in ciprofloxacin pharmacokinetic parameters during critical illness, differences in patient populations and CRRT conditions in literature reports and the absence of a consensus on dosing regimens, a prospective pharmacokinetic evaluation of ciprofloxacin during CVVHDF therapy was undertaken.

## Methods-

### Patient Demographics and Clinical Characteristics

This was an open, prospective pharmacokinetic study in a multidisciplinary, intensive care unit in a university teaching hospital. Ethics approval was obtained from the Joint Ethics Committee (St James's/AMNCH) (Reference Number 041008/7804). Clinical trial approval was granted by the Irish Medicines Boards (EudraCT Number 2004-002195-42) and the trial was registered with Current Clinical Trials (ISRCTN52722850). Consent (predominantly consent by proxy) was obtained in compliance with Helsinki declaration. Seven critically ill patients, treated concurrently with intravenous ciprofloxacin and CVVHDF therapy, were enrolled in the study. Intravenous ciprofloxacin 400 mg twice daily administered as a one hour infusion was the dosage regimen generally employed, dosing at all times was at the discretion of the physician. A dosage regimen of ciprofloxacin 400 mg once daily was also analysed for three patients, while a dosage regimen of 200 mg twice daily was also assessed in one patient. MIC susceptibility testing for pathogens isolated was not performed. Instead a representative MIC of 0.5 mg/L was employed based on an analysis of local ecology data. It should be noted that CVVHDF patients in this hospital are prescribed on average 14.3 drugs during CVVHDF, 4.7 +/-2.66 are anti-infectives.

### CVVHDF conditions

CVVHDF was performed at prescribed dialysate rates of 1 or 2 L/hr and ultrafiltration rate of 2 L/hr. This reflects the typical CVVHDF prescription of the unit. The blood flow rate was 200 ml/min, achieved using a Gambro blood pump and Hospal AN69HF haemofilter. For patients 6 and 7, CVVHDF was run heparin-free, due to coagulopathy.

### Measurement of Ciprofloxacin Concentrations

Timed serum samples were collected during each dosage interval and ultrafiltrate during 7 dosage intervals (1 per patient). Effluent fluid was collected for the entire dosage interval. The volume of each hourly batch was recorded and a 40 ml sample was taken for analysis. Aliquots from each sample were analysed for ciprofloxacin concentration and for creatinine determination. Total ciprofloxacin concentrations in serum and effluent were measured by the HPLC method of Davis et al [22], adapted for both serum and effluent fluid analysis. Quantitation was based on external standard calibration using the ratio of the peak areas of the analyte and the internal standard (β-hydroxypropyl theophylline). Replicate analysis was performed both on control samples and study samples. Ciprofloxacin hydrochloride monohydrate (1g) (gift from Bayer UK) was used to verify the concentration of the commercial infusion solution, Ciproxin®. The extraction efficiency was in excess of 80% in the concentration range 0.5-20.0 μg/ml and the between day coefficient of variation <10%. Precision was less than 5.0 R.S.D.%. The sensitivity of the assay was 0.5 μg/ml.

### Analysis of Serum Concentrations of Ciprofloxacin

Serum concentrations, from an indwelling arterial cannula, were measured immediately before the infusion was started, immediately after the infusion finished and at 2,3,4,6,8 and 12 hours post infusion where the dosage interval was 12 hr. When the prescribed dosage interval was 24 hr samples were also taken at 18 and 24 hrs. Exact sampling times were recorded. Thus $C_{pmax}$ was directly measured.

### Pharmacokinetic analysis

#### Calculating half-life and clearance

Non-compartmental pharmacokinetic methods were used. Pharmacokinetic analysis was performed using WinNonlin pharmacokinetic software, version 5.2, (Pharsight Corporation, North Carolina, U.S.A.). The terminal half-life ($t_{1/2}$) was calculated as $0.693/\lambda_z$, where $\lambda_z$ is the first order terminal elimination rate constant. The area under the plasma concentration-time curves (AUC) were calculated using the linear trapezoidal method. AUC for the study period (n = 12 or 24 hours) was used to calculate the AUC extrapolated to infinity ($AUC_{0-\infty}$) by the equation $AUC_{0-t^*} + C^*/\lambda_z$. where $C^*$ is the final plasma concentration, at the final sampling time, $t^*$. The Total Body Clearance (TBC) was calculated as $dose/AUC_{0-\infty}$ for profile 4a as this was a first dose, and as $dose/AUC_{0-\tau}$ at steady state, where $\tau$ is the dosage interval, for all other profiles except 2c, 4b and 6c, which were not at steady state.

#### Estimating clearance for profiles not at steady state

Profiles 2c, 4b and 6c did not result from initial doses, and could not be considered to be at steady state as they directly followed a change in dose or interval. For these profiles, TBC was estimated as $dose/AUC_{n0-\infty}$.

AUC $_{n0-\infty}$ in these cases was estimated as ($AUC_{0-\infty}$ $-(C^*_{(n-1)}/\lambda_{z\ (n-1)})$), where $C^*_{(n-1)}$ was the final observed concentration at the end of the preceding dose interval,

and $\lambda_{z\ (n-1)}$ was the first order terminal elimination rate constant calculated from the preceding dose interval.

#### Calculating volume of distribution at steady state ($V_{dss}$)

Because of the severity of illness body weights could not be accurately monitored, consequently parameters were not weight normalised. Volume of distribution at steady state ($V_{dss}$) for an initial dose was calculated as $TBC \times ((AUMC_{0-\infty}/AUC_{0-\infty}) - t_{inf}/2)$, where $t_{inf}$ is the duration of the infusion, and as $TBC \times (((AUMC_{0-\tau} + \tau(AUC_{0-\infty} - AUC_{0-\tau}))/AUC_{0-\tau}) - t_{inf}/2)$ from profiles at steady state. In cases where the dosing interval was changed from 24 (at steady state) to 12 hours, the first profile following the change was calculated as a 24 hour interval, with sampling ceasing at 12 hours. This was the case for profiles 6b and 7b. $V_{dss}$ was not calculated for profiles 2c, 4b and 6c as these were neither an initial dose or at steady state.

#### Calculating sieving coefficients

Sieving coefficients (S) for ciprofloxacin and creatinine were calculated from the time-matched concentrations in effluent and in serum for a single dosage interval, whereby $S_{creatinine} = C_{effluent}/C_{serum}$ and $S_{cipro} = C_{effluent}/C_{serum}$. The clearance of creatinine was calculated from $S_{creatinine}$ and the measured flow of effluent (Q) where $Cl_{creat} = S_{creat} \times Q$.

The fraction cleared by CVVHDF ($F_{CVVHDF}$) was determined from $Cl_{CVVHDF}/TBC$. The PK-PD parameters $C_{pmax}/MIC$ and $AUC_{0-24}/MIC$ were employed as predictors of the likelihood of clinical and microbiological response.

## Results

### Patients

Relevant demographic and clinical data relating to the seven patients studied are presented in Table 1. Patients were severely ill having renal failure, haemodynamic instability and coagulopathy. Six patients were prescribed ciprofloxacin for documented infection *(Pseudomonas aeruginosa, Escherichia coli)*, while one patient with suspected sepsis was prescribed ciprofloxacin empirically. The median APACHE II score was 27 (range 25-30).

### CVVHDF conditions

The actual flow rates achieved were recorded and compared with the target flow rates. The mean effluent flow rate achieved was 3.35 +/- 0.50 L/hr (Range: 2.9 - 4.0 L/hr). The mean duration of CVVHDF therapy was 9.3 +/- 3.7 days. The mean number of filters used per dosage interval was 1.1. The mean duration of use of a filter was 50.6 hours.

### Pharmacokinetic profiles

Seventeen pharmacokinetic profiles were obtained from these seven patients. The ciprofloxacin pharmacokinetic

**Table 1 Demographic and clinical data of patients on continuous veno-venous haemodiafiltration administered ciprofloxacin**

| | Sex | Age | Diagnosis | Infective pathogen | APACHE II score (initial/highest) | CVVHDF Duration(days) | ICU Mortality Outcome |
|---|---|---|---|---|---|---|---|
| 1 | M | 60 | Intestinal Obstruction, Hemicolectomy | Escherichia coli | 26 | 6 | Survived |
| 2 | F | 77 | Neutropaenic sepsis | Pseudomonas aeruginosa | 27 | 5 | Died |
| 3 | F | 68 | Intestinal obstruction, post-operative sepsis and acute renal failure | Pseudomonas aeruginosa | 28 | 14 | Survived |
| 4 | M | 47 | Acute pancreatitis, sepsis | Escherichia Coli | 25 | 14 | Survived |
| 5 | F | 71 | ESRD with severe sepsis | Empiric cover | 27 | 8 | Died |
| 6 | M | 57 | Hepatic cirrhosis with severe sepsis | Pseudomonas Aeruginosa, Enterococcus faecalis | 29 | 7 | Survived |
| 7 | M | 28 | Acute liver failure with severe sepsis | Pseudomonas aeruginosa | 30 | 11 | Survived |

parameters estimated from each patient's pharmacokinetic profile, during treatment with CVVHDF are presented in Table 2. Ciprofloxacin $t_{1/2}$ during CVVHDF was variable, ranging from 5.15 to 39.4 hours, with a median of 13.8 hours, reflecting a median elimination rate constant of 0.050 (range 0.018-0.135) $hr^{-1}$. The average $t_{1/2}$ of patients 1 and 4 (both had hepatic impairment) were 37.3 and 25.9 hours, respectively. These $t_{1/2}$ values are seven to eight times that obtained in patients with normal renal function, and were the highest obtained in the current study. Patient 4 had evidence of liver injury that may have resulted in impaired

**Table 2 Estimates of pharmacokinetic parameters obtained from multiple ciprofloxacin serum concentrations in a dosage interval using non-compartmental methods**

| Patient Profile | Dose (mg) | Dosage Interval (hours) | $T_{1/2}$ (hrs) | k ($hr^{-1}$) | $AUC_{0-\tau}$* (τ = dosage interval) (mg.hr/L) | TBC (Dose/AUC) (L/hr) | $Vd_{ss}$ (L) |
|---|---|---|---|---|---|---|---|
| 1.A | 400 | 12 | 35.2 | 0.020 | 35.4 | 11.3 | 524 |
| 1.B | 400 | 12 | 39.4 | 0.018 | 38.3 | 10.4 | 555 |
| **Mean** | | | **37.3** | **0.019** | **36.8** | **10.9** | **539** |
| 2.A | 200 | 12 | 5.15 | 0.135 | 15.2 | 13.2 | 104 |
| 2.B | 200 | 12 | 13.8 | 0.050 | 16.5 | 12.2 | 215 |
| 2.C | 400 | 12 | 12.4 | 0.056 | 51.8 | 7.72 | |
| **Mean** | | | **10.5** | **0.080** | | **11.0** | **160** |
| 3.A | 400 | 12 | 5.97 | 0.116 | 38.9 | 10.3 | 79.5 |
| 3.B | 400 | 12 | 7.50 | 0.092 | 40.2 | 10.0 | 97.3 |
| **Mean** | | | **6.73** | **0.104** | **39.5** | **10.1** | **88.4** |
| 4.A | 400 | 24 | 24.7 | 0.028 | 129 | 3.10 | 111 |
| 4.B | 400 | 12 | 27.2 | 0.026 | 81.5 | 4.91 | |
| **Mean** | | | **25.9** | **0.027** | | **4.00** | |
| 5.A | 400 | 12 | 8.44 | 0.082 | 40.4 | 9.90 | 107 |
| 5.B | 400 | 12 | 5.77 | 0.120 | 37.8 | 10.6 | 81.1 |
| 5.C | 400 | 12 | 6.80 | 0.102 | 40.9 | 9.78 | 88.2 |
| **Mean** | | | **7.00** | **0.101** | **39.7** | **10.1** | **92.2** |
| 6.A | 400 | 24 | 14.0 | 0.050 | 43.4 | 9.22 | 175 |
| 6.B | 400 | 12 | 14.7 | 0.047 | 54.0 | 7.40 | 151 |
| 6.C | 400 | 12 | 16.5 | 0.042 | 49.6 | 8.06 | |
| **Mean** | | | **15.0** | **0.046** | | **8.23** | **163** |
| 7.A | 400 | 24 | 15.1 | 0.046 | 50.6 | 7.91 | 164 |
| 7.B | 400 | 12 | 10.4 | 0.067 | 39.4 | 10.1 | 139 |
| **Mean** | | | **12.7** | **0.056** | | **9.00** | **151** |

* τ taken to be 24 hours for first profile immediately following a change in prescribed dosage interval (profiles 6b and 7b)

biliary clearance, and patient 1 had concurrent alcoholic liver disease, which may have contributed to the prolonged $t_{1/2}$. In patient 4, profile 4a, the clearance was calculated using the estimated $AUC_{0-\infty}$, as this profile was measured following the initial dose. The long half life calculated (25 h) in combination with the lower volume of distribution lead to a comparatively low estimated TBC. The $t_{1/2}$ observed in patients 3 and 5, 6.73 and 7.00 respectively, were closer to those seen in patients with normal renal function. The median TBC of ciprofloxacin was 9.90 (range 3.10-13.2) L/hr (~0.14 L/hr/kg based on a 70 kg patient). This value represents hepatic, residual renal and transintestinal ciprofloxacin clearance, in addition to ciprofloxacin clearance by the filter. The $V_{dss}$ for ciprofloxacin during CVVHDF therapy ranged from 79.5-555 L with a median of $V_{dss}$ of 125 L. The mean $C_{pmax}$ concentration following administration of 400 mg every 12 hours was 5.8 +/- 1.0 mg/L.

The clearances of ciprofloxacin and creatinine by CVVHDF are presented in Table 3. The mean clearance of ciprofloxacin by CVVHDF was 2.47 +/- 0.29 L/hr, thus the clearance of ciprofloxacin by CVVHDF was on average 26% of the TBC, reflected in the mean $F_{CVVHDF}$ of 0.26 (Table 3). This value excludes that of patient 4. In this case a significant fraction (0.74) of the clearance is calculated to have occurred via CVVHDF, and was therefore considered an atypical value.

The $S_{cipro}$ was 0.70 +/- 0.06. A simple method for estimating drug clearance through the filter, without measuring drug levels, involves using the non-protein bound fraction $(f_u)$ of ciprofloxacin as an estimate of the sieving coefficient, as it is the unbound fraction that crosses the filter. Hoffken et al [23] and Joos et al [24] have reported $f_u$ values for ciprofloxacin of 0.6 and 0.78 respectively. Applying these values to the observed flow rates in this study gives clearance estimates of 2.0 L/hr and 2.7 L/hr, which approximate the measured value of 2.47 L/hr. The sieving coefficient for creatinine (0.82 +/- 0.04) was quite similar to that estimated for ciprofloxacin. A correlation between ciprofloxacin clearance due to CVVHDF (y) and creatinine clearance by the filter (x) was observed (y = -0.29 + 1.03x, $r^2$ = 0.76) and is illustrated in Figure 1. Ciprofloxacin and creatinine clearances over time were examined in order to identify any change in filter efficiency over time. There was little variation in filter performance as the clearance of both creatinine and ciprofloxacin remaining relatively constant.

Within the observed range of effluent flow rates and CVVHDF ciprofloxacin clearance rates in the current study, there is a suggested trend ($r^2$ = 0.94) of increasing ciprofloxacin clearance with higher effluent fluid flow rates, which is illustrated in Figure 2.

### Pharmacokinetic - Pharmacodynamic parameters

The PK-PD parameters, $C_{pmax}$/MIC ratios and the ratio of $AUC_{0-24}$ /MIC, achieved with a ciprofloxacin dosing regimen of 400 mg ciprofloxacin every 12 hours are summarised in Table 4.

The median $AUC_{0-24}$/MIC ratio for patients administered Ciprofloxacin 400 mg twice daily was 161. An $AUC_{0-24}$/MIC~ > 100 has been propounded as an indicator of adequate ciprofloxacin dosing [12].

### Discussion

The pharmacokinetic parameter estimates obtained, half life [median 13.8 (range 5.15-39.4) hours], TBC [median 9.90 (range 3.10-13.2) L/hr] and median $V_{dss}$ of 125 (range 79.5-555) L illustrate the high level of inter-patient variability in ciprofloxacin disposition in critically ill patients during CVVHDF. The $t_{1/2}$ of ciprofloxacin, approximately 4 hours in patients with normal renal function, doubles in patients with severe renal impairment. In general, accumulation will not be observed with 12 hour dosing as this interval is greater than the half-life, in patients without liver dysfunction. As significant accumulation was observed with an interval of eight hours in previous studies [15,17,25] a longer dosage interval of 12 hours for patients on CVVHDF should therefore be considered. Patients 1,4,6 and 7 had

**Table 3 Ciprofloxacin and Creatinine Clearance by continuous veno-venous haemodiafiltration.**

| Patient | $Cl_{CVVHDF}$ (L/hr) | $Cl_{CREAT}$ (L/hr) | $F_{CVVHDF}$ | Measured effluent fluid rate (L/hr) | Total Body Clearance (L/hr) |
|---|---|---|---|---|---|
| 1 A | 2.8 | 2.9 | 0.25 | 4.0 | 11.3 |
| 2 C | 2.4 | 2.6 | 0.31 | 3.4 | 7.72 |
| 3 B | 2.7 | 2.9 | 0.27 | 3.9 | 9.96 |
| 4 A | 2.3 | 2.3 | 0.74 | 2.9 | 3.10 |
| 5 A | 2.2 | 2.6 | 0.22 | 3.0 | 9.90 |
| 6 C | 2.1 | 2.4 | 0.26 | 2.9 | 8.06 |
| 7 B | 2.8 | 2.9 | 0.28 | 4.0 | 10.1 |
| **Mean +/- SD** | **2.47 +/- 0.29** | **2.66 +/- 0.25** | **0.26 ± 0.03*** | **3.35 +/- 0.50** | **8.60 ± 2.7** |

* Excluding value from patient 4A

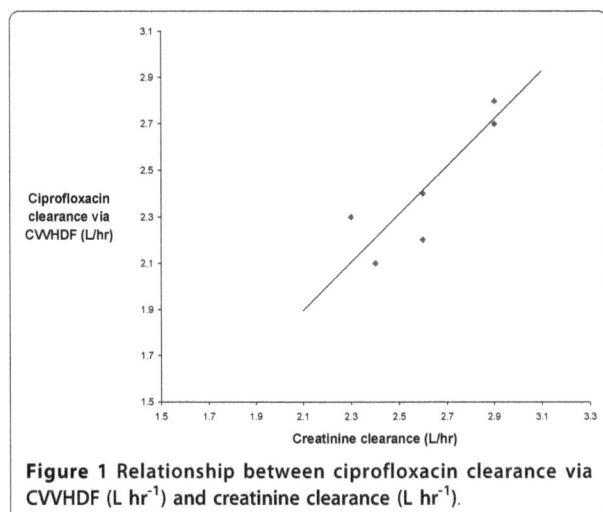

**Figure 1** Relationship between ciprofloxacin clearance via CVVHDF (L hr⁻¹) and creatinine clearance (L hr⁻¹).

**Table 4 Cpmax/MIC ratios for representative MICs for patients treated with 400 mg ciprofloxacin every 12 hours during critical illness and continuous veno-venous haemodiafiltration therapy.**

| Patient ID | Cpmax/MIC ratio (MIC = 0.5 mg/L) | $AUC_{0-24}$/MIC ratio (MIC = 0.5 mg/L) |
|---|---|---|
| 1 | 10.3 | 147 |
| 2 | 10.2 | 207 |
| 3 | 12.8 | 158 |
| 5 | 14.6 | 159 |
| 6 | 10.0 | 199 |

average half-lives varying from 13-15 hours (patients 6 and 7) to greater than 25 hours (patients 1 and 4), demonstrating the variability of pharmacokinetic profiles in this patient group, and also likely reflecting decreased hepatic clearance in these four patients.

Wallis et al [15] reported a similarly reduced ciprofloxacin clearance in six patients with renal failure, treated with 200 mg ciprofloxacin three times daily during CVVHDF therapy (0.06-0.25 L/hr/kg).

The median volume of distribution of 125 L (mean 185 +/- 155) is similar to values reported by Wallis et al [15] (mean: 135+/- 27 L) estimated from six patients treated with 200 mg every 8 hours and by Lipman et al [18] (range: 0.77 - 2.52 L/kg) for critically ill patients. The current patient sample showed greater variability: Patient 1, in particular, had a very high $V_{dss}$ of 539L. The average $V_{dss}$ for the other 6 patients was 126

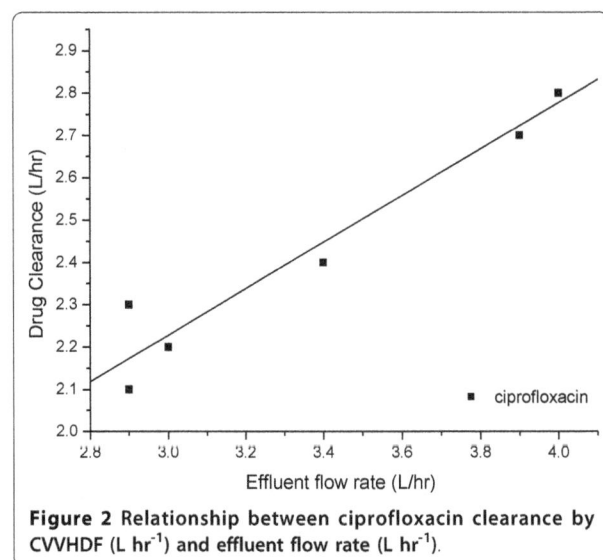

**Figure 2** Relationship between ciprofloxacin clearance by CVVHDF (L hr⁻¹) and effluent flow rate (L hr⁻¹).

+/-43L. These values compare well with those detailed above from Wallis et al [15], and probably reflect more typical $V_{dss}$ values of ciprofloxacin in this patient population. However, the high $V_{dss}$ calculated from patient 1 serves as evidence of the unpredictable drug disposition which can occur in critically ill patients, reflecting greater degrees of capillary leak in keeping with the severity of illness.

A practical and useful finding was that, within the range studied, creatinine clearance may serve as a clinical surrogate for ciprofloxacin clearance on CVVHDF. This relationship is clinically important as ciprofloxacin is not routinely assayed in most hospitals. The relationship did not decline over the life of the filter. This relationship may serve as a useful guide to dosing ciprofloxacin within this range of creatinine clearance values.

As effluent flow rates increased, there was a suggested trend of increased ciprofloxacin clearance via CVVHDF. However, there was no observed change in TBC with increasing effluent flow rate. This illustrates the varying role of compensatory and alternative elimination methods such as hepatic elimination. Further studies on this association between effluent flow rate and ciprofloxacin clearance via CVVHDF to investigate the presence of a cause-effect relationship would be beneficial and may helpfully influence dosing decisions. This is of importance in particular as increased effluent flow rates may be used for purposes other than enhancing drug clearance, and therefore TBC in such patients can be difficult to estimate in the absence of plasma concentration data and due to the varying influence of alternative elimination routes. Further insight into the effect of increasing effluent flow rate on clearance via CVVHDF is therefore desirable. Prospectively, such dosing considerations are often hampered by the discrepancy between prescribed and achieved flow rates.

CVVHDF was responsible for clearing approximately one quarter of all ciprofloxacin eliminated. Its relative contribution to ciprofloxacin TBC will be greatest in patients with concurrent hepatic and renal dysfunction, as in these patients, CVVHDF will become a proportionately more significant route. Therefore care is required in dosing patients with concurrent renal and hepatic failure/impairment to avoid accumulation of ciprofloxacin. Interestingly, clearance of ciprofloxacin via CVVH of up to 25% has been reported [21], which is similar to that observed in the current study using CVVHDF. This implies that both dialysis parameters and patient specific parameters have a role to play in the observed variability in clearance via CRRT, in addition to the CRRT method used.

There is now significant evidence that correct and timely antibiotic choices will save more lives than virtually all other ICU therapies [4,26]. A $C_{pmax}$/MIC ratio of ~>10 has been suggested [9,11] as desirable and thus a 400 mg twice daily regimen appears to achieve these target concentrations during CVVHDF therapy (Table 4), 200 mg twice daily being inadequate. For ciprofloxacin 400 mg twice daily, the median $C_{pmax}$ achieved in this study was 5.2 (range 5.0-7.3) mg/L (mean $5.8 \pm 1.0$ mg/L), which represented a median $C_{pmax}$/MIC ratio (based on an MIC of 0.5 mg/L) of 10.3. The median $AUC_{0-24}$ was 80.4 (range 70.8-104) mg.hr/L (mean $83.0 \pm 11.1$ mg.hr/L), which corresponds to a median $AUC_{0-24}$/MIC ratio of 161 (range 142-207). A suggested characteristic of adequate dosing for ciprofloxacin is an $AUC_{0-24}$/MIC ratio > 100.

Wallis et al [15] reported lower $C_{pmax}$ concentrations and $AUC_{0-24}$ values with a lower daily dose of 600 mg ciprofloxacin, compared to the 800 mg daily dose used in this study. The CVVHDF conditions in our study were similar to those reported by Wallis et al [15]. Wallis et al [15] used a dosing schedule of 200 mg every 8 hours and the mean $C_{pmax}$ concentration was 3.5 +/- 0.5 mg/L. This dosing schedule achieves on average a $C_{pmax}$/MIC ratio of 7 (based on a MIC of 0.5 mg/L). The mean $AUC_{0-24}$ achieved by the same dosing schedule of 200 mg every 8 hours was 48.3 +/- 8.7 mg.h/L, equivalent to a $AUC_{0-24}$/MIC ratio of 96.6 +/- 17.4, on the basis of a MIC value of 0.5 mg/L. Malone et al [27] reported a mean $C_{pmax}$ of 3.9 mg/L ($C_{pmax}$ /MIC ratio; 7.8) for three patients treated with 400 mg ciprofloxacin every 24 hours during CVVHDF therapy. The mean $AUC_{0-24}$ with this dosing schedule was 56.8 mg.h/L, which represents an $AUC_{0-24}$/MIC ratio of 114 (assuming an MIC of 0.5 mg/L). The CVVHDF conditions employed by Malone et al [27] were different from those used in the current work.

On the basis of these pharmacodynamic considerations, the dosing schedule utilised in this study gives better cover than previously studied dosage strategies and should serve as a pharmacokinetically and pharmacodynamically valid dose guide in the appropriate clinical circumstances.

One limitation of this work is common to all carried out in this field, that patient numbers are small, and as such the conclusions that can be drawn are limited to a very narrow patient cohort. A consideration for future research might be that a randomised crossover design could be employed to add further clarity to dosing recommendations. As both antimicrobial doses, and dialysis parameters such as flow rate, are frequently adjusted on the basis of changing clinical need in the intensive care setting, there are ethical difficulties surrounding the set up and design of such trials.

Another limitation was that liver dysfunction or impairment was not characterised in a standardised manner. However this is difficult in these patients due to blood product and vitamin K administration, particularly in septic and coagulopathic patients and also because of concurrent hepatotoxic drug administration. Similarly, the varying nature from day to day of hepatic/renal function in many critically ill patients suggest that calculations based on steady state be interpreted with caution, as clearance is likely to be variable. Furthermore, it is extremely difficult to quantify any residual renal function, and thereby contribution to the clearance, that these patients made have had.

## Conclusion
Our results suggest that a dose rate of 400 mg every 12 hours, will achieve the recommended PK-PD goals in *most* patients on CVVHDF. Twice daily dosing of ciprofloxacin maximised peak concentrations, while minimizing accumulation. Concomitant hepatic and renal dysfunction results in a prolonged elimination half-life. Creatinine clearance by the filter may be used to estimate ciprofloxacin clearance by CVVHDF (within the range studied). Thus in the absence of ciprofloxacin plasma levels, creatinine clearance by the filter could be considered as a surrogate marker for ciprofloxacin clearance in patients, this may be particularly useful when other routes of elimination are impaired.

The data suggest that drug clearance increases with increasing effluent flow rate, which in turn may require even higher ciprofloxacin dosing. This association between effluent flow rate and drug clearance requires further elucidation to determine the nature of any cause-effect relationship.

While a 400 mg dose administered at 12 hourly intervals achieved adequate $C_{pmax}$ concentrations and lower doses may result in target serum concentrations in some patients with hepatic dysfunction, given the general emergence of ciprofloxacin resistance and the wide therapeutic index of ciprofloxacin, it may be advisable to maintain the higher ciprofloxacin dose as the mainstay of therapy. The possibility of accumulation in patients where more than one elimination route is impaired should be considered and this can be addressed by extension of the dosage interval.

## Key Messages

- Ciprofloxacin 400 mg twice daily IV will achieve the recommended PK-PD goal ($AUC_{0-24}$/MIC ratio >125) in most patients on CVVHDF.
- Concomitant hepatic and renal impairment results in a prolonged ciprofloxacin elimination half life, therefore dosage interval extension may be required.
- Creatinine clearance by the filter correlates well with ciprofloxacin clearance by the filter, therefore creatinine clearance by the filter (in the range studied) may be used as a surrogate for ciprofloxacin clearance.

## List of abbreviations

APACHE II: Acute Physiology and Chronic Health Evaluation score; AUC: Area Under the Curve; AUMC: Area Under the Moment Curve; $C^*$: Final plasma concentration; $Cl_{cr}$: Clearance of creatinine; $C_{pmax}$: Maximum plasma concentration; CRRT: Continuous Renal Replacement Therapy; CVVHDF: Continuous Veno-Venous Haemodiafiltration; ESRD: End Stage Renal Disease; $F_{CVVHDF}$: Fraction cleared by continuous veno-venous haemodiafiltration; $f_u$: Non protein bound fraction; HPLC: High Performance Liquid Chromatography; ICU: Intensive Care Unit; LFTs: Liver Function Tests; MIC: Minimum Inhibitory Concentration; PK-PD: Pharmacokinetic - Pharmacodynamic; Q: Effluent flow rate; S: Sieving coefficient; $t_{1/2}$: Half life; TBC: Total Body Clearance; $t_{inf}$: Infusion duration time; $V_d$: Volume of distribution; $V_{dss}$: Volume of distribution at steady state; $\lambda_z$: First order elimination rate constant; $\tau$: Dosage interval.

## Acknowledgements

The authors acknowledge the support of the Astellas European Foundation for funds enabling purchase of the HPLC equipment employed.
The authors also acknowledge the tireless commitment of the ICU nursing staff to data collection, ongoing research and patient care.
The views expressed in this article are the personal views of the author(s).

## Author details

[1]School of Pharmacy and Pharmaceutical Sciences, Trinity College Dublin, Dublin 2, Ireland. [2]Intensive Care Medicine, Adelaide and Meath Hospital, Dublin, Incorporating the National Children's Hospital, Tallaght, Dublin 24, Ireland. [3]Pharmacy Department, Adelaide and Meath Hospital, Dublin, Incorporating the National Children's Hospital, Tallaght, Dublin 24, Ireland.

## Authors' contributions

OC, CG, MD and AS initiated and supervised the study from its inception. CD devised study protocols and completed clinical trial applications. AS and CD co-ordinated sample acquisition. AS undertook sample analysis under the supervision of OC. AS and DD completed the pharmacokinetic analysis and modelling. AS and OC authored the first draft, with review and additions by DD, MD and CG. AS, OC, CG, MD, CD and DD read and approved the final manuscript.

## Competing interests

The authors declare that they have no competing interests.

## References

1. Silva E, Angus DC: **Epidemiology of severe sepsis**. In *Twenty-five Years of Progress and Innovation in Intensive Care Medicine*. Edited by: Kuhlen R, Moreno R, Ranieri, Rhodes A. Medizinisch Wissenschaftliche Verlag; 2007:155-162.
2. Vincent JL, Rello J, Marshall J, Silva E, Anzueto A, Martin CD, Moreno R, Lipman J, Gomersall C, Sakr Y, Reinhart K, for the EPIC II Group of Investigators: **International Study of the Prevalence and Outcomes of Infection in Intensive Care Units**. *JAMA* 2009, **302(21)**:2323-2329.
3. Nseir S, Di Pompeo C, Soubrier S, Delour P, Lenci H, Roussel-Delvallez M, Onimus T, Saulnier F, Mathieu D, Durocher A: **First-generation fluoroquinolones use and subsequent emergence of multiple drug resistant bacteria in the intensive care unit**. *Crit Care Med* 2005, **33**:283-289.
4. Lipman J: **The new antibiotic treatment paradigm**. *Intensive Care Monitor* 2007, **14**:61-62.
5. Nierderman MS: **Re-examining quinolone use in the intensive care unit; Use them right or lose the fight against resistance bacteria**. *Crit Care Med* 2005, **33**:443-444.
6. Cruciani M, Bassetti D: **The fluoroquinolones as treatment for infections caused by gram-positive bacteria**. *J Antimicrobial Chemother* 1994, **33**:403-417.
7. Craig WA, Ebert S, Moffatt J: **Pharmacodynamic activity of Bay y 3118 in animal infection models**. *Abstr 33rd Interscience conference on antimicrobial agents and chemotherapy* 1993, 391.
8. Watanabe Y, Ebert S, Craig WA: **AUC/MIC ratio is unifying parameter for comparison of in vivo activity among fluoroquinolones**. *Abst 32nd interscience conference on antimicrobial agents and chemotherapy* 1992, 42.
9. Schentag JJ: **The relationship between ciprofloxacin blood concentrations, MIC values, bacterial eradication and clinical outcome in patients with nosocomial pneumonia.**Edited by: Garrad C. Ciprofloxacin iv. Defining its role in serious infection Berlin, Germany Springer-Verlag; 49-57.
10. Scaglione F: **Can PK/PD be used in everyday clinical practice?** *Int J Antimicrobial Agents* 2002, **19**:349-353.
11. Sanchez Recio MM, Colino CI, Sanchez Navarro A: **A retrospective analysis of pharmacokinetic/pharmacodynamic indices as indicators of the clinical efficacy of ciprofloxacin**. *J Antimicrob Chemother* 2000, **45**:321-328.
12. Turnidge J: **Pharmacokinetics and pharmacodynamics of fluoroquinolones**. *Drugs* 1999, **58(Suppl 2)**:29-36.
13. Pinder M, Bellomo R, Lipman J: **Pharmacological principles of antibiotic prescription in the critically ill**. *Anaesth Intensive Care* 2002, , **30**: 134-44.
14. Lipman J: **Towards better ICU antibiotic dosing**. *Crit Care Resusc* 2000, , **2**:282-9.
15. Wallis SC, Mullany DV, Lipman J, Rickard CM, Daley PJ: **Pharmacokinetics of ciprofloxacin in ICU patients on continuous veno-venous haemodiafiltration**. *Intensive Care Medicine* 2001, **27**:665-672.
16. Bayer Healthcare: **Ciproxin Infusion Summary Product Characteristics**. [http://www.medicines.ie/medicine/12239/SPC/Ciproxin+Solution+for +Infusion+2mg+ml%2c+200ml/].
17. MacGowan AP, White LO, Brown NM, Lovering AM, McMullin CM, Reeves DS: **Serum ciprofloxacin concentrations in patients with severe sepsis being treated with ciprofloxacin 200 mg i.v. bd irrespective of renal function**. *J Antimicrob Chemother* 1994, **33**:1051-1054.
18. Lipman J, Scribante J, Gous AG, Hon H, Tshukutsoane S, the Baragwanath Ciprofloxacin Study Group: **Pharmacokinetic profiles of high- dose intravenous ciprofloxacin in severe sepsis**. *Antimicrob Agents Chemother* 1998, **42**:2235-2239.
19. Vancebryan K, Guay DRP, Rotschafer JC: **Clinical pharmacokinetics of ciprofloxacin**. *Clin Pharmacokinet* 1990, **19(6)**:434-461.
20. Pea F, Viale P, Pavan F, Furlanut M: **Pharmacokinetic considerations for antimicrobial therapy in patients receiving renal replacement therapy**. *Clin Pharmacokinet* 2007, **46(12)**:997-1038.
21. Bellmann R, Egger P, Bellmann-Weiler R, Joannidis M, Dunzendorfer St, Wiedermann Ch J: **Pharmacokinetics of ciprofloxacin in patients with acute renal failure undergoing continuous venovenous haemofiltration: Influence of concomitant liver cirrhosis**. *Acta Medica Austriaca* 2002, **Heft 3**:112-116.
22. Davis JD, Aarons L, Houston BJ: **Simultaneous assay of fluoroquinolones and theophylline in plasma by high-performance liquid chromatography**. *Journal of Chromatography* 1993, **621**:105-109.
23. Hoeffken G, Lode H, Prinzing C, Borner K, Koeppe P: **Pharmacokinetics of ciprofloxacin after oral and parenteral administration**. *Antimicrob Agents Chemother* 1985, **27**:375-379.
24. Joos B, Ledergerber B, Flepp M, Bettex JD, Luthy R, Siegenthaler W: **Comparison of high-pressure liquid chromatography and bioassay for**

determination of ciprofloxacin in serum and urine. *Antimicrob Agents Chemother* 1985, **27**:353-356.

25. Davies SP, Azadian BS, Kox WJ, Brown EA: **Pharmacokinetics of ciprofloxacin and vancomycin in patients with acute renal failure treated by continuous haemodialysis.** *Nephrol Dial Transplant* 1992, **7**:848-54.

26. Kumar A, Roberts D, Wood KE, Light B, Parrillo JE, Sharma S, Suppes R, Feinstein D, Zanotti S, Taiberg L, Gurka D, Kumar A, Cheang M: **Duration of hypotension before initiation of effective antimicrobial therapy is the critical determinant of survival in human septic shock.** *Crit Care Med* 2006, **34**:1589-96.

27. Malone RS, Fish DN, Abraham E, Teitelbaum I: **Pharmacokinetics of Levofloxacin and Ciprofloxacin during Continuous Renal Replacement Therapy in Critically Ill Patients.** *Antimicrob Agents and Chemotherapy* 2001, **45**:2949-2954.

# Gastrointestinal adverse effects of varenicline at maintenance dose: a meta-analysis

Lawrence K Leung[1,2,3]*, Francis M Patafio[3] and Walter W Rosser[1,2,3]

## Abstract

**Background:** Tobacco smoking remains the leading modifiable health hazard and varenicline is amongst the most popular pharmacological options for smoking cessation. The purpose of this study is to critically evaluate the extent of gastrointestinal adverse effects of varenicline when used at maintenance dose (1 mg twice a day) for smoking cessation.

**Methods:** We conducted a meta-analysis of randomised controlled trials published in PUBMED and EMBASE according to the PRISMA guidelines. Selected studies satisfied the following criteria: (i) duration of at least 6 weeks, (ii) titrated dose of varenicline for 7 days then a maintenance dose of 1 mg twice-per-day, (iii) randomized placebo-controlled design, (iv) extractable data on adverse event - nausea, constipation or flatulence. Data was synthesized into pooled odd ratios (OR) basing on random effects model. Quality of studies was also rated as per Cochrane risk-of-bias assessment. Number need to harm (NNH) was calculated for each adverse effect.

**Results:** 98 potentially relevant studies were identified, 12 of which met the final inclusion criteria (n = 5114). All 12 studies reported adverse events on nausea, which led to an OR of 4.45 (95% CI = 3.79-5.23, $p < 0.001$; $I^2 =$ 0.06%, CI = 0%-58.34%) and a NNH of 5. Eight studies (n = 3539) contain data on constipation pooled into an OR of 2.45 (95% CI = 1.61-3.72, $p < 0.001$; $I^2 = 34.09\%$, CI = 0%-70.81%) with a NNH of 24. Finally, five studies (n = 2516) reported adverse events of flatulence, which pooled an OR of 1.74 (95% CI = 1.23-2.48, $p = 0.002$; $I^2 = 0\%$, CI = 0%- 79.2%) with a NNH of 35.

**Conclusions:** Use of varenicline at maintenance dose of 1 mg twice a day for longer than 6 weeks is associated with adverse gastrointestinal effects. In realistic terms, for every 5 treated subjects, there will be an event of nausea, and for every 24 and 35 treated subjects, we will expect an event of constipation and flatulence respectively. Family physicians should counsel patients of such risks accordingly during their maintenance therapy with varenicline.

## Background

Tobacco smoking remains the most modifiable risk factor for premature death and all-cause mortality [1], with a global estimate of 4.83 million attributable deaths in year 2000 [2]. As a result, many pharmacological agents have been developed to help patients stop tobacco smoking, some of which can be administered either nasally, orally (chewable gum or tablets) or topically (e.g., nicotine replacement patch). Amongst these agents, varenicline (branded as Champix© in UK and Canada, Chantix© in USA) has been shown to be the one of the most effective oral pharmacological agents for continued abstinence. Varenicline acts as a partial $\alpha_4\beta_2$ nicotinic acetylcholine receptor agonist in the brain to potentially decrease the degree of cravings and withdrawal symptoms during the period of smoking cessation, with effects superior to both placebos and other pharmacological agents [3]. Animal studies have found that tobacco addiction is mediated via nicotinic acetylcholine receptors (nAChRs) in the meso-limbic area of the brain that contain $\alpha_4$ and $\beta_2$ subunits. While $\alpha_4$ subunits are needed for sensitization and reinforcement to nicotinic effects and their tolerance, involvement of $\beta_2$ subunits are indispensable for development of dependence [4]. In vivo studies have shown that in the presence of nicotine, varenicline acts as a partial agonist which stimulates the release of dopamine (to ameliorate the symptoms of craving and withdrawal) and simultaneously block the

* Correspondence: leungl@queensu.ca
[1]Centre of Studies in Primary Care, Queen's University, 220 Bagot Street, Kingston Ontario, Canada K7L 5E9
Full list of author information is available at the end of the article

nicotine receptors (to reduce the likelihood of dependence)[5,6]. When compared to other mainstream pharmacotherapies (e.g., nicotine replacement therapy and bupropion), varenicline remains as the most effective choice for smoking cessation [7] and is validated by high-quality meta-analysis [8]. Nevertheless, varenicline has been associated with adverse events like headache, fatigue, sleep disorder, nausea and constipation [9,10]. Whilst risks of neuropsychiatric adverse events due to varenicline have already been reported in a polled analysis [11], the likelihood of major gastrointestinal adverse effects (such as nausea, constipation and flatulence) during maintenance phase lacks precise documentation. We hereby performed a meta-analysis of randomized double-blinded placebo-controlled trials to critically examine the relative risks of nausea, constipation and flatulence due to maintenance dose of varenicline (1 mg twice a day for at least 6 weeks) in the context of smoking cessation.

## Methods
### Eligibility criteria
Our primary interest was the reported gastrointestinal adverse-effects in using varenicline at the indicated maintenance dose (1 mg) for duration longer than six weeks. To minimise heterogeneity, we limited our scope to double-blind randomised placebo-controlled trials with comparable sample sizes and a satisfactory score from the Cochrane risk of bias assessment tool described by Higgins [12]. Eligible studies must use a one-week titrated dose (0.5 mg) of varenicline prior to maintenance dose (1 mg twice a day), and contain at least one extractable adverse gastrointestinal event of nausea, constipation or flatulence.

### Search strategy
A literature search of published medical reports was performed in all languages from PUBMED (from 1947 to December 2010), EMBASE (from 1947 to December 2010) and All EBM Reviews using the OVID Portal of Queen's University, Kingston, Ontario. Abstracts were initially obtained using keywords of "smoking cessation" AND "varenicline. They were further narrowed down by imposing keywords of "human" AND "controlled trial". Manual searches of references and review articles supplemented the computerized search.

### Study selection, data extraction and quality assessment
Two reviewers (LL and FP) worked independently and went over the initial search for abstracts that satisfied the keywords as mentioned in the search strategy section. They then adopted a simple form to select trials that satisfied the eligibility criteria stated above. Evaluation of selected studies were performed independently by each reviewer according to the Cochrane risks of bias tool [12]

in regards to the quality of study, randomization protocol, adequacy of concealment and blinding and, rigor of follow-up for dropouts. Information was extracted and tabulated in spreadsheet regarding the demography of the study population, duration of study, the types of adverse events, the number of affected subjects taking varenicline and placebo respectively and finally a numeric score for the Cochrane risk of bias. Spreadsheets were compared and any disagreement was discussed and resolved to reach mutual consensus.

### Statistical Analysis
All data were synthesized in a meta-analysis and odds ratios (OR) were calculated with appropriate confidence intervals (CI) basing on the number of subjects reporting the relevant adverse effects in the study. Where necessary, the value of 1 was added to any arm with zero outcome event according to the Sheele +1 rule [13]. The random effects analysis model as described by DerSimonian and Laird [14] was adopted instead of the fixed effects model to account for extra variance due to heterogeneous samples drawn from a wide population [15]. Forest plots [16] were generated basing on OR for each gastrointestinal symptom of nausea, constipation and flatulence. Basing on the values of OR and the baseline risks of adverse effects, the number needed to harm (NNH) was also calculated which gives a realistic idea of the likelihood of the adverse effects. Funnel plots [17] were displayed as a reference for possible publication bias. To assess heterogeneity across included studies, we adopted the Cochran Q-statistic [18] and the $I^2$ index [19,20] with 95% confidence intervals. We assumed a $p$-value of less than 0.10 for the Cochran Q-statistic and an $I^2$ index of greater than 50% as a threshold of heterogeneity. Statistical advice was provided by data analyst at our Centre of Studies in Primary Care.

## Results
### Study description
1431 abstracts were identified using keywords of "smoking cessation" AND "varenicline", which were reduced to 108 abstracts when imposing extra keywords of "human" AND "controlled trial" with supplementation from reference lists of included abstracts. 10 duplicates were removed and 82 abstracts were further excluded on grounds of having no placebo control group, combined mixed treatments, no relevant gastrointestinal adverse events data, or duplication trial publication or report. 16 relevant full text paper publications were then retrieved for potential inclusion. After imposing the eligibility criteria as described, only 12 studies were deemed eligible upon which mutual consensus was reached between the reviewers after discussion and comparison of the data spreadsheets. Using the 2009 PRISMA

checklist [21] (Additional File 1), all 27 items were present and identified scored. A flow diagram of the literature search and selection process according to the PRISMA format [21] was given in Figure 1, and the included studies were tabulated in Table 1. From the 12 studies, 2,622 patients were randomly assigned to receive varenicline (oral dose of 1 mg twice per day), and 2,492 patients were randomly assigned to receive placebo. Total sample size per study ranged from 248 to 714 and three studies had a total size of greater than 500. Except for the study by Tashkin et al. [22] which specifically targeted patients with COPD, all other studies recruited subjects from the general population. One

trial used varenicline for 6 weeks [23] while another for 52 weeks [24], the rest used 12 weeks. All but one study [23] employed the standard low-dose titration regime before using the 1 mg twice per day dosage. There was no exclusion as for the type of tobacco used by smokers in all trials except for the study by Fagerstrom et al. [9] which recruited subjects using smokeless tobacco.

**Assessment of study quality**

All 12 studies achieved a score of at least 4 out of 6, using the Cochrane risk of bias assessment [12] (See table 1) and was considered satisfactory with mutual agreement between the two reviewers. After consultation with our

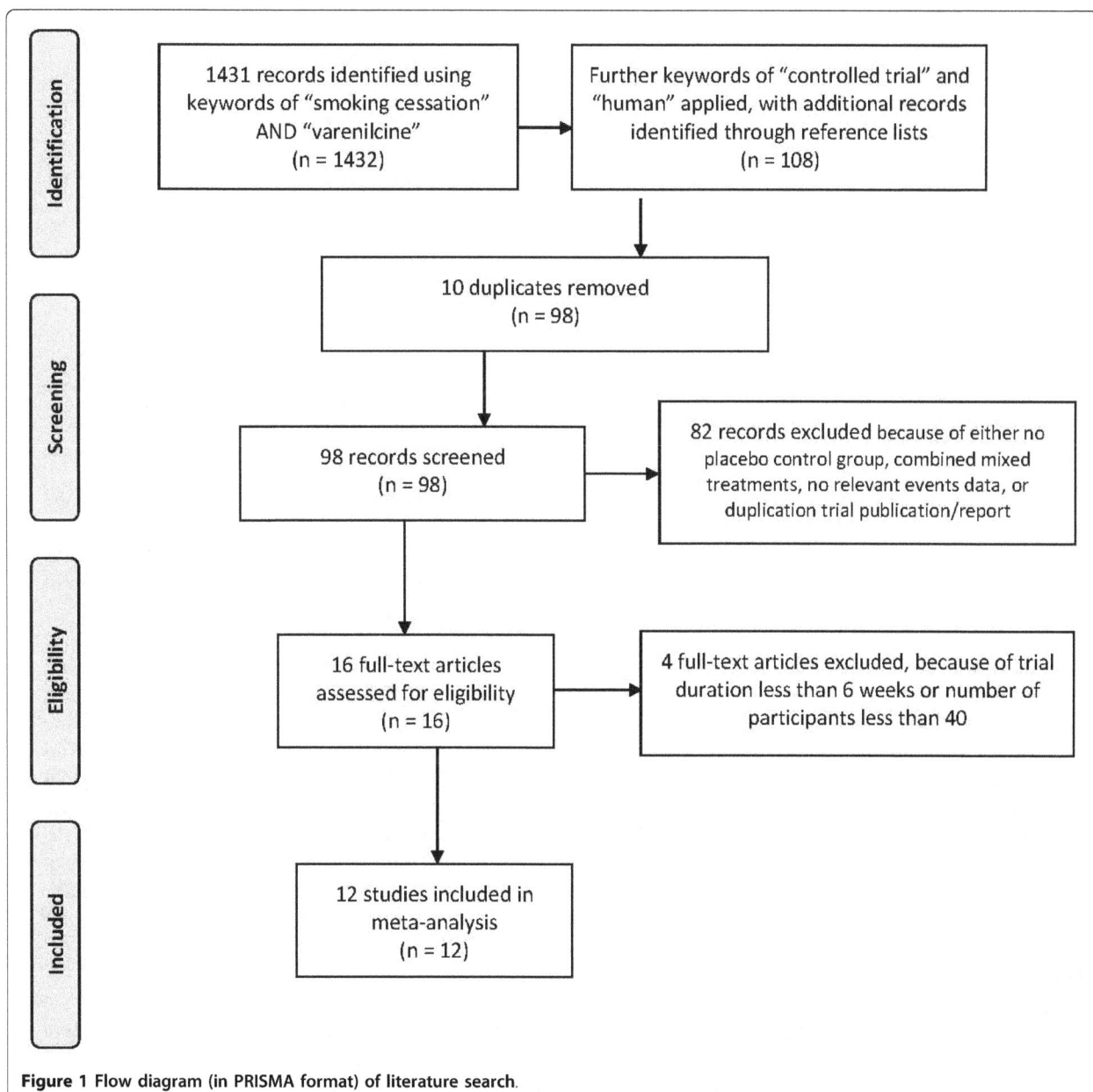

**Figure 1 Flow diagram (in PRISMA format) of literature search.**

**Table 1 Summary of the 12 studies included for meta-analysis**

| Study | Total Sample Size (n) | Adverse effects[¥] | Mean Age | % Male | Trial Duration with 1 mg BID dose(Weeks) | Size of Trial group | Size of Control Group | Cochrane risk of bias assessment[§] | | | | | | |
|---|---|---|---|---|---|---|---|---|---|---|---|---|---|---|
| | | | | | | | | P | Q | R | S | T | U | Overall score |
| Gonzales et al (2006)[32] | 696 | A, B, C | 42.55 | 52.05 | 12 | 352 | 344 | 1 | 1 | 1 | 1 | 1 | 1 | 6/6 |
| Jorenby et al (2006)[29] | 685 | A, B, C | 43.45 | 56.65 | 12 | 344 | 341 | 1 | 1 | 1 | 1 | 1 | 0 | 5/6 |
| Oncken et al (2006)[27] | 259 | A, B, C | 41.1 | 50.2 | 12 | 130 | 129 | 1 | 1 | 1 | 1 | 0 | 0 | 4/6 |
| Nides et al (2006)[25] | 248 | A, B | 41.7 | 51.2 | 6 | 125 | 123 | 1 | 1 | 0 | 1 | 1 | 0 | 4/6 |
| Nakamura et al(2007)[30] | 310 | A, B | 40 | 77.6 | 12 | 156 | 154 | 1 | 1 | 1 | 1 | 1 | 1 | 6/6 |
| Tsai et al (2007)[28] | 250 | A, B | 40.3 | 88.8 | 12 | 126 | 124 | 1 | 1 | 0 | 1 | 1 | 0 | 4/6 |
| Williams et al (2007)[26] | 377 | A, B, C | 47.7 | 48.6 | 52 | 251 | 126 | 1 | 1 | 0 | 1 | 1 | 0 | 4/6 |
| Niaura et al (2008)[34] | 312 | A | 41.8 | 51.9 | 12 | 157 | 155 | 1 | 1 | 1 | 1 | 1 | 0 | 5/6 |
| Wang et al (2009)[33] | 333 | A | 38.7 | 96.7 | 12 | 165 | 168 | 1 | 1 | 0 | 1 | 1 | 0 | 4/6 |
| Rigotti et al (2010)[31] | 714 | A, B | 56.45 | 78.7 | 12 | 355 | 359 | 1 | 1 | 0 | 1 | 1 | 1 | 5/6 |
| Fagerstrom et al(2010)[8] | 431 | A | 43.9 | 89.3 | 12 | 213 | 218 | 1 | 1 | 1 | 1 | 1 | 1 | 6/6 |
| Tashkin et al (2010)[24] | 499 | A, C | 57.2 | 62.3 | 12 | 248 | 251 | 1 | 1 | 0 | 1 | 1 | 0 | 4/6 |

[¥]A = Nausea, B = Constipation, C-Flatulence.

[#]Denote use of 1-week low-dose titration treatment.

[§]Cochrane risk of bias assessment: P = Allocation sequence adequately generated?; Q = Allocation adequately concealed?; R = Knowledge of allocated intervention adequately concealed?; S = incomplete outcome data adequately addressed?; T = Reports free of selective outcome reporting?; U = study free of other factors leading to high risk of bias?; 1 = item positive; 0 = negative or unknown.

statistician, the random effects model was adopted for subsequent analysis.

## Outcome Measures

### Nausea

All 12 studies [9,22-32] reported adverse effects of nausea with a total sample size of 5114. Out of the total 2622 subjects randomized to varenicline, 826 reported nausea; of the 2492 subjects taking placebo, 232 had nausea. The pooled OR was 4.45 (95% confidence levels [CI] of 3.79-5.23, $p < 0.001$) with a non-significant Cochrane Q-statistic of 11.01 ($p = 0.443$) and an $I^2$ index of 0.06% (95% confidence levels of 0% - 58.34%). With a baseline risk of nausea at 9.3%, the number need to harm (NNH) is 5. The Forest plot was shown in Figure 2 and funnel plot in Additional File 2.

### Constipation

8 studies [23-30] reported adverse effects of constipation with a total sample size of 3539. 146 of 1839 subjects in the varenicline group and 53 of 1700 in the control group reported adverse effects of constipation. The pooled OR was 2.45 (95% confidence levels [CI] of 1.61-3.72, $p <$ 0.001) with a non-significant Cochrane Q-statistic of 10.62 ($p = 0.156$) and an $I^2$ index of 34.09% (95% confidence levels of 0% - 70.81%). The baseline risk of constipation is 3.1%, yielding a NNH of 24. The Forest plot was shown in Figure 3 and the funnel plot in Additional File 2.

### Flatulence

5 studies [22,24,25,27,30] were included reporting adverse effects of flatulence with a total sample size of 2516 subjects. 102 of 1325 subjects in the varenicline group and 50 of 1191 in the control group reported adverse effects of flatulence. The pooled OR was 1.74 (95% confidence levels [CI] of 1.23-2.48, $p = 0.002$) with a non-significant Cochrane Q-statistic of 1.82 ($p = 0.768$) and an $I^2$ index of 0% (95% confidence levels of 0% - 79.2%). With a baseline risk of flatulence at 4.2%, the NNH is 35. The Forest plot was shown in Figure 4 and the funnel plot in Additional File 2.

## Discussion

Our meta-analysis data confirms that using varenicline at maintenance dose of 1 mg twice per day for a period of more than 6 weeks is significantly associated with

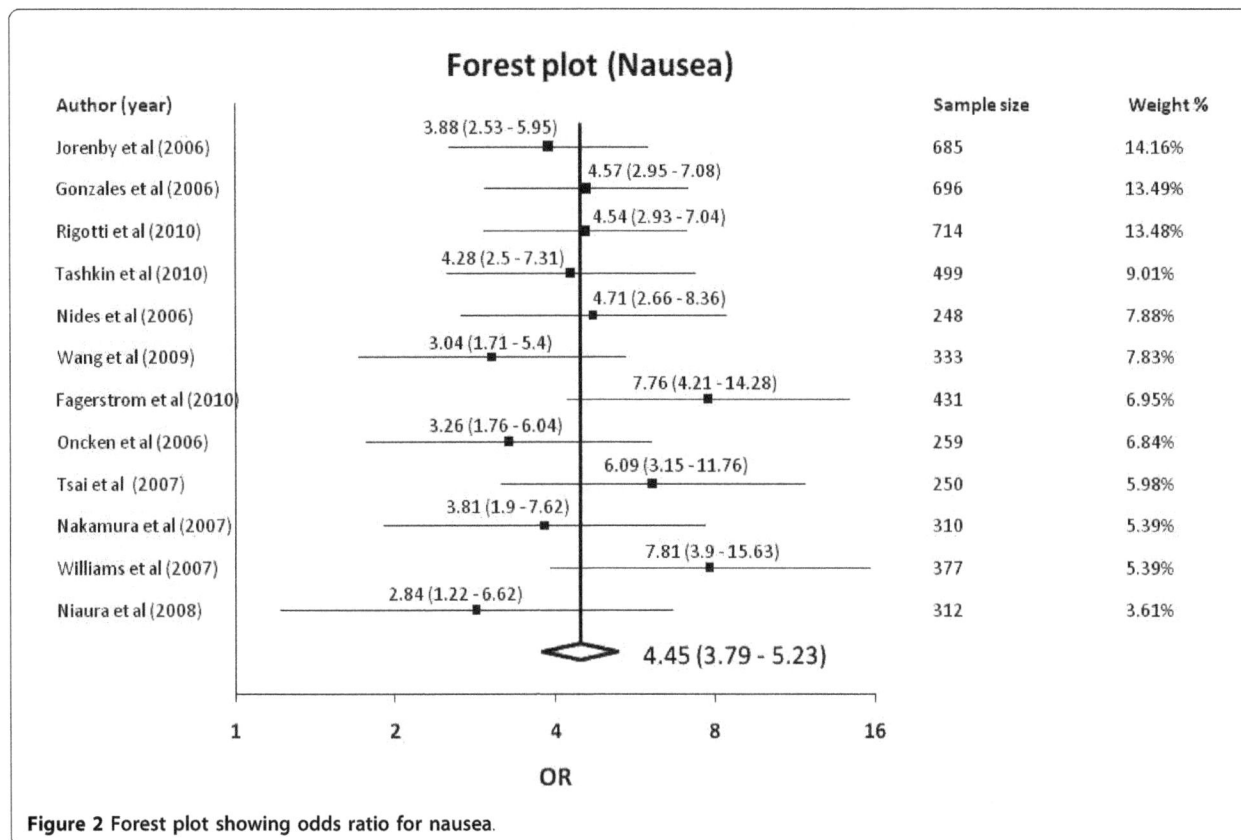

**Figure 2** Forest plot showing odds ratio for nausea.

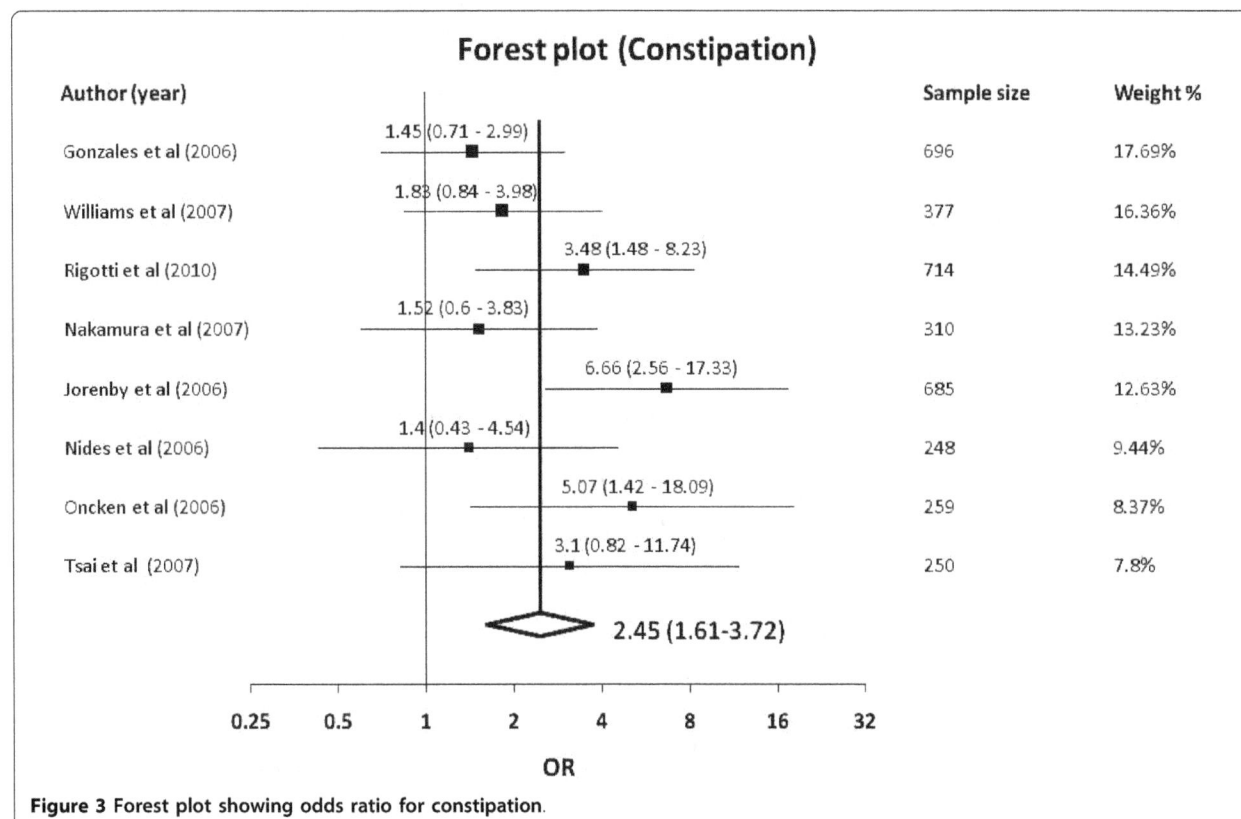

**Figure 3** Forest plot showing odds ratio for constipation.

## Forest plot (Flatulence)

| Author (year) | | Sample size | Weight % |
|---|---|---|---|
| Williams et al (2007) | 1.34 (0.66 - 2.71) | 377 | 25.02% |
| Tashkin et al (2010) | 1.43 (0.69 - 2.99) | 499 | 22.87% |
| Gonzales et al (2006) | 2.01 (0.93 - 4.36) | 696 | 20.67% |
| Jorenby et al (2006) | 2.57 (1.12 - 5.92) | 685 | 17.81% |
| Oncken et al (2006) | 1.94 (0.75 - 5.02) | 259 | 13.63% |

1.74 (1.23 - 2.48)

0.5   1   2   4   8

OR

**Figure 4** Forest plot showing odds ratio for flatulence.

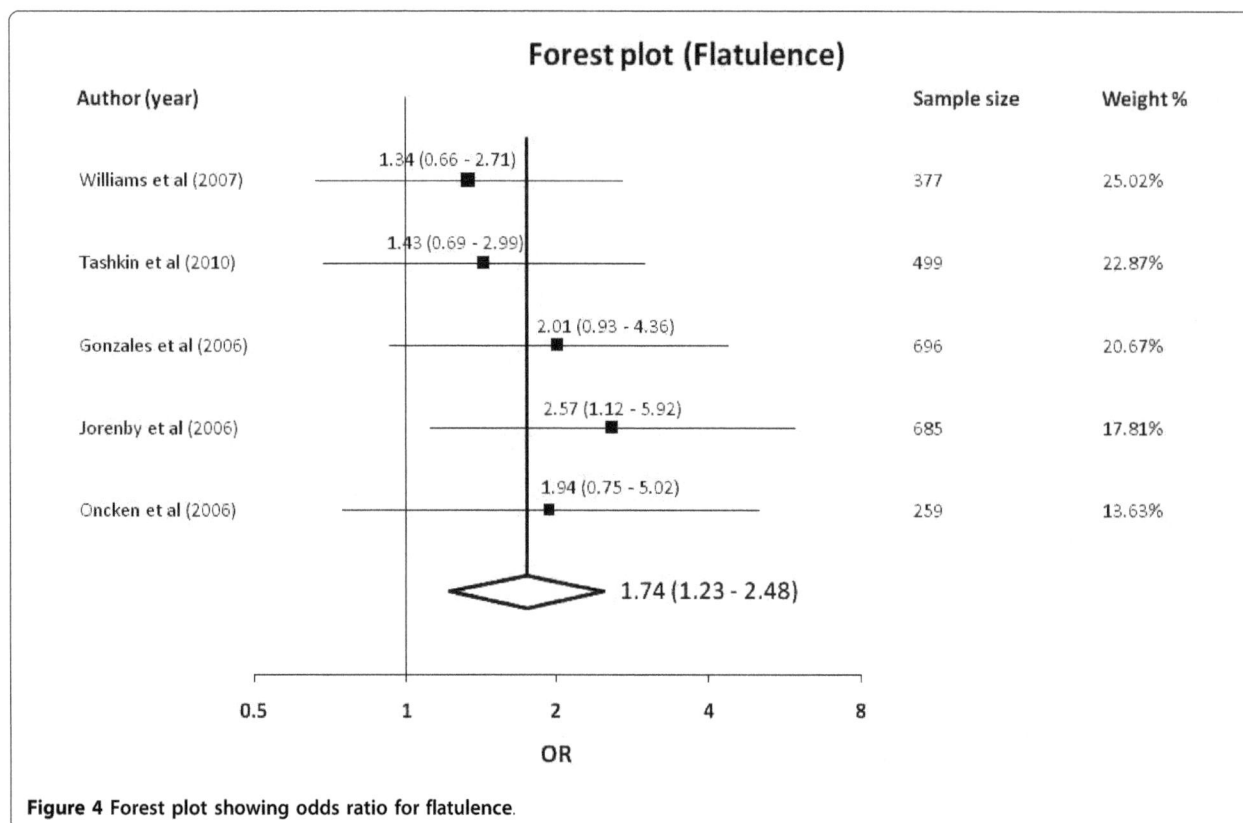

adverse effects of nausea and, to a lesser extent, constipation and flatulence. Using pooled odds ratios (OR) and subsequently translating them to number need to harm (NNH), we showed that for nausea, constipation and flatulence, the NNH is 5, 24 and 35 respectively. Such numbers provide clinicians with a realistic picture of the likelihood for gastrointestinal adverse effects when prescribing varenicline as a drug of choice for smoking cessation. As the commonest gastrointestinal adverse effect, nausea accounts for failure of varenicline treatment amongst 1.8% to 7.6% of our study population [24,26,27,30,31]. The effects of nausea usually peak around 4 weeks of treatment and becoming less thereafter [24]. No similar discontinuation rates due to effects of constipation or flatulence have been reported.

### Limitation of studies

Our study has two limitations. Gastrointestinal adverse effects like nausea and flatulence are primarily subjective feelings which are difficult to quantify, despite crude stratification into mild, moderate or severe in several studies. Definition for constipation is also not standardised as per Rome criteria [33] amongst the included studies in terms of bowel frequency or patient's difficulty in defecation. They may constitute data heterogeneity across studies in our meta-analysis.

The second limitation is the potential of publication bias. Our search strategy only isolated full-length published trials with sufficient population sizes to maintain statistical significance. In addition, we excluded studies with populations less than 40. However adoption of the random effects model in meta-analysis will help compensate irregularities due to small and potentially negative studies that we have excluded. Our funnel plots do not show obvious asymmetry (Additional File 2), suggesting the low likelihood of publication bias in our analysis. Thus said, the visual asymmetry of funnel plots should not be used to confirm the extent of publication bias [34], especially when the number of studies is small [35]. The $I^2$ index suggests very low heterogeneity across studies for both nausea and flatulence (both at 0%) and slightly higher but still acceptable heterogeneity for constipation (34%)[20]. Like the Cochran Q-statistic, the $I^2$ index is known to have limitations with its power affected by the actual number of included studies [36].

### Conclusions

Varenicline is one of the most preferred pharmacological options for smoking cessation and gastrointestinal adverse effects have been mentioned but not documented precisely. Our comprehensive meta-analysis on randomised double-blind placebo-controlled trials concluded that in realistic terms, use of varenicline at the indicated maintenance dose (1 mg twice per day) for longer than 6 weeks will lead to one adverse event of nausea for every 5 treated subjects, one event of constipation for every treated 24 subjects and one event of flatulence for every 35 treated subjects. These data will better enable clinicians in counseling patients when using varenicline for smoking cessation both in facilitating and reinforcing optimal smoking cessation rate.

## Conflict of interests

The authors declare that they have no competing interests.

## Additional material

Additional file 1: PRISMA 2009 Checklist for the meta-analysis study. All items in the 2009 PRISMA checklist are considered and verified against the page of the original manuscript.

Additional file 2: Funnel plots showing bias of studies for adverse effects of (a)nausea, (b)constipation, (c)flatulence. File contains the funnel plots of various studies basing on the odds ratio, as categorised by the adverse effects of nausea, constipation and flatulence respectively.

## Author details

[1]Centre of Studies in Primary Care, Queen's University, 220 Bagot Street, Kingston Ontario, Canada K7L 5E9. [2]Department of Family Medicine, Queen's University, 220 Bagot Street, Kingston Ontario, Canada K7L 5E9. [3]School of Medicine, Queen's University, Kingston General Hospital, 18 Stuart Street, Kingston Ontario, Canada K7L 3N6.

## Authors' contributions

LL and FP designed the review and performed the literature search. LL performed the analysis and generation of the graphic plots. LL and FP analysed and interpreted the data and both contributed to the drafting of the manuscript. WR provided comments and advice on the overall study. ALL authors have read and approved the submitted version for publication.

## References

1.  Peto R, Lopez AD, Boreham J, Thun M, Heath C Jr, Doll R: **Mortality from smoking worldwide**. *Br Med Bull* 1996, **52**(1):12-21.
2.  Ezzati M, Lopez AD: **Regional, disease specific patterns of smoking-attributable mortality in 2000**. *Tob Control* 2004, **13**(4):388-395.
3.  Keating GM, Lyseng-Williamson KA: **Varenicline: a pharmacoeconomic review of its use as an aid to smoking cessation**. *Pharmacoeconomics* 2010, **28**(3):231-254.
4.  Foulds J: **The neurobiological basis for partial agonist treatment of nicotine dependence: varenicline**. *Int J Clin Pract* 2006, **60**(5):571-576.
5.  Rollema H, Chambers LK, Coe JW, Glowa J, Hurst RS, Lebel LA, Lu Y, Mansbach RS, Mather RJ, Rovetti CC, *et al*: **Pharmacological profile of the alpha4beta2 nicotinic acetylcholine receptor partial agonist varenicline, an effective smoking cessation aid**. *Neuropharmacology* 2007, **52**(3):985-994.
6.  Coe JW, Brooks PR, Vetelino MG, Wirtz MC, Arnold EP, Huang J, Sands SB, Davis TI, Lebel LA, Fox CB, *et al*: **Varenicline: an alpha4beta2 nicotinic receptor partial agonist for smoking cessation**. *J Med Chem* 2005, **48**(10):3474-3477.
7.  Garrison GD, Dugan SE: **Varenicline: a first-line treatment option for smoking cessation**. *Clin Ther* 2009, **31**(3):463-491.
8.  Mills EJ, Wu P, Spurden D, Ebbert JO, Wilson K: **Efficacy of pharmacotherapies for short-term smoking abstinence: a systematic review and meta-analysis**. *Harm Reduct J* 2009, **6**:25.
9.  Fagerstrom K, Gilljam H, Metcalfe M, Tonstad S, Messig M: **Stopping smokeless tobacco with varenicline: randomised double blind placebo controlled trial**. *BMJ* 2010, **341**:c6549.
10. Fagerstrom K, Nakamura M, Cho HJ, Tsai ST, Wang C, Davies S, Ma W, Lee TC, Russ C: **Varenicline treatment for smoking cessation in Asian populations: a pooled analysis of placebo-controlled trials conducted in six Asian countries**. *Curr Med Res Opin* 2010, **26**(9):2165-2173.
11. Tonstad S, Davies S, Flammer M, Russ C, Hughes J: **Psychiatric adverse events in randomized, double-blind, placebo-controlled clinical trials of varenicline: a pooled analysis**. *Drug Saf* 2010, **33**(4):289-301.
12. Higgins JAD: **Assessing risk of bias in included studies**. *Cochrane handbook for systematic reviews of interventions*. 1 edition. John Wiley and Sons; 2008, 187-241.
13. Sheehe PR: **Combination of log relative risk in retrospective studies of disease**. *Am J Public Health Nations Health* 1966, **56**(10):1745-1750.
14. DerSimonian R, Laird N: **Meta-analysis in clinical trials**. *Control Clin Trials* 1986, **7**(3):177-188.
15. Fleiss JL: **The statistical basis of meta-analysis**. *Stat Methods Med Res* 1993, **2**(2):121-145.
16. Lewis S, Clarke M: **Forest plots: trying to see the wood and the trees**. *BMJ* 2001, **322**(7300):1479-1480.
17. Egger M, Davey Smith G, Schneider M, Minder C: **Bias in meta-analysis detected by a simple, graphical test**. *BMJ* 1997, **315**(7109):629-634.
18. Cochran WG: **The combination of estimates from different experiments**. *Biometrics Vol* 1954, **10**:101-129.
19. Higgins JP, Thompson SG: **Quantifying heterogeneity in a meta-analysis**. *Stat Med* 2002, **21**(11):1539-1558.
20. Higgins JP, Thompson SG, Deeks JJ, Altman DG: **Measuring inconsistency in meta-analyses**. *BMJ* 2003, **327**(7414):557-560.
21. Liberati A, Altman DG, Tetzlaff J, Mulrow C, Gotzsche PC, Ioannidis JP, Clarke M, Devereaux PJ, Kleijnen J, Moher D: **The PRISMA statement for reporting systematic reviews and meta-analyses of studies that evaluate healthcare interventions: explanation and elaboration**. *BMJ* 2009, **339**: b2700.
22. Tashkin DP, Rennard S, Hays JT, Ma W, Lawrence D, Lee TC: **Effects of Varenicline on Smoking Cessation in Mild-to-Moderate COPD: A Randomized Controlled Trial**. *Chest* 2010.
23. Nides M, Oncken C, Gonzales D, Rennard S, Watsky EJ, Anziano R, Reeves KR: **Smoking cessation with varenicline, a selective alpha4beta2 nicotinic receptor partial agonist: results from a 7-week, randomized, placebo- and bupropion-controlled trial with 1-year follow-up**. *Arch Intern Med* 2006, **166**(15):1561-1568.
24. Williams KE, Reeves KR, Billing CB Jr, Pennington AM, Gong J: **A double-blind study evaluating the long-term safety of varenicline for smoking cessation**. *Curr Med Res Opin* 2007, **23**(4):793-801.
25. Oncken C, Gonzales D, Nides M, Rennard S, Watsky E, Billing CB, Anziano R, Reeves K: **Efficacy and safety of the novel selective nicotinic acetylcholine receptor partial agonist, varenicline, for smoking cessation**. *Arch Intern Med* 2006, **166**(15):1571-1577.
26. Tsai ST, Cho HJ, Cheng HS, Kim CH, Hsueh KC, Billing CB Jr, Williams KE: **A randomized, placebo-controlled trial of varenicline, a selective alpha4beta2 nicotinic acetylcholine receptor partial agonist, as a new therapy for smoking cessation in Asian smokers**. *Clin Ther* 2007, **29**(6):1027-1039.
27. Jorenby DE, Hays JT, Rigotti NA, Azoulay S, Watsky EJ, Williams KE, Billing CB, Gong J, Reeves KR: **Efficacy of varenicline, an alpha4beta2 nicotinic acetylcholine receptor partial agonist, vs placebo or sustained-release bupropion for smoking cessation: a randomized controlled trial**. *JAMA* 2006, **296**(1):56-63.
28. Nakamura M, Oshima A, Fujimoto Y, Maruyama N, Ishibashi T, Reeves KR: **Efficacy and tolerability of varenicline, an alpha4beta2 nicotinic acetylcholine receptor partial agonist, in a 12-week, randomized, placebo-controlled, dose-response study with 40-week follow-up for smoking cessation in Japanese smokers**. *Clin Ther* 2007, **29**(6):1040-1056.
29. Rigotti NA, Pipe AL, Benowitz NL, Arteaga C, Garza D, Tonstad S: **Efficacy and safety of varenicline for smoking cessation in patients with cardiovascular disease: a randomized trial**. *Circulation* 2010, **121**(2):221-229.

30. Gonzales D, Rennard SI, Nides M, Oncken C, Azoulay S, Billing CB, Watsky EJ, Gong J, Williams KE, Reeves KR: **Varenicline, an alpha4beta2 nicotinic acetylcholine receptor partial agonist, vs sustained-release bupropion and placebo for smoking cessation: a randomized controlled trial.** *JAMA* 2006, **296(1)**:47-55.
31. Wang C, Xiao D, Chan KP, Pothirat C, Garza D, Davies S: **Varenicline for smoking cessation: a placebo-controlled, randomized study.** *Respirology* 2009, **14(3)**:384-392.
32. Niaura R, Hays JT, Jorenby DE, Leone FT, Pappas JE, Reeves KR, Williams KE, Billing CB: **The efficacy and safety of varenicline for smoking cessation using a flexible dosing strategy in adult smokers: a randomized controlled trial.** *Curr Med Res Opin* 2008, **24(7)**:1931-1941.
33. Drossman DA: **Rome III: the new criteria.** *Chin J Dig Dis* 2006, **7(4)**:181-185.
34. Terrin N, Schmid CH, Lau J: **In an empirical evaluation of the funnel plot, researchers could not visually identify publication bias.** *J Clin Epidemiol* 2005, **58(9)**:894-901.
35. Song F, Khan KS, Dinnes J, Sutton AJ: **Asymmetric funnel plots and publication bias in meta-analyses of diagnostic accuracy.** *Int J Epidemiol* 2002, **31(1)**:88-95.
36. Ioannidis JP, Patsopoulos NA, Evangelou E: **Uncertainty in heterogeneity estimates in meta-analyses.** *BMJ* 2007, **335(7626)**:914-916.

# Comparative *in vitro* study of the antimicrobial activities of different commercial antibiotic products of vancomycin

Jorge A Diaz[1†], Edelberto Silva[1*†], Maria J Arias[2] and María Garzón[1]

## Abstract

**Background:** One of the most critical problems about antimicrobial therapy is the increasing resistance to antibiotics. Previous studies have shown that there is a direct relation between erroneous prescription, dosage, route, duration of the therapy and the antibiotics resistance. Other important point is the uncertainty about the quality of the prescribed medicines. Some physicians believe that generic drugs are not as effective as innovator ones, so it is very important to have evidence that shows that all commercialized drugs are suitable for therapeutic use.

**Methods:** Microbial assays were used to establish the potency, the Minimal Inhibitory Concentrations (MICs), the Minimal Bactericidal Concentration (MBCs), the critical concentrations, and the production of spontaneous mutants that are resistant to vancomycin.

**Results:** The microbial assay was validated in order to determine the Vancomycin potency of the tasted samples. All the products showed that have potency values between 90 - 115% (USP requirement). The products behave similarly because the MICs, The MBCs, the critical concentrations, the critical concentrations ratios between standard and samples, and the production of spontaneous mutants don't have significant differences.

**Conclusions:** All products analyzed by microbiological tests, show that both trademarks and generics do not have statistical variability and the answer of antimicrobial activity Show also that they are pharmaceutical equivalents.

## Background

Pharmaceutical products, especially antibiotics, must comply with standards of quality, efficacy and reliability, attributes that are determined by various authorities [[1,2], and [3]]. A discussion about the quality and efficacy of generic antibiotics has taken place in recent decades. This discussion has included presentations in congress and research articles in which the authors have shown that some products do not meet regulatory standards [4,5] and that their behavior is not similar in animal models [6,7]

Some antibiotics must be analyzed using biological assays (e.g., penicillin, amikacyn, vancomycin, and neomycin) [2]. These products are measured by their potency or biological activity compared against an international standard. Therefore, the commercial products must be similar in composition to the international reference standard [7]. With antibiotics like vancomycin, if the commercial products do not fulfill the requirements of pharmacopeia, their behavior and performance could put a patient's health in danger.

Biological assays and other analytical procedures must be validated before they are applied in the analysis of the content of the antibiotic under study because, otherwise, neither the information or data generated nor conclusions obtained will be reliable [3]. Our worry arises from the fact that some researchers confuse a "gold standard" with an international reference standard for quantification. A gold standard is something that is a defined commercial product used as reference of performance in comparative studies. It is not a reference standard, but another commercial product with its own variation. Gold standards are established for purposes of bioequivalence and bioavailability studies [2], but in the case of IV antibiotics, the bioavailability is 100%, and therefore, pharmacodynamic

---

* Correspondence: esilvag@unal.edu.co
† Contributed equally
[1]Universidad Nacional de Colombia, Facultad de Ciencias, Departamento de Farmacia, Laboratorio de Asesorías e Investigaciones en Microbiología, 472. Ciudad Universitaria. Carrera 30 Calle 45. A.A.14490. Bogotá D. C. Colombia
Full list of author information is available at the end of the article

studies must be supported with validated analytical results [2].

Our group has been focusing on developing validated techniques using proper international reference standards to evaluate the content or potency of commercial antibiotics. These techniques can be used in performance studies like those for the determination of a Minimal Inhibitory Concentration (MIC), Minimal Lethal Concentration, Critical Concentration and production of Spontaneous Mutants [8,9].

This paper presents the results for the evaluation of commercial products of vancomycin to describe some issues that are important in the evaluation of antibiotics.

## Methods
### Microorganisms
THE UNITED STATES PHARMACOPOEIA XXVII states that spores of *Bacillus subtilis* ATCC 6633 are the source of this microorganism used to develop a microbiological assay for evaluating the potencies of vancomycin products. For MIC and MBC studies, we used *Acinetobacter baumanii* strains 59, 139, 147 and 173, *Enterococcus gallinarum, Streptococcus faecalis* ATC 29212, a nosocomial strain 319623 and a vancomycin-sensitive strain, *Escherichia coli* strains 39, 50 and 69, *Klebsiella pneumoniae* strains 1, 43, 63, 65 and 207, *Pseudomonas aeruginosa* strains 42, 74, 151, 157, and HE1, *Staphylococcus aureus* strains 287, 291 and ATCC 25923, and *Morganella morganii* HE2. All of the microorganisms were grown in Mueller Hinton (MH) broth (incubated at 35°C for 24 h). Each strain was then plated on MH agar to obtain isolated colonies, which were then used to make larger cultures in MH medium. The cultures were harvested with cryopreservation broth. A portion of each was kept in a cryovial at -70°C, and the other portion was used to prepare a suspension with 25% transmittance at 600 nm (25%T) to develop *in vitro* assays. These suspensions were kept in cryovials at - 70°C.

### Analytical Bioassay
An analytical bioassay was established and validated for vancomycin. First, the proper concentration range was determined, and then the linearity, precision, specificity and stability of the compound in question were assessed [2,3]. All of the samples were evaluated with this analytical bioassay under the chosen conditions.

### Minimal Inhibitory Concentration (MIC) and Minimal Bactericidal Concentration (MBC)
Assays to assess these parameters were developed in two parts. (1) **Preparation of inocula:** the number of colony forming units (CFUs) was determined for each suspension at 25%T to prepare inocula of 1-5 × 10⁶ CFUs/ml.

(2) **MIC and MBC determination by micro-dilution:** samples were diluted to 2 mg/ml for evaluation. Using a multichannel pipette, 100 µl Mueller Hinton Broth was placed in each well of a 96-well ELISA plate, with 200 µl in column 12. Next, 100 µl of the antibiotic solution (2 mg/ml) was placed in the first column and thoroughly mixed by pipetting. From these wells, 100 µl was added to the second column and mixed, and this procedure was repeated up to column 10, after which the 100-µl portion was discarded. Columns 11 and 12 were positive and negative controls, respectively. Each row (A to H) represented a different sample to be analyzed. Each inoculum (100 µl) was then pipetted into each microplate, which was incubated at 37°C for 24 h. Growth in the wells was assessed. The lowest dilution showing no growth, the first dilution with growth, and the two controls were plated onto MH agar. The **MIC** was defined as the lowest dilution that showed no growth on the ELISA plate but showed growth on MH agar. The **MBC** was defined as the lowest dilution that did not show growth on either the ELISA plate or MH agar [10].

### Critical Concentration (CC)
The CC was determined similarly to the analytical bioassay. The inocula for **MIC** and **MBC** determinations and two-fold serial dilutions of each sample from 993 to 31,03 µg/ml were used (The batch of Vancomycin USP standard has a potency of 99300 µg per vial). The halo of inhibition was measured, and the crown length (X) was calculated (the inhibition halo diameter minus the reservoir diameter divided by 2). The log concentration vs. $X^2$ was plotted, and a linear regression ($y = mx + b$) was applied. The y-intercept ($b$) is equivalent to the log of the CC [10].

### Spontaneous mutants
Spontaneous mutation was analyzed similarly to the analytical bioassay. Again, the inocula for the **MIC** and **MBC** determinations were used. Specific microorganisms and dilutions were selected after determinations of critical concentrations. On each plate, a dilution of the USP standard and samples of the same concentration were used.

### Samples
Commercial products purchased from the pharmacies of different hospitals in Bogotá, D. C. Colombia, were analyzed. They included trademarked products and generic products of vancomycin. All of the samples had declared contents of 500mg. They were all diluted in sterile water in 100 ml volumetric flasks. The solutions were divided into 5-ml fractions for storage at -70°C and were diluted to **1** mg/ml to develop the analytical bioassays.

## Statistical Analysis

All the assays were performed three times, and the statistical tool of Microsoft Excel® was applied to analyze the dates.

## Results

### Analytical Bioassay

The United Stated Pharmacopoeia XXVII recommends *Bacillus subtilis* ATCC 6633 as the biological organism to use to develop the analytical bioassay for vancomycin products. Figure 1 shows the results of this bioassay.

### *Determination of concentration range, incubation time and culture medium pH*

Ten concentrations were used to determine the concentration range (two-fold dilutions from 1005 to 1.96 μg/ml, because this batch of Vancomycin USP standard has a potency of 100500 μg/vial). Table 1 shows that the best linearity was in the range between C3 and C8 (251.25 to 7.85 μg/ml) ($R^2$ = 0.9907, Figure 2).

The assay required an 8 to 10 h incubation time at 37°C. This incubation is shorter than many common assays, which require between 18 and 24 h.

The results for Vancomycin show that a pH of 6.4 or 6.5 is optimal because growth was abundant and homogenous, and inhibition haloes were well defined at this pH (Table 2).

### *Linearity*

In Tables 3 and 4, the concentration of antibiotic correlates well with the diameter of the zone of inhibition.

From this point on, the selected concentrations will be designated C1 to C6 for clarity.

**Table 1 Evaluation of the range of concentrations for Vancomycin (USP standard)**

| Concentration Range | | Equation | | |
|---|---|---|---|---|
| From | To | Slope | Intercept | $R^2$ |
| C1 | C6 | 2.462680435 | 6.415123505 | 0.996221756 |
| C2 | C7 | 2.324635129 | 7.259328533 | 0.989384179 |
| **C3** | **C8** | **2.270224777** | **7.362386326** | **0.990682625** |
| C4 | C9 | 2.367915749 | 6.864768679 | 0.98750859 |

Cited on page 6

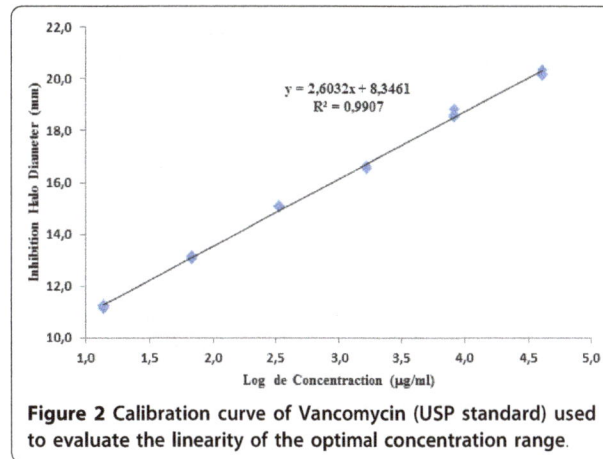

**Figure 2** Calibration curve of Vancomycin (USP standard) used to evaluate the linearity of the optimal concentration range.

**Table 2 Evaluation of the pH effect on linearity**

| pH | Equation | $R^2$ | Incubation Time |
|---|---|---|---|
| 5.4 | y = 1.8463x + 14.882 | 0.9806 | 8 hours |
| 5.9 | y = 2.3895x + 19.128 | 0.9898 | 8 hours |
| **6.4** | **y = 1.5517x + 11.817** | **0.9977** | **8 hours** |
| **6.5** | **y = 2.134x + 7.4113** | **0.9975** | **8 hours** |
| 7 | y = 1.7824 + 11.212 | 0.9794 | 9 hours |
| 7.5 | y = 1.875x + 11.009 | 0.9663 | 10 hours |
| 8 | y = 2.3651x + 9.3311 | 0.9763 | 11 hours |

Cited on page 6.

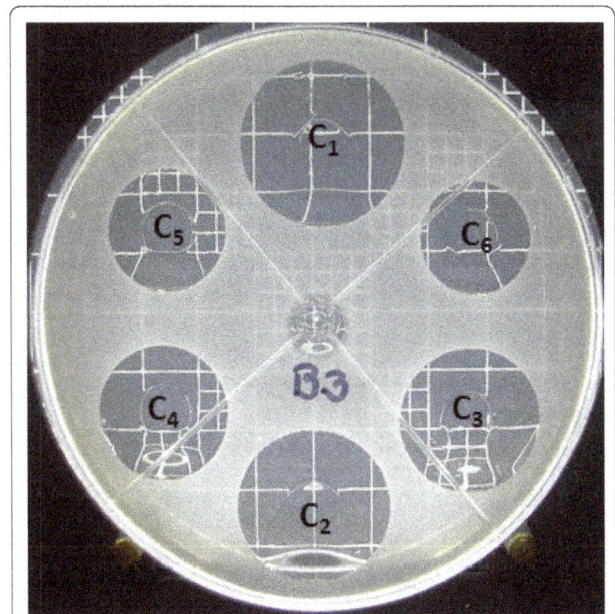

**Figure 1** Bioassay of Vancomycin (USP standard) against *Bacillus subtilis* ATCC 6633.

**Table 3 Evaluation of the linearity of Vancomycin**

| Test | HYPOTHESIS | Experimental t | Theoretical t | Decision |
|---|---|---|---|---|
| Slope | $H_0$: m = 0<br>$H_1$: m ≠0 | 19.7 | 2.120 | Reject $H_0$ |
| Intercept | $H_0$: b = 0<br>$H_1$: b ≠0 | 125.3 | 2.120 | Reject $H_0$ |
| Correlation | $H_0$: R = 0<br>$H_1$: R ≠ 0 | 67.5 | 2.120 | Reject $H_0$ |

Cited on page 6.

**Table 4 Regression analysis by analysis of variance (ANOVA)**

| Test | HYPOTHESIS | Experimental t | Theoretical t | Decision |
|---|---|---|---|---|
| Regression | $H_0$: There is no regression<br>$H_1$: There is regression | 146.6 | 4.670 | Reject $H_0$ |
| Deviation from Linearity | $H_0$: There is no deviation from linearity<br>$H_1$: There is a deviation from linearity | -3.0 | 3.71 | Accept $H_0$ |

Cited on page 6.

### Precision

The reproducibility and between-day precision of our assays were evaluated in several ways. Reproducibility was studied by determining the coefficient of variation, which was less than 1% and was acceptable for analytical assays in the pharmaceutical industry (Table 5).

The between-day precision was also analyzed. Analysis of variance (ANOVA) showed that, for the antibiotic evaluated, the results of assays performed on different days did not significantly differ (Table 6).

### Stability

The stability of each compound during the experimental period was verified. Solutions of vancomycin in water and phosphate buffer, pH 4.5 (1005 µg/ml; USP Standard), were incubated at 37°C, 18°C and 4°C, and samples were taken after 24, **48**, and 86 hours or seven and fifteen days of incubation. The samples (Vancomycin Standard Solution) under different treatments, were diluted fromC1 to C6 to perform the relation Log Concentration vs. Halo Diameter Inhibition, and the results were plotted and compared to reveal any reduction in antibiotic activity (i.e., a decrease in the diameter of the zone of inhibition).

From the equation $y = mx + b$, where $y$ represents the inhibition zone diameter and $x$ represents the log of the concentration, changes in the value of $b$ indicate changes in activity. If there is no change in the intercept, the antibiotic is stable. If the value of $b$ decreases, this trend indicates instability or a loss of activity.

The solutions showed a slight decrease in the intercept values after 24 h of at each storage temperature (Tables 7 and 8). From this result, it appears that the molecule remained stable during our assays (48 hours at

37°C). Therefore, the assay results reflect the exact potency of the product.

### Specificity

To test specificity, solutions of the antibiotics were incubated at 50°C. The vancomycin solutions lost a small amount of activity (3% to 4%) after 15 days, but after 30 days, there was no longer any activity, meaning that vancomycin was the only molecule in solution responsible for the antimicrobial activity (Table 9).

### Sample analysis

The samples were analyzed with the previously validated assay. The results were quantified using the statistical method described by Hewitt (1977). Table 10 shows the content of vancomycin in the samples purchased, and in each case, the values fulfill the criteria laid out by USP XXV II for intravenous vancomycin: "**...Contents no less than 90% and no more than 115% of Vancomycin, calculated on anhydrous base of the quantity registered of Vancomycin**".

### Minimal inhibitory and bactericidal concentrations

Using the previously described methods, the samples were analyzed in groups of seven per plate, and each plate was inoculated with a single bacterial strain. The first row of the plate contained the USP standard; the other seven rows contained the samples. Figure 3 shows the results for vancomycin products. The plates showed the same performance for the standard as for the samples.

Growth was inhibited at the same concentration of each sample. After transfer onto MH agar, there was no growth in concentrations C1 to C5 or C12, but there was growth in C6 to C11. This result means that the antibiotic has an

**Table 5 Reproducibility of assays using Vancomycin (Cochran Test)**

| Concentration (mg/ml) | 251.25 | 165.63 | 62.85 | 31.41 | 15.70 | 7.85 |
|---|---|---|---|---|---|---|
| Standard deviation | 0.096 | 0.076 | 0.237 | 0.084 | 0.100 | 0.270 |
| Variance Coefficient (%) | 0.4759 | 0.408422 | 1.4576 | 0.559623 | 0.7061 | 2.2425 |
| Variance ($S^2$) | 0.0092 | 0.00583 | 0.0113 | 0.00707 | 0.0099 | 0.01213 |
| Sum ($S^2$) | | | | | | 0.05544 |

Cited on page 6.

**Table 6 ANOVA of the between-day precision of assays using Vancomycin**

| Concentration | Experimental F | Theoretical F | Decision |
|---|---|---|---|
| C1 | 0.041 | 4.96 | Accept $H_0$ |
| C2 | 0.047 | 4.96 | Accept $H_0$ |
| C3 | 0.069 | 4.96 | Accept $H_0$ |
| C4 | 0.093 | 4.96 | Accept $H_0$ |
| C5 | 0.128 | 4.96 | Accept $H_0$ |
| C6 | 0.182 | 4.96 | Accept $H_0$ |

Cited on page 6.

**Table 7 Stability of Vancomycin in water for injection at 4°C, 18°C and 37°C**

| Time | 4°C | | | 18°C | | | 37°C | | |
|---|---|---|---|---|---|---|---|---|---|
| | Slope | Intercept | $R^2$ | Slope | Intercept | $R^2$ | Slope | Intercept | $R^2$ |
| 0 h | 1.5177 | 12.556 | 0.9913 | 1.5177 | 12.556 | 0.9913 | 1.5177 | 12.556 | 0.9913 |
| 24 h | 1.5305 | 12.543 | 0.9908 | 1.5241 | 12.518 | 0.9916 | 1.5063 | 12.5210 | 0.9900 |
| 48 h | 1.522 | 12.544 | 0.9919 | 1.518 | 12.501 | 0.9926 | 1.4936 | 12.495 | 0.9924 |
| 86 h | 1.5224 | 12.509 | 0.9916 | 1.5178 | 12.461 | 0.9924 | 1.4981 | 12.4720 | 0.9928 |
| 7 days | 1.5165 | 12.4780 | 0.9919 | 1.5217 | 12.342 | 0.9935 | 1.4742 | 12.3040 | 0.9904 |
| 15 days | 1.5247 | 12.3460 | 0.9921 | 1.5041 | 12.273 | 0.9923 | 1.4425 | 12.1980 | 0.9916 |

Cited on page 7.

MBC but no MIC. The MBC is C5 for the USP standard and for all the samples. For all of the samples, using all of the microorganisms evaluated, the results showed that the samples had the same performances at each repetition of the assay (Table 11 includes results for only some samples as an illustration).

### Critical concentration (CC)

The CC is the minimum concentration that inhibits microorganism growth. It occurs at the limit of the inhibition halo. It is a measure of a microorganism's sensitivity and can be different from the MIC, which is determined under different conditions. The CC can be defined mathematically as $Ln(CC) = Ln(C_O) - X^2/DT_O$, where CC is the critical concentration, $C_O$ is the antibiotic concentration in the reservoir, X is the length of the crown (see above), D is the diffusion coefficient, and $T_O$ is the critical time. The intercept of a plot of Ln $(C_O)$ vs. $X^2$ is the Ln of CC [7].

Figure 4 shows the different behaviors of the microorganisms tested with the vancomycin standard. In Figures 4A and 4B, the microorganisms exhibited growth of spontaneous mutants. Figure 4C shows a microorganism resistant to vancomycin, and, finally, Figures 4D, E and 4F correspond to microorganisms with well-defined haloes, allowing for a comparison of the performances of the products tested for development. A well-defined inhibition halo was the selection criterion for evaluating CCs. For the CC assays, *E. faecalis*, *E. faecalis* ATCC 29212, *E. faecalis* 319623, *A. baumanii* 59, *E. gallinarum*, *P. aeruginosa* 43 and 74, *S. aureus* 281, 291 and

ATCC 25923 were selected. Figure 5 shows the correlation of $X^2$ with the log of antibiotic concentration. The regression equation is $y = 0.0353x + 0.9297$, and $b$ is therefore 0.9287. The CC is equivalent to antilog (0.9297), i.e., 8.506 μg/ml.

The CC values for the different vancomycin products showed no significant differences, meaning that the products behaved in similar ways against the different microorganisms tested (Table 12). On this basis, the generic products meet all of the quality standards applied to the pharmaceutical products and perform as well as the newest versions of these products.

In addition, the ratio between the sample CCs and standard CCs are similar to the ratios of antibiotic contents. In other words, all samples perform the same with regard to their antimicrobial activities *in vitro* (Table 13).

### Spontaneous mutants

It was noted in the previous assays that some strains produced spontaneous mutants (Figure 4A), as indicated by the appearance of colonies within the inhibition halo. Therefore, an assay to assess spontaneous mutation was developed with appropriate concentrations of antibiotics. Each experimental setup included an agar plate inoculated with a test strain. Of the six reservoirs, two contained standard solutions and the other four contained sample solutions. The numbers of mutants produced by the standard and sample solutions were counted after incubation.

For the spontaneous mutant assays, the strains selected were *S. aureus* 291 as a control strain (showing no production of spontaneous mutants) and *A. baumanii* 54 and

**Table 8 Stability of Vancomycin in phosphate buffer, pH 4**

| Time | 4°C | | | 18°C | | | 37°C | | |
|---|---|---|---|---|---|---|---|---|---|
| | Slope | Intercept | $R^2$ | Slope | Intercept | $R^2$ | Slope | Intercept | $R^2$ |
| 0 h | 1.4807 | 12.799 | 0.9916 | 1.4807 | 12.799 | 0.9916 | 1.4807 | 12.799 | 0.9916 |
| 24 h | 1.4910 | 12.7640 | 0.9917 | 1.4833 | 12.764 | 0.9917 | 1.5195 | 12.5150 | 0.9916 |
| 48 h | 1.487 | 12.733 | 0.9924 | 1.4747 | 12.716 | 0.9928 | 1.509 | 12.497 | 0.9922 |
| 86 h | 1.4787 | 12.7260 | 0.9933 | 1.4701 | 12.689 | 0.9927 | 1.5057 | 12.4700 | 0.9915 |
| 7 days | 1.4804 | 12.6510 | 0.9925 | 1.4766 | 12.571 | 0.9931 | 1.4966 | 12.3800 | 0.9922 |
| 15 days | 1.4826 | 12.5170 | 0.9937 | 1.4566 | 12.505 | 0.9932 | 1.4887 | 12.2510 | 0.9926 |

Cited on page 7.

**Table 9 Stability of Vancomycin in phosphate buffer, pH 4**

| Time | Phosphate Buffer, pH 4.5 | | | Water For Injection | | |
|---|---|---|---|---|---|---|
| | Slope | Intercept | R$^2$ | Slope | Intercept | R$^2$ |
| 0 h | 1.4807 | 12.799 | 0.9916 | 1.5177 | 12.556 | 0.9913 |
| 24 h | 1.5268 | 12.4310 | 0.9909 | 1.5059 | 12.4640 | 0.9905 |
| 48 h | 1.4924 | 12.479 | 0.9912 | 1.4907 | 12.409 | 0.993 |
| 86 h | 1.4894 | 12.4530 | 0.9914 | 1.4939 | 12.3520 | 0.9930 |
| 7 days | 1.4515 | 12.3970 | 0.9869 | 1.4569 | 12.3230 | 0.9897 |
| 15 days | 1.4226 | 12.3060 | 0.9855 | 1.4343 | 12.2370 | 0.9907 |
| 30 days | NDA | | | NDA | | |

ND: Non detectable activity.

Cited on page 7.

*E. gallinarum* as mutant producing strains. After statistical analysis, the results (Table 14) showed no significant differences between the products in the production of spontaneous mutants for any of the strains tested (Figure 6).

**Table 10 Potency of the commercial samples of vancomycin**

| Samples | Potency |
|---|---|
| 1 | |
| 2 | 0.995 |
| 3 | 1.012 |
| 4 | 1.005 |
| 5 | 1.100 |
| 6 | 0.936 |
| 7 | 1.124 |
| 8 | 1.032 |
| 9 | |
| 10 | 1.064 |
| 11 | |
| 12 | 1.019 |
| 13 | 1.023 |
| 14 | 1.150 |
| 15 | 1.108 |
| 16 | 0.9859 |
| 17 | 1.107 |
| 18 | 1.047 |
| 19 | |
| 20 | 0.981 |
| 21 | 1.019 |
| 22 | 1.011 |
| 23 | |
| 24 | 1.003 |
| 25 | 1.023 |
| 26 | 1.011 |
| 27 | 0.961 |
| 28 | |
| 29 | 1.062 |
| 30 | |

Cited on pages 7 and 9.

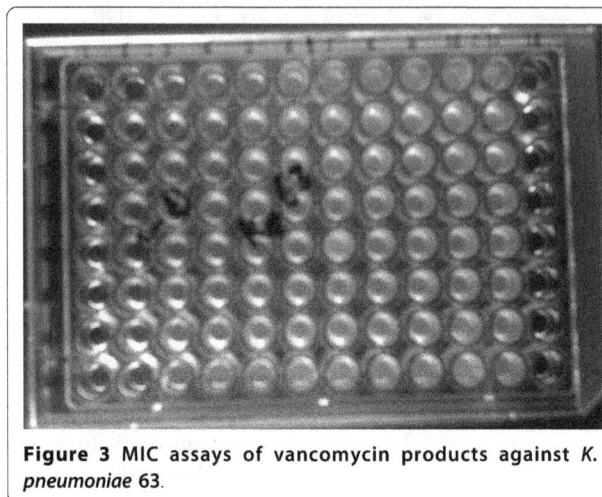

**Figure 3 MIC assays of vancomycin products against *K. pneumoniae* 63.**

## Discussion

Despite the fact that USP Pharmacopoeia assesses the bioassay conditions for vancomycin evaluation, the bioassay was validated following the suggestions of the

**Table 11 Determination of MICs and MBCs for Vancomycin (USP standard)**

| Microorganism | MIC (µg/ml) | | | MBC (µg/ml) | | |
|---|---|---|---|---|---|---|
| | Std | M1 | M2 | Std | M1 | M2 |
| *A. baumanii* 59 | 62.06 | 62.06 | 62.06 | 124.13 | 124.13 | 124.13 |
| *A. baumanii* 139 | 124.13 | 124.13 | 124.13 | 248.25 | 248.25 | 248.25 |
| *A. baumanii* 147 | 993 | 993 | 993 | ND | ND | ND |
| *A. baumanii* 173 | 62.06 | 62.06 | 62.06 | 124.13 | 124.13 | 124.13 |
| *E. faecalis* | 1.93 | 1.93 | 1.93 | 3.88 | 3.88 | 3.88 |
| *E. faecalis* ATCC 29212 | 7.76 | 7.76 | 7.76 | 15.52 | 15.52 | 15.52 |
| *E. faecalis* 319623 | 62.06 | 62.06 | 62.06 | 124.13 | 124.13 | 124.13 |
| *E. gallinarum* | ND | ND | ND | 124.13 | 124.13 | 124.13 |
| *E. coli* 39 | 124.13 | 124.13 | 124.13 | 248.25 | 248.25 | 248.25 |
| *E. coli* 50 | 124.13 | 124.13 | 124.13 | 248.25 | 248.25 | 248.25 |
| *E. coli* 69 | 496.50 | 496.50 | 496.50 | 993.00 | 993.00 | 993.00 |
| *K. pneumoniae* 1 | ND | ND | ND | 496.50 | 496.50 | 496.50 |
| *K. pneumoniae* 43 | 496.5 | 496.5 | 496.5 | 993.00 | 993.00 | 993.00 |
| *K. pneumoniae* 63 | 993.00 | 993.00 | 993.00 | ND | ND | ND |
| *K. pneumoniae* 65 | 993.00 | 993.00 | 993.00 | ND | ND | ND |
| *K. pneumoniae* 207 | 496.00 | 496.00 | 496.00 | 993.00 | 993.00 | 993.00 |
| *Ps. aeruginosa* 42 | 1.94 | 1.94 | 1.94 | 3.88 | 3.88 | 3.88 |
| *Ps. aeruginosa* 74 | 1.94 | 1.94 | 1.94 | 3.88 | 3.88 | 3.88 |
| *Ps. aeruginosa* 151 | 993.00 | 993.00 | 993.00 | ND | ND | ND |
| *Ps. aeruginosa* 157 | 993.00 | 993.00 | 993.00 | ND | ND | ND |
| *Ps. aeruginosa* HE1 | 993.00 | 993.00 | 993.00 | ND | ND | ND |
| *St. Aureus* 287 | 1.94 | 1.94 | 1.94 | 3.88 | 3.88 | 3.88 |
| *St. Aureus* 291 | 1.94 | 1.94 | 1.94 | 3.88 | 3.88 | 3.88 |
| *St. Aureus* ATCC 25923 | 1.94 | 1.94 | 1.94 | 3.88 | 3.88 | 3.88 |
| *M. morganii* HE2 | 496.50 | 496.50 | 496.50 | 993.00 | 993.00 | 993.00 |

Cited on pages 7 and 9.

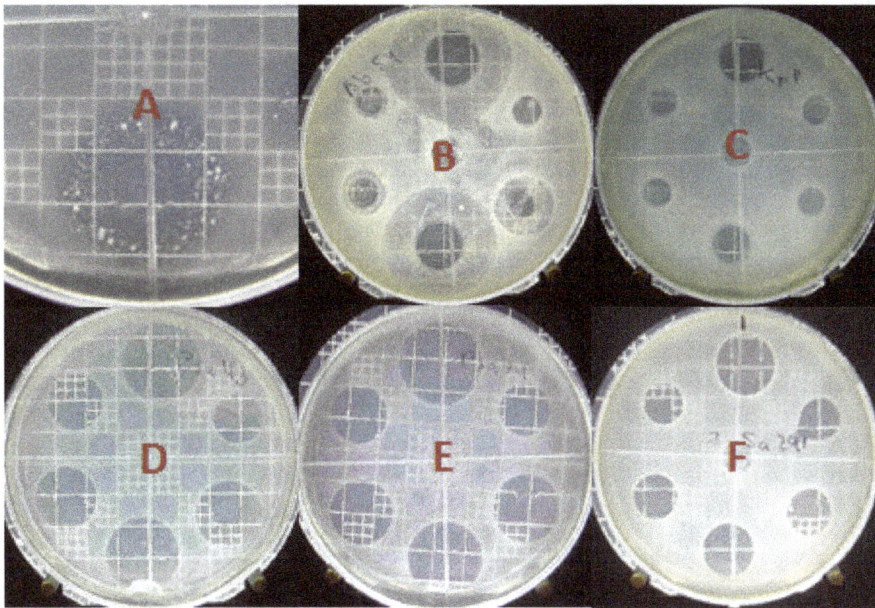

**Figure 4** Zones of inhibition produced by Vancomycin against (A) *E. gallinarum*, (B) *A. baumanii* 54, (C) *K. pneumoniae* 1, (D) *P. aeruginosa* 43, (E) *P. aeruginosa* 74 and (F) *S. aureus* 291.

specialized literature [1-3], to assure the certainty of results concerning the sample contents. The experiment to evaluate assay performance showed that it fulfilled the assay requirements (linearity, repeatability, precision). In the assay, the best linearity was shown over the range of 251.25 µg/ml to 7.85 µg/ml, i.e., the correlation was the highest ($R^2 = 0.9907$). The reproducibility and between-day precision of both assays had coefficients of variation less than 1%, and ANOVA showed no significant differences at any concentration. Antibiotic activity remained stable over the course of the assay at the selected temperature. Finally, the inhibition assay results were due only to the molecules evaluated. In conclusion,

the assay was exact and accurate with reproducible results.

Our results were generally similar to those of Zuluaga et al. (2009), but with some differences. Zuluaga et al. (2009) proposed a comparison of the performances of all samples by linear correlation against the performance of the original compound to determine pharmaceutical equivalence. This approach is problematic because the commercial products exhibit some differences in their potency. The USP Pharmacopoeia XXVII states **"...Contents no less than 90% and no more than 115% of Vancomycin, calculated on anhydrous base of the quantity registered of Vancomycin"**, are acceptable. Therefore, if we use a reference element for which there is uncertainty about its content, a sample could be assessed against different potencies. For example, if the commercial sample has 90% of the potency of Vancomycin, the potency of the sample under study will be overvalued, but if the reference sample has 115% of the potency, the sample under study will be undervalued. Finally, we strongly recommend that an antibiotic must be evaluated against an international reference standard by established and validated bioassays using an appropriate test microorganism and conditions. Then, the conclusions about the samples contents will be certain.

Analyses of commercial versions of the antibiotics tested (brand-name and generic products) indicate that all of the samples can be considered pharmaceutical equivalents because they all fulfill the standards of the USP Pharmacopoeia (Table 10). In the study by Zuluaga

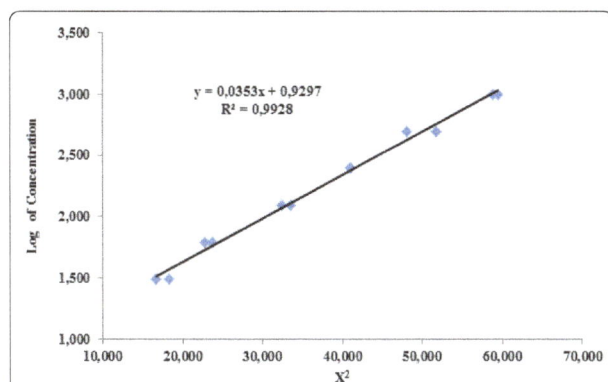

**Figure 5** Determination of critical concentration of Vancomycin against *P. aeruginosa* 74.

**Table 12 Critical concentrations (μg/ml) of different samples of Vancomycin against various microorganisms.**

| Sample | E. f. | E. f. 29212 | E. f. 319623 | A. b. 59 | E. g. | P. a. 43 | P. a. 74 | S. a. 281 | S. a. 291 | S. a. 25923 |
|---|---|---|---|---|---|---|---|---|---|---|
| Standard | 13.251 | 14.098 | 26.733 | 7.712 | 14.725 | 10.932 | 8.586 | 9.951 | 12.473 | 13.108 |
| M2 | 13.332 | 14.173 | 26.826 | 7.735 | 14.850 | 10.988 | 8.646 | 10.044 | 12.558 | 13.164 |
| M3 | 13.050 | 14.170 | 26.505 | 7.759 | 14.993 | 10.977 | 8.745 | 10.032 | 12.764 | 13.410 |
| M4 | 13.166 | 14.041 | 26.630 | 7.670 | 15.076 | 10.870 | 8.635 | 9.991 | 12.682 | 13.202 |
| M5 | 12.961 | 14.566 | 26.160 | 8.305 | 14.798 | 11.716 | 9.474 | 10.941 | 13.753 | 14.662 |
| M6 | 14.495 | 13.338 | 28.017 | 7.355 | 13.974 | 10.308 | 8.016 | 9.280 | 11.725 | 12.324 |
| M7 | 12.523 | 14.237 | 26.540 | 7.856 | 16.029 | 12.348 | 9.666 | 11.143 | 14.076 | 14.729 |
| M8 | 13.441 | 13.627 | 27.530 | 8.053 | 15.008 | 11.248 | 8.903 | 10.138 | 13.220 | 13.440 |
| M13 | 13.052 | 14.193 | 26.574 | 8.003 | 14.955 | 11.146 | 8.908 | 10.306 | 12.713 | 13.489 |
| M14 | 13.792 | 15.904 | 28.612 | 8.481 | 15.291 | 12.621 | 9.897 | 11.480 | 14.454 | 15.286 |
| M15 | 13.791 | 15.673 | 27.431 | 8.190 | 15.700 | 11.969 | 9.500 | 11.015 | 13.820 | 14.539 |
| M16 | 13.483 | 14.326 | 26.535 | 7.698 | 14.991 | 10.743 | 8.458 | 9.795 | 12.363 | 12.986 |
| M17 | 13.720 | 15.128 | 27.261 | 8.068 | 15.794 | 12.163 | 9.519 | 11.006 | 13.786 | 14.510 |
| M18 | 13.697 | 14.790 | 26.915 | 7.720 | 15.196 | 11.671 | 8.965 | 10.384 | 13.427 | 13.807 |
| M20 | 13.568 | 14.405 | 27.117 | 7.660 | 14.535 | 10.760 | 8.506 | 9.835 | 12.249 | 12.886 |
| M21 | 13.192 | 14.632 | 26.985 | 7.857 | 16.048 | 11.178 | 8.759 | 10.091 | 12.625 | 13.413 |
| M22 | 14.067 | 13.946 | 26.536 | 7.774 | 15.571 | 11.309 | 8.741 | 10.057 | 12.769 | 13.437 |
| M24 | 13.334 | 14.046 | 26.701 | 7.856 | 14.655 | 10.895 | 8.639 | 10.016 | 12.418 | 13.125 |
| M26 | 13.882 | 14.592 | 26.519 | 7.638 | 15.409 | 11.116 | 8.739 | 10.038 | 12.671 | 13.299 |
| M27 | 12.741 | 13.544 | 25.775 | 7.474 | 14.126 | 10.499 | 8.326 | 9.612 | 12.200 | 12.595 |
| M29 | 13.571 | 14.008 | 26.770 | 8.274 | 15.281 | 11.105 | 9.143 | 10.404 | 12.998 | 13.887 |

Cited on pages 8 and 10

**Table 13 Ratios of sample CC/standard CC for Vancomycin**

| SAMPLE | MICROORGANISMS | | | | | | | | | | Ratio Median | Potency |
|---|---|---|---|---|---|---|---|---|---|---|---|---|
| | E. f. | E. f. 29212 | E. f. 319623 | A. b. 59 | E. g. | P. a. 43 | P. a. 74 | S. a. 281 | S. a. 291 | S. a. 25923 | | |
| Standard | | | | | | | | | | | | |
| M2 | 1.006 | 1.005 | 1.003 | 1.003 | 1.008 | 1.005 | 1.007 | 1.009 | 1.007 | 1.004 | 1.006 | 0.995 |
| M3 | 0.985 | 1.005 | 0.991 | 1.006 | 1.018 | 1.004 | 1.018 | 1.008 | 1.023 | 1.023 | 1.008 | 1.012 |
| M4 | 0.994 | 0.996 | 0.996 | 0.995 | 1.024 | 0.994 | 1.006 | 1.004 | 1.017 | 1.007 | 1.003 | 1.005 |
| M5 | 0.978 | 1.033 | 0.979 | 1.077 | 1.005 | 1.072 | 1.103 | 1.100 | 1.103 | 1.119 | 1.057 | 1.100 |
| M6 | 1.094 | 0.946 | 1.048 | 0.954 | 0.949 | 0.943 | 0.934 | 0.933 | 0.940 | 0.940 | 0.968 | 0.936 |
| M7 | 0.945 | 1.010 | 0.993 | 1.019 | 1.089 | 1.130 | 1.126 | 1.120 | 1.128 | 1.124 | 1.068 | 1.124 |
| M8 | 1.014 | 0.967 | 1.030 | 1.044 | 1.019 | 1.029 | 1.037 | 1.019 | 1.060 | 1.025 | 1.024 | 1.032 |
| M13 | 0.985 | 1.007 | 0.994 | 1.038 | 1.016 | 1.020 | 1.038 | 1.036 | 1.019 | 1.029 | 1.018 | 1.023 |
| M14 | 1.041 | 1.128 | 1.070 | 1.100 | 1.038 | 1.155 | 1.153 | 1.154 | 1.159 | 1.166 | 1.116 | 1.150 |
| M15 | 1.041 | 1.112 | 1.026 | 1.062 | 1.066 | 1.095 | 1.106 | 1.107 | 1.108 | 1.109 | 1.083 | 1.108 |
| M16 | 1.018 | 1.016 | 0.993 | 0.998 | 1.018 | 0.983 | 0.985 | 0.984 | 0.991 | 0.991 | 0.998 | 0.986 |
| M17 | 1.035 | 1.073 | 1.020 | 1.046 | 1.073 | 1.113 | 1.109 | 1.106 | 1.105 | 1.107 | 1.079 | 1.107 |
| M18 | 1.034 | 1.049 | 1.007 | 1.001 | 1.032 | 1.068 | 1.044 | 1.044 | 1.076 | 1.053 | 1.041 | 1.047 |
| M20 | 1.024 | 1.022 | 1.014 | 0.993 | 0.987 | 0.984 | 0.991 | 0.988 | 0.982 | 0.983 | 0.997 | 0.981 |
| M21 | 0.996 | 1.038 | 1.009 | 1.019 | 1.090 | 1.023 | 1.020 | 1.014 | 1.012 | 1.023 | 1.024 | 1.019 |
| M22 | 1.062 | 0.989 | 0.993 | 1.008 | 1.057 | 1.035 | 1.018 | 1.011 | 1.024 | 1.025 | 1.022 | 1.011 |
| M24 | 1.006 | 0.996 | 0.999 | 1.019 | 0.995 | 0.997 | 1.006 | 1.006 | 0.996 | 1.001 | 1.002 | 1.003 |
| M26 | 1.048 | 1.035 | 0.992 | 0.990 | 1.046 | 1.017 | 1.018 | 1.009 | 1.016 | 1.015 | 1.019 | 1.011 |
| M27 | 0.962 | 0.961 | 0.964 | 0.969 | 0.959 | 0.960 | 0.970 | 0.966 | 0.978 | 0.961 | 0.965 | 0.961 |
| M29 | 1.024 | 0.994 | 1.001 | 1.073 | 1.038 | 1.016 | 1.065 | 1.046 | 1.042 | 1.059 | 1.036 | 1.062 |

**Table 14 Spontaneous mutant production in the diffusion gel assay for vancomycin products**

| Sample | Mutants of *A. baumanii* 54 | | Mutants of *E. gallinarum* | |
|---|---|---|---|---|
| | Median | σ | Median | σ |
| Standard | 106.17 | 1.47 | 96.500 | 5.089 |
| M2 | 111.00 | 1.00 | 100.667 | 2.082 |
| M3 | 104.33 | 1.53 | 98.333 | 1.528 |
| M4 | 106.67 | 2.08 | 104.667 | 5.686 |
| M5 | 103.67 | 0.58 | 99.000 | 2.000 |
| M6 | 109.00 | 1.00 | 96.000 | 2.000 |
| M7 | 110.67 | 1.53 | 100.667 | 1.155 |
| M8 | 108.67 | 1.53 | 98.667 | 1.155 |
| M10 | 104.00 | 1.73 | 95.667 | 1.528 |
| M12 | 110.67 | 1.53 | 93.333 | 2.517 |
| M13 | 106.33 | 1.53 | 94.000 | 3.000 |
| M14 | 106.67 | 2.52 | 101.000 | 1.000 |
| M15 | 110.67 | 1.15 | 99.333 | 1.155 |
| M17 | 105.33 | 1.15 | 93.667 | 3.786 |
| M18 | 104.33 | 2.08 | 96.000 | 1.000 |
| M20 | 109.33 | 1.53 | 100.667 | 0.577 |
| M22 | 112.00 | 1.00 | 103.000 | 3.000 |
| M24 | 105.33 | 1.53 | 96.000 | 1.000 |
| M26 | 109.33 | 1.53 | 100.667 | 0.577 |
| M27 | 112.00 | 1.00 | 103.000 | 3.000 |
| M29 | 105.33 | 1.53 | 96.000 | 1.000 |
| F | 10.026 | | 4.424 | |
| Prob. | 0.001 | | 0.005 | |
| VCF | 1.706 | | 1.706 | |

Cited on page 9

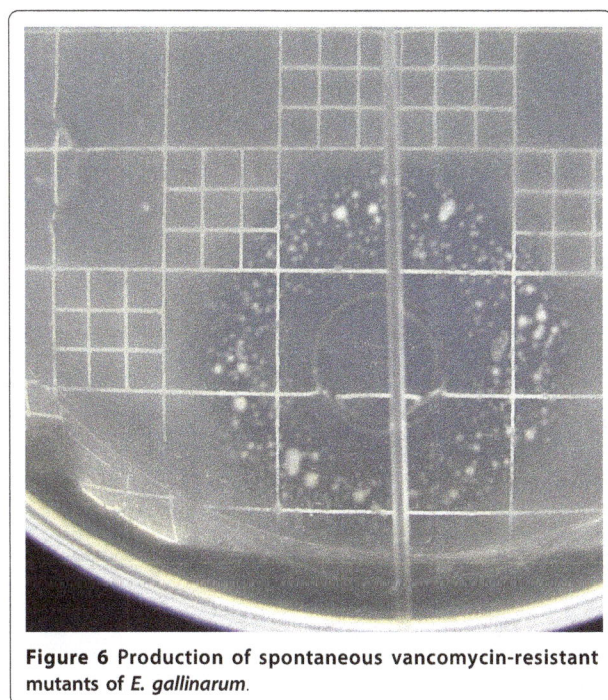

**Figure 6** Production of spontaneous vancomycin-resistant mutants of *E. gallinarum*.

et al. (2009), the performance of all samples was similar to the innovator, and the results were accurate and reproducible, which means that all of the producers of this antibiotic are using similar parameters to manufacture their products.

The MIC and MBC results obtained with different pathogenic strains showed no differences between samples (Tables10 and 11), which is probably because the samples were pharmaceutical equivalents. We conclude that generic and novel products perform equally well. In other words, the generic products evaluated in this study fulfill the requirements to be considered for use in antimicrobial therapy.

We also designed an assay to determine critical concentrations using a few selected strains to confirm that all of the generic products evaluated were effective in antimicrobial therapy. The results showed no significant differences among samples (Table 12). Moreover, the ratios between the CC of the standard and those of the different samples were similar to their potency levels (Tables 13).

Along the same lines, an assay was designed to determine the production of spontaneous mutants in diffusion gel assays. The results again showed that all the samples behaved similarly, leading us to conclude that none of the samples studied markedly differ in their antimicrobial activities. That is, generic and brand name products that comply with the international specifications for manufacturing pharmaceutical products behave similarly to novel products.

Our results are different from those of other studies [5,6]. Those studies were conducted using the newest product as a "standard of comparison," but the researchers did not take into account that a commercial product may have a range of content between 90% and 120%. Consequently, there would be great variability in the results with respect to the performance of the antibiotic. For instance, if the novel drug product has a hypothetical content of 120% relative to the declared content on the label, and the generic product has a hypothetical content of 90%, then the effective content of the generic product would be 75% (90/120) of the novel drug. This scenario could produce misleading results because although both products fulfill the content requirements, the first is at the upper limit and the second at the lower limit.

It has been proposed that generic antibiotics behave differently from innovator products against pathogenic microorganisms [5,6]. This is possible if the generic antibiotic does not fulfill the quality standards for that pharmaceutical product (e.g., purity or content). For instance, contaminants in generic drugs could interfere with their antibiotic activities.

Vesga et al (2009) reported that none of the vancomycin products have differences in *in vitro* assays; they had no differences in potency, MIC or MBC. Also, in time-kill curves and single-dose serum Pharmacokinetics (PK) in infected mouse there were no differences. However, the pharmacodynamic study had very odd results; the products tested did not behave like the innovator *in vitro*. We think that these results should be reanalyzed or retested because at the lower concentration, the generics have a better antimicrobial activity than the innovator, but in the higher concentrations, these behaviors change. The free antibiotic in the serum is the only chemical responsible for the antimicrobial activity and they showed in the PK model that all of the antibiotics diffuse into the blood in an equivalent way; so, they should behave against the same microorganism in an equivalent way.

## Conclusions
All of the samples analyzed by standardized, microbiological methods fulfill the requirements for content according to USP XXVII. They all show the same antimicrobial behavior because they have similar MIC, MBC and CC values and produce similar numbers of mutants.

### Abbreviations
MIC: Minimal Inhibitory Concentration; MBC: Minimal Bactericidal Concentration; CC: Critical Concentration; C1: Concentration 1; C2: Concentration 2; C10: Concentration 10; *A. b.: Acinetobacter baumanii; S. f.: Streptococcus faecalis; E. g.: Enterococcus gallinarum; E. c.: Escherichia coli; K. p.: Klebsiella pneumonia; P. a.: Pseudomonas aeruginosa; S. a.: Staphylococcus aureus;* M1: Sample 1; M2: Sample 2, ...

### Acknowledgements
The authors wish to express their gratitude to VITALIS PHARMACEUTICAL, for its support of this collaborative research, a joint venture between Vitalis S.A. and the National University of Colombia.

### Author details
[1]Universidad Nacional de Colombia, Facultad de Ciencias, Departamento de Farmacia, Laboratorio de Asesorías e Investigaciones en Microbiología, 472. Ciudad Universitaria. Carrera 30 Calle 45. A.A.14490. Bogotá D. C. Colombia.
[2]Vitalis Pharmaceutical, Proyectos Especiales, Carrera 7 No 156-80. Oficina No 1104. Bogotá D. C. Colombia.

### Authors' contributions
MG, a student at the National University of Colombia, jointly developed a process to validate the quantitative assay for vancomycin for their theses in Pharmaceutical Chemistry. MJA was the project administrator and contributed to article redaction. JAD and ES conceived the study, obtained necessary funding, designed and directed the execution and analysis of data, edited the manuscript and approved it for publication.
All the authors read and are in agreement with the whole all of article text.

### Competing interests
Diaz and Silva received financial support for lectures from Vitalis S. A. to participate in national scientific meetings in Colombia. The present study was a joint venture between the Science Faculty of National University of Colombia and Vitalis Pharmaceutical. And was also financed by Vitalis Pharmaceutical.

### References
1. CENTERS FOR DISEASE CONTROL AND PREVENTION, FOOD AND DRUG ADMINISTRATION, NATIONAL INSTITUTES OF HEALTH. A Public Health Action Plan to Combat Antimicrobial Resistance;[http://www.cdc.gov/drugresistance/pdf/2010/Interagency-Action-Plan-PreClearance-03-2011.pdf].
2. THE UNITED STATES PHARMACOPOEIA. XXVII. *Biological test and assays* Pharmacopoeia Convention Inc Bronx New York USA; 1883, 358.
3. INTERNATIONAL CONFERENCE ON HARMONISATION OF TECHNICAL REQUIREMENTS FOR REGISTRATION OF PHARMACEUTICALS FOR HUMAN USE. *Validation of Analytical Procedures: Text and Methodology. Q2 (R1). Current Step 4 version. Parent Guideline dated 27 October 1994 (Complementary Guideline on Methodology dated 6 November 1996 incorporated in November 2005)* .
4. Jones RN, Fritsche TR, Moet GJ: **In vitro potency evaluations of various piperacillin/tazobactam generic products compared with the contemporary branded (Zosyn®, Wyeth) formulation.** *Diagnostic Microbiology and Infectious Disease* 2008, **61**:76-79.
5. Moeta JGary, Wattersa AAmy, Sadera SHelio, Jonesx NRonald: **Expanded studies of piperacillin/Tazobactam formulations: variations among branded product lots and assessment of 46 generics lots.** *Diagnostic Microbiology and Infectious Disease* 2009, **65**:319-322.
6. Zuluaga AF, Agudelo M, Rodriguez CA, Vesga O: **Application of microbiological assay to determine pharmaceutical equivalence of generic intravenous antibiotics.** *BMC Clinical Pharmacology* 2009, **9**:1.
7. Vesga O, Agudelo M, Salazar BE, Rodriguez CA, Zuluaga F: **Generic products of vancomycin fail in vivo despite being pharmaceutical equivalents of the innovator.** *Antimicrob Agents Chemother* 2010, **54**:3271-3279.
8. Melendez P, Diaz J, Silva E, Gonzales P, Gonzalez P, Moreno E, Amaya P, Serrato N, Saenz E: **Estudio comparativo de la actividad antimicrobiana de diferentes presentaciones comerciales de antibióticos de administración intravenosa a través de métodos** *in vitro. Revista Colombiana de Ciencias Químico-Farmacéuticas* 2005, **34**.
9. Silva E, Diaz JA, Arias MJ, Hernadez AP, De La Torre A: **Comparative in vitro study of the antimicrobial activities of different commercial antibiotic products for intravenous administration.** *BMC Clinical Pharmacology* 2010, **10**:3.
10. Lorian V, (Ed.): **Antibiotics in Laboratory Medicine.** Williams & Wilkins. Baltimore; 1980, 95-98.

# 5

# Microneedle pretreatment enhances the percutaneous permeation of hydrophilic compounds with high melting points

Jessica Stahl[*], Mareike Wohlert and Manfred Kietzmann

**Abstract**

**Background:** Two commercially available microneedle rollers with a needle length of 200 μm and 300 μm were selected to examine the influence of microneedle pretreatment on the percutaneous permeation of four non-steroidal anti-inflammatory drugs (diclofenac, ibuprofen, ketoprofen, paracetamol) with different physicochemical drug characteristics in Franz-type diffusion cells. Samples of the receptor fluids were taken at predefined times over 6 hours and were analysed by UV–VIS high-performance liquid-chromatography. Histological examinations after methylene blue application were additionally performed to gather information about barrier disruption.

**Results:** Despite no visible pores in the *stratum corneum*, the microneedle pretreatment resulted in a twofold (200 μm) and threefold higher (300 μm) flux through the pretreated skin samples compared to untreated skin samples for ibuprofen and ketoprofen ($LogK_{ow} > 3$, melting point < 100°C). The flux of the hydrophilic compounds diclofenac and paracetamol ($logK_{ow} < 1$, melting point > 100°C) increased their amount by four (200 μm) to eight (300 μm), respectively.

**Conclusion:** Commercially available microneedle rollers with 200–300 μm long needles enhance the drug delivery of topically applied non-steroidal anti-inflammatory drugs and represent a valuable tool for percutaneous permeation enhancement particularly for substances with poor permeability due to a hydrophilic nature and high melting points.

**Keywords:** Transdermal drug delivery, Microneedles, $logK_{ow}$, Melting point, Non-steroidal anti-inflammatory drug, *In vitro* permeation study, Physical penetration enhancement

## Background

The topical transdermal administration of systemically active drugs represents a convenient alternative to systemic administration via oral route in both humans and animals with many advantages like the avoidance of the first-pass hepatic metabolism, enzymatic degradation and side effects in the gastro-intestinal tract. The outmost layer of the epidermis, the *stratum corneum*, plays a key role in the skin barrier concerning the intrusion of foreign substances from the environment and transepidermal water loss (TEWL) [1]. It is composed of keratin containing corneocytes embedded in a lipid rich matrix, which acts like a kit-substance and mainly comprises ceramides, free fatty acids and cholesterol [2]. Substances applied onto the skin surface, thereby, can pass this complex structure by different routes. Although the tortuous pathway between the corneocytes is likely to be the main route through the *stratum corneum*, it can be bypassed by orifices and glands, both of which can account for a large part of the body surface [1]. However, transdermal drug delivery is severely limited to a small percentage of drugs due to physicochemical drug characteristics and barrier properties of the skin. Therefore, considerable effort has been put into the development of sophisticated new transdermal drug delivery systems to overcome the skin barrier. Besides chemical permeation enhancers [3] and electrical techniques of enhancement like iontophoresis and electroporation [4-6], systems like

* Correspondence: xjessica.stahl@tihoannover.de
Department of Pharmacology, Toxicology and Pharmacy, University of Veterinary Medicine Hannover, Foundation, Buenteweg 17, Hannover 30559, Germany

patches and microneedles have been developed for a convenient and effective transdermal drug delivery [7]. Microneedle technology has been established to perforate the skin barrier without inducing pain or bleeding, as the needles are too short to stimulate the nerves and to damage blood vessels in the dermis [8,9]. The needles are made of silicon, glass, metal, polymers or sugar with sizes ranging from sub-micron to millimetres to form microscopic holes that allow enhanced drug delivery [10]. Unlike skin abrasion the microneedle application represents a safe, efficient and controllable alternative for increasing transdermal drug delivery [11].

Over the past few years, four different designs such as "poke and patch" [12], "coat and poke", "poke and release" [13,14], and "poke and flow" [15] have been fabricated which have already been established for macromolecules like insulin or vaccines [9,12].

The easiest approach of using microneedles is to employ solid microneedles to form a pore in the skin, through which compounds can pass out of the topical formulation [16]. Therefore, two different techniques are disposable: Firstly, solid microneedle arrays are pressed onto the skin or scraped on the skin and secondly, rollers with attached microscopic needles are rolled over the skin. The pores produced by either method are alike, whereby the rollers are easier to use [17]. *In vitro* examinations with solid microneedles have increased skin permeability for substances ranging from nanomaterials to proteins [12,18] concurrent with an increase in the TEWL [10,19].

In the present study, two commercially available microneedle rollers with different needle lengths (200 μm and 300 μm) were utilised with the aim to determine the efficiency of skin perforation and to describe their influence on the permeation of several topically applied non-steroidal anti-inflammatory drugs with different physico-chemical drug characteristics in an *in vitro* setup. Moreover, histological staining was performed to characterise the degree of skin perforation after microneedle pretreatment.

## Methods
### Chemicals
All reagents used in the present study were of the highest purity available. Diclofenac (molecular weight (MW): 296 g/mol, logK$_{o/w}$: 0.7, melting point (MP): 284°C), ketoprofen (MW: 254 g/mol, logK$_{o/w}$: 1.8, MP: 94°C), ibuprofen (MW: 206 g/mol, logK$_{o/w}$: 3.97, MP: 76°C), and paracetamol (acetaminophen; MW: 151 g/mol, logK$_{o/w}$: 0.46, MP: 170°C) [20] were obtained from Sigma-Aldrich (Steinheim, Germany). Methanol was purchased from Applichem GmbH (Darmstadt, Germany). All other reagents were obtained from Merck (Darmstadt, Germany).

### Animal skin
The skin was obtained from bovine udders, all of which were harvested from Holstein Friesian cows which died at a slaughterhouse for food production, and the cleaned skin samples were stored at - 20°C until use. After thawing at room temperature split skin samples with a thickness of 600 μm ± 50 μm were produced using an electrical microtome (Zimmer, Eschbach, Germany), whereby damaged skin samples were excluded from the study [21].

### Skin perforation by microneedles
Two different microneedle rollers were used (200 μm needle length and 300 μm needle length), both of which possessed of 192 titanium needles (Medik8, London, United Kingdom, Figure 1) in a cylindrical arrangement. Prior to the experiment split skin samples with appropriate size of 2 x 2 cm were incubated in phosphate buffered saline (PBS) for 30 minutes. They were placed on a styropor panel and fixed with needles beyond the subsequent diffusion area of the skin samples before the microneedle rollers were rolled in four axes radial over the skin surface (Figure 1 C).

### Light microscopy
Visualisation of the produced pores was performed by light microscopy. The skin samples were treated with the microneedles as mentioned above and were incubated with saturated methylene blue solution in PBS for 120 minutes. The skin samples were forthwith examined under the light microscope to count the amount of needles pores within the diffusion area. Afterwards, they were frozen and cut in 10 μm thick sections with a cryostat.

### *In-vitro* permeation
The diffusion experiments were performed in Franz-type diffusion cells obtained from PermeGear (Riegelsville, PA, USA) with a receptor chamber of approximately 12 ml and a diffusion area of approximately 1.77 cm². Sonicated PBS was used as receptor fluid. One ml of the following 80% saturated solution in PBS was applied onto the skin samples immediately (within 5 minutes) after pore production: diclofenac 2.6 mg/ml, ibuprofen 23.4 mg/ml, ketoprofen 2.4 mg/ml, paracetamol 17.5 mg/ml. The donor chambers were covered with parafilm® (American Can Company, Baltimore, USA) and were checked for precipitation of the compounds during the whole experiment. Aliquots were taken from the receptor fluid and replaced by the same amount of fresh PBS at 0, 0.5, 1, 2, 4, and 6 hours. Each treatment (untreated control, 200 μm microneedle, and 300 μm microneedle) was performed in duplicate per animal (n = 6).

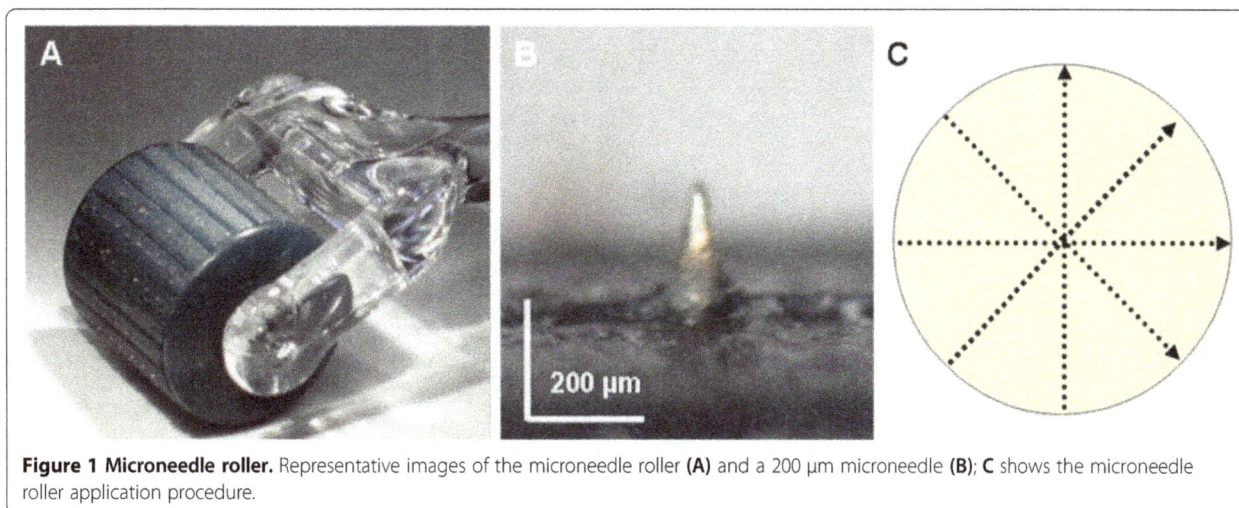

**Figure 1 Microneedle roller.** Representative images of the microneedle roller **(A)** and a 200 μm microneedle **(B)**; **C** shows the microneedle roller application procedure.

## Analysis

The receptor fluid samples (100 μl) were analysed by high-performance liquid-chromatography, the methodology of which has derived from recent studies [22]. The following components were obtained from Beckman (Fullerton, CA, USA): autosampler 507, pump 126, and UV–VIS detector 168. The separation took place on a reversed phase column (LiChroCART 125–4, LiChrospher 100 RP-18e, 5 μm (Merck, Darmstadt, Germany)), which was maintained at 40°C. The mobile phase consisted of 80% methanol and 20% McIlvaine citrate buffer (pH 2.2) for both diclofenac and ibuprofen, of 60% methanol and 40% McIlvaine citrate buffer for ketoprofen, and of 15% methanol and 85% McIlvaine citrate buffer for paracetamol. The detection was performed at 282 nm (diclofenac), 238 nm (ibuprofen), 260 nm (ketoprofen) and 245 nm (paracetamol), respectively.

## Data analysis

The results of the diffusion experiment are expressed as mean and standard error. The linear part of the gradient of the permeation curve (time vs. concentration in the receptor fluid) represents the maximum flux $J_{max}$ (μg/cm²/h) and is employed to calculate the apparent permeability coefficient $P_{app}$ (cm/s) according to Niedorf et al. 2008 [23]. Differences between control samples and pretreated skin samples were evaluated by Friedman test followed by Dunn´s multiple comparison test (GraphPad Prism 4.01 (GraphPad Software Inc., San Diego, USA). A 0.05 significance level was adopted.

## Results

The microneedle application results in an enhanced permeation of all applied compounds compared to untreated skin (Figure 2). In skin samples pretreated with the 300 μm microneedles a significant higher permeation was found than in the untreated skin samples, by which the maximum flux ($J_{max}$) and the $P_{app}$-value are up to 3-fold (ketoprofen, ibuprofen) to 7-fold (diclofenac) and 8-fold (paracetamol) higher in the microneedle treated skin samples (Table 1) and hence result in higher recoveries after microneedle pretreatment.

The correlation of physicochemical drug characteristics with the enhancement of the permeation reveals that substances with low lipophilicity ($R^2 = 0.73$) and high melting points ($R^2 = 0.76$) benefit from microneedle application, while there is no correlation of the microneedle pretreatment to the molecular weight ($R^2 = 0.01$).

Although no visible pores are detectable by light microscopy directly after puncturing the skin, the methylene blue application reveals the existence of barrier damage after microneedle treatment (Figure 3 A and B), which is also detectable in histological sections (Figure 3 C and D). The density of the microscopic holes was approximately 48 pores/cm².

## Discussion

In the present study, two commercially available microneedle rollers with different needle lengths have been utilised to overcome the natural skin barrier. A staining method was employed to determine the ability of the microneedles to invade into the skin, and diffusion experiments with several non-steroidal anti-inflammatory drugs were performed to investigate the ability of microneedles to enhance transdermal drug delivery of non-steroidal anti-inflammatory drugs.

At first, the capability of the microneedle rollers to disrupt the skin barrier could be confirmed by the blue staining under the light microscope. Methylene blue is a dye with a molecular mass of 320 g/mol with a high affinity to proteins. The latter characteristic results in the fact that after application of methylene blue solution onto physiological intact skin no dye can be found in deeper skin layers. Thus, the methylene blue staining

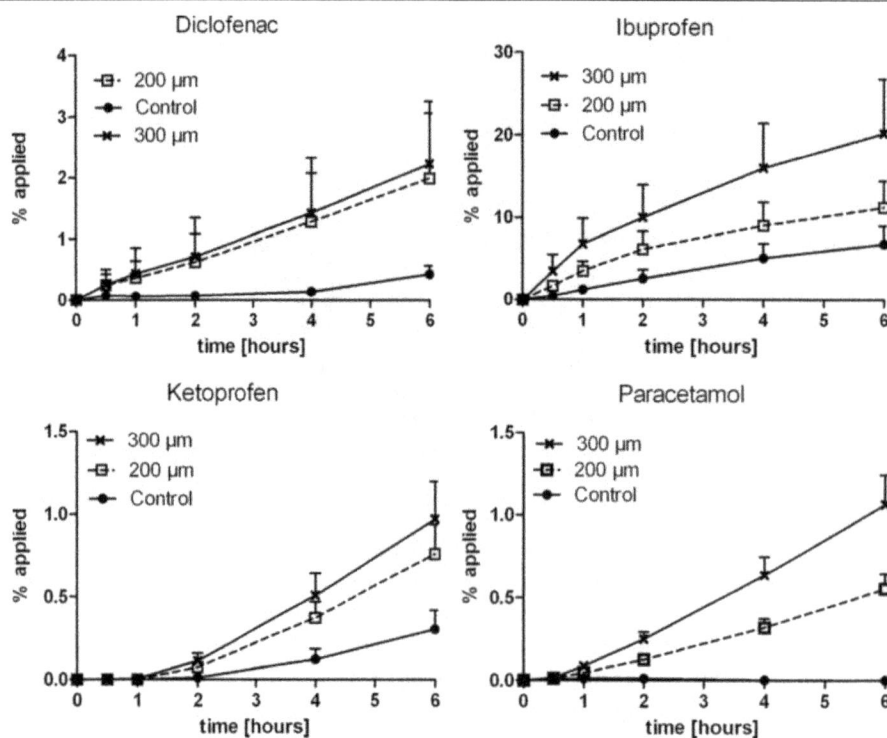

**Figure 2 Permeation profile.** Permeation of diclofenac, ibuprofen, ketoprofen and paracetamol through bovine udder skin samples following pretreatment with 200 µm and 300 µm microneedles in comparison to untreated control skin (n = 5–6); mean + SEM.

made the non visible pores after microneedle pretreatment detectable.

As the needle assembly, the geometry and the velocity insertion of the microneedles treatment [24] severely influence the penetration depth and the pore size, a direct comparison between various types of microneedles should be made with caution. However, in accordance with former studies which demonstrated that 150 µm long needles do not form measurable wholes in the skin [10], the 200 µm and 300 µm needles show similarly manners. As a result of an *in vitro*-study, information about pain or bleeding could not be determined. Since no alterations in the deeper skin layers have been observed (Figure 3 C and D), it is likely that the needles used in the present study can not cause any pain or bleeding, and recent studies in humans have demonstrated that microneedles were applied to human skin in a painless manner [8,25].

Moreover, the ability of microneedles to enhance skin permeability of non-steroidal anti-inflammatory drugs was verified by *in vitro*-diffusion experiments with bovine split skin. The application of two types of microneedles resulted in altered permeation rates for both needle lengths, yet only the 300 µm-microneedle roller led to a statistical significant higher permeation rate for all test compounds. This may be due to the considerable barrier disruption produced by the 300 µm needles and may be adjusted by increasing amounts of pores of the 200 µm needles. However, higher amounts of pores intensify skin permeability only for a certain extent [26]. For microbiological risk assessment, an *in vitro*-study has been performed after microneedle administration by Donnelly et al. 2009 [27]. It has been shown that microneedle induced holes in the *stratum corneum* result in significant less microbial penetration than hypodermic needles

**Table 1 Permeation parameters**

| Parameter | Substance | | | | | | | | | | | |
|---|---|---|---|---|---|---|---|---|---|---|---|---|
| | Diclofenac | | | Ibuprofen | | | Ketoprofen | | | Paracetamol | | |
| | Control | 200 µm | 300 µm | Control | 200 µm | 300 µm | Control | 200 µm | 300 µm | Control | 200 µm | 300 µm |
| $J_{max}$ (µg/cm²/h) | 1.72 | 8.75 | 11.55 | 167.78 | 368.69 | 431.52 | 1.03 | 2.36 | 2.99 | 2.58 | 9.97 | 19.42 |
| $10^{-6}$ $P_{app}$ (cm/s) | 0.18 | 0.93 | 1.24* | 1.92 | 4.21 | 5.27* | 0.12 | 0.28 | 0.35* | 0.04 | 0.16 | 0.31* |
| Recovery (%) | 0.49 | 3.17 | 3.54 | 6.76 | 11.15 | 17.75 | 0.30 | 0.76 | 0.96 | 0.14 | 0.55 | 1.06 |

Mean permeation parameters following substance application to bovine skin; * = p<0.05 (microneedle versus control), n = 5–6.

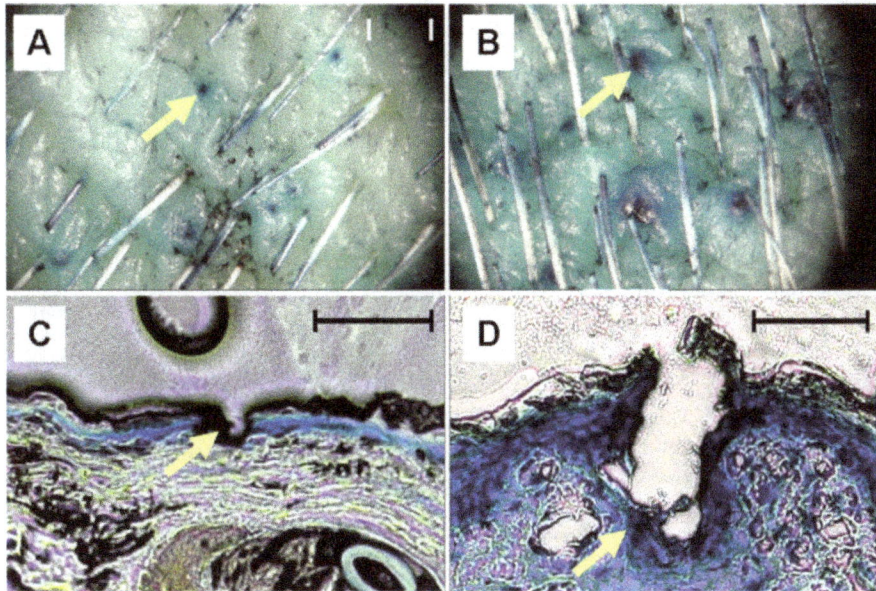

**Figure 3 Microneedle treatment.** Light microscopic images of bovine skin treated with microneedles of 200 μm **(A)** and 300 μm **(B)** needle lengths after topical administration of methylene blue solution for 6 hours; the arrows show the punctured areas with methylene blue penetration into deeper skin layers. C and D show histological images of perforated skin samples **(C:** 200 μm, **D:** 300 μm) after administration of methylene blue on the microneedle pretreated skin samples; the arrows show the punctured areas with methylene blue penetration into deeper skin layers. The bars represent 500 μm.

and no microorganisms crossed the viable epidermis after microneedle pretreatment. Thus, it is likely that microneedle application in an appropriate manner will not result in either local or systemic infections in immune-competent individuals as far as the microneedles are manufactured under aseptic or sterile conditions [27].

Recent *in vitro*-examinations about permeation enhancement of topically applied substances in microneedle treated skin revealed a permeation enhancement up to 2 times for the hydrophilic acetylsalicylic acid [28], whereas the previous study demonstrated permeation enhancements up to 3–8 times depending on the substance lipophilicity. But it has to be taken into consideration that the manner of application of the needles complicates a direct comparison between different examinations as well as the skin type used (full thickness skin vs. split skin) [10].

In order to obtain information about the influence of physicochemical drug characteristics on drug enhancement by microneedles, non-steroidal anti-inflammatory drugs with different molecular weights, lipophilicities and melting points were chosen. Despite the application of 80% saturated solutions for each compound, different levels of permeation enhancement were obtained. In contrast to a comparative study with different particle sizes which demonstrated that small sizes were more effective in drug delivering into the horny layer [10] the present study did not reveal a correlation between

permeation enhancement and molecular weight. However, a higher permeation enhancement was observed for more hydrophilic compounds like paracetamol and diclofenac compared to the lipophilic drugs ibuprofen and ketoprofen. This may be due to the effect that hydrophilic substances, that bypass the lipophilic *stratum corneum* e.g. by a microscopic pore, partition faster into the hydrophilic skin layers compared to lipophilic compounds [7,10,29-34]. Once a hydrophilic drug has bypassed the lipophilic *stratum corneum* a fast permeation into the receptor fluid can be assumed, since the dermis does not represent a distinct barrier for hydrophilic compounds [35].

Another important physicochemical drug characteristic in transdermal drug delivery is the melting point of the applied compound [36,37]. Substances with low melting points exhibit a high solubility in epidermal lipids, which in turn provides a higher thermodynamic activity for percutaneous permeation. Hence, it is not surprising that the present study reveals a higher permeation enhancement for substances with high melting points (diclofenac and paracetamol), both of which can bypass the *stratum corneum* lipids through the pores produced by the microneedles.

Previous *in vivo*-investigations performed by Bal et al. 2008 [38] showed that under non occlusive conditions the pores remained open for a few hours, which can be enhanced up to 72 hours by performance of occlusive conditions [39]. Since the present study was conducted under occlusive conditions, it is likely that the pores have been open for the entire experiment. Furthermore, barrier disruption can result in a fast substance influx into the deeper skin layer with depot formation. This depot can release the substance into the blood or lymphatic system *in vivo*.

## Conclusion

The present study demonstrates the ability of 200 μm and 300 μm long microneedles to interrupt the main skin barrier and to enhance transdermal drug delivery of topically applied non-steroidal anti-inflammatory drugs especially with a hydrophilic nature and high melting points by orders of magnitude. This transdermal delivery approach is easy to employ, minimally invasive and represents an appealing method with great potential for other applications.

**Competing interests**
The authors declare that they have no competing interests.

**Acknowledgements**
The authors acknowledge the help given by Bettina Blume with respect to the acquisition of the bovine udder skin and Theiss Wystemp and Victoria Garder for technical help.

**Authors' contributions**
JS designed the study, conducted the histological examinations, contributed to the analysis, interpreted results and drafted the manuscript. MW participated in the diffusion experiments. MK participated in the study design development. All authors read and approved the final manuscript.

## References

1. Hadgraft J: **Skin, the final frontier 32.** *IntJPharm* 2001, **224:**1–18.
2. Lampe MA, Burlingame AL, Whitney J, Williams ML, Brown BE, Roitman E, Elias PM: **Human stratum corneum lipids: characterization and regional variations 3.** *JLipid Res* 1983, **24:**120–130.
3. Williams AC, Barry BW: **Skin absorption enhancers.** *Crit Rev Ther Drug Carrier Syst* 1992, **9:**305–353.
4. Singh J, Singh S: **Transdermal iontophoresis: effect of penetration enhancer and iontophoresis on drug transport and surface characteristics of human epidermis.** *Curr Probl Dermatol* 1995, **22:**179–183.
5. Srinivasan V, Higuchi WI, Sims SM, Ghanem AH, Behl CR: **Transdermal iontophoretic drug delivery: mechanistic analysis and application to polypeptide delivery.** *J Pharm Sci* 1989, **78:**370–375.
6. Escobar-Chavez JJ, Bonilla-Martinez D, Villegas-Gonzalez MA, Revilla-Vazquez AL: **Electroporation as an efficient physical enhancer for skin drug delivery.** *J Clin Pharmacol* 2009, **49:**1262–1283.
7. Henry S, McAllister DV, Allen MG, Prausnitz MR: **Microfabricated microneedles: A novel approach to transdermal drug delivery.** *J Pharm Sci* 1998, **87:**922–925.
8. Kaushik S, Hord AH, Denson DD, McAllister DV, Smitra S, Allen MG, Prausnitz MR: **Lack of pain associated with microfabricated microneedles.** *Anesth Analg* 2001, **92:**502–504.
9. Prausnitz MR, Mikszta JA, Cormier M, Andrianov AK: **Microneedle-based vaccines.** *Curr Top Microbiol Immunol* 2009, **333:**369–393.
10. Badran MM, Kuntsche J, Fahr A: **Skin penetration enhancement by a microneedle device (Dermaroller) *in vitro*: dependency on needle size and applied formulation.** *Eur J Pharm Sci* 2009, **36:**511–523.
11. Wu Y, Qiu Y, Zhang S, Qin G, Gao Y: **Microneedle-based drug delivery: studies on delivery parameters and biocompatibility.** *Biomed Microdevices* 2008, **10:**601–610.
12. Martanto W, Davis SP, Holiday NR, Wang J, Gill HS, Prausnitz MR: **Transdermal delivery of insulin using microneedles *in vivo*.** *Pharm Res* 2004, **21:**947–952.
13. Ito Y, Hagiwara E, Saeki A, Sugioka N, Takada K: **Feasibility of microneedles for percutaneous absorption of insulin.** *Eur J Pharm Sci* 2006, **29:**82–88.
14. Lee JW, Park JH, Prausnitz MR: **Dissolving microneedles for transdermal drug delivery.** *Biomaterials* 2008, **29:**2113–2124.
15. Martanto W, Moore JS, Kashlan O, Kamath R, Wang PM, O'Neal JM, Prausnitz MR: **Microinfusion using hollow microneedles.** *Pharm Res* 2006, **23:**104–113.
16. Prausnitz MR: **Microneedles for transdermal drug delivery.** *Adv Drug Deliv Rev* 2004, **56:**581–587.
17. Zhou CP, Liu YL, Wang HL, Zhang PX, Zhang JL: **Transdermal delivery of insulin using microneedle rollers *in vivo*.** *Int J Pharm* 2010, **392:**127–133.
18. McAllister DV, Wang PM, Davis SP, Park JH, Canatella PJ, Allen MG, Prausnitz MR: **Microfabricated needles for transdermal delivery of macromolecules and nanoparticles: fabrication methods and transport studies.** *Proc Natl Acad Sci U S A* 2003, **100:**13755–13760.
19. Verbaan FJ, Bal SM, van den Berg DJ, Groenink WH, Verpoorten H, Luttge R, Bouwstra JA: **Assembled microneedle arrays enhance the transport of compounds varying over a large range of molecular weight across human dermatomed skin.** *J Control Release* 2007, **117:**238–245.
20. *ChemIDPlus advance*. http://chem.sis.nlm.nih.gov/chemidplus/.
21. Ludewig T, Michel G, Gutte G: **Histological and histochemical investigations on the structure of udder skin of cattle with special reference to changes during *in vivo* udder perfusion models.** *Dtsch Tierarztl Wochenschr* 1996, **103:**501–505.
22. Stahl J, Niedorf F, Kietzmann M: **The correlation between epidermal lipid composition and morphologic skin characteristics with percutaneous permeation: an interspecies comparison of substances with different lipophilicity.** *J Vet Pharmacol Ther* 2011, **34:**502–507.
23. Niedorf F, Schmidt E, Kietzmann M: **The automated, accurate and reproducible determination of steady-state permeation parameters from percutaneous permeation data.** *Altern Lab Anim* 2008, **36:**201–213.
24. Verbaan FJ, Bal SM, van den Berg DJ, Dijksman JA, van Hecke M, Verpoorten H, van den Berg A, Luttge R, Bouwstra JA: **Improved piercing of microneedle arrays in dermatomed human skin by an impact insertion method.** *J Control Release* 2008, **128:**80–88.
25. Mikszta JA, Alarcon JB, Brittingham JM, Sutter DE, Pettis RJ, Harvey NG: **Improved genetic immunization via micromechanical disruption of skin-barrier function and targeted epidermal delivery.** *Nat Med* 2002, **8:**415–419.
26. Gomaa YA, Morrow DI, Garland MJ, Donnelly RF, El-Khordagui LK, Meidan VM: **Effects of microneedle length, density, insertion time and multiple applications on human skin barrier function: assessments by transepidermal water loss.** *Toxicol In Vitro* 2010, **24:**1971–1978.
27. Donnelly RF, Singh TR, Tunney MM, Morrow DI, McCarron PA, O'Mahony C, Woolfson AD: **Microneedle arrays allow lower microbial penetration than hypodermic needles *in vitro*.** *Pharm Res* 2009, **26:**2513–2522.
28. Park JH, Choi SO, Seo S, Choy YB, Prausnitz MR: **A microneedle roller for transdermal drug delivery.** *Eur J Pharm Biopharm* 2010, **76:**282–289.
29. Oh JH, Park HH, Do KY, Han M, Hyun DH, Kim CG, Kim CH, Lee SS, Hwang SJ, Shin SC, Cho CW: **Influence of the delivery systems using a microneedle array on the permeation of a hydrophilic molecule, calcein.** *Eur J Pharm Biopharm* 2008, **69:**1040–1045.
30. Herkenne C, Naik A, Kalia YN, Hadgraft J, Guy RH: **Ibuprofen Transport into and through Skin from Topical Formulations: In Vitro-In Vivo Comparison 1.** *J Invest Dermatol* 2006, **127:**135–142.
31. Kasting G, Smith R, Cooper E, Shroot B, Schaefer H: *Effect of lipid solubility and molecular size on percutaneous absorption. In Pharmacology and the Skin. Volume 1.* Basel: Karger; 1987:138–153.
32. Nielsen JB, Nielsen F, Sorensen JA: *In vitro* **percutaneous penetration of five pesticides–effects of molecular weight and solubility characteristics 3.** *AnnOccupHyg* 2004, **48:**697–705.
33. Nielsen JB: **Percutaneous penetration through slightly damaged skin.** *Arch Dermatol Res* 2005, **296:**560–567.
34. Henry S, McAllister DV, Allen MG, Prausnitz MR: **Microfabricated microneedles: A novel approach to transdermal drug delivery.** *J Pharm Sci* 1999, **88:**948.

35.  Singh TR, Garland MJ, Cassidy CM, Migalska K, Demir YK, Abdelghany S, Ryan E, Woolfson AD, Donnelly RF: **Microporation techniques for enhanced delivery of therapeutic agents.** *Recent Pat Drug Deliv Formul* 2010, **4**:1–17.

36.  Fiala S, Brown MB, Jones SA: **Dynamic in-situ eutectic formation for topical drug delivery.** *J Pharm Pharmacol* 2011, **63**:1428–1436.

37.  Stott PW, Williams AC, Barry BW: **Mechanistic study into the enhanced transdermal permeation of a model beta-blocker, propranolol, by fatty acids: a melting point depression effect.** *Int J Pharm* 2001, **219**:161–176.

38.  Bal SM, Caussin J, Pavel S, Bouwstra JA: ***In vivo* assessment of safety of microneedle arrays in human skin.** *Eur J Pharm Sci* 2008, **35**:193–202.

39.  Banga AK: **Microporation applications for enhancing drug delivery.** *Expert Opin Drug Deliv* 2009, **6**:343–354.

# 6

# Adverse drug reactions to antiretroviral therapy (ARVs): incidence, type and risk factors in Nigeria

George I Eluwa[1,2*], Titilope Badru[2] and Kesiena J Akpoigbe[3]

## Abstract

**Background:** Data on adverse drug reactions (ADRs) related to antiretroviral (ARV) use in public health practice are few indicating the need for ART safety surveillance in clinical care.

**Objectives:** To evaluate the incidence, type and risk factors associated with adverse drug reactions (ADRs) among patients on antiretroviral drugs (ARV).

**Methods:** Patients initiated on ARVs between May 2006 and May 2009 were evaluated in a retrospective cohort analysis in three health facilities in Nigeria. Regimens prescribed include nucleoside backbone of zidovudine (AZT)/lamivudine (3TC), stavudine (d4T)/3TC, or tenofovir (TDF)/3TC in combination with either nevirapine (NVP) or efavirenz (EFV). Generalized Estimating Equation (GEE) model was used to identify risk factors associated with occurrence of ADR.

**Results:** 2650 patients were followed-up for 2456 person-years and reported 114 ADRs (incidence rate = 4.6/100 person-years).There were more females 1706(64%) and 73(64%) of the ADRs were reported by women. Overall, 61 (54%) of ADRs were reported by patients on AZT with 54(47%) of these occurring in patients on AZT/NVP. The commonest ADRs reported were pain 25(30%) and skinrash 10(18%). Most ADRs were grade 1(39%) with only 1% being life threatening (grade 4). Adjusted GEE analysis showed that ADR was less likely to occur in patients on longer duration of ART compared to the first six months on treatment; 6-12 months AOR 0.38(95% CI:0.16-0.91) and 12-24 months AOR 0.34(95% CI:0.16-0.73) respectively. Compared to patients on TDF, ADR was less likely to occur in patients on d4T and AZT AOR 0.18(95% CI 0.05-0.64) and AOR 0.24(95% CI:0.7-0.9) respectively. Age, gender and CD4 count were not significantly associated with ADRs.

**Conclusion:** ADRs are more likely to occur within the first six months on treatment. Close monitoring within this period is required to prevent occurrence of severe ADR and improve ART adherence. Further research on the tolerability of tenofovir in this environment is recommended.

**Keywords:** Adverse drug reactions, ADR, Antiretroviral, Zidovudine, Stavudine, Tenofovir, HIV/AIDS, Nigeria, Incidence, Risk factors

## Background

The concerted efforts of developed nations and international organizations have significantly reduced the impact of the HIV epidemic in developing countries by providing the means to scale up care and treatment. Millions of eligible HIV infected patients have access to life prolonging antiretroviral (ARV) drugs. This has led to appreciable decrease in HIV related morbidity and mortality [1-4]. Like most chronically administered drugs, ARVs have documented toxicities and adverse effects. ADRs range from mild to life threatening with short and long term effects, however little is known about the adverse drug reactions (ADR) of ARVs in many HIV programs in the public health sector of developing countries [2]. The spectrum of adverse effects associated with ARVs may vary between developed and developing countries [5]. Variance in psychological and socioeconomic support of HIV positive patients in the public health sector of developing

* Correspondence: dreluwag@gmail.com
[1]Department of Operations Research, HIV/AIDS Program. Population Council, Nigeria. Plot 759, Cadastral Zone AO, Off Constitution Avenue, Central Business District, Abuja, Nigeria
Full list of author information is available at the end of the article

countries coupled with co-morbidities make monitoring ADRs to antiretroviral a necessity. Studies on the incidence of ADR from developing and developed countries have reported incidence of ADR among patients on ARVs to range between 11%-35.9% [6,7] with incidence as high as 54% [8] in the presence of opportunistic infection. Incidence of severe ADR has been reported to be as high as 10% [6] with a study observing an incidence rate of 8 per 100 person years [4]. The long term effects of ARTs are largely unknown but ongoing research provides insights into some ADRs of ARV [9]. These include peripheral neuropathy and lipodystrophy associated with stavudine,[3,4] anaemia associated with zidovudine [10,11] and nevirapine based hepatotoxicity and rash [12-22]. Incidence of hepatotoxicity was observed to be 16% and 8% for patients on NVP and EFV respectively [23] while incidence of anaemia ranged from 3- 12% among patients on zidovudine in developing countries including Nigeria [5].

There is substantial evidence linking treatment success to adherence to ARVs [4,15]. However adherence to treatment is closely linked to adverse drug reactions [4,9,15]. It is thus imperative that clinicians clearly understand ADRs, readily recognize them in patients and manage them effectively. Most studies on ADRs are clinical trials and represent a select group of cohort; however studies of large cohorts of unselected patients are more suited [4] to inform on the situation of ADRs in actual clinical practice of the public health sector.

Nigerian operates a universal health care system which supports the provision of primary, secondary and tertiary levels of health services [24]. Primary health care is funded by the local government, while secondary and tertiary level care is funded by the state and federal government respectively. Delivery of healthcare is decentralized to the state level, leading to much variation in resources and funding. In 2004, Nigeria received over $400 million dollars in funding to scale up ART and part of this fund was implemented by Family Health International under the Global HIV/AIDS Initiative Nigeria (GHAIN) project. This resulted in the influx of ART into the country on a large scale.

Admission into the GHAIN supported ART program represents the typical approach to ART care and treatment in public health setting. Typically it starts with the HIV counselling and testing and determination of the patients HIV status using rapid test kits. The eligibility for ARV is established using clinical staging and CD4 count (stage I or II with CD4 count < 350 or Stage IV irrespective of CD4 for adults; CD4 < 25% for children less than 11 months and CD4 less than 20% for children between the ages of 12-35 months) as per the Nigerian national guidelines [25]. Drugs, laboratory testing and clinical consultation are provided free of charge.

There are no known studies to the best of our knowledge that provides reliable information on the adverse drug reactions to ART in Nigeria. This study is the largest cohort study conducted in Nigeria and one of the largest cohort studies in West Africa and thus presents complementary information on ADRs in ART care and treatment. The purpose of this paper was to estimate the incidence of known ADRs and to determine risk factors associated with ADRs among HIV positive patients on ARVs.

## Methods
This study was a retrospective cohort analysis of prescription events that were routinely monitored for all patients on ART at the study sites.

### Study sites
The study was conducted at three public hospitals - two secondary level hospitals (Maitama District Hospital, Abuja, and Calabar General Hospital, Calabar) and one tertiary level hospital (Federal Medical Center, Owo). Collectively, they serve over 3000 HIV/AIDS patients with support from the Global HIV/AIDS Initiative, Nigeria (GHAIN), a USAID funded program managed by Family Health International (FHI). Like most public hospitals, the three sites serve mostly uninsured population and operate in an environment characterized by low staff morale, shortage of staff, irregular supply of commodities and weak management systems in general. GHAIN's support to the sites included infrastructure renovations in the clinical area, laboratory and pharmacy, laboratory equipment, training on HIV related topics, provision of job aids, supply of drugs and strengthening the M&E system. An electronic medical record system, the Lafiya Management Information System (LAMIS) was established in these sites since 2007.

### Study population and sample
The cohort included all patients who were initiated on ART between May 2006 and May 2009 and had at least one follow up clinical visit after commencing ARVs between May 2009 and May 2010. Once eligible for ARVs, all patients are initiated on combination antiretroviral therapy consisting of a nucleoside backbone of zidovudine (AZT)/lamivudine (3TC), stavudine (d4T)/ 3TC, or tenofovir (TDF)/3TC in combination with either nevirapine (NVP) or efavirenz (EFV). Any ARV regimen outside these groups was classified as others. Thereafter, the patient was reviewed monthly for two months. At each appointment, adherence counselling was provided. The patient was subsequently given two monthly prescriptions if found tolerant and adherent to the medication. Baseline CD4, haematology and chemistry test are conducted for all patients and follow up

laboratory test scheduled at 3 months and 6 monthly or as determined by the physician. Ethical approval was obtained from the National Health Research Ethics Committee, Nigeria.

## Data collection and management

Active ADR screening commenced in May 2009 under the GHAIN project, however passive screening of ADR had been ongoing and data captured on the patient's ART care card was designated as either yes/no, though details of the ADR was not captured. GHAIN developed a structured ADR screening form modified from World Health Organization and closely related to the ADR form used by the National Food and Drug Agency (NAFDAC). The ADR screening form was designed to identify 38 ADRs that occurred in different organ systems, namely skin and appendages, musculoskeletal system, cardiovascular/respiratory system, central and peripheral nervous system, gastrointestinal/hepato-biliary/renal system, metabolic/endocrine system and systemic signs/symptoms. It also allowed for grading of the ADR reported and documents any intervention provided. ADRs were graded on a four point scale using the W.H.O. severity grading [26]; Grade 1 was classified as "mild" and no limitation of daily activities; Grade 2 classified as "moderate" with mild to moderate limitation of activities; Grade 3 classified as "severe" with marked limitation of activities and Grade 4 classified as "life threatening" with extreme limitation of activities and significant medical intervention.

Clinicians and pharmacist were trained on the content and use of the form by the Medical Services Department of FHI in collaboration with Howard University Continuation Education project (HUCE PACE). They were required to use the form on all patients on ARV at every clinical visit. Each visit screened for an ADR is captured as a yes/no (i.e. yes if an ADR is reported) and binary outcome of 1 was designated if the screening yielded an ADR (i.e. value of 0 if no ADR was reported). All ADRs reported were reviewed by a pharmacovigilance committee (PVC) in each of the sites. Each site had its own PVC which is made up of physicians, pharmacists and laboratory scientists. This committee was responsible for establishing causality of any ADR reported. LAMIS generated an ADR report which provided details of current ART regimen, concomitant medication taken by the patient and most current laboratory parameters of each patient. This information was evaluated per case and causality established before the ADR report is sent to the National pharmacovigilance center under the jurisdiction of the National Agency for Food and Drug Administration and Control. The LAMIS also captured sociodemographic information of each patient such as age, sex and physical

address including local government area. All patients clinical encounter (clinical visit, drug refill, laboratory tests) including ADRs were entered into the LAMIS database daily. Data from the LAMIS is backed up daily and domiciled at a central server in a secure location within the hospital. Every month, the data were reviewed by the health facility records officer for completeness and issues identified are discussed at the monthly Multi-LAMIS Evaluation Group (MLEG) meeting. This group was a facility based health management group that worked as a program support group and aimed to ensure program and data ownership and increased data use at the facility level. Members included all cadres of health staff; clinician, pharmacist, nurses, lab scientist, record officers e.t.c.

## Toxicity definition

We used the WHO definition of ADR as any response to a medicine which is noxious and unintended, and which occurs at doses normally used in man [27]. ADRs were evaluated using standard clinical signs and symptoms.

## Data availability

Each LAMIS supported site had three full time data clerks that supported data entry at multiple service delivery areas; general clinic, pharmacy, laboratory and tuberculosis clinic. Patients' data were captured daily and when back log of data occurred, they were captured by the end of the week.

## Statistical analysis

Data from the LAMIS was exported to STATA 10 software (Stata Corporation, College Station, Texas). Follow up data were censored as of May $31^{st}$ 2010. Descriptive and univariate analysis were performed on quantitative data. Median values were used to group CD4 count. Other risk factors include W.H.O. clinical stage, age, sex, duration on treatment and type of regimen prescribed. The Wilcoxon sign rank test was used to compare changes in continuous variables while chi square ($\chi^2$) test was used to test the statistical significance of categorical variables by regimen group. Given the multiple screening of ADR per person, generalized estimating equation (GEE) with logit link was used to determine risk factors associated with ADRs [28,29]. Independence correlation structure was used to account for repeated observations from ADR screening on the same patient over time.

The incidence rate of ADR was expressed as the number of patients with at least one occurrence of the given event per 100 person years [10]. Incidence rate was calculated by time to event method. Patients experiencing an ADR drug reaction were censored at the first occurrence of an ADR. Patients who died, stopped treatment or transferred out to another treatment facility were also censored at time of event. Patients not experiencing any ADR were censored at the end of the observation period. Total time of observation contributed by each patient was summed up to obtain total person years of observation. A $p$-value < 0.05 was considered to be significant for all test conducted.

## Results

### Baseline characteristics

4103 patients initiated ART between May 2006 and May 2009. 1453 were excluded from the analysis (Figure 1) because they had no clinical visits in the observation period. During the one year of observation period 2,650 patients had 13,479 clinical visits, an average of five visits per patient. Table 1 shows the baseline characteristics of the study population. There were more females 1706 (64%) than males 944 (36%).

The median interval between follow up visits was 2 months (IQR 1.8-2.7). About 80% of the patients were between the ages of 15-46 years, median age was 32 years (IQR 27-40). Clinically, 725 (28%) patients were diagnosed with Stage I disease at initiation. 2139 (81%)

patients had at least one CD4 count done during the period under observation. The median baseline CD4 count was 172 cells/µL (IQR 85 - 275). It doubled during follow up, to a median CD4 count of 354 cells/µL (IQR 223 - 517) [p < 0.001].

Of the 2650 patients, 1374 (52%) were on zidovudine based regimen, 1223 (46%) on stavudine based regimen, 46 (1.7%) on tenofovir based regimen and 7 (< 1%) on other regimen. Of the 13, 479 clinical visits, 10,084 (75%) were screened for an ADR and 114 (1.13%) visits reported an ADR.

### Distribution of ADRs

Table 2 shows onset of ADR and distribution by specific characteristics. Of the 114 ADRs reported 83 (73%) had their specific detail collected and 15 patients (28%) reported at least 2 ADRs. Forty-six (45%) of the 114 reported ADRs occurred between 12-24 months on treatment. Sixty-one ADRs (54%) occurred with patients on zidovudine based regimen, 50(44%) with patients on stavudine based regimen and 3 (3%) with patients on tenofovir based regimen.

The ADR screening program implemented by the GHAIN project routinely screened 38 adverse drug

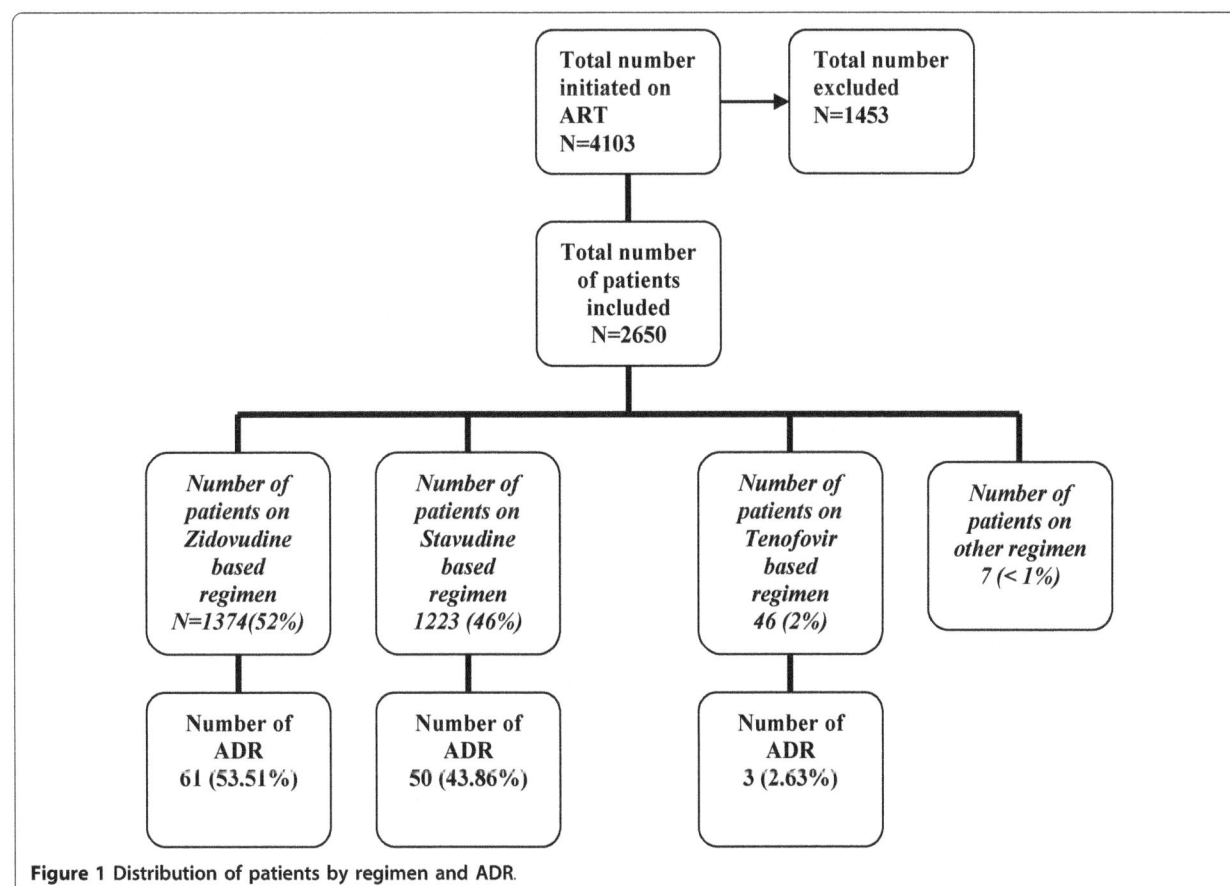

**Figure 1** Distribution of patients by regimen and ADR.

**Table 1 Baseline Characteristics of Study Population**

| Variable | % (n) |
|---|---|
| **Sex** | |
| Female | 64.38 (1,706) |
| Male | 35.62 (944) |
| **Age (years)** | |
| < 15 | 6.26 (144) |
| 16-45 | 80.0 (2120) |
| > 45 | 13.74 (364) |
| **Baseline CD4** | |
| < = 200 | 58.72 (1556) |
| 200 - 350 | 26.68 (707) |
| > 350 | 14.60 (387) |
| Median baseline CD4 (IQR) | 172 (85-275) |
| **Baseline WHO Staging\*** | |
| Stage I | 27.36 (725) |
| Stage II | 26.60 (705) |
| Stage III | 40.23 (1066) |
| Stage IV | 4.08 (108) |
| **ART Regimen** | |
| **NRTI Backbone** | |
| Zidovudine based | 51.85 (1374) |
| Stavudine based | 46.15 (1223) |
| Tenofovir based | 1.74 (46) |
| Others | 0.26 (7) |
| **NNRTI Backbone** | |
| Nevirapine_based | 80.04 (2121) |
| Efavirenze_based | 19.96 (529) |

\* Total do not add up to 114 due to missing data

**Table 2 Onset and Distribution of ADR**

**Onset of Adverse Drug Reaction From ART Initiation\* (n = 102)**

| Onset of ADR | n (%) |
|---|---|
| 0-3 months | 8 (7.84) |
| 3-6 months | 14 (13.73) |
| 6-12 months | 22 (21.57) |
| 12-24 months | 46 (45.10) |
| 24-36 months | 10 (9.80) |
| > 36 months | 2 (1.96) |
| **ADR distribution by age (n = 114)** | |
| < 15 years | 0 |
| 16-45 years | 97 (85.09) |
| > 45 years | 17 (14.91) |
| **ADR distribution by gender (n = 114)** | |
| Male | 41 (35.96) |
| Female | 73 (64.04) |

\* Total do not add up to 114 due to missing data

reactions and of these 18 (50%) were reported. For severity of ADRs, most of the ADRs reported were Grade 1 (39%), Grade 2 and 3 ADRs were 32% and 28% respectively, while 1% of ADRs was found to be life threatening. Amongst those that reported an ADR, no change in regimen was documented.

**Incidence of ADRs**

Patients were followed up for a total of 2456 person-years yielding an incidence rate (IR) of 4.6/100 person-years. Overall incidence of ADR by nucleoside backbone was 4.4%, 4.1% and 6.5% for patients on AZT, d4T and TDF based regimen respectively while by non-nucleoside base, incidence was 4.2% and 4.9% for patients on nevirapine and efavirenz respectively.

Table 3 shows the incidence rates of reported ADR by regimen group. Pain/tingling/numbness was the most common ADR reported (30%) with an IR of 2.1 and 0.1 per 100 person-years among patients on d4T and AZT based regimen respectively, followed by skin rash (18%) with an IR of 2.6, 0.5 and 0.6 per 100 person years among patients on TDF, d4T and AZT respectively.

**Risk factors for ADR**

Table 4 shows risk factors associated with ADRs. The adjusted GEE analysis showed that patients on longer duration of treatment had decreased odds of developing an ADR compared to patients in their first six months on treatment, 6-12 months (AOR 0.38, 95% CI 0.16-0.91, $P = 0.03$), 12-24 months (AOR 0.35, 95% CI 0.16-0.73, $P = 0.005$), 24-36 months (AOR 0.37, 95% CI 0.14-0.96, $P = 0.05$). With TDF based regimen as the reference, patients on d4T (AOR 0.18, CI 0.05-0.64, p = 0.009) and AZT (AOR 0.24, CI 0.07-0.904, p = 0.034) were less likely to report an ADR. Age (AOR 1.27, CI 0.59-2.77, p = 0.544) gender (AOR 0.83, 0.43-1.57, p = 0.562) and CD4 count (AOR 0.93, CI 0.51-1.70, p = 0.816) were not significantly associated with developing an ADR.

**Discussion**

The likelihood of developing an adverse drug reaction was highest in the first six months of commencing antiretroviral therapy. Xavier et al. [4] proffered an explanation that early occurrence of ADRs is an expression of a mechanism of intrinsic intolerance rather than of a time-dependent toxic accumulation process. Close monitoring of patients within this time frame is thus imperative to prevent the occurrence of severe ADRs, improve adherence as well as improve documentation of ADRs. However 45% of the reported ADRs occurred within 12-24 months of commencing ARVs. This calls for the need to intensify long term ADR monitoring in patients on ARV. Some studies have proposed time-dependent

**Table 3 Incidence Rates of ADR by Regimen per 100 person-years of Treatment**

| Specific ADR by Organ System | AZT_based (n) | d4T_based (n) | TDF_based (n) | Total (%) |
|---|---|---|---|---|
| **Gastrointestinal** | | | | |
| Abdominal pain | - | 0.09 (1) | - | 1 (1.20) |
| Diarrhea | 0.32 (4) | - | - | 4 (4.82) |
| Dyspepsia | 0.08 (1) | - | - | 1 (1.20) |
| Nausea & Vomiting | 0.24 (3) | - | - | 3 (3.61) |
| **Cardiovascular/Respiratory System** | | | | |
| Chest pain | - | 0.09 (1) | - | 1 (1.20) |
| Cough | - | 0.09 (1) | - | 1 (1.20) |
| **Skin and Appendages** | | | | |
| Pruritus | 0.24 (3) | 0.61 (7) | - | 10 (12.05) |
| Steven Johnson syndrome | 0.08 (1) | - | - | 1 (1.20) |
| Skin rash | 0.64 (8) | 0.52 (6) | 2.56 (1) | 15 (18.07) |
| **Central and Peripheral Nervous System** | | | | |
| Headache | 0.08 (1) | 0.09 (1) | - | 2 (2.41) |
| Dizziness | 0.08 (1) | 0.44 (5) | - | 6 (7.23) |
| Insomnia | 0.16 (2) | - | - | 2 (2.41) |
| Nightmare | 0.08 (1) | 0.09 (1) | - | 2 (2.41) |
| Pain/Tingling/Numbness | 0.08 (1) | 2.09 (24) | - | 25 (30.12) |
| **Musculoskeletal System** | | | | |
| Myalgia | 0.08 (1) | - | - | 1 (1.20) |
| **Systemic Signs/Symptoms** | | | | |
| Rigor | 0.08 (1) | - | - | 1 (1.20) |
| Fatigue | 0.08 (1) | - | - | 1 (1.20) |
| Fever | 0.08 (1) | - | - | 1 (1.20) |
| **Total** | **34** | **48** | **1** | **83** |

**Table 4 Generalized Estimating Equation Analysis for Risk Factors Associated with ADR**

| Variables | N (%) | Unadjusted OR | p | Adjusted OR | p |
|---|---|---|---|---|---|
| **Gender** | | | | | |
| Female | 1706 (64.4) | | | | |
| Male | 944 (35.6) | 1.11(0.71-1.73) | 0.663 | 0.83 (0.43-1.57) | 0.562 |
| **Age (years)** | | | | | |
| 15-45 | 2120 (85.3) | | | | |
| > 45 | 364 (14.7) | 0.81(0.48-1.36) | 0.422 | 1.27 (0.59-2.77) | 0.544 |
| **Regimen** | | | | | |
| TDF_based | 46 (1.7) | | | | |
| AZT_based | 1374 (52.0) | 0.56 (0.18-1.75) | 0.319 | 0.24 (0.07-0.90) | 0.034 |
| D4T_based | 1223 (46.3) | 0.33 (0.10-1.03) | 0.057 | 0.18 (0.05-0.64) | 0.009 |
| **Duration on treatment (months)** | | | | | |
| 0-6 | 21 (0.79) | | | | |
| 6-12 | 79 (2.98) | 0.54 (0.33-0.89) | 0.02 | 0.38 (0.16-0.91) | 0.03 |
| 12-24 | 259 (47.5) | 0.25 (0.15-0.41) | < 0.001 | 0.35 (0.16-0.73) | 0.005 |
| 24-36 | 952 (35.9) | 0.16 (0.08-0.34) | < 0.001 | 0.37 (0.14-0.96) | 0.042 |
| **CD4 cell count cells/μL** | | | | | |
| < 350 | 950 (44.8) | | | | |
| > 350 | 1180 (55.2) | 1.08 (0.6-2.0) | 0.791 | 0.93 (0.51-1.70) | 0.816 |

toxic accumulation as the mechanism of developing an ADR long after commencing medication. Thus monitoring for ADR should be an ongoing process as we have both early onset and late onset ADRs. Adding a laboratory component to the ADR screening would go a long way in determining biochemical markers that would help to improve patient management. However from a programmatic aspect in a resource constrained environment, having sound knowledge of the risk factors or common ADRs associated with different ARV regime can help focus scarce resources to managing ADRs in these settings.

Since adverse drug reactions are the single most common reason for poor adherence to treatment, identifying risk factors for the occurrence of ADRs is of crucial importance to optimize the initial choice of ARVs regimen before initiating therapy and to adapt the pace of surveillance to each unique situation [4]. Our study showed no difference in reported ADR between men and women, however Bonfati et al [7]. observed that women experienced significantly greater number of adverse effects compared to men. Though the population of patients on tenofovir based regimen was small compared to AZT and d4T, our data shows that patients on AZT or d4T were less likely to report an ADR than those on TDF. A multisite trial in Africa, found tenofovir therapy to be associated with 1.3% rate of significant nephrotoxicity which was comparable to other regimen,[5,30] thus showing no significant toxicity difference between tenofovir and other regimens. This raises a sentinel sign that perhaps drug response to TDF in this setting is not in conformity with the results from other studies where drug profile of TDF has been superior over AZT and d4T. A closer look at the drug profile and toxicity of TDF is urgently needed to better understand its tolerance in patients in this setting. Furthermore, the most common side effect of tenofovir is renal impairment as measured by reduced creatinine clearance,[31] thus as tenofovir replaces d4T as the nucleoside backbone of choice in HIV treatment, laboratories in resource poor settings must be strengthened to able to conduct this test.

Incidence of anaemia was low at 4% and occurred exclusively in patients on AZT. This is similar to other studies conducted in Nigeria, Coˆ te d'Ivoire, Haiti and India that observed anaemic rates of 3%-12% [5,32-38]. The incidence of skin toxicity (18%) is similar to that in other reports,[15,17] though some reports have observed low incidence of skin toxicity,[10,31] however the incidence of Steven-Johnson syndrome (1%) was similar to other reports which reported less than 5% [14-17]. Most of the reported ADRs (71%) were mild to moderate and self limiting in nature while 1% were life threatening.

This suggests good tolerance level to ARVs in general. While other studies have associated low CD4 count at treatment initiation as a risk factor for ADR [5], our study did not show any association between CD4 cell count and clinical stage with ADRs.

Our study takes strength in its large sample size. This is the largest cohort of patients who have been surveyed in Nigeria for ADR using active surveillance. It also presents ADR outcomes in a large public health program and more closely presents treatment outcomes that are more generalizable than clinical studies. Finally data in this study was of good quality giving the scale of the program and its routine nature of collection. Mathieu Forster et al. [39] assessed data quality for ART services in low income countries by evaluating the availability of six key variables (age, sex, W.H.O clinical staging at baseline and follow-up, CD4 count and year of ART initiation) and calculating the proportion of missing data to determine the quality of data and the median was found to be 10.9%. The median of the percentages of missing variables was 0% for all sites surveyed.

This study has some limitations. The study included patients who had initiated ART before active surveillance of ADR commenced. Though this provided information on long term adverse effects, we may have missed early onset ADR from these patients. The small sample size of patients on tenofovir based regimen limits our ability to compare ADR reported by this group with other regimen groups. Also the ADR screening tool was structured and thus, does not allow details of unknown ADR to be captured and graded, thus the study was confined to report on known ADRs only. Finally, not all ADRs reported had their complete details collected and graded. Thus the specific ADRs in this study are most likely under reported.

## Conclusion

Incidence rate (4.6/100 person years) of ADRs is low amongst patients on ARVs. Active screening of ADRs has increased the documentation of the occurrence of these events and should be scaled up to all facilities providing comprehensive care to HIV patients. Improving quality of care to patients by providing ADR screening provides an avenue for early identification and subsequently treatment of adverse drug reactions. Further evaluation of patients on tenofovir would be beneficial in documenting adverse drug reactions related to tenofovir as well as its tolerability. Finally more field based studies in resource constrained settings should be conducted and ADRs related to ARVs evaluated and compared to ADRs observed from clinical trials. This will provide valuable insight in the incidence, prevalence and type of ADRs associated with ARVs.

## Acknowledgements
Support for this paper was provided by FHI Global HIV/AIDS Initiative in Nigeria with funds from the U.S. President's Emergency Plan for AIDS Relief (PEPFAR) through U.S. Agency for International Development (USAID) Cooperative Agreement No. 620-A-00-04-00-122-00

## Author details
[1]Department of Operations Research, HIV/AIDS Program. Population Council, Nigeria. Plot 759, Cadastral Zone AO, Off Constitution Avenue, Central Business District, Abuja, Nigeria. [2]Department of Health Policy and Management, Diadem Consults Ltd, Abuja, Nigeria. [3]Society for Family Health, Abuja, Nigeria.

## Authors' contributions
GE conceived the study, performed the statistical analysis and drafted the manuscript. KA drafted the manuscript and provided critical review of the article. TB participated in study design, performed statistical analysis and reviewed the article. All authors read and approved the final manuscript

## Competing interests
The author declares that they have no competing interests.

## References
1. Detels R, Muñoz A, McFarlane G, Kingsley LA, Margolick JB, Giorgi J, Schrager LK, Phair JP: **Effectiveness of potent antiretroviral therapy on time to AIDS and death in men with known HIV infection duration.** *AIDS Cohort Study Investigators JAMA* 1998, **280**:1497-1503.
2. Hogg RS, Yip B, Kully C, Craib KJ, O'Shaughnessy MV, Schechter MT, Montaner JS: **Improved survival among HIV infected patients after initiation of triple drug antiretroviral regimens.** *CMAJ* 1999, **160(Suppl 5)**:659-665.
3. Palella FJ Jr, Delaney KM, Moorman AC, Loveless MO, Fuhrer J, Satten GA, Aschman DJ, Holmberg SD: **Declining morbidity and mortality among patients with advanced human imunodeficiency virus infection. HIV outpatient Study Investigators.** *N Engl J Med* 1998, **338**:853-860.
4. Duval X, Journot V, Leport C, Chêne G, Dupon M, Cuzin L, May T, Morlat P, Waldner A, Salamon R, Raffi F, Antiprotease Cohort (APROCO) Study Group: **Incidence of and risk factors for adverse drug reactions in a prospective cohort of HIV infected adults initiating protease inhibitor containing therapy.** *Infectious Dis Soc Am* 2004, **39**:248-255.
5. Subbaraman R, Chaguturu SK, Mayer KH, Flanigan TP, Kumarasamy N: **Adverse effects of highly active antiretroviral therapy in developing countries.** *Clin Infectious Dis* 2007, **45**:1093-1101.
6. Patrice S, Juste MA, Ambroise A, Eliacin L, *et al*: **Early versus standard antiretroviral therapy for HIV infected adults in Haiti.** *N Engl J Med* 2010, **363**:257-265.
7. Bonfanti P, Valsecchi L, Parazzini F, Carradori S, Pusterla L, *et al*: **Incidence of adverse reactions in HIV patients treated with protease inhibitors: a cohort study.** *JAIDS* 2000, **23**:236-245.
8. Dean GL, Edwards SG, Ives NJ, Matthews G, Fox EF, Navaratne L, Fisher M, Taylor GP, Miller R, Taylor CB, de Ruiter A, Pozniak AL: **Treatment of tuberculosis in HIV infected persons in the era of highly active antiretroviral therapy.** *AIDS* 2002, **16**:75-83.
9. World Health Organization: **Pharmacovigilance for antiretrovirals in resource poor countries. medicines policy and standards.** *Geneva, World Health Organization* 2007.
10. Laurent C, Bourgeois A, Mpoudi-Ngolé E, Ciaffi L, Kouanfack C, Mougnutou R, Nkoué N, Calmy A, Koulla-Shiro S, Delaporte E: **Tolerability and effectiveness of first line regimens combining nevirapine and lamivudine plus zidovudine or stavudine in Cameroon.** *AIDS Res Human Retroviruses* 2008, **24(Suppl 3)**:393-399.
11. Pollard RB, Robinson P, Dransfield K: **Safety profile of nevirapine, a nonnucleoside reverse transcriptase inhibitor for the treatment of human immunodeficiency virus infection.** *Clin Ther* 1998, **20**:1071-1092.
12. (DHHS), U. S. D. o. H. a. H. S: **Guidelines for the use of antiretroviral agents in HIV-1 infected adults and adolescents.** *Panel on antiretroviral guidelines for adults and adolescents* 2006.
13. Gazzard B, Bernard AJ, Boffito M, Churchill D, Edwards S, Fisher N, Geretti AM, Johnson M, Leen C, Peters B, Pozniak A, Ross J, Walsh J, Wilkins E, Youle M: **British HIV association (BHIVA) guidelines for the treatment of HIV infected adults with antiretroviral therapy.** *HIV Med* 2006, **7(Suppl 8)**:487-503.
14. Colebunders R, Kamya MR, Laurence J, Kambugu A, Byakwaga H, Songa Mwebaze P, Muganzi Muganga A, Katwere M, Katabira E, Muganzi A: **First-line antiretroviral therapy in Africa, how evidence based are our recommendations?** *AIDS Rev* 2005, **7(Suppl 3)**:148-154.
15. Montessori V, Press N, Harris M, Akagi L, Montaner JSG: **Adverse effects of antiretroviral therapy for HIV infection.** *Can Med Assoc Licensors* 2004, **170(Suppl 2)**:229-238.
16. Jamisse L, Balkus J, Hitti J, Gloyd S, Manuel R, Osman N, Djedje M, Farquhar C: **Antiretroviral associated toxicity among HIV 1 seropositive pregnant women in Mozambique receiving nevirapine based regimens.** *J Acquir Immune Defic Syndr* 2007, **44(Suppl 4)**:371-376.
17. Phanuphak N, Apornpong T, Teeratakulpisarn S, Chaithongwongwatthana S, Taweepolcharoen C, Mangclaviraj S, Limpongsanurak S, Jadwattanakul T, Eiamapichart P, Luesomboon W, Apisarnthanarak A, Kamudhamas A, Tangsathapornpong A, Vitavasiri C, Singhakowinta N, Attakornwattana V, Kriengsinyot R, Methajittiphun P, Chunloy K, Preetiyathorn W, Aumchantr T, Toro P, Abrams EJ, El-Sadr W, Phanuphak P: **Nevirapine associated toxicity in HIV-infected Thai men and women, including pregnant women.** *Br HIV Assoc* 2007, **8**:357-366.
18. Dieterich DT, Love J, Stern JO: **Drug-induced liver injury associated with the use of nonnucleoside reverse-transcriptase inhibitors.** *Clin Infect Dis* 2004, **38(Suppl 2)**:S80-S89.
19. Baylor MS, Johann-Liang R: **Hepatotoxicity associated with nevirapine use.** *J Acquir Immune Defic Syndr* 2004, **35**:538.
20. Stern JO, Robinson PA, Love J, Lanes S, Imperiale MS, Mayers DL: **A comprehensive hepatic safety analysis of nevirapine in different populations of HIV-infected patients.** *J Acquir Immune Defic Syndr* 2003, **34**:S21-S33.
21. de Maat MM, ter Heine R, van Gorp EC, Mulder JW, Mairuhu AT, Beijnen JH: **Case series of acute hepatitis in a non-selected group of HIV-infected patients on nevirapine containing antiretroviral treatment.** *AIDS* 2003, **17**:2209-2214.
22. Martínez E, Blanco JL, Arnaiz JA, Pérez-Cuevas JB, Mocroft A, Cruceta A, Marcos MA, Milinkovic A, García-Viejo MA, Mallolas J, Carné X, Phillips A, Gatell JM: **Hepatotoxicity in HIV infected patients recieving nevirapine containing antiretroviral therapy.** *AIDS* 2001, **15**:1261-1268.
23. Sulkowski MS, Thomas DL, Mehta SH, Chaisson RE, Moore RD: **Hepatotoxicity associated with nevirapine or efavirenz containing antiretroviral therapy:role of hepatitis C and B infections.** *Hepatology* 2003, **1**:35.
24. Asuzu MC: **The necessity for a health systems reform in Nigeria.** *J Community Med & Primary Health Care* 2000, **16**:1-3.
25. Federal Ministry of Health Abuja, Nigeria: **National guidelines for HIV/AIDS treatment and care in adolescents and adults.** 2010.
26. World Health Organization: **Antiretroviral therapy for HIV infection in adults and adolescents: recommendations for a public health approach.** *WHO* 2006, 28 [http://www.who.int/hiv/pub/guidelines/artadultguidelines. pdf], (accessed December 3rd, 2011).
27. World Health Organization: **Assuring safety of preventive chemotherapy interventions for neglected tropical diseases. practical advice for national programme managers on the prevention, detection and management of serious adverse effects.** *WHO* 2011, 1 [http://whqlibdoc. who.int/publications/2011/9789241502191_eng.pdf], (accessed December 3rd, 2011).
28. Liang KY, Zeger SL: **Longitudinal data analysis using generalized linear models.** *Biometrica* 1986, **73**:13-22.
29. Liang KY, Zeger SL: **Regression analysis for correlated data.** *Annu Rev Publ Health* 1993, **14**:43-68.
30. Reid A, Walker S, Ssali F, Munderi P, Gilks C: **Glomerular dysfunction and associated risk factors following initiation of ART in adults with HIV infection in Africa [abstract THAB0105].** *International AIDS Society* 2006.
31. Forna F, Liechty CA, Solberg P, Asiimwe F, Were W, Memin J, Behumbiize P, Tong T, Brooks JT, Weidle PJ: **Clinical toxicity of highly active antiretroviral therapy in a home-based AIDS care program in rural Uganda.** *J Acquir Immune Defic Syndr* 2007, **44(Suppl 4)**:456-462.

32. Kumarasamy N, Lai A, Cecelia AJ, *et al*: Toxicities and adverse events following generic HAART in south Indian HIV-infected individuals [abstract P189]. *Proceedings of the 7th International Congress on Drug Therapy and HIV Infection (Glasgow, United Kingdom)* 2004.

33. Idoko JA, Akinsete L, Abalaka AD, Keshinro LB, Dutse L, Onyenekwe B, Lhekwaba A, Njoku OS, Kehinde MO, Wambebe CO: A multicentre study to determine the efficacy and tolerability of a combination of nelfinavir (VIRACEPT), zalcitabine (HIVID) and zidovudine in the treatment of HIV infected Nigerian patients. *West Afr J Med* 2002, 21:83-86.

34. Moh R, Danel C, Sorho S, Sauvageot D, Anzian A, Minga A, Gomis OB, Konga C, Inwoley A, Gabillard D, Bissagnene E, Salamon R, Anglaret X: Haematological changes in adults receiving a zidovudine-containing HAART regimen in combination with cotrimoxazole in Coˆ te d'Ivoire. *Antivir Ther* 2005, 10:615-624.

35. Shah I: Adverse effects of antiretroviral therapy in HIV-1 infected children. *J Trop Pediatr* 2006, 52:244-248.

36. Severe P, Leger P, Charles M, Noel F, Bonhomme G, Bois G, George E, Kenel-Pierre S, Wright PF, Gulick R, Johnson WD Jr, Pape JW, Fitzgerald DW: Antiretroviral therapy in a thousand patients with AIDS in Haiti. *N Engl J Med* 2005, 353:2325-2334.

37. Bygrave H, Kranzer K, Hilderbrand K, Jouquet G, Goemaere E, Vlahakis N, Triviño L, Makakole L, Ford N: Renal safety of tenofovir containing first line regimen: experience from an antiretroviral cohort in rural Lesotho. *PLoS One* 2011, 6(Suppl 3):e17609.

38. Lucas GM, Moore RD: Highly active antiretroviral therapy in a large urban clinic: risk factors for virologic failure and adverse drug reactions. *Ann Intern Med* 1999, 131(Suppl 2):81-87.

39. Forster M, Bailey Christopher, Brinkhof WGMartin: Electronic medical record systems, data quality and loss to follow-up: survey of antiretroviral therapy programs in resource-limited settings. *Bull World Health Organization* 2008, 86:939-947.

# 7

# Pharmacokinetics of high-dose oral thiamine hydrochloride in healthy subjects

Howard A Smithline[1,4*], Michael Donnino[2] and David J Greenblatt[3]

## Abstract

**Background:** High dose oral thiamine may have a role in treating diabetes, heart failure, and hypermetabolic states. The purpose of this study was to determine the pharmacokinetic profile of oral thiamine hydrochloride at 100 mg, 500 mg and 1500 mg doses in healthy subjects.

**Methods:** This was a randomized, double-blind, single-dose, 4-way crossover study. Pharmacokinetic measures were calculated.

**Results:** The $AUC_{0-10\ hr}$ and Cmax values increased nonlinearly between 100 mg and 1500 mg. The slope of the $AUC_{0-10\ hr}$ vs dose, as well as the $C_{max}$ vs dose, plots are steepest at the lowest thiamine doses.

**Conclusion:** Our study demonstrates that high blood levels of thiamine can be achieved rapidly with oral thiamine hydrochloride. Thiamine is absorbed by both an active and nonsaturable passive process.

**Trial Registration:** ClinicalTrials.gov: NCT00981877

## Background

Thiamine, vitamin $B_1$, was isolated in 1926 and synthesized in 1936. Its importance for preventing illness was known as early as the turn of the century. Thiamine requirements are related to energy metabolism; specifically, 0.33 mg of thiamine are required for every 4400 kJ of energy. For adults the DRI of thiamine is between 1.1 and 1.4 mg per day. The primary active form of the vitamin, thiamine diphosphate (ThDP), is also known as thiamine pyrophosphate (TPP). ThDP is a necessary cofactor for enzymes related to carbohydrate metabolism: pyruvate dehydrogenase (PDH), $\alpha$-ketoglutarate dehydrogenase, and transketolase.

Thiamine, vitamin $B_1$, is not synthesized by humans and is not stored in large quantities in humans [1]. One of its phosphorylated forms, thiamine diphosphate, also known as thiamine pyrophosphate, is the primary active form of the vitamin. Thiamine diphosphate is a necessary co-factor for several enzymes involved in the glycolytic pathway, citric acid cycle, pentose phosphate pathway, and degradation of branched chain amino acids.

Thiamine is used to treat various genetic disorders linked to the above metabolic pathways and thiamine deficiency syndromes (beriberi and Wernicke-Korsakoff syndrome). Oral thiamine may also have a role in treating some of the pathophysiologic conditions associated with diabetes, heart failure, and hypermetabolic states [2-5].

The optimum dosing for these beneficial effects is unknown. Rare side effects of thiamine have been attributed to allergic reactions. And although, ganglionic blockade can occur at extremely high intravenous doses, oral dosing of 3 g per day and higher have been used for extended periods of time without deleterious effects [6-8].

Free thiamine is taken-up by the body by a saturable transport system in the proximal small intestine that was thought to severely limit the amount of thiamine that can be absorbed by a single oral dose [9-11]. For this reason, alternate forms of thiamine (S-acyl thiamine derivatives and lipid-soluble thiamine disulfide derivatives), that are more absorbable by the body, had been developed [12]. However, free thiamine may be taken-up by the body by both a saturable active transport system and a nonsaturable passive process. Thus high doses of thiamine hydrochloride may be absorbable.

* Correspondence: howard.smithline@baystatehealth.org
[1]Department of Emergency Medicine, Tufts University School of Medicine and Baystate Medical Center, Springfield, MA, USA
Full list of author information is available at the end of the article

There is very limited pharmacokinetic data of oral thiamine at doses that are typically used and virtually no data on high-dose oral thiamine. The purpose of this study was to determine the pharmacokinetic profile of oral thiamine hydrochloride between 100 mg and 1500 mg in healthy subjects.

## Methods

### Subjects

The Institutional Review Board at Baystate Medical Center approved this study. All subjects provided written informed consent prior to participation. Fourteen healthy subjects consented to be in the study (2 dropped out on the first study day). Screening procedures included a medical history, physical exam, hematologic profile, blood chemistries, pregnancy test, and urine analysis. Subjects were not taking any medications nor were they taking any dietary or herbal supplements.

### Study design and procedures

Subjects participated in a randomized, double-blind, single-dose, 4-way crossover study with a minimum of 1 week elapsing between trials. The 4 treatment groups were:

1. Placebo
2. 100 mg thiamine hydrochloride
3. 500 mg thiamine hydrochloride
4. 1500 mg thiamine hydrochloride

Subjects fasted overnight except for water. In the morning they had a blood sample drawn followed by a standardized breakfast. After 1 hour they were administered the study medication. Additional blood specimens were obtained immediately prior to the study medication and at 0.5, 1, 1.5, 2, 3, 4, 5, 6, 8, and 10 hours after taking the study medication. Subjects received a standardized lunch after the 6-hour blood draw. All blood specimens were drawn in duplicate (for plasma and whole blood assays) in 3 mL lavender-top vacutainers® containing $K_2$EDTA. They were immediately placed in an ice bath and protected from the light. One vacutainer® of each pair was centrifuged at 3000 RPM for 20 min at 4°C to separate the plasma. The plasma sample and whole blood sample were then frozen at -70°C.

### Study medication

Thiamine tablets each containing 100 mg of thiamine hydrochloride were used (Amneal Pharmaceuticals). These were placed intact into opaque capsules. Identical capsules containing sucrose tablets were used as placebo such that the same number of capsules were used for each trial.

### Analysis of blood specimens

Quest Diagnostics analyzed all specimens for total thiamine using HPLC [4]. At Quest Diagnostics, plasma was deproteinized and then incubated with acid phosphatase to convert thiamine phosphate esters to free thiamine. The free thiamine was then oxidized to thiochrome by the addition of alkaline potassium ferricyanide. Depending on the age of the column and the temperature of the room, thiochrome retention time varied from 2.5 to 3.0 min. The mixture was injected to a Supelco (Bellefonte, PA, USA) high-performance liquid chromatographic column (7.5 cm³ 4.6 mm, particle size 3 mm) connected to a high-performance liquid chromatographic system using a Hitachi (Pleasant, CA, USA) pump, autosampler, and fluorescent detector (excitation wavelength 365 nm, emission wavelength 440 nm). The mobile phase was 75 mmol/L of potassium phosphate at pH 7.5 with 25% methanol. The flow rate was set at 1.0 mL/min. Through this process, the thiochrome was then separated from other interfering substances and then measured fluorometrically. The amount of total thiamine in an unknown sample is proportional to the amount of thiochrome formed. The limit of quantification is 7 nmol/L. The assay range is 7 to 450 nmol/L. Samples with values above this range were diluted. The coefficient of variation for both the plasma and whole blood thiamine assays was calculated from the data collected in this study.

### Pharmacokinetic and statistical analysis

The thiamine levels were corrected by subtracting the baseline value. The baseline value was calculated as the average of the -1-hour and 0-hour values. Net systemic exposure to thiamine in each subject in each trial was quantitated using the area under the whole blood or plasma concentration curve from time zero through 10 hours after dosage ($AUC_{0-10 \text{ hr}}$). This was calculated using the cubic splines method. The overall effect of treatment condition (thiamine dose) on $AUC_{0-10 \text{ hr}}$ in blood and plasma was tested using analysis of variance (ANOVA) for repeated measures. This was followed by the Student-Newman-Keuls procedure, nonparametric form, for evaluating all pairwise comparisons of the mean $AUC_{0-10 \text{ hr}}$ values for the dosage groups. The peak thiamine concentration ($C_{max}$) and the time to peak thiamine concentration ($T_{max}$) were also calculated. Finally, half-life ($t_{1\backslash2}$) values were calculated where the terminal phase appeared log-linear.

The relative impact of active and passive absorption were assessed by comparing the $AUC_{0-10 \text{ hr}}$ vs dose for 0 mg to 100 mg, 100 mg to 500 mg, and 500 mg to 1500 mg doses using multilevel mixed-effects linear regression. This was then repeated for $C_{max}$ vs dose.

The data from the placebo trials was used to calculate the coefficient of variation for both the plasma and whole blood assays using the logarithmic method. The coefficient of variation for plasma was 0.15 and the coefficient of variation for whole blood was 0.11.

Stata statistical software version 11 was used for all calculations.

## Results

Fourteen subjects consented to be in the study. Of these, 2 dropped out because of poor venous access during the 1st trial and their data are not included in this analysis. Table 1 lists the demographics of the subjects. Table 2 shows the pharmacokinetic values for the whole blood and plasma thiamine measures.

Figures 1 and 2 show whole blood and plasma thiamine concentrations vs time plots for each thiamine dose. The overall effect of dose was significant (Plasma: ANOVA $p < 0.001$; Whole Blood: ANOVA $p < 0.001$). Additionally, the mean $AUC_{0-10 \; hr}$ for each dose was also significantly different from the others (Student-Newman-Keuls procedure, $p < 0.05$).

Figures 3 and 4 show semi-log plots of the terminal phase of thiamine concentration vs time plots for each thiamine dose for whole blood and plasma. The plots suggest that the terminal phase of thiamine concentration vs time for the 1500 mg dose (whole blood) as well as the 500 mg and 1500 mg doses (plasma) are log-linear. The half-life was calculated for these doses: $4.78 \pm 2.02$ hrs (1500 mg, whole blood), $3.92 \pm 2.24$ hrs (500 mg, plasma), and $2.97 \pm 1.05$ hrs (1500 mg, plasma).

## Table 1 Demographics

| | |
|---|---|
| Age (years) | 29 (10) |
| Weight (kg) | 87 (20) |
| Gender | |
| Female | 64% |
| Male | 36% |
| Race | |
| White | 79% |
| Black | 21% |
| Ethnicity | |
| Hispanic | 36% |
| Non-Hispanic | 64% |
| Hemoglobin (g/dL) | 15 (4) |
| Sodium (mmol/L) | 139 (2) |
| Potassium (mmol/L) | 4.1 (0.3) |
| Chloride (mmol/L) | 102 (2) |
| Bicarbonate (mmol/L) | 27 (2) |
| Glucose (mg/dL) | 92 (9) |
| BUN (mg/dL) | 13 (3) |
| Creatinine (mg/dL) | 0.8 (0.2) |

values are either mean (SD) or percentages

## Table 2 Pharmacokinetic Values

| PARAMETER | THIAMINE DOSE | | |
|---|---|---|---|
| | 100 mg | 500 mg | 1500 mg |
| $AUC_{0-10 \; hr}$ (nmol/Liter × hours) | | | |
| whole blood | 214 ± 69 | 623 ± 178 | 2046 ± 1222 |
| plasma | 177 ± 62 | 612 ± 257 | 2059 ± 1415 |
| $C_{max}$ (nmol/Liter) | | | |
| whole blood | 40 ± 11 | 95 ± 27 | 385 ± 188 |
| plasma | 39 ± 13 | 113 ± 42 | 397 ± 250 |
| $T_{max}$ (hours) | | | |
| whole blood | 3.43 ± 1.69 | 4.14 ± 1.57 | 4.14 ± 0.90 |
| plasma | 3.14 ± 1.05 | 3.18 ± 0.98 | 4.27 ± 1.01 |

All values are presented as mean ± standard deviation. $p < 0.05$ for all pairwise comparisons (plasma and whole blood values were analyzed separately)

Figures 5 and 6 show the $AUC_{0-10 \; hr}$ vs thiamine dose plots for whole blood and plasma. Figures 7 and 8 show the $C_{max}$ vs thiamine dose plots for whole blood and plasma. These plots suggest that the slope is steepest between 0 mg and 100 mg doses of thiamine. This was then tested in separate multilevel mixed effects models and the results are shown in Table 3. The steepest slope is between 0 mg and 100 mg suggesting that while active and passive transport probably occur at all doses, active and transport is more dominant at lower thiamine doses compared to higher thiamine doses. The lack of reaching statistical significance comparing the 0 mg - 100 mg to the 500 mg - 1500 mg segment should be interpreted cautiously because of the small sample size of this study.

## Discussion

The mechanism of how thiamine is absorbed has been somewhat controversial. One group of researchers concluded that thiamine is only absorbed by a saturable active transport mechanism in the proximal small intestine; however other researchers have shown that thiamine is also absorbed by a passive process [13]. Several studies by Thomson demonstrated that a maximum amount between 4.8 and 8.3 mg of thiamine could be absorbed by a single oral dose of thiamine hydrochloride. In these studies, subjects were given a single dose oral thiamine between 1 and 20 mg [9-11]. In another study, Morrison, found that very little thiamine was excreted in urine when doses above 2.5 mg were given orally [14]. This saturable active transport mechanism has been attributed to two carriers, thiamine transporter-1 and thiamine transporter-2.

Using a study design where thiamine was infused directly into the lumen of the small intestine, Hoyumpa demonstrated that thiamine was absorbed by an active process at low concentrations (0.2 to 2.0 μM) and by a

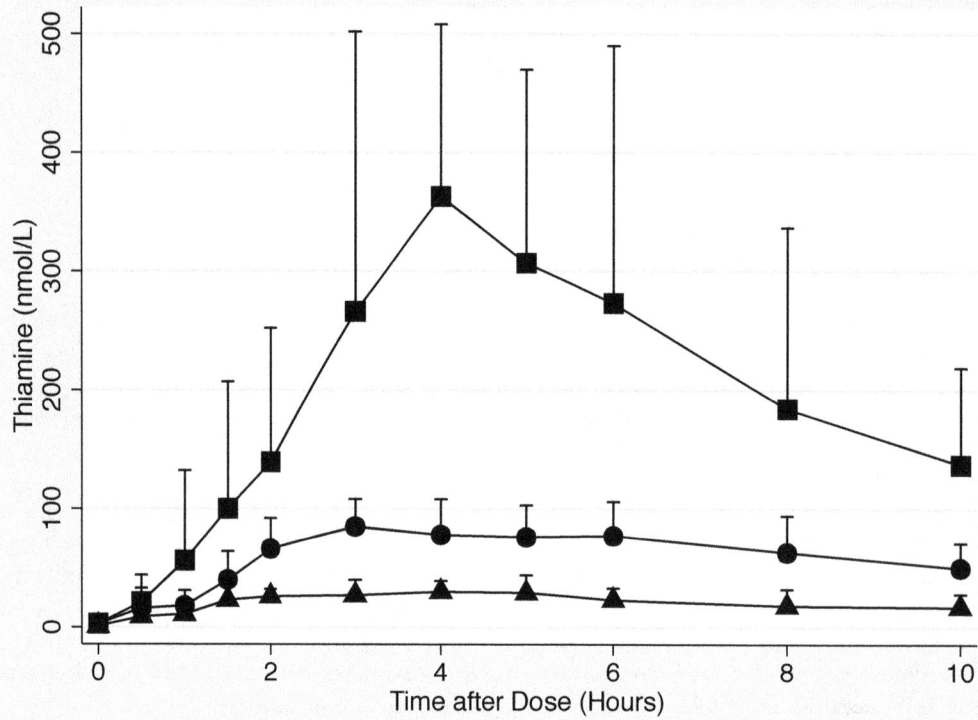

**Figure 1 Oral Thiamine Whole Blood Concentration vs Time Plot**. The concentration of thiamine in plasma from 0 hour to 10 hours after 100 mg (♦), 500 mg (●) and 1500 mg (■) of oral thiamine. Error bars are standard deviations.

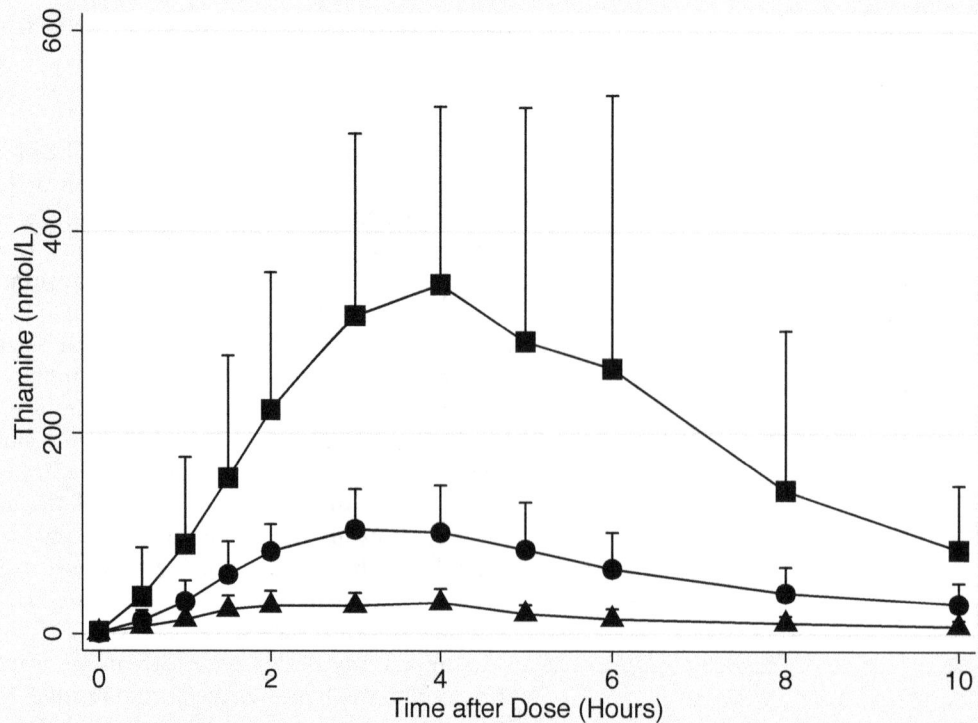

**Figure 2 Oral Thiamine Plasma Concentration vs Time Plot**. The concentration of thiamine in whole blood from 0 hour to 10 hours after 100 mg (♦), 500 mg (●) and 1500 mg (■) of oral thiamine. Error bars are standard deviations.

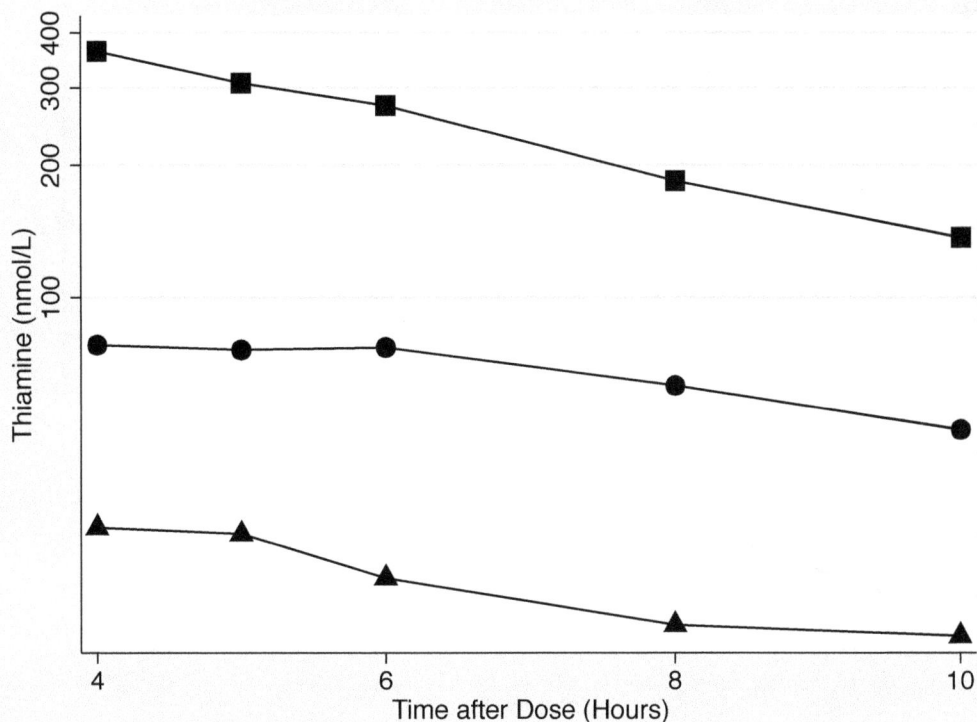

**Figure 3 Semi-log Plot of the Terminal Phase of Oral Thiamine Whole Blood Concentration vs Time**. The concentration of thiamine in whole blood from 4 hour to 10 hours after 100 mg (♦), 500 mg (●) and 1500 mg (■) of oral thiamine.

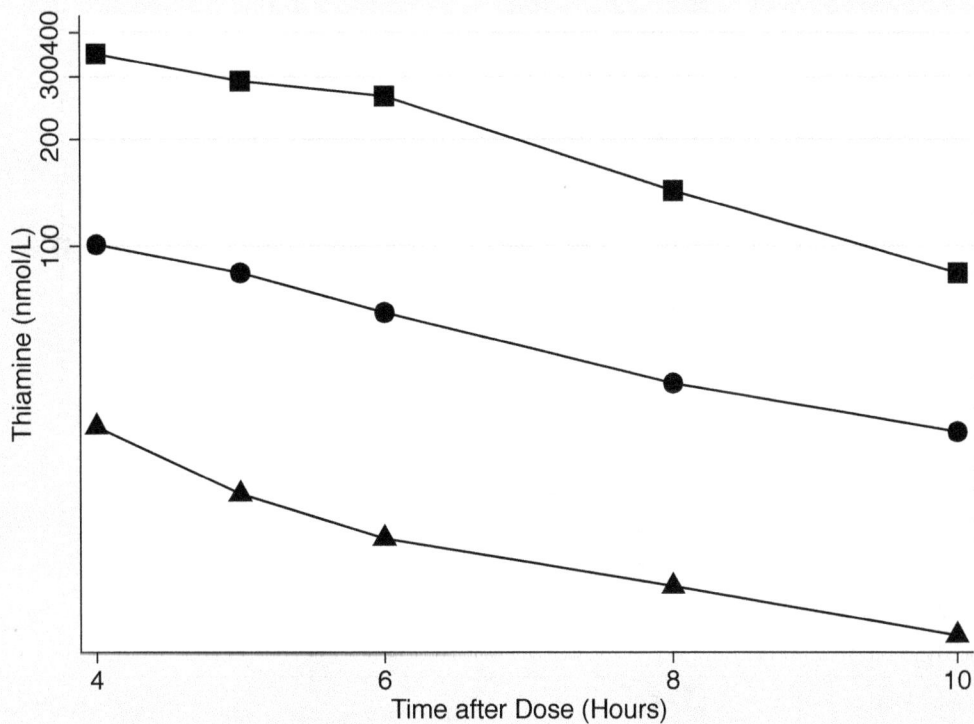

**Figure 4 Semi-log Plot of the Terminal Phase of Oral Thiamine Plasma Concentration vs Time**. The concentration of thiamine in plasma from 4 hour to 10 hours after 100 mg (♦), 500 mg (●) and 1500 mg (■) of oral thiamine.

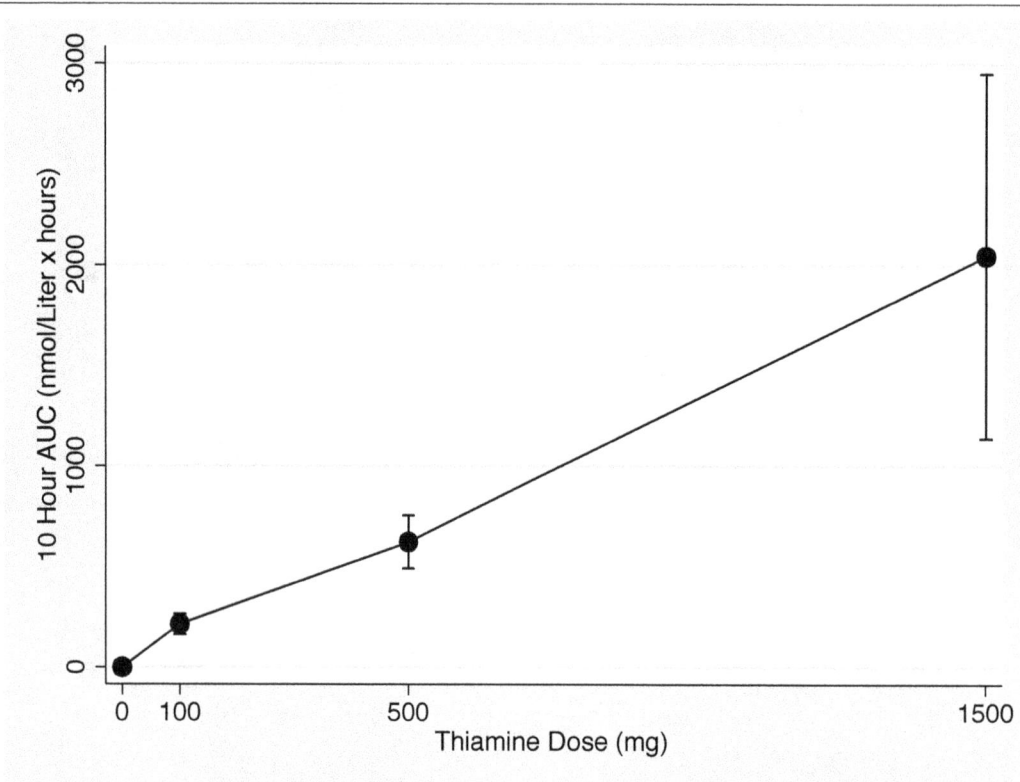

**Figure 5 Whole Blood 0 to 10 Hour AUC vs Thiamine Dose Plot**. The mean area under the curve values for whole blood thiamine measures from time 0 hour to time 10 hours vs thiamine dose after 0 mg, 100 mg, 500 mg and 1500 mg of oral thiamine. Error bars are 95% confidence intervals.

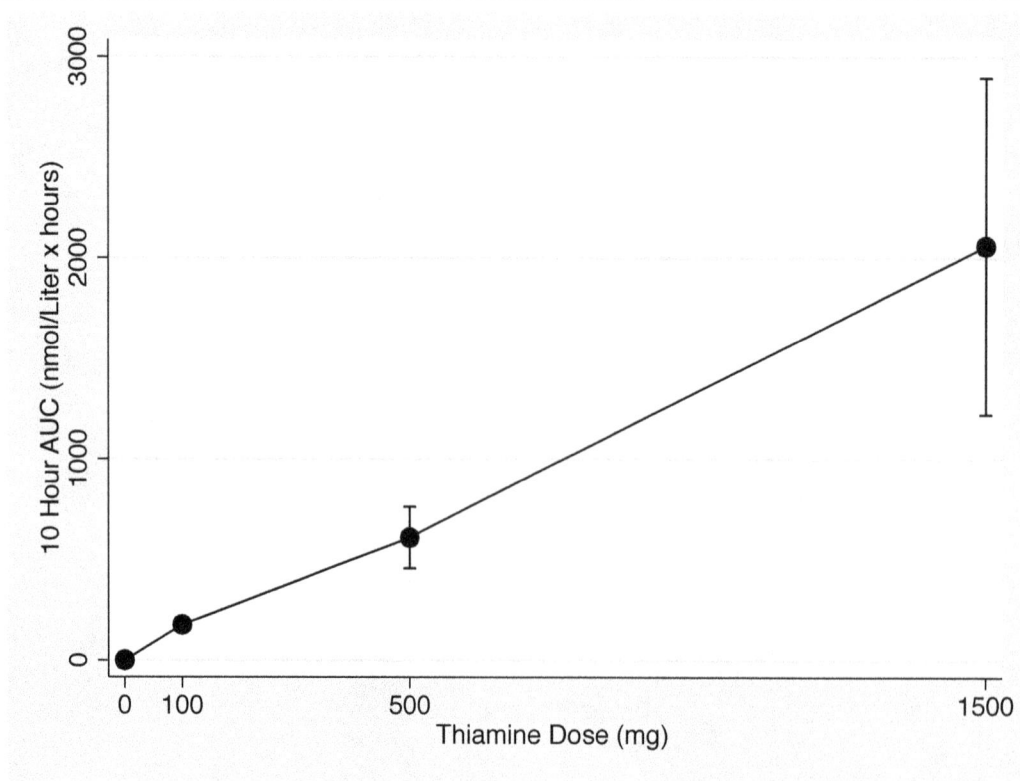

**Figure 6 Plasma 0 to 10 Hour AUC vs Thiamine Dose Plot**. The mean area under the curve values for plasma thiamine measures from time 0 hour to time 10 hours vs thiamine dose after 0 mg, 100 mg, 500 mg and 1500 mg of oral thiamine. Error bars are 95% confidence intervals.

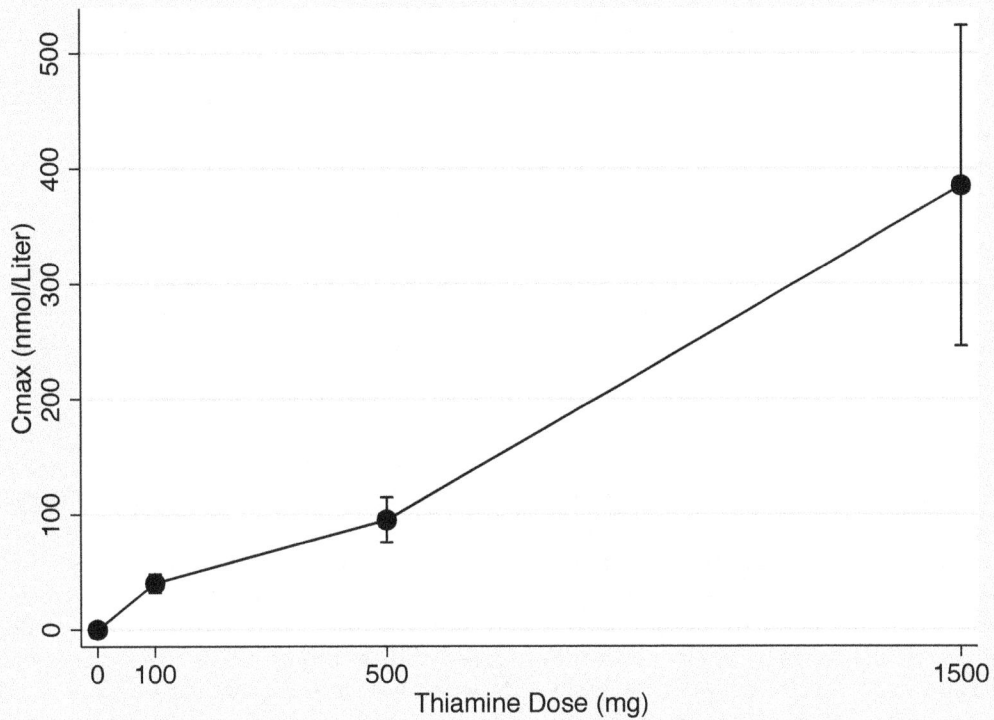

**Figure 7 Whole Blood C$_{max}$ vs Thiamine Dose Plot**. The mean maximum whole blood thiamine concentration between time 0 hour and time 10 hours vs thiamine dose after 0 mg, 100 mg, 500 mg and 1500 mg of oral thiamine. Error bars are 95% confidence intervals.

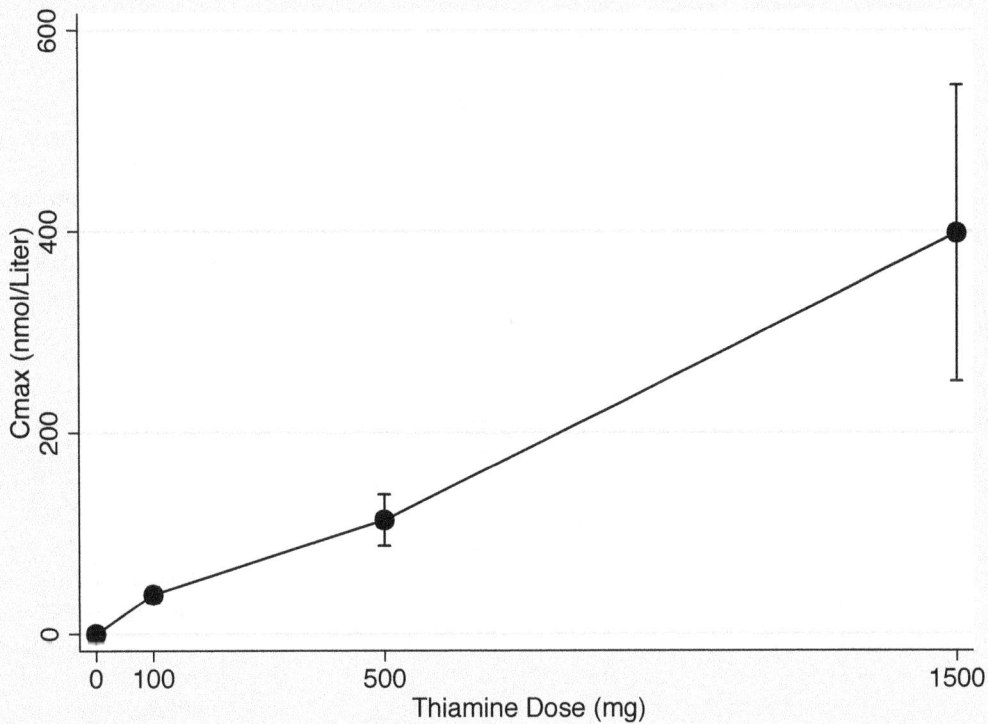

**Figure 8 Plasma C$_{max}$ vs Thiamine Dose Plot**. The mean maximum whole blood thiamine concentration between time 0 hour and time 10 hours vs thiamine dose after 0 mg, 100 mg, 500 mg and 1500 mg of oral thiamine. Error bars are 95% confidence intervals.

**Table 3 Comparison of Slopes for 0 to 10 Hour AUC vs Thiamine Dose**

| Segment | AUC$_{0-10\ hr}$ | | C$_{max}$ | |
|---|---|---|---|---|
| | Slope | *p*-value* | Slope | *p*-value* |
| 0 to 100 mg | | | | |
|    whole blood | 2.14 | | 0.40 | |
|    plasma | 1.76 | | 0.39 | |
| 100 mg to 500 mg | | | | |
|    whole blood | 1.02 | < 0.01 | 0.14 | < 0.01 |
|    plasma | 1.09 | 0.06 | 0.18 | < 0.01 |
| 500 mg to 1500 mg | | | | |
|    whole blood | 1.42 | 0.06 | 0.29 | 0.03 |
|    plasma | 1.45 | 0.40 | 0.29 | 0.08 |

*Compared to the 0 to 100 mg segment

passive process at higher concentrations (5.0 to 50.0 µM) [15-18]. This was also found in an in vitro study [19]. Thomson found a linear relationship between urinary excretion and oral dose of thiamine between 10 and 50 mg [20]. This is further supported by Weber who gave a single dose of oral thiamine to 3 subjects (50, 100, or 200 mg) and found that the subject given the largest oral dose also had the highest plasma thiamine levels [21]. Although, the design of this study and its small sample size limits any conclusions.

Studies to determine the optimal dosing of thiamine for various conditions have not been performed and dosing recommendations appear to be based on limited data. Thiamine deficiency syndromes are typically initially treated with intravenous thiamine between 100 mg once a day and 500 mg three times a day [22,23]. Oral dosing of thiamine up to 100 mg/kg divided three times a day have been reported to be required to treat children with genetic abnormalities of pyruvate dehydrogenase. Children with these abnormalities who were not improved by taking thiamine, may have been treated with an inadequate dosage [24]. In studies of Alzheimer's disease, subjects were treated with 1000 mg of oral thiamine hydrochloride three times a day for 2 to 12 months without any reports of adverse effects [7,25,26]. In a separate experiment, subjects were titrated up to 8000 mg per day over a 1-year period. The only side effects reported were nausea and indigestion in 2 subjects when they reached 7000 and 7500 mg per day [7]. There have been several clinical trials of thiamine derivatives for a variety of disorders that used doses between 300 and 900 mg per day in divided doses for periods up to 3 months. No side effects were reported in these studies [2,27-29].

Alternate forms of oral thiamine (S-acyl thiamine derivatives and lipid-soluble thiamine disulfide derivatives) have been developed because they have a much higher bioavailability than thiamine hydrochloride [12].

Thiamine hydrochloride has been estimated to have a bioavailability between 3.7% and 5.3% [21,30]. However, it is not clear that these thiamine derivatives are needed. First, tissue uptake is highly variable across different tissues and different derivatives [12]. Second, oral thiamine hydrochloride when given over a 1-week period produce blood levels that approach those obtained by intramuscular and intravenous administration [31,32]. Finally, in vitro studies that have compared thiamine to thiamine derivatives have generally found them to have similar effects [33-38]. In studies where a thiamine derivative was thought to be superior to thiamine hydrochloride, the difference could be completely explained by differences in bioavailability [39-41].

This study has demonstrated that the absorption mechanism is not saturable up to 1500 mg. Our results are consistent with a combination of passive and active transport. The active transport plays a larger role in thiamine absorption at lower doses compared to higher doses. These results contradict the results found by Thomson but is consistent with the animal studies done by Hoyumpa. The constant difference between plasma and whole blood thiamine levels is consistent with a rapid equilibrium between red blood cells and plasma.

This study was limited in that we did not measure tissue levels of thiamine nor did we measure biological effects of high dose oral thiamine hydrochloride. Additionally, while no side effects were reported, this study was not designed to detect adverse events. Our calculation of the coefficient of variation has additional limitations. It includes error related to the analytic method in addition to error related to biologic variation as well as all of the steps between obtaining the blood and its preparation prior to analysis. A greater understanding of the absorption process could have determined if we studied a larger number of thiamine doses and followed the subjects for a longer period of time.

## Conclusions

In conclusion, our study demonstrates that high blood levels of thiamine can be achieved rapidly with oral thiamine hydrochloride. Thiamine is absorbed by both an active and unsaturable passive transport mechanism up to 1500 mg.

### Acknowledgements

I'd like to acknowledge Richard Barus, Fidela S. J. Blank, Ryan Coute, Jerold S. Harmatz, Sarah J. Parent, Jennifer Stetkiewicz, and Paul Visintainer for their help with this study.
Funding
Society for Academic Emergency Medicine Scholarly Sabbatical Grant

### Author details

[1]Department of Emergency Medicine, Tufts University School of Medicine and Baystate Medical Center, Springfield, MA, USA. [2]Department of Emergency Medicine, Harvard University School of Medicine and Beth Israel Deaconess Medical Center, Boston, MA, USA. [3]Program in Pharmacology and Experimental Therapeutics, Tufts University School of Medicine and Tufts Medical Center, Boston, MA, USA. [4]Baystate Medical Center, 759 Chestnut Street, Springfield, MA 01199, USA.

### Authors' contributions

HAS made substantial contributions to conception and design, acquisition of data, analysis and interpretation of data, drafting the manuscript. MD made substantial contributions to analysis and interpretation of data and revised the manuscript critically for important intellectual content. DJG made substantial contributions to conception and design, analysis and interpretation of data, and revised the manuscript critically for important intellectual content. All authors read and approved the final manuscript.

### Competing interests

The authors declare that they have no competing interests.

### References

1. Young RC, Blass JP: **Iatrogenic nutritional deficiencies.** *Annu Rev Nutr* 1982, **2**:201-227.
2. Balakumar P, Rohilla A, Krishan P, Solairaj P, Thangathirupathi A: **The multifaceted therapeutic potential of benfotiamine.** *Pharmacol Res* 2010, **61**:482-488.
3. Donnino M, Carney E, Cocchi M, Barbash I: **Thiamine deficiency in critically ill patients with sepsis.** *J Crit Care* 2010, **25**:576-581.
4. Donnino MW, Cocchi MN, Smithline H, Carney E, Chou PP, Salciccioli J: **Coronary artery bypass graft surgery depletes plasma thiamine levels.** *Nutrition* 2010, **26**:133-136.
5. Soukoulis V, Dihu JB, Sole M, Anker SD, Cleland J, Fonarow GC, Metra M, Pasini E, Strzelczyk T, Taegtmeyer H, Gheorghiade M: **Micronutrient deficiencies an unmet need in heart failure.** *J Am Coll Cardiol* 2009, **54**:1660-1673.
6. Hartung E, Freye E: **The effect of thiamine on the contractile responses of the isolated heart muscle.** *Acta Vitaminol Enzymol* 1980, **2**:3-5.
7. Meador K, Loring D, Nichols M, Zamrini E, Rivner M, Posas H, Thompson E, Moore E: **Preliminary findings of high-dose thiamine in dementia of Alzheimer's type.** *J Geriatr Psychiatry Neurol* 1993, **6**:222-229.
8. Wolfson SK, Ellis S: **Thiamine: toxicity and ganglionic blockade.** *Fed Proc* 1954, **13**:418.
9. Thomson AD, Baker H, Leevy CM: **Patterns of 35S-thiamine hydrochloride absorption in the malnourished alcoholic patient.** *J Lab Clin Med* 1970, **76**:34 45.
10. Thomson AD: **Mechanisms of vitamin deficiency in chronic alcohol misusers and the development of the Wernicke-Korsakoff syndrome.** *Alcohol Alcohol Suppl* 2000, **35**:2-7.
11. Thomson AD, Leevy CM: **Observations on the mechanism of thiamine hydrochloride absorption in man.** *Clin Sci* 1972, **43**:153-163.
12. Volvert ML, Seyen S, Piette M, Evrard B, Gangolf M, Plumier JC, Bettendorff L: **Benfotiamine, a synthetic S-acyl thiamine derivative, has different mechanisms of action and a different pharmacological profile than lipid-soluble thiamine disulfide derivatives.** *BMC Pharmacol* 2008, **8**:10.
13. Davis R, Icke G: **Clinical chemistry of thiamin.** In *Advances in Clinical Chemistry* Edited by: Elsevier 1983, **23**:93-140.
14. Morrison AB, Campbell JA: **Vitamin absorption studies. I. Factors influencing the excretion of oral test doses of thiamine and riboflavin by human subjects.** *J Nutr* 1960, **72**:435-440.
15. Hoyumpa AM, Breen KJ, Schenker S, Wilson FA: **Thiamine transport across the rat intestine. II. Effect of ethanol.** *J Lab Clin Med* 1975, **86**:803-816.
16. Hoyumpa AM, Strickland R, Sheehan JJ, Yarborough G, Nichols S: **Dual system of intestinal thiamine transport in humans.** *J Lab Clin Med* 1982, **99**:701-708.
17. Hoyumpa AM, Middleton HM, Wilson FA, Schenker S: **Thiamine transport across the rat intestine. I. Normal characteristics.** *Gastroenterol* 1975, **68**:1218-1227.
18. Hoyumpa AM: **Characterization of normal intestinal thiamin transport in animals and man.** *Ann NY Acad Sci* 1982, **378**:337-343.
19. Zielinska-Dawidziak M, Grajek K, Olejnik A, Czaczyk K, Grajek W: **Transport of high concentration of thiamin, riboflavin and pyridoxine across intestinal epithelial cells Caco-2.** *J Nutr Sci Vitaminol* 2008, **54**:423-429.
20. Thomson AD, Frank O, Baker H, Leevy CM: **Thiamine propyl disulfide: absorption and utilization.** *Ann Intern Med* 1971, **74**:529-534.
21. Weber W, Kewitz H: **Determination of thiamine in human plasma and its pharmacokinetics.** *Eur J Clin Pharmacol* 1985, **28**:213-219.
22. Thomson AD: **The Royal College of Physicians report on alcohol: guidelines for managing Wernicke's Encephalopathy in the accident and emergency department.** *Alcohol Alcohol* 2002, **37**:513-521.
23. Wrenn KD, Murphy F, Slovis CM: **A toxicity study of parenteral thiamine hydrochloride.** *Ann Emerg Med* 1989, **18**:867-870.
24. Barnerias C, Saudubray JM, Touati G, De Lonlay P, Dulac O, Ponsot G, Marsac C, Brivet M, Desguerre I: **Pyruvate dehydrogenase complex deficiency: four neurological phenotypes with differing pathogenesis.** *Dev Med Child Neurol* 2010, **52**:e1-e9.
25. Blass JP, Gleason P, Brush D, DiPonte P, Thaler H: **Thiamine and Alzheimer's disease. A pilot study.** *Arch Neurol* 1988, **45**:833-835.
26. Nolan KA, Black RS, Sheu KF, Langberg J, Blass JP: **A trial of thiamine in Alzheimer's disease.** *Arch Neurol* 1991, **48**:81-83.
27. Alkhalaf A, Klooster A, van Oeveren W, Achenbach U, Kleefstra N, Slingerland RJ, Mijnhout GS, Bilo HJ, Gans RO, Navis GJ, Bakker SJ: **A double-blind, randomized, placebo-controlled clinical trial on benfotiamine treatment in patients with diabetic nephropathy.** *Diabetes Care* 2010, **33**:1598-1601.
28. Stracke H, Gaus W, Achenbach U, Federlin K, Bretzel RG: **Benfotiamine in diabetic polyneuropathy (BENDIP): results of a randomised, double blind, placebo-controlled clinical study.** *Exp Clin Endocrinol Diabetes* 2008, **116**:600-605.
29. Thornalley PJ: **The potential role of thiamine (vitamin B1) in diabetic complications.** *Curr Diabetes Rev* 2005, **1**:287-298.
30. Tallaksen CME, Sande A: B?hmer T, Bell H, Karlsen J: **Kinetics of thiamin and thiamin phosphate esters in human blood, plasma and urine after 50 mg intravenously or orally.** *Eur J Clin Pharmacol* 1993, **44**:73-78.
31. Baines M, Bligh JG, Madden JS: **Tissue thiamin levels of hospitalised alcoholics before and after oral or parenteral vitamins.** *Alcohol Alcohol* 1988, **23**:49-52.
32. Royer-Morrot MJ, Zhiri A, Paille F, Royer RJ: **Plasma thiamine concentrations after intramuscular and oral multiple dosage regimens in healthy men.** *Eur J Clin Pharmacol* 1992, **42**:219-222.
33. Babaei-Jadidi R, Karachalias N, Ahmed N, Battah S, Thornalley PJ: **Prevention of incipient diabetic nephropathy by high-dose thiamine and benfotiamine.** *Diabetes* 2003, **52**:2110-2120.
34. Beltramo E, Berrone E, Buttiglieri S, Porta M: **Thiamine and benfotiamine prevent increased apoptosis in endothelial cells and pericytes cultured in high glucose.** *Diabetes Metab Res Rev* 2004, **20**:330-336.
35. Beltramo E, Nizheradze K, Berrone E, Tarallo S, Porta M: **Thiamine and benfotiamine prevent apoptosis induced by high glucose-conditioned extracellular matrix in human retinal pericytes.** *Diabetes Metab Res Rev* 2009, **25**:647-656.

36.  Berrone E, Beltramo E, Solimine C, Ape AU, Porta M: **Regulation of intracellular glucose and polyol pathway by thiamine and benfotiamine in vascular cells cultured in high glucose.** *J Biol Chem* 2006, **281**:9307-9313.

37.  Karachalias N, Babaei-Jadidi R, Kupich C, Ahmed N, Thornalley PJ: **High-dose thiamine therapy counters dyslipidemia and advanced glycation of plasma protein in streptozotocin-induced diabetic rats.** *Ann N Y Acad Sci* 2005, **1043**:777-783.

38.  Karachalias N, Babaei-Jadidi R, Rabbani N, Thornalley PJ: **Increased protein damage in renal glomeruli, retina, nerve, plasma and urine and its prevention by thiamine and benfotiamine therapy in a rat model of diabetes.** *Diabetologia* 2010, **53**:1506-1516.

39.  Frank T, Bitsch R, Maiwald J, Stein G: **High thiamine diphosphate concentrations in erythrocytes can be achieved in dialysis patients by oral administration of benfotiamine.** *Eur J Clin Pharmacol* 2000, **56**:251-257.

40.  Greb A, Bitsch R: **Comparative bioavailability of various thiamine derivatives after oral administration.** *Int J Clin Pharmacol Ther* 1998, **36**:216-221.

41.  Stracke H, Hammes HP, Werkmann D, Mavrakis K, Bitsch I, Netzel M, Geyer J, Kopcke W, Sauerland C, Bretzel RG, Federlin KF: **Efficacy of benfotiamine versus thiamine on function and glycation products of peripheral nerves in diabetic rats.** *Exp Clin Endocrinol Diabetes* 2001, **109**:330-336.

# What can we learn from consumer reports on psychiatric adverse drug reactions with antidepressant medication? Experiences from reports to a consumer association

Andreas Vilhelmsson[1*], Tommy Svensson[2], Anna Meeuwisse[3] and Anders Carlsten[4]

## Abstract

**Background:** According to the World Health Organization (WHO) the cost of adverse drug reactions (ADRs) in the general population is high and under-reporting by health professionals is a well-recognized problem. Another way to increase ADR reporting is to let the consumers themselves report directly to the authorities. In Sweden it is mandatory for prescribers to report serious ADRs to the Medical Products Agency (MPA), but there are no such regulations for consumers. The non-profit and independent organization Consumer Association for Medicines and Health, KILEN has launched the possibility for consumers to report their perceptions and experiences from their use of medicines in order to strengthen consumer rights within the health care sector. This study aimed to analyze these consumer reports.

**Methods:** All reports submitted from January 2002 to April 2009 to an open web site in Sweden where anyone could report their experience with the use of pharmaceuticals were analyzed with focus on common psychiatric side effects related to antidepressant usage. More than one ADR for a specific drug could be reported.

**Results:** In total 665 reports were made during the period. 442 reports concerned antidepressant medications and the individual antidepressant reports represented 2392 ADRs and 878 (37%) of these were psychiatric ADRs. 75% of the individual reports concerned serotonin-reuptake inhibitor (SSRI) and the rest serotonin-norepinephrine reuptake inhibitor (SNRI). Women reported more antidepressant psychiatric ADRs (71%) compared to men (24%). More potentially serious psychiatric ADRs were frequently reported to KILEN and withdrawal symptoms during discontinuation were also reported as a common issue.

**Conclusions:** The present study indicates that consumer reports may contribute with important information regarding more serious psychiatric ADRs following antidepressant treatment. Consumer reporting may be considered a complement to traditional ADR reporting.

## Background

The World Health Organization (WHO) argues that the cost of adverse drug reactions (ADRs) in the general population (in developed countries) is high [1]. Pharmacoeconomic studies from 1997 and 1998 have estimated that ADRs may lead to an additional $1.56 to $4 billion in direct hospital costs per year in the United States [2-4]. These estimations are however uncertain and in most countries the extent of this expenditure has not been measured. The reporting of potential ADRs by healthcare professionals is supported by WHO and their Drug Monitoring Programme [5], and under-reporting by health professionals is a well-recognized problem by the WHO [6]. Another way to increase ADR reporting could be to let the consumers themselves report directly to the authorities.

One important step towards consumer reporting of ADRs was recently taken by the European Parliament,

* Correspondence: andreas.vilhelmsson@nhv.se
[1]Nordic School of Public Health (NHV), Box 121 33, SE-402 42 Gothenburg, Sweden
Full list of author information is available at the end of the article

who in September 2010 voted in favor for a new pharmacovigilance legislation to ensure greater patient safety and to improve public health [7,8]. This was later cleared by the European Council in December 2010 [9]. The new legislation came into force on 1 January 2011 but will not apply until July 2012 [7,9]. Member States will then have to adopt these changes in order to harmonize national adverse event systems, and one important change to the current law foresees the inclusion of direct patient reporting (DPR) of adverse events [10]. Some mean that this will mark the beginning of a new chapter in drug safety [11]. The WHO acknowledges that it is not always easy to recognize ADRs (which may act through the same physiological and pathological pathways as different diseases) and proposes a step-wise procedure to assessing possible drug-related ADRs [6]. Therefore, the organization proclaims consumer reporting to be of great importance in order to safeguard a pharmacovigilance that will help each patient to receive optimum therapy, and on a population basis will lead to ensure the acceptance and effectiveness of public health programmes [12].

Consumers in both the Netherlands and Denmark have had the possibility to report ADRs to their authorities since 2003. Different studies have shown that ADRs reported by patients has the potential to increase knowledge about the possible harm of medicines [10]. A Danish study of reports to the Danish Medicines Agency (DKMA) showed for instance that patients are more likely to report ADRs from the nervous and psychiatric system than are health professionals [13]. A Dutch study indicated that patients seem to report different experiences compared to healthcare professionals regarding ADRs from antidepressants [14], and that patients now take great interest in their drug use and often search for more information about their own medication and often focus on ADRs [15]. Withdrawal symptoms are according to an English study described in a clearer way by consumer reports compared to how it was done by the National drug regulatory agencies [16]. However, very few studies have compared 'real life' reports made by patients and health professionals about antidepressants [10,14,16,17]. Previous research in the Netherlands and in Denmark has also suggested that consumer experiences should be included in the evaluation of antidepressant treatment in clinical practice [14], and in systematic drug surveillance systems [13].

In the Nordic countries sales of antidepressants has increased up to four fold since the middle of the nineties [1], and the sales has now stabilized [18] (Table 1). In Sweden in 2010 approximately 8.1% of the population did purchase an antidepressant drug and more than five million prescriptions of antidepressants were dispensed to almost 760 000 patients (66% were women) [19]. In

**Table 1 Sales of antidepressants (N06A) in the Nordic Countries during 1995-2008 in DDD*/1000 inhabitants per day [1,35]**

|  | Denmark | Finland | Iceland | Norway | Sweden |
|---|---|---|---|---|---|
| 1995 | 18.3 | 20.3 | 33.0 | 22.5 | 27.8 |
| 2000 | 34.7 | 35.5 | 70.5 | 41.0 | 48.8 |
| 2004 | 55.2 | 49.9 | 91.9 | 52.4 | 64.6 |
| 2005 | 59.9 | 52.1 | 94.8 | 51.8 | 66.1 |
| 2006 | 64.7 | 55.5 | 92.6 | 52.7 | 69.7 |
| 2007 | 69.9 | 61.1 | 95.4 | 54.8 | 72.1 |
| 2008 | 73.4 | 63.9 | 94.7 | 55.1 | 73.7 |

* Defined Daily Doses according to WHO classification

2009 the estimated sales for antidepressants in Sweden were almost 70 million Euros [20]. Increased use may be followed by a higher incidence of adverse drug reactions (ADRs) and pharmacovigilance is therefore considered important aiming to make the best use of medicines for the treatment or prevention of disease [12]. In a societal perspective increased knowledge of this kind is of great importance. In Sweden drug-related problem may account for as much as 12% of hospital admissions [21] and the medical burden of fatal ADRs is estimated to occur in 3% of all deaths [22]. Antidepressants drugs are commonly implicated in FADRs [23].

In Sweden it is mandatory for prescribers to report potential serious ADRs to the Medical Products Agency (MPA) [24]. There are however no such regulations for consumers. Despite the possibility for consumers to report potential ADRs to the MPA the number of incoming reports is quite few. The information about how patients perceive their treatment with antidepressants and their perception of ADRs is scarce. The non-profit and independent organization Consumer Association for Medicines and Health, KILEN has launched the possibility for consumers to report their perceptions and experiences from their use of medicines in order to strengthen consumer rights within the health care sector. KILEN established a consumer database already in 1997 to collect consumer reports mainly focusing on benzodiazepines and antidepressants. KILEN was created in 1992 but their co-workers had already a long history of working with pharmaceutical drug dependency when it in the 1960s became clear that the new benzodiazepines were causing dependency and harm. Since 2002 it has also been possible to report experiences with medicines to KILEN through a web based report form (http://www.kilen.org). These reports have not yet been scrutinized and analyzed. Hence, this study aimed to analyze these consumer reports.

## Methods

All reports submitted from January 2002 to April 2009 to KILEN's internet-based reporting system in Sweden were analyzed. Main focus in the study was common ADRs related to antidepressant usage. According to WHO an ADR is defined as a response to a medicine which is noxious and unintended, and which occurs at doses normally used in man whilst an adverse event or experience is defined as any untoward medical occurrence that may present during treatment with a medicine but which does not necessarily have a causal relationship with this treatment [6].

A report in the KILEN material was defined as one individual's reported experience with a drug and an ADR was equal to one single reported effect connected to a specific drug. The report form items included user information (age, sex, location and condition of health), the story about the treatment (medical history, drugs, doses and reactions). It was also possible to give a longer description of the experience as free text. In this study we chose to analyze age, sex, drug reported and ADRs. More than ADR related to the same drug could be submitted. The reported ADRs to KILEN were compiled and coded in a similar way to those listed in the Swedish Physicians' Desk Reference, FASS. FASS is building on the Summary of Product Characteristics (SPC) from the pharmaceutical companies. KILEN personnel using the database software FileMaker did this coding.

The drugs in reports were coded according to therapeutic groups [Anatomical Therapeutic Chemical (ATC) system] [25] and types of reported ADRs (system organ classes) [26]. The ATC Classification with Defined Daily Doses (ATC/DDD) system classifies therapeutic drugs and the purpose of the system is to serve as a tool for drug utilization research in order to improve quality of drug use [25]. In the ATC classification system, the drugs are divided into different groups according to the organ or system on which they act and their chemical, pharmacological and therapeutic properties [25]. This system is also valid for the Swedish Physicians' Desk Reference, FASS. The ADRs in FASS are classified according to MedDRA system organ class where reactions are reported corresponding to their frequency (Very common = >10%, Common = 1-10%, Less common = 0.1-1%, Rare = 0.01-0.1%, Very rare = <0.01%, Unknown frequency). Data submitted to KILEN are not handled to the regulatory authorities like the MPA. The project was approved by the ethics board in Gothenburg, Sweden (No. 319-10).

## Results

In total 665 individuals submitted reports on ADRs to a specific drug and 469 of these concerned antidepressants. Fifteen different antidepressant drugs were reported but for eight of these antidepressants too little information (≤10 individual reports) was available. The

442 individual antidepressant reports included in the study represented 2392 ADRs and of these were 878 psychiatric ADRs (37%) (Table 2). 75% of the individual reports concerned serotonin-reuptake inhibitor (SSRI) and 25% a serotonin-norepinephrine reuptake inhibitor (SNRI). The most reported antidepressants to KILEN were: Sertraline (26%), Citalopram (24%), Venlafaxine (18%), Paroxetine (13%), Mirtazapine (8%) Fluoxetine (6%), and Escitalopram (5%). Sertraline and Citalopram were the most common antidepressants according to both reports (116 and 107), total ADRs (626 and 570) and psychiatric ADRs (226 and 226) (Table 2). Women were responsible for 323 of the submitted reports compared to men with 98 reports. 21 individuals did not report their gender and eight individuals did not submit their age. Of the psychiatric ADRs were women responsible for 622 (70.8%) and men 208 (23.7%), whilst 5.5% did not report their gender (Table 3). The distribution of ADRs per report was quite even between women (5.4) and men (5.2). A majority (34.5%) of the antidepressant psychiatric ADRs were reported by consumers within the age group 30-39 years of age (women 26.8% and men 6%) (Table 3). Also age groups 15-29 years of age (23.6%) and 40-49 years of age (22.1%) were common reporting groups. Several reports to KILEN included withdrawal symptoms, where one fourth to one third of psychiatric ADRs were reported during discontinuation (Table 4). Women were responsible for a majority of the reports within the different antidepressants (65.3-82.7%) compared to men (12.2-28.9%) (Table 5). Only Mirtazapine was more evenly reported (52.1 compared to 43.5%).

The most frequently reported psychiatric ADRs to KILEN were anxiety, a sensation of unreality, insomnia, uneasiness/nervousness, irritability, aggressiveness, suicidal behavior, and depression (Table 2). The most common ADR was anxiety (4.2-7.9%). Insomnia was reported for all antidepressants to KILEN (2.3-6.1%). The ADR uneasiness/nervousness was reported for five antidepressants (2.3-2.8%). Experiencing a sensation of unreality was a common ADR in four analyzed antidepressants (2.8-6.2%). Depression was a reported psychiatric ADR in three antidepressants (2.1-3.5%). Irritability, aggressiveness was a reported psychiatric ADR for six antidepressants (2.1-3.5%). Suicidal behavior was a reported psychiatric ADR for all antidepressants in the KILEN material (1.9-3.2).

## Discussion

The KILEN material showed reports of potentially serious psychiatric ADRs. Some psychiatric ADRs were more reported with certain antidepressants but anxiety, insomnia and suicidal behavior were reported for all drugs. But do these consumer reports differ according

**Table 2 Reports and ADRs of antidepressant medication to an open web site according to the system organ class of psychiatric system[1]**

| Antidepressant ATC code N06A | Reports (N) Total = 442 | ADRs (N) Total = 2392 | Psychiatric ADRs (N) Total = 878 | ADRs/report | Most common psychiatric ADR (%) |
|---|---|---|---|---|---|
| Sertraline[a] N06AB06 | 116 | 626 | 226 | 5.4 | Anxiety 5.9 Sensation of unreality 4.0 Insomnia 3.0 Uneasiness/nervousness 2.6 Irritability, aggressiveness 2.2 Suicidal behavior 1.9 |
| Citalopram[a] N06AB04 | 107 | 570 | 226 | 5.3 | Anxiety 7.9 Insomnia 3.7 Sensation of unreality 2.8 Suicidal behavior 2.5 Uneasiness/nervousness 2.5 Depression 2.1 Irritability, aggressiveness 2.1 |
| Venlafaxine[b] N06AX16 | 78 | 505 | 171 | 6.5 | Anxiety 4.2 Suicidal behavior 3.2 Uneasiness/nervousness 2.8 Sensation of unreality 2.8 Insomnia 2.4 |
| Paroxetine[a] N06AB05 | 58 | 327 | 121 | 5.6 | Anxiety 5.2 Irritability, aggressiveness 3.4 Suicidal behavior 3.1 Insomnia 2.3 Depression 2.1 |
| Mirtazapine[b] N06AX11 | 34 | 131 | 46 | 3.9 | Anxiety 6.9 Insomnia 6.1 Irritability, aggressiveness 3.1 Suicidal behavior 2.3 Uneasiness/nervousness 2.3 |
| Fluoxetine[a] N06AB03 | 28 | 120 | 39 | 4.3 | Anxiety 5.0 Irritability, aggressiveness 2.5 Suicidal behavior 2.5 Insomnia 2.5 |
| Escitalopram[a] N06AB10 | 21 | 113 | 49 | 5.4 | Anxiety 7.1 Sensation of unreality 6.2 Insomnia 5.3 Depression 3.5 Irritability, aggressiveness 3.5 Suicidal behavior 2.7 Uneasiness/nervousness 2.7 |

[1]According to ATC classification system, the drugs are divided into different groups according to the organ or system on which they act and their chemical, pharmacological and therapeutic properties.
[a]Selective serotonin reuptake inhibitor (SSRI)
[b]Serotonin-norepinephrine reuptake inhibitor (SNRI)

to information found in the Summary of Product Characteristics (SPC)? If we compare reports to KILEN between the years 2002-2009 with FASS 2004 [27] and FASS 2009 [28] we take in consideration that it often takes years before new ADRs are published in FASS.

FASS is the most used tool for health care professionals in Sweden to use when prescribing drugs and therefore of interest in a comparison with consumer reports. ADR information in FASS is mainly based on information from the pharmaceutical companies and a somewhat

**Table 3 Consumer reported psychiatric ADRs (N = 878) to KILEN according to age and gender (N) and (%)**

| Gender | Age group | | | | | | | | |
| | 15-29 | 30-39 | 40-49 | 50-59 | 60-69 | 70-79 | 80-89 | No age | Total |
|---|---|---|---|---|---|---|---|---|---|
| Female | 150 (17.1) | 235 (26.8) | 151 (17.2) | 42 (4.8) | 17 (1.9) | 10 (1.1) | - | 17 (1.9) | 622 (70.8) |
| Male | 46 (5.2) | 53 (6.0) | 64 (7.3) | 30 (3.4) | 10 (1.1) | - | 3 (0.3) | 2 (0.2) | 208 (23.7) |
| Not given | 9 (1.0) | 16 (1.8) | 14 (1.6) | - | - | - | - | 9 (1.0) | 48 (5.5) |
| Total | 550 (23.6) | 804 (34.5) | 515 (22.1) | 242 (10.4) | 85 (3.6) | 23 (1.0) | | 44 (1.9) | 878 |

good correspondence to the consumers' reports is expected. However, the consumer reports gave another perspective of experiences with antidepressants. The consumer reports to KILEN contained more potentially serious psychiatric ADRs that are not always listed in FASS, especially experiencing a sensation of unreality, irritability, aggressiveness, suicidal thoughts, and depression. Anxiety was the most reported psychiatric ADR to KILEN for all antidepressants but for some substances anxiety is not listed at all in one version of FASS, but listed as common in the other.

This result goes well in accordance with previous research that consumer/patient reporting does add value to professional reports of ADRs by identifying possible new reactions [13,14,29,30]. For instance was a sensation of unreality an important psychiatric ADR among the consumer reports to KILEN, but is not listed at all as an ADR in FASS. Withdrawal symptoms in connection with discontinuation of antidepressants medication was reported to KILEN but is not always mentioned in FASS, and when it is mentioned it is generally regarded as rare [27,28]. This is worth considering since a study by Tint and colleagues (2008) showed that withdrawal symptoms of antidepressants in depressed patients could be associated with worsening depression symptoms and increasing suicidal ideation [31].

Consumer reporting may be one way of picking up harms that are missed in clinical trials, where for instance the KILEN material introduces a common self reported harm in experiencing a sensation of unreality. The new legislation in the EU-countries to stimulate a systematic consumer reporting can therefore be an important step to take, and hopefully will also the newly

established consumer reporting system to the Swedish Medical Product Agency lead to a safer prescription culture. Since the start in 2008 and up until November 2010 the agency has received over 4000 consumer reports, according to the MPA. There is however a major uneven distribution due to the vaccination campaign during the A(H1N1) pandemic in 2009. Research has also shown that educating general practitioners (GPs) to focus on ADRs improved the ADR reporting [32]. This is particularly serious since only five percent of doctors are estimated to participate in any pharmacovigilance system [33]. Educating physicians more in pharmacology or an active involvement of pharmacists when prescribing medication may therefore be one way to minimize ADRs and thereby increase safety. Maybe increased consumer reporting can lead to an increase in ADR reporting from health professionals. Distribution of start packages of antidepressant medication can also be one important aspect in a safer prescription culture and an important step in minimizing ADRs through better follow-up. However, as Danish research suggests, can consumer ADR report might act as whistleblowers of new and previously undetected ADRs, but if the quality of the reports is questionable they may bring too much noise rather than valuable information to the pharmacovigilance systems [34].

Gender is also an important issue to highlight since the sales of antidepressants are almost twice as high among women compared to men in all age groups [35]. Women reported ADRs to KILEN in a much higher degree, between three to four times more often than men, and sometimes more within certain age groups. Especially women 30-39 years of age was a large

**Table 4 Reported antidepressant psychiatric ADRs to KILEN during different stages of treatment**

| Type of reported psychiatric adverse drug reaction and frequency (N) | During treatment (%) | During discontinuation treatment (%) | After treatment (%) |
|---|---|---|---|
| Anxiety (139) | 40 | 34 | 26 |
| Sensation of unreality (57) | 54 | 25 | 21 |
| Insomnia (72) | 54 | 28 | 18 |
| Uneasiness/nervousness (50) | 50 | 30 | 20 |
| Irritability/aggressiveness (45) | 49 | 33 | 18 |
| Suicidal behaviour (59) | 68 | 19 | 13 |
| Depression (20) | 25 | 45 | 30 |

**Table 5 Internet reported antidepressant psychiatric ADRs to KILEN according to age and gender (%)**

| | Sertraline | Citalopram | Venlafaxine | Paroxetine | Mirtazapine | Fluoxetine | Escitalopram |
|---|---|---|---|---|---|---|---|
| Gender | | | | | | | |
| Female | 67.3 | 82.7 | 68.4 | 67.8 | 52.1 | 71.8 | 65.3 |
| Male | 27.8 | 16.4 | 21.6 | 28.9 | 43.5 | 25.6 | 12.2 |
| Age group | | | | | | | |
| 15-29 | 26.5 | 12.4 | 20.5 | 33.1 | 37.0 | 30.8 | 26.5 |
| Female | 16.8 | 9.7 | 15.8 | 24.0 | 37.0 | 30.8 | 10.2 |
| Male | 7.1 | 2.6 | 4.1 | 9.1 | - | - | 12.2 |
| 30-39 | 45.5 | 39.8 | 27.5 | 30.6 | 14.0 | 17.9 | 28.6 |
| Female | 27.4 | 36.7 | 27.5 | 23.1 | - | 2.6 | 28.6 |
| Male | 13.3 | 2.2 | - | 5.0 | 14.0 | 15.4 | - |
| 40-49 | 12.8 | 27.9 | 38.6 | 28.1 | 4.6 | 38.5 | 40.8 |
| Female | 11.8 | 21.2 | 19.3 | 13.2 | 2.3 | 35.9 | 24.5 |
| Male | 0.9 | 6.6 | 15.8 | 14.9 | 2.3 | 2.6 | - |
| 50-59 | 7.5 | 12.4 | 5.5 | 3.3 | 26.4 | 2.6 | 2.0 |
| Female | 2.6 | 8.4 | 3.6 | 3.3 | 11.1 | 2.6 | 2.0 |
| Male | 4.9 | 4.0 | 1.9 | - | 15.3 | - | - |
| 60-69 | 4.9 | 3.5 | - | 1.6 | 14.9 | - | - |
| Female | 4.0 | 2.6 | - | 1.6 | - | - | - |
| Male | 0.9 | 0.9 | - | - | 14.9 | - | - |
| 70-79 | 2.0 | - | - | - | - | - | - |
| Female | 2.0 | - | - | - | - | - | - |
| Male | - | - | - | - | - | - | - |
| 80-89 | - | - | - | - | - | 7.7 | - |
| Female | - | - | - | - | - | - | - |
| Male | - | - | - | - | - | 7.7 | - |
| No age given | 0.8 | 4.0 | 7.9 | 3.9 | 3.1 | 2.5 | 2.1 |

frequently reporting group, but also younger women (15-29 years of age) was a common group. This may be an effect of that maybe women to a higher degree turn to non-profit organizations for help. It can also be an effect of women tending to have a higher risk of ADRs than men, which increases with age and increased numbers of drugs prescribed [36]. Citalopram was in particular a commonly reported antidepressant medication by women answering for almost 83% of the psychiatric ADRs for this drug. Both suicidal behavior and depression, which are more frequently associated with women, were commonly reported psychiatric ADRs for Citalopram in the KILEN material. There is an almost two-fold higher occurrence of lifetime prevalence of major depressive disorder and anxiety disorders in females than in males [37], and older women with a previous history of treatment by a psychiatrist may have an increased risk of becoming long-term users of antidepressants [38]. Since depression was a highly reported psychiatric ADR during discontinuation in the KILEN material it may be of importance to include consumer reports when prescribing the drug of choice for instance depression.

However, this study does have several limitations. There is for instance the question of potential problems with polypharmacy, with an unknown interaction between psychotropic drugs, for instance different antidepressants and anxiolytics. As indicated by a Swedish study the prevalence of polypharmacy, as well as the mean number of dispensed drugs per individual, increased for instance year-by-year in Sweden 2005-2008 [39]. Hence we cannot know for sure if the reported consumer reports do contain specific psychiatric ADRs for one antidepressant drug alone or if it is a combined effect due to other drugs. Some of the antidepressants have quite few reports (Mirtazapine, Fluoxetine and Escitalopram) and therefore it is not possible to draw any conclusions for each medication. It is a strength with the KILEN material that consumers are asked to fill in the report form concerning other medications as well, but it is still difficult to know if the reported ADR is a result of a specific medication or the combination of a number of medications. This is however not unique for KILEN but also valid for the report form from the MPA. Nevertheless, consumer reporting may make an important contribution in gaining information about unknown drug interactions. The KILEN data was based on spontaneous consumer reports and thereby a selected material, which may enhance a negative view of antidepressant medication. Despite these limitations the study is still of value since the material gives us unique information of consumer reporting in Sweden.

## Conclusions

The present study indicates that consumer reporting may contribute with important information. Consumer reporting may be considered a complement to traditional ADR reporting.

### Acknowledgements

This study has received funding from Stiftelsen Kempe-Carlgrenska Fonden, Stiftelsen Lars Hiertas Minne and Elsa Lundberg och Greta Flerons fond för studier av läkemedelsbiverkan. The sponsors had no role in the study design; in the collection, analysis, and interpretation of data; in the writing of the manuscript; and in the decision to submit the article for publication. The researchers were independent from the funders. The authors would like to thank Lena Westin, Jan Albinsson and Kersti Andersson at KILEN for providing the research material. Kersti Andersson has also provided with valuable help in organizing the data. The authors would also like to thank Eva Lesén (Nordic School of Public Health) for valuable comments on a previous version of this paper.
Disclaimer
The opinions or assertions contained herein are the private views of the authors and are not to be construed as official or reflecting the views of the Medical Products Agency.

### Author details

[1]Nordic School of Public Health (NHV), Box 121 33, SE-402 42 Gothenburg, Sweden. [2]Department of Behavioural Sciences and Learning, Linkoping University, Linkoping, Sweden. [3]School of Social Work, Lund University, Lund, Sweden. [4]Medical Products Agency, Uppsala, Sweden.

### Authors' contributions

AV and AC were responsible for study concept and design. AV acquired the data. AV and AC interpreted the data. AV drafted the manuscript and all authors contributed with critical revisions of the manuscript. All authors read and approved the final manuscript.

### Competing interests

The authors declare that they have no competing interests.

### References

1. Nordic Medico-Statistical Committee (NOMESCO): *Medicines Consumption in the Nordic Countries 2004-2008* Copenhagen; 2010.
2. Lazarou J, Pomeranz BH, Corey PN: **Incidence of adverse drug reactions in hospitalized patients: a meta-analysis of prospective studies.** *JAMA* 1998, **279**:1200-1205.
3. Classen DC, Pestonik SL, Evans RS, Lloyd JF, Burke JP: **Adverse drug events in hospitalized patients: excess length of stay, extra costs, and attributable mortality.** *JAMA* 1997, **277(4)**:301-306.
4. Bates DW, Spell N, Cullen DJ, Burdick E, Laird N, Petersen LA, Small SD, Sweitzer BJ, Leape LL: **The costs of adverse drug events in hospitalized patients.** *JAMA* 1997, **277(4)**:307-311.
5. World Health Organization (WHO): *The importance of pharmacovigilance: an essential tool* Geneva; 2002.
6. World Health Organization (WHO): *Safety of medicines-a guide to detecting and reporting of adverse drug reactions. Why health professionals need to take action* Geneva; 2002.
7. **Pharmacovigilance - Major developments.** [http://ec.europa.eu/health/human-use/pharmacovigilance/developments/index_en.htm#].
8. Regulation (EU) No 1235/2010 of the European Parliament and of the Council. *Official Journal of the European Union* [http://eur-lex.europa.eu/LexUriServ/LexUriServ.do?uri=OJ:L:2010:348:0001:0016:EN:PDF], L 348/1.
9. Waller P: **Getting to grips with the new European Union pharmacovigilance legislation.** *Pharmacoepidemiology and drug safety* 2011, **20**:544-549.
10. Herxheimer A, Crombag MR, Alves TL: *Direct patient reporting of adverse drug reactions. A twelve-country survey & literature review* Health Action International (HAI) (Europe). Amsterdam; 2010.
11. Borg JJ, Aislaitner G, Pirozynski M, Mifsud S: **Strengthening and rationalizing pharmacovigilance in the EU: where is Europe heading to?** *Drug Saf* 2011, **34(3)**:187-197.
12. World Health Organization (WHO): *The safety of medicines in public health programmes: Pharmacovigilance an essential tool* Geneva; 2006.
13. Aagaard L, Nielsen LH, Hansen EH: **Consumer reporting of adverse drug reactions. A retrospective analysis of the Danish adverse drug reaction database from 2004 to 2006.** *Drug Saf* 2009, **32(11)**:1067-1074.
14. van Geffen ECG, van der Wal SW, van Hulten R, de Groot MCH, Egberts ACG, Heerdink ER: **Evaluation of patients' experiences with antidepressants reported by means of a medicine reporting system.** *Eur J Clin Pharmacol* 2007, **63**:1193-1199.
15. van Grootheest K, van Puijenbroek EP, de Jong-van den Berg LTW: **Do pharmacists' reports of adverse drug reactions reflect patients' concerns?** *Pharm World Sci* 2004, **26**:155-159.
16. Medawar C, Herxheimer A: **A comparison of adverse drug reaction reports from professionals and users, relating to risk of dependency and suicidal behaviour with paroxetine.** *Int J Risk & Safety in Medicine* 2003, **16**:5-19.
17. Herxheimer A, Mintzes B: **Antidepressants and adverse effects in young patients: uncovering the evidence.** *CMAJ* 2004, **170(4)**:487-489.
18. Nordic Medico-Statistical Committee (NOMESCO): *Health Statistics in the Nordic Countries 2006* Copenhagen; 2008.
19. The National Board of health and Welfare: *Official statistics of Sweden. Statistics-Health and Medical Care. Pharmaceuticals-statistics for 2010* Stockholm; 2011.
20. The National Board of health and Welfare: *Official statistics of Sweden. Statistics-Health and Medical Care. Pharmaceuticals-statistics for 2009* Stockholm; 2010.
21. Mjörndal T, Danell Boman M, Hägg S, Bäckström M, Wiholm BE, Wahlin A, Dahlqvist R: **Adverse drug reactions as a cause for admissions to a department of internal medicine.** *Pharmacoepidemiol Drug Saf* 2002, **11**:65-72.
22. Jönsson AK, Hakkarainen KM, Spigset O, Druid H, Hiselius A, Hägg S: **Preventable drug related mortality in a Swedish population.** *Pharmacoepidemiol Drug Saf* 2010, **19(2)**:211-215.
23. Wester K, Jönsson AK, Spigset O, Druid H, Hägg S: **Incidence of fatal adverse drug reactions: a population based study.** *Br J Clin Pharmacol* 2008, **65(4)**:573-579.
24. Bäckström M, Mjörndal T, Dahlqvist R: **Under-reporting of serious adverse drug reactions in Sweden.** *Pharmacoepidemiol Drug Saf* 2004, **13**:483-487.
25. WHO Classification: *The Anatomical Therapeutic Chemical Classification System with Defined Daily Doses (ATC/DDD)* [http://www.who.int/classifications/atcddd/en/], [Online] 2010. [Citat: den 8 May 2010.].
26. MedDRA. [http://www.meddramsso.com], (last accessed 16 August 2001 [password required]..
27. **Läkemedelsföreningen, LIF (The Swedish Association of the Pharmaceutical Industry).** *Farmacevtiska specialiteter i Sverige 2004 (FASS 2004) (Pharmaceutical Specialties in Sweden-Swedish Physicians Desk Reference)* Stockholm, Elanders; 2004.
28. **Läkemedelsföreningen, LIF (The Swedish Association of the Pharmaceutical Industry).** *FASS.se för förskrivare (FASS.se for prescribers)* [http://www.fass.se].
29. Egberts TCG, Smulders M, de Koning FHP, Meyboom RHB, Leufkens HGM: **Can adverse drug reactions be detected earlier? A comparison of reports by patients and professionals.** *BMJ* 1996, **313**:530-531.
30. Blenkinsopp A, Wilkie P, Wang M, Routledge PA: **Patient reporting of suspected adverse drug reactions: a review of published literature and international experience.** *Br J Clin Pharmacol* 2006, **63(2)**:148-156.
31. Tint A, Haddad PM, Anderson IM: **The effect of rate of antidepressant tapering on the incidence of discontinuation symptoms: a randomised study.** *J Psychopharmacol* 2008, **22(3)**:330-332.

32. Passier A, ten Napel M, van Grootheest K, van Puijenbroek E: **Reporting of adverse drug reactions by general practioners. A questionnaire-based study in the Netherlands.** *Drug Saf* 2009, **32(10)**:851-858.

33. World Health Organization (WHO): *The importance of pharmacovigilance: safety monitoring of medicinal products* Geneva; 2002.

34. Aagaard L, Hansen EH: **Consumers' reports of suspected adverse drug reactions volunteered to a consumer magazine.** *Br J Clin Pharmacol* 2010, **69(3)**:317-318.

35. Nordic Medico-Statistical Committee (NOMESCO): *Medicines Consumption in the Nordic Countries 1999-2003* Copenhagen; 2004.

36. Zopf Y, Rabe C, Neubert A, Gaßmann KG, Rascher W, Hahn EG, Brune K, Dormann H: **Women encounter ADRs more often than do men.** *Eur J Clin Pharmacol* 2008, **64**:999-1004.

37. Breslau N, Schultz L, Peterson E: **Sex differences in depression: a role for preexisting anxiety.** *Psychiatry Research* 1995, **58**:1-12.

38. Meijer WEE, Heerdink ER, Leufkens HGM, Herings RMC, Egberts ACG, Nolen WA: **Incidence and determinants of long-term use of antidepressants.** *Eur J Clin Pharmacol* 2004, **60**:57-61.

39. Hovstadius B, Hovstadius K, Astrand B, Petersson G: **Increasing polypharmacy - an individual-based study of the Swedish population 2005-2008.** *BMC Clinical Pharmacology* 2010, **10(16)**.

# 9

# Low rates of hepatotoxicity among Asian patients with paracetamol overdose: a review of 1024 cases

Abd-Rahman Marzilawati[1,2], Yen-Yew Ngau[2] and Sanjiv Mahadeva[1*]

## Abstract

**Background:** The metabolism of paracetamol in Asians is thought to differ from Westerners. Detailed clinical features of paracetamol -induced hepatotoxicity among Asians remains largely unreported.

**Methods:** A retrospective review of adult cases with paracetamol overdose over a five-year duration was performed in two of the largest public institutions in this country. Prevalence and predictive factors for hepatotoxicity were determined.

**Results:** Data on 1024 patients (median age 23 years, 82.0% female, ethnic groups: Malays 40.8%, Chinese 20.9% , Indian 33.2%) were obtained from January 2005 to December 2009. The median amount of paracetamol ingestion was 10.0 (IQR 5.0 - 15.0) g and the median serum paracetamol level was 274.80 (IQR 70.0 - 640.0) μmol/L at presentation. 75 (7.3%) patients developed hepatotoxicity. 23/ 55 (41.8%) patients who had ingested > 10 g of paracetamol and had a delayed (> 24 hour) administration of N-acetyl cystine (NAC) developed hepatotoxicity. No patients developed acute liver failure nor suffered any mortality (0%). Independent predictors for hepatotoxicity were identified as Malay (OR 2.22, 95% CI = 1.13-4.37) and Chinese (OR 3.26, 95% CI = 1.55-6.84) ethnicity, paracetamol dose > 10 g (OR 2.61, 95% CI = 1.53-4.46), prolonged duration of time from paracetamol ingestion to hospital presentation (> 24 hours OR 10.71, 95% CI = 3.46-33.15) and prolonged duration of time from paracetamol ingestion to NAC administration (> 24 hours OR 9.02, 95% CI = 2.97-27.45).

**Conclusions:** Paracetamol-induced hepatotoxicity rates in a multi-ethnic Asian population was low at 7.3%. Mortality and morbidity were non-existent despite high doses of paracetamol ingestion and delayed presentations to hospital.

**Keywords:** Paracetamol, Acetaminophen, Hepatotoxicity, Acute liver failure, N-acetyl cysteine, Asian

## Background

Paracetamol, or acetaminophen, overdose is a common means of self-poisoning worldwide due its wide availability and accessibility. It has been reported as the most common drug overdose either accidentally or unintentionally in the United Kingdom (UK), Europe, United States (US), and Australasia [1-3]. Paracetamol overdose is recognised to cause a range of hepatic damage from mild to severe hepatotoxicity, leading to acute liver failure (ALF) and death, despite the availability of antidote therapy. ALF resulting from paracetamol overdose has been extensively reported in the UK, US, France, Canada and Australia [4,5]. ALF due to paracetamol overdose

has been reported to be most common in the U.K. (60-75% of ALF aetiology), but less frequent in the U.S. (approximately 20% of ALF aetiology) and even lower in certain parts of Europe (2% of ALF aetiology in France) [4,6]. However, in recent years, the incidence of paracetamol-induced ALF cases in the US has increased exponentially [7].

In a recent review article on the differences in aetiopathogenesis of ALF between Western and Eastern populations, it was reported that viral hepatitis remained the commonest cause of ALF in Asians. Paracetamol overdose resulting in ALF was believed to be infrequent in Asia due to differences in healthcare cultural practices and lack of availability of over-the-counter drugs [8]. Whilst the latter fact may be true in lesser developed countries, many rapidly developing Asian nations have a

* Correspondence: sanjiv@ummc.edu.my
[1]Division of Gastroenterology, Department of Medicine, University of Malaya, Kuala Lumpur, Malaysia
Full list of author information is available at the end of the article

wide availability of over-the-counter drugs and cultural practices which are similar to the West. To date, two reports from small sample-sized studies in Hong Kong and Penang, Malaysia, have only demonstrated low rates of paracetamol-induced hepatotoxicity ranging from 2 - 6% [9,10]. Details on predictive factors for paracetamol-induced hepatotoxicity among Asians remain uncertain. This study aimed to examine the prevalence of hepatotoxicity in a large sample of adults with paracetamol overdose in a multi-ethnic Asian population, and determine predictive factors for hepatotoxicity in these patients.

## Methods
### Study design and data collection
Approval from the University Malaya Medical Centre (UMMC) ethics committee was obtained prior to the conduct of this study. In Malaysia, the majority of our urban population is concentrated in the capital, Kuala Lumpur. The UMMC, a 900-bedded hospital and the General Hospital of Kuala Lumpur (GHKL), a 1000-bedded institution, are the two oldest and largest public institutions in the city. Both UMMC and GHKL have an estimated 110, 000 and 150,000 admissions to their Emergency Departments on an annual basis respectively (local institutional statistics 2008, unpublished). A retrospective review of clinical records was performed in both these centres for a five-year duration from 2005 to 2009. The International Classification and Diagnosis (ICD) 9 and 10 coding systems were used to identify individuals with paracetamol overdose from the Medical Records units of both institutions. All patients aged ≥ 18 years of age who had a diagnosis of paracetamol overdose from ICD 9 and 10 coding system were included.

Information obtained from the medical records included the following: basic demography, timings of paracetamol overdose, presentation to Emergency Departments and administration of N-Acetylcysteine (NAC), estimated doses of paracetamol ingested based on patient's recall, concomitant ingestion of other drugs, alcohol, history of psychiatric disorders and numbers of overdose attempts. All blood investigations during this period were available in both institutions' computerised laboratory database and the following data were collected: serum paracetamol level, liver function tests, pH, coagulation profile and renal profile. The main outcomes in terms of duration of hospital stay and survival (i.e. discharged or died in hospital) were also available from both institutions' computerised data system.

### Definitions
Hepatotoxicity was defined by a peak serum alanine transaminase (ALT) level > 1000 IU/L, in accordance with previous accepted nomenclature in the literature

[11]. ALF was defined as the presence of coagulopathy (INR > 1.5) together with hepatic encephalopathy within 8–26 weeks of onset of symptoms in a patient without any prior liver disease [12].

### Statistics
All results were analysed using the Statistical Package for Social Scientists (SPSS version 19.0, USA). Continuous variables were expressed as means with a standard deviation or medians where appropriate. Categorical data were expressed as proportions. Continuous data were analysed using Student's t-test, Mann–Whitney –U test and Kruskal Wallis test where appropriate. Categorical data were analysed with chi-square test or Fischer's exact test where appropriate. Significant associations with hepatotoxicity identified at univariate analysis were subsequently analysed in a multivariate analysis to identify independent predictors of hepatotoxicity. Predictive factors were expressed as odds ratios with a 95% confidence interval. Statistical significance was defined as a p value of <0.05.

## Results
Between January 2005 to December 2009, a total of 1,410 cases were identified as paracetamol overdose according to ICD 9 or ICD 10 coding systems in both UMMC and HKL. 386 cases were excluded due to a combination of missing medical records, coding misclassification and age < 18 years. 1024 cases of medical records were finally available for analysis. The incidence of paracetamol overdoses from January 2005 to December 2009 in UMMC and KLGH are highlighted in Figure 1. In general, there had been an increase in incidence in both institutions from 2005 to 2006, with a steady rate of paracetamol overdose cases in the last 4 years. More cases of paracetamol overdose had been admitted to UMMC (n = 583) compared to KLGH (n = 441) during the period of study.

### Clinical characteristics of paracetamol overdose patients
Demographic and clinical data of the study population are highlighted in Table 1. The median age of adults with paracetamol overdose was 23 years, 840 (82.0%) patients were female and the major ethnic group consisted of Malays (n = 418, 40.8%). Paracetamol overdose resulted from deliberate self-harm in 885 (81.7%) cases, unintentional overdose in 198 (18.3%) cases and alcohol co-ingestion was not common (n = 46, 4.2%). The clinical presentation of patients with paracetamol poisoning consisted mainly of gastrointestinal tract symptoms. 859 (79.3%) of patients received NAC for their paracetamol overdose.

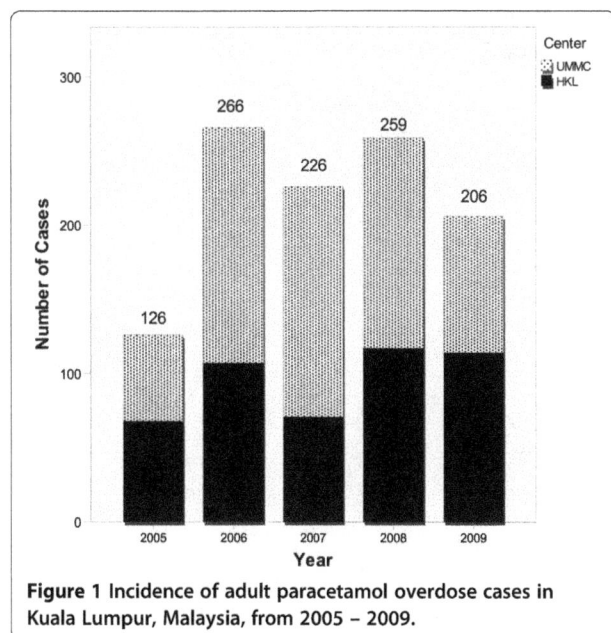

**Figure 1 Incidence of adult paracetamol overdose cases in Kuala Lumpur, Malaysia, from 2005 – 2009.**

## Table 1 Demographic and clinical data on paracetamol overdose patients

| Category | n | (%) |
|---|---|---|
| Age (median, IQR) years | 23.00 (20.00 to 28.00) | – |
| Gender | | |
| Male | 184 | 18.0 |
| Female | 840 | 82.0 |
| Races | | |
| Malay | 418 | 40.8 |
| Chinese | 214 | 20.9 |
| Indian | 340 | 33.2 |
| Others | 52 | 5.1 |
| Previous History of Drug Overdose | 99 | 9.7 |
| Previous History of paracetamol Overdose | 82 | 8.0 |
| Previous Psychiatry History | 107 | 10.4 |
| Drug Co-ingestion | | |
| Alcohol | 45 | 4.4 |
| Benzodiazepine | 11 | 1.1 |
| Antidepressant | 3 | 0.3 |
| Anticonvulsant | 2 | 0.2 |
| Clinical features | | |
| Nausea | 298 | 29.1 |
| Vomiting | 576 | 56.2 |
| Abdominal Pain | 333 | 32.5 |
| Drowsiness | 149 | 14.6 |
| Loss of Consciousness | 8 | 0.8 |
| Circumstances | | |
| Deliberate | 836 | 81.6 |
| Unintentional | 188 | 18.4 |
| Treatment received | | |
| Charcoal | 425 | 41.5 |
| Gastric Lavage | 486 | 47.5 |
| N-Acetylcysteine | 859 | 79.3 |

### Clinical details of paracetamol overdose

The median amount of paracetamol ingestion in 1024 patients was 10.0 (IQR 5.0 - 15.0) g and the median serum paracetamol level was 274.80 (IQR 70.0 - 640.0) μmol/L at presentation. The median duration from paracetamol ingestion to hospital presentation was 4.5 (IQR 2.3 - 11.5) hours. There was a median duration of 6.50 (IQR 2.5 - 14.0) hours from timing of paracetamol ingestion to NAC administration, whilst timing from hospital presentation to NAC administration was a median of 1.5 (IQR 0.0 to 4.1) hours, indicating that there was little delay in the administration of NAC at presentation to the emergency units in both hospitals. Most patients were admitted for a median of 3 days, ranging from 2 – 4 days.

### Hepatotoxicity rates and clinical outcome

75 (7.3%) patients with paracetamol overdose developed hepatotoxicity, i.e. a peak serum ALT ≥ 1000 IU/L. 124 (12.1%) patients had a moderately raised peak serum ALT (66–999 IU/L) whilst the remaining 825 (80.6%) had normal liver function tests. 146 (14.3%) cases had an INR ≥ 1.5 but none of the patients with hepatotoxicity developed acute liver failure. 24/ 149 patients with mild drowsiness or stupor at presentation had an INR > 1.5. However, 10 of these patients had alcohol intoxication and the remainder had co-ingestion or either benzodiazepines or antidepressants. All 1024 patients with paracetamol overdose were discharged well following hospitalisation. 542 patients had ingested > 10 g of paracetamol, but only 61 (11.3%) developed hepatotoxicity. Among these 542 cases, 23/ 55 (41.8%) patients who had a delayed (> 24 hours) administration of NAC developed hepatotoxicity.

### Predictive factors for paracetamol-induced hepatotoxicity

Potential risk factors for paracetamol-induced hepatotoxicity were evaluated by univariate analysis (Table 2). Demographically, no specific age nor gender groups were found to have a risk of hepatotoxicity. However, a significant association with hepatotoxicity was observed with ethnicity (ethnic Indians 3.8% vs ethnic Malays 8.6% vs ethnic Chinese 12.1%). Clinically, a paracetamol dose of > 10 g was associated with hepatotoxicity (11.3% > 10 g vs 2.7% < 10 g, p < 0.001), together with a prolonged duration of time from paracetamol ingestion to hospital presentation (1.8% < 3.9 hours vs 8.6% 4–24 hours vs 32.4% > 24 hours) and duration of time from paracetamol ingestion to NAC administration (1.9% < 3.9 hours vs 8.7% 4–24 hours vs 34.8% > 24 hours) (Table 2).

**Table 2 Risk factors for paracetamol-induced hepatotoxicity in study patients**

| Category | Hepatotoxicity | | Unadjusted OR | 95% CI | p value | Adjusted OR | 95% CI | p value |
|---|---|---|---|---|---|---|---|---|
| | Yes n = 75 | No n = 949 | | | | | | |
| Age(years) | | | | | | | | |
| <20 | 18(5.9) | 288 (94.5) | 1.00 | | 0.33 | 1.00 | | 0.31 |
| 21-30 | 47(8.4) | 510(91.6) | 1.48 | 0.84-2.59 | 0.18 | 1.41 | 0.75 - 2.63 | 0.29 |
| >30 | 10(6.2) | 151(93.8) | 1.06 | 0.48-2.35 | 0.89 | 0.82 | 0.34 - 2.00 | 0.67 |
| Gender | | | | | | | | |
| Female | 60 (7.1) | 780 (92.9) | 1.00 | | | | | |
| Male | 15 (8.2) | 169 (91.8) | 1.15 | 0.64 - 2.08 | 0.64 | NA | NA | NA |
| Race | | | | | | | | |
| Indian | 13 (3.8) | 327 (96.2) | 1.00 | | 0.002 | 1.00 | | 0.007 |
| Malay | 36 (8.6) | 382 (91.4) | 2.31 | 1.23-4.34 | 0.009 | 2.22 | 1.13 - 4.37 | 0.023 |
| Chinese | 26 (12.1) | 188 (87.9) | 3.39 | 1.73-6.64 | <0.001 | 3.26 | 1.55 - 6.84 | 0.002 |
| PCM# Dose (g) | | | | | | | | |
| <10 | 12(2.7) | 436(97.3) | 1.00 | | | 1.0 | | |
| >10 | 61(11.3) | 481(88.7) | 2.59 | 1.68-3.99 | <0.001 | 2.61 | 1.53 - 4.46 | <0.001 |
| Alcohol Co-ingestion | | | | | | | | |
| Yes | 3(6.7) | 42(93.3) | 1.00 | | | | | |
| No | 72(7.4) | 907 (92.6) | 1.11 | 0.34-3.67 | 0.87 | NA | NA | NA |
| BZDP* Co-ingestion | | | | | | | | |
| No | 73(7.2) | 940(92.8) | 1.00 | | | | | |
| Yes | 2(18.2) | 9(81.8) | 2.95 | 0.63-13.91 | 0.17 | 3.20 | 0.60 - 17.68 | 0.18 |
| Time from PCM Ingestion to Hospital Presentation (hours) | | | | | | | | |
| <3.9 | 9(1.9) | 454(98.1) | 1.00 | | <0.001 | 1.00 | | <0.001 |
| 4.0-24.0 | 43(8.7) | 452(91.3) | 5.00 | 2.42-10.34 | <0.001 | 3.45 | 1.60 - 7.43 | 0.001 |
| >24.1 | 23(34.8) | 43(65.2) | 25.50 | 11.17-58.24 | <0.001 | 10.71 | 3.46 - 33.15 | <0.001 |
| Time from PCM Ingestion to NAC administration (hours) | | | | | | | | |
| <3.9 | 5(1.5) | 332(98.5) | 1.00 | | <0.001 | 1.00 | | <0.001 |
| 4.0-24.0 | 41(6.8) | 560(93.2) | 4.95 | 1.94-12.62 | 0.001 | 2.94 | 1.07 - 8.00 | 0.037 |
| >24.1 | 29(34.1) | 56(65.9) | 36.31 | 13.54-97.40 | <0.001 | 9.02 | 2.97 - 27.43 | <0.001 |

\# PCM - paracetamol.
\* BZDP - benzodiazepines.

Independent predictors of paracetamol-induced hepatotoxicity, explored by logistic regression analysis, were found to include the following: Malay (OR 2.22, 95% CI = 1.13-4.37) and Chinese (OR 3.26, 95% CI = 1.55-6.84) ethnicity, paracetamol dose > 10 g (OR 2.61, 95% CI = 1.53-4.46), prolonged duration of time from paracetamol ingestion to hospital presentation (4–24 hours OR 3.45, 95% CI = 1.60-7.43; > 24 hours OR 10.71, 95% CI = 3.46-33.15) and prolonged duration of time from paracetamol ingestion to NAC administration (4–24 hours OR 2.94, 95% CI = 1.07-8.00; > 24 hours OR 9.02, 95% CI = 2.97-27.45).

## Discussion

This retrospective study represents one of the largest case series of paracetamol overdoses that has been reported to date. The duration of 5 years demonstrated little variation in admission patterns (apart from the first year) and there had been no major changes in the medical management of paracetamol overdose during this period. As all cases of poisoning in this country are solely managed in public institutions, the data from this study is fairly representative of the population from the largest city in this country. Furthermore, the general Malaysian urban population consists of 3 major ethnic groups, i.e. Malays, Chinese and Indians [13]. Hence, our study has relevance to other populations in Asia as well.

In this study, we have demonstrated that despite significant numbers of paracetamol overdose over a 5-year duration, only 7.3% of this multi-ethnic Asian adult population developed hepatotoxicity and no (i.e. n = 0) patients developed ALF following paracetamol overdose. Our results are in concurrence with previous reviews that paracetamol overdose is a rare cause of ALF in Asians. It is noteworthy that > 50% of patients who ingested > 10 g of paracetamol and had a delayed (> 24 hours after paracetamol ingestion) administration of NAC did not develop hepatotoxicity. Whilst the usual characteristics of paracetamol pharmacology such as cumulative dose and delayed timing of NAC administration predicted hepatotoxicity, this study identified that ethnicity, particularly those of Malay (OR 2.22) and Chinese (OR 3.26), were independent determinants of hepatotoxicity. The latter fact may suggest, but does not confirm, that ethnic differences in paracetamol metabolism may contribute towards paracetamol-induced hepatotoxicity.

We have compared our case series with previous publications and summarised the salient features in Table 3. Paracetamol-induced hepatotoxicity rates, using a similar definition as ours, in Western patients have been reported to range from 15% to 36% [5,9,10,14-22]. The only exception was a study from Edinburgh, UK, which reported a 4% rate of hepatotoxicity among 987 patients with paracetamol overdose, but patients who presented > 15 hours post paracetamol ingestion had been excluded [21]. Paracetamol overdose had a mortality rate of up to 7% despite NAC administration, although mortality rates have declined over time due to successful liver transplantation in many centres. In contrast to Caucasian patients in Western studies, two publications from Asia and a single study from the Caribbean have reported hepatotoxicity rates ranging from 2% to 7% [9,10,19]. Acute liver failure was not a feature and no mortality had been reported in the latter case series. The data from our large case series of 1024 patients appears to mirror the findings from these earlier smaller sample-sized studies.

A possible explanation for the lower hepatotoxicity rates in non-Western studies may be explained by the cumulative dose of paracetamol ingested by individuals. The minimal amount of paracetamol known to cause toxicity in adults is approximately 7.5 g and liver toxicity is usually associated with paracetamol doses of > 10 g [23]. In our study, we estimated that 52% of patients had ingested > 10 g of paracetamol and the median dose in our population was 10 g. In several of the studies that have been reported from Western centres, the mean or median doses of paracetamol ingested have been reported to be higher, although not in all [17,21,22]. The mean/ median doses of paracetamol ingested in studies from the U.K., U.S. and Denmark have been reported as 15 g, 18 g and 25 g respectively (Table 3). However, other studies on Caucasian populations with similar median paracetamol doses (to ours) still reported higher hepatotoxicity rates of 14 - 31% (Table 3). An additional point is that NAC administration in our patients was based on normalised dosing. Asian patients may have inadvertently received higher NAC doses compared to Western patients of a higher averaged body weight.

An alternative explanation for an increased paracetamol-induced hepatotoxicity among Western patients may be related to alcohol co-ingestion. Chronic alcohol exposure is recognised to increase short term toxicity from paracetamol overdose by 2 to 3 fold increase in hepatic content of cytochrome P4502E1, the major isoform responsible for the generation of the toxic metabolite from paracetamol [24]. About 25% of Western patients with paracetamol overdose were documented to have a regular alcohol consumption and excessive alcohol co-ingestion with paracetamol overdose was reported in 20-40% of cases [14,15,18]. In contrast, the rate of alcohol co-ingestion was only 4.2% in our study and 10 - 17% in other Asian studies [10,19].

Variation in the timing of NAC administration may be another explanation for differences in hepatotoxicity

**Table 3 Summary of studies that have examined hepatotoxicity rates in patients with paracetamol overdose**

| Author | Year | Location | n | Hepatotoxicity % | Survival % | Paracetamol Dose |
|---|---|---|---|---|---|---|
| Proudfoot [22] | 1970 | Edinburgh, U.K. | 41 | 39% | 97.6% | 39% > 15 g |
| Schiodt [14] | 1997 | Texas, U.S. | 71 | 32% | 93% | Median = 17.6 g 93% > 4 g |
| Hawton [17] | 1996 | Oxford, U.K. | 80 | 31% | NA | 69% > 12.5 g |
| Gyamlani [15] | 2001 | New York, USA | 93 | 16% | 98% | NA |
| James [16] | 2008 | USA | 157 | 15% (1.3% ALF) | 100% | Mean 18 g |
| Ayonrinde [5] | 2005 | Australia | 188 | 14% | 100% | Median = 12 g |
| Mohd-Zain [9] | 2006 | Penang, Malaysia | 165 | 7.3% | 100% | 38% > 10 g |
| Current study | 2011 | Kuala Lumpur , Malaysia | 1024 | 7.5% | 100% | Median 10 g (54.3% > 10 g) |
| Chan [10] | 1993 | Hong Kong | 104 | 6% | 100% | Median 5 g 6.7% > 10 g |
| Mills [19] | 2008 | Jamaica | 49 | 2% | 100% | Range 2–30 g |
| Schmidt [18] | 2002 | Copenhagen, Denmark | 737 | No data on hepatotoxicity (0.9% ALF) | 99.9% | Median 25 g |

rates between studies. Delayed administration of NAC to patients with potentially toxic doses of paracetamol is a recognised risk factor for hepatotoxicity, an observation that was also demonstrated in our study. Patients with paracetamol overdose who had received NAC > 24 hours after paracetamol ingestion in our study were 10.4 times more likely to develop hepatotoxicity compared to those who received NAC earlier. Among our study cases, 92% of patients received NAC within 24 hours. Unfortunately, data on the timing of NAC administration has not been reported widely in the literature, and further comparisons have not been possible. However, it is notable that despite 80% of patients receiving NAC within 24 hours of paracetamol overdose a 14% hepatotoxicity rate (i.e. double the rate in our study) was reported in a recent Australian study [5].

Pharmacogenetic variation in the metabolism of paracetamol between Caucasians and Orientals has previously been studied [25]. In a study comparing urinary excretion of paracetamol metabolites in 125 Caucasians and 33 ethnic Chinese, heterogeneity in the conversion of paracetamol cysteine conjugates (toxic paracetamol metabolites) to mercapturate via N-acetylation had been demonstrated. Adults with Chinese ethnicity demonstrated relatively extensive glucuronidation but lower sulfation in paracetamol metabolism, when compared to Caucasians. Whilst clinical relevance of this variation in metabolic pathways remains uncertain, it is possible that intrinsic differences in the pharmacogenetics of paracetamol metabolism may be a major reason for differences in hepatotoxicity between Asians and Caucasians.

## Conclusions

This study has obvious limitations in the light of its' retrospective design. Nevertheless, its' large sample size, representative study population and accurate capture of computerised laboratory data are its' major strengths. We have demonstrated that the rates of hepatotoxicity among 1024 Asian patients with paracetamol overdose is low at 7.3%. Although differences in the clinical characteritics of paracetamol overdose between Western and Asian patients are recognised, it is possible that intrinsic differences in paracetamol metabolism may be a contributory factor as well. Our data supports the findings from a recent study demonstrating that N-acetyl cysteine therapy is not cost-effective in the management of Asian patients with paracetamol overdose [26], and treatment algorithms developed in the West may not be appropriate in the East.

### Competing interests
The authors declare that they have no competing interests.

### Authors' contributions
ARM collected the data, performed initial data analysis and drafted the manuscript. NYY provided administrative support. SM conceived and designed the study, performed final data analysis and helped to draft the manuscript. All authors read and approved the final manuscript.

### Acknowledgements
We would like to thank the University of Malaya Short Term Research Grant for their partial funding in the conduct of this study.

### Author details
[1]Division of Gastroenterology, Department of Medicine, University of Malaya, Kuala Lumpur, Malaysia. [2]Department of Medicine, Hospital Kuala Lumpur, Kuala Lumpur, Malaysia.

### References

1.  Gunnell D, Hawton K, Murray V, Garnier R, Bismuth C, Fagg J, Simkin S: **Use of paracetamol for suicide and non-fatal poisoning in the UK and France: are restrictions on availability justified?** *J Epidemiol Community Health* 1997, **51**(2):175–179.
2.  Robinson D, Smith AM, Johnston GD: **Severity of overdose after restriction of paracetamol availability: retrospective study.** *BMJ* 2000, **321**(7266):926–927.
3.  Ostapowicz G, Fontana RJ, Schiodt FV, Larson A, Davern TJ, Han SH, McCashland TM, Shakil AO, Hay JE, Hynan L, *et al*: **Results of a prospective study of acute liver failure at 17 tertiary care centers in the United States.** *Ann Intern Med* 2002, **137**(12):947–954.
4.  Ostapowicz G, Lee WM: **Acute hepatic failure: a Western perspective.** *J Gastroenterol Hepatol* 2000, **15**(5):480–488.
5.  Ayonrinde OT, Phelps GJ, Hurley JC, Ayonrinde OA: **Paracetamol overdose and hepatotoxicity at a regional Australian hospital: a 4-year experience.** *Intern Med J* 2005, **35**(11):655–660.
6.  O'Grady JG, Schalm SW, Williams R: **Acute liver failure: redefining the syndromes.** *Lancet* 1993, **342**(8866):273–275.
7.  Larson AM, *et al*: **Acetaminophen induced acute liver failure: results of a United States multicenter, prospective study.** *Hepatology* 2005, **42**:1364–1372.
8.  Acharya SK, Batra Y, Hazari S, Choudhury V, Panda SK, Dattagupta S: **Etiopathogenesis of acute hepatic failure: Eastern versus Western countries.** *J Gastroenterol Hepatol* 2002, **17**(Suppl 3):S268–S273.
9.  Mohd Zain ZFAI, Ab Rahman AF: **Characteristics and outcomes of paracetamol poisoning cases at a general hospital in Northern Malaysia.** *Singapore Med J* 2006, **47**(2):134–137.
10. Chan TY, Chan AY, Critchley JA: **Paracetamol poisoning and hepatotoxicity in Chinese–the Prince of Wales Hospital (Hong Kong) experience.** *Singapore Med J* 1993, **34**(4):299–302.
11. McClain CJPS, Barve S, Devalarja R, Shedlofsky S: **Acetaminophen hepatotoxicity: An update.** *Curr Gastroenterol Rep* 1999, **1**(1):42–49.
12. Lee WM, Squires RH Jr, Nyberg SL, Doo E, Hoofnagle JH: **Acute liver failure: Summary of a workshop.** *Hepatology* 2008, **47**(4):1401–1415.
13. DoSM: **Population Distribution and Basic Demographic Characteristics.** In *The 2000 Population and Housing Census of Malaysia Putrajaya*; 2000.
14. Schiodt FV, Rochling FA, Casey DL, Lee WM: **Acetaminophen toxicity in an urban county hospital.** *N Engl J Med* 1997, **337**(16):1112–1117.
15. Gyamlani GG, Parikh CR: **Acetaminophen toxicity: suicidal vs. accidental.** *Crit Care* 2002, **6**(2):155–159.
16. James LP, Capparelli EV, Simpson PM, Letzig L, Roberts D, Hinson JA, Kearns GL, Blumer JL, Sullivan JE: **Acetaminophen-associated hepatic injury: evaluation of acetaminophen protein adducts in children and adolescents with acetaminophen overdose.** *Clin Pharmacol Ther* 2008, **84**(6):684–690.
17. Hawton K, Ware C, Mistry H, Hewitt J, Kingsbury S, Roberts D, Weitzel H: **Paracetamol self-poisoning. Characteristics, prevention and harm reduction.** *Br J Psychiatry* 1996, **168**(1):43–48.
18. Schmidt LE, Dalhoff K: **The effect of regular medication on the outcome of paracetamol poisoning.** *Aliment Pharmacol Ther* 2002, **16**(8):1539–1545.
19. Mills MO, Lee MG: **Acetaminophen overdose in Jamaica.** *West Indian Med J* 2008, **57**(2):132–134.
20. Brotodihardjo AE, Batey RG, Farrell GC, Byth K: **Hepatotoxicity from paracetamol self-poisoning in western Sydney: a continuing challenge.** *Med J Aust* 1992, **157**(6):382–385.

21. Waring WS, Robinson OD, Stephen AF, Dow MA, Pettie JM: **Does the patient history predict hepatotoxicity after acute paracetamol overdose?** *QJM* 2008, **101**(2):121–125.
22. Proudfoot AT, Wright N: **Acute paracetamol poisoning.** *Br Med J* 1970, **3**(5722):557–558.
23. Rumack BH, Peterson RC, Koch GG, Amara IA: **Acetaminophen overdose. 662 cases with evaluation of oral acetylcysteine treatment.** *Arch Intern Med* 1981, **141**(3 Spec No):380–385.
24. Prescott LF: **Paracetamol, alcohol and the liver.** *Br J Clin Pharmacol* 2000, **49**(4):291–301.
25. Patel M, Tang BK, Kalow W: **Variability of acetaminophen metabolism in Caucasians and Orientals.** *Pharmacogenetics* 1992, **2**(1):38–45.
26. Senarathna SG, Sri Ranganathan S, Buckley N, Fernandopulle R: **A cost effectiveness analysis of the preferred antidotes for acute paracetamol poisoning patients in Sri Lanka.** *BMC Clin Pharmacol* 2012, **12**(1):6.

# 10

# Effect of exenatide on the pharmacokinetics of a combination oral contraceptive in healthy women: an open-label, randomised, crossover trial

Prajakti A Kothare[1*], Mary E Seger[1], Justin Northrup[1], Kenneth Mace[1], Malcolm I Mitchell[1] and Helle Linnebjerg[2]

## Abstract

**Background:** Consistent with its effect on gastric emptying, exenatide, an injectable treatment for type 2 diabetes, may slow the absorption rate of concomitantly administered oral drugs resulting in a decrease in maximum concentration ($C_{max}$). This study evaluated the drug interaction potential of exenatide when administered adjunctively with oral contraceptives, given their potential concomitant use.

**Methods:** This trial evaluated the effect of exenatide co-administration on single- and multiple-dose pharmacokinetics of a combination oral contraceptive (ethinyl estradiol [EE] 30 µg, levonorgestrel [LV] 150 µg [Microgynon 30®]). Thirty-two healthy female subjects participated in an open-label, randomised, crossover trial with 3 treatment periods (oral contraceptive alone, 1 hour before exenatide, 30 minutes after exenatide). Subjects received a single dose of oral contraceptive on Day 8 of each period and QD doses on Days 10 through 28. During treatment periods of concomitant usage, exenatide was administered subcutaneously prior to morning and evening meals at 5 µg BID from Days 1 through 4 and at 10 µg BID from Days 5 through 22. Single- (Day 8) and multiple-dose (Day 22) pharmacokinetic profiles were assessed for each treatment period.

**Results:** Exenatide did not alter the bioavailability nor decrease daily trough concentrations for either oral contraceptive component. No substantive changes in oral contraceptive pharmacokinetics occurred when oral contraceptive was administered 1 hour before exenatide. Single-dose oral contraceptive administration 30 minutes after exenatide resulted in mean (90% CI) $C_{max}$ reductions of 46% (42-51%) and 41% (35-47%) for EE and LV, respectively. Repeated daily oral contraceptive administration 30 minutes after exenatide resulted in $C_{max}$ reductions of 45% (40-50%) and 27% (21-33%) for EE and LV, respectively. Peak oral contraceptive concentrations were delayed approximately 3 to 4 hours. Mild-to-moderate nausea and vomiting were the most common adverse events observed during the trial.

**Conclusions:** The observed reduction in $C_{max}$ is likely of limited importance given the unaltered oral contraceptive bioavailability and trough concentrations; however, for oral medications that are dependent on threshold concentrations for efficacy, such as contraceptives and antibiotics, patients should be advised to take those drugs at least 1 hour before exenatide injection.

**Trial registration:** ClinicalTrials.gov: NCT00254800.

**Keywords:** exenatide twice daily, pharmacokinetics, oral contraceptive

* Correspondence: kotharep@yahoo.com
[1]Eli Lilly and Company, Lilly Corporate Center, Indianapolis, IN, USA
Full list of author information is available at the end of the article

## Background

Exenatide, a 39-amino acid peptide and antidiabetic agent known as a glucagon-like peptide-1 receptor agonist, has multiple glucoregulatory actions which are similar to those of endogenous glucagon-like peptide-1. In the European Union, it is an adjunctive therapy for patients with type 2 diabetes who are suboptimally controlled with metformin, a sulphonylurea, a thiazolidinedione, and combinations of metformin plus a sulphonylurea or metformin plus a thiazolidinedione. In the United States, exenatide is indicated as an adjunct to diet and exercise to improve glycaemic control in adults with type 2 diabetes mellitus. Following a subcutaneous dose (5 or 10 µg BID), exenatide is rapidly absorbed with a time to peak concentration ($T_{max}$) of approximately 2 hours, has a terminal half-life ($t_{1/2}$) of 2.4 hours [1], and is predominantly eliminated by passive renal mechanisms [2]. Exenatide has been shown to reduce fasting and postprandial glucose by the combined contribution of glucose-dependent insulin secretion, suppression of glucagon secretion, and slowing of gastric emptying [3-5]. There is evidence that this treatment also reduces appetite [6] and energy intake [7].

Consistent with its pharmacological effect of slowing gastric emptying, exenatide may reduce the rate of absorption of concomitantly administered oral drugs. Drug-drug interaction studies with digoxin [8], warfarin [9], lovastatin [10], and lisinopril [11] have demonstrated that concomitant exenatide treatment reduced the maximum plasma concentrations ($C_{max}$) and delayed the $T_{max}$ for these drugs, both of which are consistent with slowing of gastric emptying. Reductions in overall exposure (area under the curve [AUC]) were only observed in the exenatide-lovastatin interaction study. However, given the known pharmacokinetic characteristics of exenatide, the potential for a CYP3A induction was considered unlikely and the observed results were considered to be related to incomplete characterization of the single-dose lovastatin AUC following exenatide dosing. Acetaminophen [12], a marker of gastric emptying, was studied with exenatide to understand how the relative timing of exenatide administration might change the magnitude of pharmacokinetic effects observed for orally administered drugs. In addition, this prior study provided information on the optimal timing for administration of other concomitant oral medications. Changes in the acetaminophen profile were not evident when acetaminophen was given 1 hour prior to the exenatide dose as the absorption process for acetaminophen had likely been completed before the onset of exenatide action. However, a reduced $C_{max}$ and delayed $T_{max}$ were observed when acetaminophen was given after exenatide administration; the magnitude of changes was greatest 1 to 2 hours after exenatide administration.

The present study evaluated the drug-drug interaction potential of exenatide with a widely used concomitantly administered combination oral contraceptive (OC) consisting of ethinyl estradiol (EE) and levonorgestrel (LV). The study included a treatment period in which OC was administered 30 minutes after exenatide, such that the anticipated time of peak exposure of the oral contraceptive would coincide with the maximum effect of slowed gastric emptying. A second treatment period with OC administered 1 hour before exenatide was also included. No interaction would be expected during the second treatment period, as OC absorption was likely to be completed prior to the onset of exenatide action. The interaction was assessed after single, as well as multiple doses of OC to maximise pharmacokinetic information generated from the study.

## Methods

### Subjects

This study was conducted at 1 clinical study center in the United Kingdom. The protocol was approved by the Independent Ethics Committee Plymouth, UK, and was conducted in accordance with the 1975 Declaration of Helsinki, as revised in 2000 [13], and the European Commission's directive on clinical research (2001/20/CE) [14]. Before enrollment, all subjects provided written informed consent. Subjects were required to be taking an OC prior to study entry and be healthy pre-menopausal females, 18 to 45 years old, with a BMI between 19 to 35 kg/m$^2$. Subjects were excluded from the study if they had diabetes mellitus or had received implanted contraceptives for 6 months or injectable contraceptives for 12 months prior to the study. Grapefruit was restricted within 7 days and concomitant drug therapies that could induce or inhibit CYP3A were not permitted within 14 days before the first drug administration. In case of mild intercurrent illness during the study, ibuprofen and/or anti-emetic medications that would not affect gastrointestinal motility were allowed at the discretion of the investigator. Lifestyle habits of eligible subjects, such as smoking, alcohol consumption, diet, and exercise, were not altered during the study.

### Study design

This was an open-label, 3-period, 3-sequence, randomised crossover study in healthy female subjects who were using OCs prior to study entry (clinicaltrials.gov registration: NCT00254800). The primary objective was to evaluate the effect of exenatide on the multiple-dose PK of a combination oral contraceptive (EE and LV) administered 1 hour before and 30 minutes after the exenatide dose. Up to 40 subjects were to be enrolled to ensure that approximately 18 subjects completed the study. Comparing OC alone and OC administered 1 hour before exenatide, a sample size of 18 subjects was estimated to provide approximately 90% power to demonstrate that the 90% CI of the ratio of geometric means for AUC (EE or LV) would be contained within the interval (0.80, 1.25). This sample size estimate was based on an intra-subject coefficient of variation of 15%.

The OC combination product (Microgynon 30®) consisted of EE, 30 µg and LV, 150 µg. Prior to starting the active dosing period, screening was conducted over 2 visits. The purpose of the first screening visit, approximately 2 months prior to admission, was to initiate a run-in period either to convert to the study OC or to synchronise the OC cycle within a cohort of subjects. The second screening visit occurred approximately 21 days prior to the first day of dosing to confirm study eligibility.

Each subject participated in 3 treatment periods, each of 28 days duration: OC alone, OC 1 hour before exenatide, and OC approximately 30 minutes after exenatide. Exenatide was self-administered 15 minutes prior to the morning and evening meals at 5 µg BID on Days 1 through 4 and increased to 10 µg BID on Days 5 through 22. Subjects received a single dose of OC on Day 8 of each treatment period; dosing was omitted on Day 9 to allow for single-dose PK sampling. Subsequently, once-daily doses of OC were resumed on Days 10 through 28. Given that exenatide was administered 15 minutes before meals, OC was administered either 75 minutes before the meal (ie, 1 hour before exenatide) or 15 minutes after the meal (ie, 30 minutes after exenatide), depending on the treatment period. In the OC alone arm, all multiple OC doses and the majority of the single OC doses were given approximately 75 minutes before the meal.

During each treatment period after the first dose of the OC (Day 8), venous blood samples (4 mL each) were taken pre-dose, and at 0.5, 1, 1.5, 2, 2.5, 3, 3.5, 4, 4.5, 5, 6, 8, 10, 12, 16, 24 and 48 hours post-dose. Blood samples were also taken following multiple doses of the OC (Day 22) pre-dose, and at 0.5, 1, 1.5, 2, 2.5, 3, 3.5, 4, 4.5, 5, 6, 8, 10, 12, 16 and 24 hours post-dose. At a minimum, subjects were admitted to the Clinical Research Unit (CRU) on Day 7, resident on Day 8, and discharged on Day 9, then admitted again on Day 21, resident on Day 22, and discharged on Day 23. Subjects were required to attend the CRU on Days 10 and 28 as outpatients. At the investigator's discretion, subjects could be resident in the CRU or attend as outpatients after the first exenatide dose (Day 1) and upon dose increases to 10 µg (Day 5).

### Bioanalytical methods

Human plasma PK samples obtained during this study were analysed at PPD, Richmond, VA, USA. The samples were analysed for EE and LV using validated liquid chromatography with tandem mass spectrometric methods [15]. The lower limit of quantification was 2.00 pg/mL for EE and 50.0 pg/mL for LV; the upper limit of

quantification was 200 pg/mL for EE and 12500 pg/mL for LV and. The intra-assay accuracy (% relative error) during partial validation ranged from -4.24% to 0.992% for LV and from 0.233% to 2.96% for EE. The intra-assay precision (% relative standard deviation) during partial validation ranged from 6.30% to 8.67% for LV and from 4.63% to 12.1% for EE.

### Pharmacokinetic assessments

Plasma EE and LV pharmacokinetics were characterised by noncompartmental methods of analysis using WinNon-Lin Professional Version 5.0.1 (Pharsight, Cary, NC). Plasma concentrations for each OC component were plotted semi-logarithmically against time following single (Day 8) or multiple doses (Day 22). The maximum concentration after single or multiple doses ($C_{max}$ or $C_{max, ss}$) and the corresponding time of maximum concentration ($T_{max}$ or $T_{max, ss}$) were identified from the observed data. After a single dose, the area under the concentration-time curve up to the last sampling time point ($AUC_{0-t, last}$) was calculated and extrapolated to infinity ($AUC_{0-\infty}$) using the log-linear trapezoidal rule. Following multiple-dose administration of the OC, the area under the curve over the 24-hour post-dose interval ($AUC_{0-\tau, ss}$) was calculated on Day 22. Additionally, concentrations were tabulated at the 24-hour post-dose scheduled time points following single and multiple doses. These 24-hour post-dose concentrations are referred to as daily trough concentrations in the remainder of the document.

### Statistical methods

The statistical analysis included all data from subjects who received at least 1 dose of drug, and who had evaluable PK data. The primary PK parameters analysed statistically for EE and LV were $AUC_{0-\infty}$ and $C_{max}$ following single-dose administration (Day 8) and $AUC_{0-\tau, ss}$ and $C_{max, ss}$ following multiple-dose administration (Day 22). In addition, OC trough concentrations on Day 8 and Day 22 were analysed. PK parameters were log-transformed (base e) prior to analysis. Single- (Day 8) and multiple-dose (Day 22) PK profiles of EE and LV were assessed separately. A linear mixed-effects model was applied that included subject as a random effect, and treatment, period, and sequence as fixed effects. The differences between treatments and the control (OC alone) were back-transformed to yield the ratio of the LS geometric mean for each PK parameter relative to the control treatment, and the corresponding 90% CI. An interaction was concluded when the 90% CI for the ratio of the LS geometric mean was not contained within the pre-specified interval (0.80, 1.25). Inter-and intra-subject variability estimates were derived from the mixed-effects model. $T_{max}$ was analysed separately for Day 8 and Day 22 using the nonparametric Wilcoxon rank sum test.

## Safety assessments

Safety was assessed by recording spontaneously reported adverse events and was evaluated at scheduled intervals by physical examination, vital sign measurement (including sitting blood pressure and heart rate), body weight assessments, clinical laboratory tests (including serum biochemistry, hematology, and urinalysis), and 12-lead electrocardiogram recordings.

## Results

### Subjects

A total of 38 healthy female subjects entered the study, 32 of these subjects were randomly assigned to 1 of the 3 sequences. Of the 38 subjects who entered the study, 20 completed the 3 treatment periods, and 18 subjects were withdrawn from the study. The mean (SD) age, weight and body mass index (BMI) for the 32 subjects assigned to treatment were 28 (6.8) years, 69.0 (9.3) kg and 25.1 (3.2) kg/m², respectively. The majority (n = 31) of subjects were Caucasian. Twelve subjects were smokers.

Six subjects were withdrawn during the lead-in period, prior to being randomly assigned to a sequence. Four of these 6 subjects withdrew their consent during the run-in period because they were unable to participate on the required study dates. One subject was withdrawn due to appendicitis. One subject was withdrawn due to protocol non-compliance. The other 12 subjects were withdrawn after being assigned to treatment: 10 subjects due to adverse events and 2 subjects due to withdrawal of consent. Two of the 12 subjects were withdrawn when OC was given alone, 5 when OC was given 1 hour before exenatide, and 5 when OC was given 30 minutes after exenatide.

### Safety and tolerability

No break-through bleeding was reported during the study. The incidence of adverse events considered to be related to OC was generally similar across all treatments. An increase in the incidence of adverse events overall was observed with concomitant administration of exenatide and OC compared to administration of OC alone. The majority of subjects experienced adverse events considered to be related to exenatide. Overall, nausea and vomiting were reported by 91% and 81% of subjects, respectively. All cases of nausea were mild or moderate in severity. One case of vomiting was considered to be severe. Twenty subjects received concomitant medication for the treatment and/or prophylaxis of nausea and vomiting, and 6 subjects were withdrawn from the study due to mild or moderate nausea or vomiting. The incidence of vomiting was higher when the OC was administered 30 minutes after exenatide (74%), compared to 58% when administered 1 hour before

exenatide; however, these incidences were not statistically different.

Seventeen subjects (53%) in the study reported skin-related adverse events, including injection-site rash (11 subjects) and skin rash (8 subjects). The skin-related adverse events were considered by the investigator to be related to exenatide in all but one of the cases. Two subjects were withdrawn from the study due to rash.

There were no clinically important trends in the serum biochemistry, hematology, urinalysis, blood pressure, heart rate, or 12-lead electrocardiogram data from baseline in each treatment period to follow-up.

### Pharmacokinetics

For subjects who discontinued the study prior to completion of all 3 treatment periods, pharmacokinetics (PK) data generated in other completed periods were included in the PK assessments. Although some subjects experienced vomiting on PK-assessment days, none of these data were excluded from analyses as their concentrations at a scheduled time point were within the pre-specified outlier threshold of 3 standard deviations from the mean for the remainder of concentrations at that time point.

### Single-dose pharmacokinetics

Mean plasma concentration time profiles following single-dose administration EE and LV are shown in Figures 1 (EE) and 2 (LV). Mean plasma concentration time profiles associated with OC given 1 hour before exenatide were similar to those observed with OC alone. Mean plasma EE and plasma LV concentration time profiles following OC administration 30 minutes after exenatide were characterised by a reduced $C_{max}$ and delayed $T_{max}$.

Statistical comparisons for single-dose PK parameters are shown in Table 1 (EE) and Table 2 (LV). Consistent with the graphical evaluations, concomitant exenatide

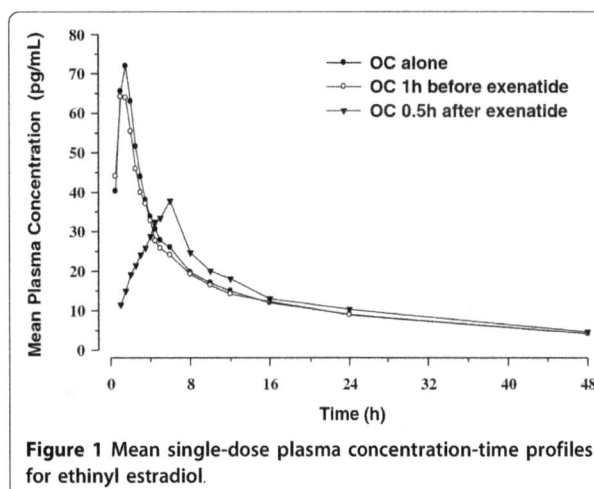

Figure 1 Mean single-dose plasma concentration-time profiles for ethinyl estradiol.

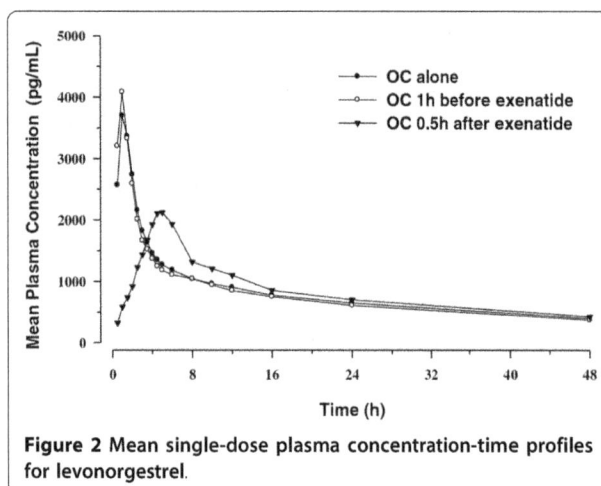

**Figure 2** Mean single-dose plasma concentration-time profiles for levonorgestrel.

administration did not alter the bioavailability (as measured by $AUC_{0-\infty}$) of EE or LV, as the 90% confidence intervals (CI) for the ratios of the least-squares (LS) geometric means were contained within the pre-specified "no effect" range (0.8 to 1.25). Administration of OC 1 hour before exenatide did not result in a change in $C_{max}$ for either EE or LV, but administration of OC 30 minutes after exenatide resulted in reductions in $C_{max}$ of 46% and 41% for EE and LV, respectively, compared to OC given alone. These reductions in $C_{max}$ were accompanied by median $T_{max}$ increases of 4.05 and 3.75 hours for EE and LV, respectively. No differences in trough concentrations of either EE or LV were observed when OC was administered 1 hour before exenatide. Increases in trough concentrations for both EE (24%) and LV (15%) were observed when OC was administered 30 minutes after exenatide.

### Multiple-dose pharmacokinetics
Mean plasma concentration time profiles following repeated daily dosing (Day 22) are presented in Figures 3 (EE) and 4 (LV). Similar to the single-dose PK evaluations, results from the multiple-dose PK assessments demonstrated that administration of OC 30 minutes after exenatide reduced $C_{max}$ and delayed $T_{max}$ for both EE and LV compared with OC given alone. As with the single-dose period, PK differences following repeated daily dosing were mainly evident in the absorptive phase. When OC was given 1 hour before exenatide, no changes in the OC PK profiles were observed.

Between-treatment statistical comparisons for multiple-dose PK parameters are shown in Table 1 (EE) and Table 2 (LV). As with the single-dose data, regardless of timing of exenatide administration relative to OC dosing, no changes in bioavailability ($AUC_{0-\tau, ss}$) of either EE or LV were observed after concomitant repeated daily administration of OC and exenatide. Compared to OC

given alone, repeated daily administration of OC 1 hour before exenatide resulted in a small reduction in EE $C_{max}$ of approximately 15% but did not alter LV $C_{max}$. Reductions in $C_{max}$ were more notable when the OC was administered 30 minutes after exenatide. Repeated daily doses of OC given 30 minutes after exenatide reduced EE and LV $C_{max}$ by 45% and 27%, respectively, compared with OC given alone. Median $T_{max}$ was also delayed by 3 hours and 3.5 hours for EE and LV, respectively, compared with OC alone. As observed in the single-dose results, increases in trough concentrations for both EE (20%) and LV (11%) were observed when OC was administered 30 minutes after exenatide. No differences in trough concentrations of EE or LV were observed when OC was administered 1 hour before exenatide.

### Discussion
In this pharmacokinetic drug-interaction study, co-administration with exenatide did not affect mean plasma AUC of EE and LV under single- or multiple-dose conditions. Furthermore, no decreases in trough concentrations were observed. Additionally, no substantive changes in PK profiles were observed when the OC was administered 1 hour before exenatide. A small effect was observed (90% CI; 0.78, 0.93) in $C_{max}$ when OC was administered alone, however, as the lower confidence bound is close to 0.8, this shift is not likely to be of clinical relevance. Reductions in peak OC concentrations, accompanied by delayed $T_{max}$, were observed with OC administered 30 minutes after exenatide. This effect of exenatide on OC absorption would be expected, due to its action to slow gastric emptying, and is consistent with prior drug-drug interaction studies of exenatide with other orally administered drugs [8-12].

Drug-drug interaction studies with oral contraceptives are generally conducted to understand the potential for concomitantly administered drugs to induce or inhibit cytochrome P450 isoenzyme (CYP) mediated oxidative metabolism of EE [16]. While EE is metabolised by both CYP3A-mediated oxidative metabolism and Phase II metabolism, including glucuronidation and sulfation, the most clinically relevant metabolic pathway is induction or inhibition of CYP3A. Drugs that decrease EE bioavailability via CYP3A induction may potentially result in reduced OC efficacy. The observation that OC AUC concentrations were unaltered in this study confirmed that exenatide does not induce CYP3A. However, the clinical relevance of $C_{max}$ reductions seen in the study (up to 46% for EE and 41% for LV) requires additional consideration.

Reports of large inter-subject variability in concentrations of OCs, with several-fold differences in serum concentrations likely due to inter-individual differences in first-pass metabolism, have been described in the

**Table 1 Ethinyl Estradiol Single- and Multiple-dose Pharmacokinetics: Comparison of Mean Pharmacokinetic Parameters Across Treatments**

| | | Single Dose | | Multiple Dose | |
|---|---|---|---|---|---|
| | | LS Geometric Mean | Comparison to OC alone: Ratio (90% CI) | LS Geometric Mean | Comparison to OC alone: Ratio (90% CI) |
| AUC (pg·h/mL) | OC alone | 718.89 | - | 761.06 | - |
| | 1 h before exenatide | 691.69 | 0.96 (0.91, 1.02) | 716.70 | 0.94 (0.88, 1.01) |
| | 0.5 h after exenatide | 692.56 | 0.96 (0.91, 1.02) | 734.01 | 0.96 (0.90, 1.04) |
| $C_{max}$ (pg/mL) | OC alone | 72.18 | - | 102.15 | - |
| | 1 h before exenatide | 65.49 | 0.91 (0.83, 0.99) | 87.09 | 0.85 (0.78, 0.93) |
| | 0.5 h after exenatide | 38.64 | 0.54 (0.49, 0.58) | 56.32 | 0.55 (0.50, 0.60) |
| 24-h concentration (pg/mL) | OC alone | 8.27 | - | 14.64 | - |
| | 1 h before exenatide | 8.13 | 0.98 (0.92, 1.05) | 15.03 | 1.03 (0.95, 1.11) |
| | 0.5 h after exenatide | 10.25 | 1.24 (1.16, 1.33) | 17.52 | 1.20 (1.10, 1.30) |
| $T_{max}$ median (range) (h) | OC alone | - | 1.50 (0.50-2.50) | - | - |
| | 1 h before exenatide | - | 1.50 (0.50-2.00) | - | - |
| | 0.5 h after exenatide | - | 6.00 (2.00-6.13) | - | - |
| $t_{1/2}$ geometric mean (range) (h) | OC alone | - | 19.5 (13.8-32.1) | - | - |
| | 1 h before exenatide | - | 18.9 (14.0-30.1) | - | - |
| | 0.5 h after exenatide | - | 17.4 (8.78-31.9) | - | - |

literature. Goldzieher et al. [17] have reported that differences in EE concentrations have been shown to vary between ethnic groups, as well as across study sites and, even for a given individual, EE AUCs can vary by almost a factor of 4. This same study group has also reported the existence of high intra- and inter-subject variability in the pharmacokinetics of progestins such as LV [17]. Thus, the magnitude of $C_{max}$ reduction observed in the present study was likely within the inherent PK variability of the OC components.

The current study did not measure OC pharmacodynamics (eg, follicle-stimulating hormone or luteinizing hormone concentrations); therefore, a direct within-study clinical relationship with the observed $C_{max}$ reduction cannot be derived. Importantly, no break-through bleeding was reported. Break-through bleeding may be associated with low concentrations of estrogen-progestin [16,18].

A review of prescription labeling indicates that drug interactions with OCs are deemed to be clinically important, and dosage adjustments are thereby recommended, only when associated with a significant reduction in OC AUC. However, there does not appear to be a well-accepted minimum threshold concentration for pharmacological activity. Importantly, in this study OC AUC was unchanged. Furthermore, trough concentrations did not decrease in the presence of exenatide suggesting that sub-therapeutic concentrations were unlikely.

In the absence of conclusive literature on the exposure-efficacy relationships of OCs, other aspects of OC PK/PD were considered to help understand the possible clinical relevance of the $C_{max}$ decrease observed in the present study. In food-effect studies, OC $C_{max}$ reductions of up to 40% are commonly observed without changes in AUC. Despite this potential effect of food on $C_{max}$, OCs are generally recommended to be taken without regard to food [19], suggesting that PK changes observed in this study are not likely to be clinically relevant. In the current study, the effect of food consumption on the OC PK cannot be clearly differentiated from the effects of exenatide; however, these data reflect conditions under which the 2 drugs are likely to be co-administered, given that exenatide is to be administered within an hour of meals. Thus, in consideration of indirect evidence from food-effect studies, the large inherent variability in OC concentrations, and the

**Table 2 Levonorgestrel Single- and Multiple-dose Pharmacokinetics: Comparison of Mean Pharmacokinetic Parameters Across Treatments**

| | | Single Dose | | Multiple Dose | |
|---|---|---|---|---|---|
| | | LS Geometric Mean | Comparison to OC alone: Ratio (90% CI) | LS Geometric Mean | Comparison to OC alone: Ratio (90% CI) |
| AUC (pg·h/mL) | OC alone | 55698.79 | - | 72974.62 | - |
| | 1 h before exenatide | 53530.64 | 0.96 (0.90, 1.03) | 72952.67 | 1.00 (0.92, 1.09) |
| | 0.5 h after exenatide | 60591.89 | 1.09 (1.01, 1.17) | 76344.29 | 1.05 (0.96, 1.14) |
| $C_{max}$ (pg/mL) | OC alone | 3882.56 | - | 6598.95 | - |
| | 1 h before exenatide | 4061.86 | 1.05 (0.94, 1.16) | 6657.22 | 1.01 (0.92, 1.10) |
| | 0.5 h after exenatide | 2284.25 | 0.59 (0.53, 0.65) | 4800.68 | 0.73 (0.67, 0.79) |
| 24-h concentration (pg/mL) | OC alone | 600.88 | - | 2136.51 | - |
| | 1 h before exenatide | 571.47 | 0.95 (0.89, 1.02) | 2173.05 | 1.02 (0.93, 1.11) |
| | 0.5 h after exenatide | 691.10 | 1.15 (1.07, 1.23) | 2367.68 | 1.11 (1.01, 1.21) |
| $T_{max}$ median (range) (h) | OC alone | - | 1.00 (0.50-2.07) | - | - |
| | 1 h before exenatide | - | 0.92 (0.50-1.50) | - | - |
| | 0.5 h after exenatide | - | 4.75 (3.00-6.02) | - | - |
| $t_{1/2}$ geometric mean (range) (h) | OC alone | - | 33.6 (20.0-78.5) | - | - |
| | 1 h before exenatide | - | 32.1 (19.8-55.7) | - | - |
| | 0.5 h after exenatide | - | 32.6 (17.9-72.4) | - | - |

fact that product labeling suggests changes in OC dosage only in the presence of large changes in OC AUC alone, we conclude that the PK changes observed in the present study are not likely to have clinical implications.

Concomitant administration of exenatide and a combination OC to healthy female subjects resulted in a high incidence of gastrointestinal adverse events. This study used 4-day dose initiation at 5 µg BID, rather than 4 weeks as recommended for exenatide dosing [20], and

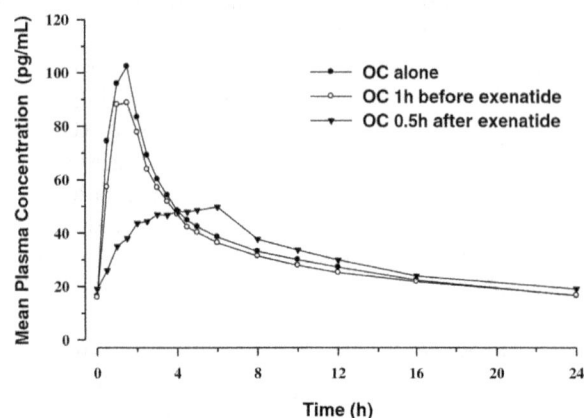

**Figure 3** Mean steady-state plasma concentration-time profiles for ethinyl estradiol.

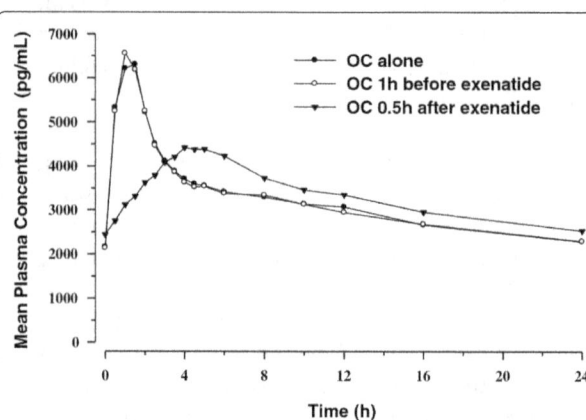

**Figure 4** Mean steady-state plasma concentration-time profiles for levonorgestrel.

this may have contributed to the poor tolerability. Furthermore, cross-study comparisons have suggested that exenatide administration may result in a higher incidence of gastrointestinal adverse events in healthy subjects compared with patients with type 2 diabetes [8]. More specifically, the high incidence of nausea and vomiting observed in the present drug-drug interaction study has not been observed in large clinical trials of exenatide-treated patients with type 2 diabetes [21-24]. Additionally, although there were no unexpected adverse events observed in this study, the incidence of skin-related adverse events among exenatide-treated subjects (53%) was higher than the incidence observed in previous clinical studies [21-24].

## Conclusions

This study evaluated the potential effect of subcutaneously administered exenatide (10 µg BID) on the single and multiple doses pharmacokinetics of a combination OC (EE/LV). No pharmacokinetic interaction was observed when the OC was administered an hour prior to exenatide treatment. However, administration of the OC 30 minutes after exenatide therapy was associated with a reduced $C_{max}$ with a delayed $T_{max}$ of EE and LV. The observed reduction in $C_{max}$ is likely of limited importance as co-administration of exenatide did not cause significant changes in the overall bioavailability of EE or LV after single or multiple doses. For oral medications that are dependent on threshold concentrations for efficacy, such as contraceptives and antibiotics, patients should be advised to take those drugs at least 1 hour before exenatide injection.

### Acknowledgements
The contributing coauthors would like to thank the clinical trial investigators and their staffs at the participating research sites, Shobha Reddy for her assistance with the analyses, and Laura Bean Warner of i3Statprobe for her assistance with preparing this manuscript.

### Author details
[1]Eli Lilly and Company, Lilly Corporate Center, Indianapolis, IN, USA. [2]Eli Lilly and Company, Lilly Research Center, Earl Wood Manor, Windlesham, Surrey GU20 6PH, UK.

### Authors' contributions
PAK, MES, HL, MM, and KM participated in the design of the study. PAK, HL, MES, and JN have been involved in drafting the manuscript. All authors have participated in the analysis and interpretation of data, and the critical revision for important intellectual content. All authors approved the version to be published.

### Competing interests
This study was sponsored by Amylin Pharmaceuticals, Inc. and Eli Lilly and Company. Sponsors were involved in the study design, protocol development, and the collection, review, and analysis of the data. Authors are employees of Eli Lilly and Company.

### References
1. Reddy S, Park S, Fineman M, Jay L, Carter M, Reynolds L, Sanburn N, Kothare PA: Clinical pharmacokinetics of exenatide in patients with type 2 diabetes [abstract]. AAPS J 2005, 7:M1285.
2. Copley K, McCowen K, Hiles R, Nielsen LL, Young A, Parkes DG: Investigation of exenatide elimination and its in vivo and in vitro degradation. Curr Drug Metabol 2006, 7:367-374.
3. Kolterman OG, Buse JB, Fineman MS, Gaines E, Heintz S, Bicsak TA, Taylor K, Kim D, Aisporna M, Wang Y, Baron AD: Synthetic exendin-4 (exenatide) significantly reduces postprandial and fasting plasma glucose in subjects with type 2 diabetes. J Clin Endocrinol Metab 2003, 88:3082-3089.
4. Kolterman OG, Kim DD, Shen L, Ruggles JA, Nielsen LL, Fineman MS, Baron AD: Pharmacokinetics, pharmacodynamics, and safety of exenatide in patients with type 2 diabetes mellitus. Am J Health Syst Pharm 2005, 62:173-181.
5. Linnebjerg H, Park S, Kothare PA, Trautmann ME, Mace K, Fineman M, Wilding I, Nauck M, Horowitz M: Effect of exenatide on gastric emptying and relationship to postprandial glycemia in type 2 diabetes. Regul Pept 2008, 151:123-129.
6. Verdich C, Flint A, Gutzwiller JP, Näslund E, Beglinger C, Hellström PM, Long SJ, Morgan LM, Holst JJ, Astrup A: A meta-analysis of the effect of glucagon-like peptide-1 (7-36) amide on ad libitum energy intake in humans. J Clin Endocrinol Metab 2001, 86:4382-4389.
7. Edwards CM, Stanley SA, Davis R, Brynes AE, Frost GS, Seal LJ, Ghatei MA, Bloom SR: Exendin-4 reduces fasting and postprandial glucose and decreases energy intake in healthy volunteers. Am J Physiol Endocrinol Metab 2001, 281:E155-E161.
8. Kothare PA, Soon DK, Linnebjerg H, Park S, Chan C, Yeo A, Lim M, Mace KF, Wise SD: Effect of exenatide on the steady-state pharmacokinetics of digoxin. J Clin Pharmacol 2005, 45:1032-1037.
9. Soon D, Kothare PA, Linnebjerg H, Park S, Yuen E, Mace KF, Wise SD: Effect of exenatide on the pharmacokinetics and pharmacodynamics of warfarin in healthy Asian men. J Clin Pharmacol 2006, 46:1179-1187.
10. Kothare PA, Linnebjerg H, Skrivanek Z, Reddy S, Mace K, Pena A, Han J, Fineman M, Mitchell M: Exenatide effects on statin pharmacokinetics and lipid response. Int J Clin Pharmacol Ther 2007, 45:114-120.
11. Linnebjerg H, Kothare P, Park S, Mace K, Mitchell M: The effect of exenatide on lisinopril pharmacodynamics and pharmacokinetics in patients with hypertension. Int J Clin Pharmacol Ther 2009, 47:651-658.
12. Blase E, Taylor K, Gao HY, Wintle M, Fineman M: Pharmacokinetics of an oral drug (acetaminophen) administered at various times in relation to subcutaneous injection of exenatide (exendin-4) in healthy subjects. J Clin Pharmacol 2005, 45:570-577.
13. Zhang H, Cui D, Wang B, Han YH, Balimane P, Yang Z, Sinz M, Rodrigues AD: Pharmacokinetic drug interactions involving 17[alpha]-ethinylestradiol: a new look at an old drug. Clin Pharmacokinet 2007, 46:133-157.
14. Goldzieher JW, Stanczyk FZ: Oral contraceptives and individual variability of circulating levels of ethinyl estradiol and progestins. Contraception 2008, 78:4-9.
15. Hall SD, Wang Z, Huang SM, Hamman MA, Vasavada N, Adigun AQ, Hilligoss JK, Miller M, Gorski JC: The interaction between St John's wort and an oral contraceptive. Clin Pharmacol Ther 2003, 74:525-535.
16. Boyd RA, Zegarac EA, Eldon MA: The effect of food on the bioavailability of norethindrone and ethinyl estradiol from norethindrone acetate/ethinyl estradiol tablets intended for continuous hormone replacement therapy. J Clin Pharmacol 2003, 43:52-58.
17. Byetta (package insert). San Diego, CA: Amylin Pharmaceuticals, Inc; 2008 [http://documents.byetta.com/Byetta_PI.pdf].
18. Buse JB, Henry RR, Han J, Kim DD, Fineman MS, Baron AD: Exenatide-113 Clinical Study Group: Effects of exenatide (exendin-4) on glycemic control over 30 weeks in sulfonylurea-treated patients with type 2 diabetes. Diabetes Care 2004, 27:2628-2635.
19. DeFronzo RA, Ratner RE, Han J, Kim DD, Fineman MS, Baron AD: Effects of exenatide (exendin-4) on glycemic control and weight over 30 weeks in metformin-treated patients with type 2 diabetes. Diabetes Care 2005, 28:1092-1100.
20. Kendall DM, Riddle MC, Rosenstock J, Zhuang D, Kim DD, Fineman MS, Baron AD: Effects of exenatide (exendin-4) on glycemic control over 30 weeks in patients with type 2 diabetes treated with metformin and a sulfonylurea. Diabetes Care 2005, 28:1083-1091.

21. Klonoff DC, Buse JB, Nielsen LL, Guan X, Bowlus CL, Holcombe JH, Wintle ME, Maggs DG: **Exenatide effects on diabetes, obesity, cardiovascular risk factors and hepatic biomarkers in patients with type 2 diabetes treated for at least 3 years.** *Curr Med Res Opin* 2008, **24**:275-286.
22. World Medical Association Declaration of Helsinki: **ethical principles for medical research involving human subjects.** *JAMA* 2000, **284**:3043-3045.
23. **Directive 2001/20/EC of the European Parliament and of the Council of 4 April 2001.** The European Parliament and the Council of the European Union;[http://www.ema.europa.eu/ema/index.jsp?curl=pages/includes/document/document_detail.jsp?webContentId=WC500011204&murl=menus/document_library/document_library.jsp&mid=WC0b01ac058009a3dc].
24. Li W, Li YH, Li AC, Zhou S, Naidong W: **Simultaneous determination of norethindrone and ethinyl estradiol in human plasma by high performance liquid chromatography with tandem mass spectrometry-experiences on developing a highly selective method using derivatization reagent for enhancing sensitivity.** *J Chromatogr B Analyt Technol Biomed Life Sci* 2005, **825**:223-232.

# 11

# Impact of information letters on the reporting rate of adverse drug reactions and the quality of the reports: a randomized controlled study

Marie-Louise Johansson[1], Staffan Hägg[2] and Susanna M Wallerstedt[1*]

## Abstract

**Background:** Spontaneous reporting of adverse drug reactions (ADRs) is an important method for pharmacovigilance, but under-reporting and poor quality of reports are major limitations. The aim of this study was to evaluate if repeated one-page ADR information letters affect (i) the reporting rate of ADRs and (ii) the quality of the ADR reports.

**Methods:** All 151 primary healthcare units in the Region Västra Götaland, Sweden, were randomly allocated (1:1) to an intervention (n = 77) or a control group (n = 74). The intervention consisted of one-page ADR information letters administered at three occasions during 2008 to all physicians and nurses in the intervention units. The number of ADR reports received from the 151 units was registered, as was the quality of the reports, which was defined as high if the ADR was to be reported according to Swedish regulations, that is, if the ADR was (i) serious, (ii) unexpected, and/or (iii) related to the use of new drugs and not labelled as common in the Summary of Product Characteristics. A questionnaire was administered to evaluate if the ADR information letter had reached the intended recipient.

**Results:** Before the intervention, no significant differences in reporting rate or number of high quality reports could be detected between the randomization groups. In 2008, 79 reports were sent from 37 intervention units and 52 reports from 30 control units (mean number of reports per unit ± standard deviation: 1.0 ± 2.5 vs. 0.7 ± 1.2, P = 0.34). The number of high quality reports was higher in intervention units than in control units (37 vs. 15 reports, 0.5 ± 0.9 vs. 0.2 ± 0.6, P = 0.048). According to the returned questionnaires (n = 1,292, response rate 57%), more persons in the intervention than in the control group had received (29% vs. 19%, P < 0.0001) and read (31% vs. 26%, P < 0.0001) an ADR information letter.

**Conclusions:** This study suggests that repeated ADR information letters to physicians and nurses do not increase the ADR reporting rate, but may increase the number of high quality reports.

## Background

Clinical trials contribute greatly to knowledge on drug safety. However, uncommon adverse drug reactions (ADRs) and ADRs in certain patient groups not included in clinical trials, e.g. children and older people with many concomitant diseases and medications, cannot be expected to be detected in these trials. Hence post-marketing surveillance on effects of drugs in clinical practice is essential and spontaneous reporting of ADRs

has shown to be an important method to increase drug safety knowledge [1]. In Sweden, physicians, dentists, and nurses are obliged to report (i) serious ADRs, (ii) ADRs not mentioned in the summary of product characteristics (SPC), (iii) ADRs related to the use of new drugs (≤ 2 years on the market) except those labelled as common in the SPC, and (iv) ADRs which incidence seems to increase [2]. Reports concerning the three first points may be most important as far as pharmacovigilance is concerned since they may result in relevant ADR signals, defined as reported information on a possible causal relationship between a drug and an adverse event, the relationship being unknown or incompletely documented

* Correspondence: susanna.wallerstedt@pharm.gu.se
[1]Department of Clinical Pharmacology and Regional Pharmacovigilance Centre, Sahlgrenska University Hospital, Gothenburg, Sweden
Full list of author information is available at the end of the article

previously [3]. Thus, the reporting of ADRs ideally should be focused on such ADRs.

A major limitation of the spontaneous reporting system is that only a small part of all ADRs are reported [4]. A review shows that factors associated with under-reporting include ignorance (only severe ADRs need to be reported), diffidence (fear of appearing ridiculous for reporting merely suspected ADRs), lethargy (e.g. lack of interest or time), indifference (one case from an individual doctor does not contribute to medical knowledge), insecurity (causality between a drug and an adverse event is hard to determine), and complacency (only safe drugs are allowed on the market) [5]. Hence, methods to improve the reporting rate of ADRs could address one or more of these obstacles. Ignorance, diffidence, indifference, insecurity, and complacency can be defeated by education and distribution of drug safety information; methods which have been shown to increase the ADR reporting rate [6-9]. Education may also have positive effects on lethargy, but availability of clinical research assistants may be more effective as far as this obstacle is concerned [10]. Methods which reward individual reporters could also be interesting alternatives to increase the reporting, e.g. lottery tickets [11] or detailed feedback [12]. In addition, allowing other categories of reporters could be beneficial, e.g. nurses [13] and patients/consumers [14].

The methods mentioned above differ in efforts and costs, and there is a need for additional easily managed methods to improve ADR reporting which can be maintained over time without too much efforts or costs. Such a method may be distribution of written information. We have previously shown that such information via e-mail had no apparent effect on the reporting of ADRs, although an increase in the reporting rate in general was noted [8]. From our own experience, we know that e-mails are often overlooked and thus the effect on information via this route, although cheap and easily managed, may have limited effects. In the present study, we hypothesized that written information in the format of a letter administered to health care personnel may have a larger impact on the reporting rate. Indeed, a previous time series analysis has shown positive effects on reporting rate when an ADR bulletin was administered quarterly to physicians [7]. To the best of our knowledge, however, the impact of written ADR information letters administered to healthcare personnel on reporting of ADRs has previously not been evaluated in a randomized controlled study. Moreover, knowledge lacks on the impact of such information on which ADRs are reported, an aspect which is important since some ADRs are more valuable in the pharmacovigilance work, as previously mentioned. The aim of the present study was thus to evaluate if repeated ADR information letters administered to physicians and nurses in primary healthcare

units through the secretary of the unit can affect (i) the reporting rate of ADRs and (ii) the quality of the ADR reports.

## Methods

All 151 primary healthcare units in the Region Västra Götaland, Sweden, were randomly allocated (1:1) to an intervention or a control group. A primary healthcare unit generally consists of several general practitioners and nurses who serve patients in a limited geographic area, although patients may choose to attend another unit at their convenience. The units were expected to report ADRs to various extents. Furthermore, in 2007, 63 of the units were included in a randomized controlled trial of repeated e-mails with ADR information [8]. Hence, the allocation was stratified according to number of ADR reports in 2007 and whether or not the unit had received the repeated drug safety e-mails. A person not involved in the study and without knowledge about the study protocol performed the randomization procedure.

The intervention consisted of a one-page ADR information letter which was sent to the secretary of each unit with an instruction letter that it should be distributed to all physicians and nurses at the unit. The number of letters supplied for each unit was estimated based on publicly available information on the staffing of the units, and the secretary was instructed to copy the information letter if more letters were needed.

The ADR information letters were constructed by the authors of this study, who, at the time of the study, all worked at the regional pharmacovigilance centre which serves the Region Västra Götaland. The letters consisted of (i) the heading "ADR Information Letter", (ii) a current case report of an ADR and (iii) instructions on what and how to report [see Additional files 1, 2 and 3]. The letters were sent in January, May, and September 2008.

ADR reports from the included primary healthcare units were extracted from the SWEdish Drug Information System (SWEDIS), the Swedish ADR database where all ADR reports are registered, after being assessed for e.g. causality and seriousness according to the definitions by the World Health Organization [3]. The number of reports from each primary healthcare unit was thus registered, as was the quality of the report, which was defined as high if the ADR was to be reported according to the Swedish regulations on ADR reporting, that is, if the ADR was (i) serious, (ii) unexpected, that is, not labelled in the SPC, and/or (iii) related to the use of new drugs ($\leq$ 2 years on the market) and not labelled as common in the SPC. Trained and experienced staff working at the regional pharmacovigilance centre conducted the assessments.

In January 2009, questionnaires were supplied to the secretaries of the intervention and the control units, to be distributed to all physicians and nurses, using a procedure similar to the one described above. The questionnaire included questions as to whether the ADR information letter had been received and read [see Additional file 4]. The questionnaire was to be answered anonymously, and questionnaires administered to intervention and control units differed in the first letter of one word (capital or lower case), in order to distinguish the origin of the returned questionnaire (intervention or control unit).

## Statistics

Statistical analyses were conducted using SPSS 14.0. Mann-Whitney test was used for between-group comparisons of number of reports per unit. A P-value < 0.05 was considered significant. Where appropriate mean (standard deviation) and median (interquartile range [IQR]) was used.

## Results

A total of 77 primary healthcare units were randomly allocated to the intervention group, and the remaining 74 units to the control group. As for characteristics of the randomized units, the median (IQR) numbers of physicians and nurses working at intervention units were 6 (4-7) and 9 (7-13), respectively. The corresponding numbers for the control units were 5 (4-7) and 9 (6-13), respectively. The reporting rate the year before the intervention was 62 reports from 32 (42%) intervention units, and 55 reports from 31 (42%) control units (mean number of reports per unit ± standard deviation (SD): 0.8 ± 1.4 vs.0.74 ± 1.1, P = 0.93). The number of reports per unit ranged from 0 to 8 (intervention) and 0 to 4 (control). There was no statistically significant difference in the number of high quality reports reported by the intervention and control units (n = 30 vs. n = 19, 0.4 ± 0.8 vs. 0.3 ± 0.6, P = 0.21).

In 2008, a total of 131 reports were received from the participating healthcare units; 79 reports were sent from 37 intervention units and 52 reports from 30 control units (mean number of reports per unit ± SD: 1.0 ± 2.5 vs. 0.7 ± 1.2, P = 0.34, Table 1). The number of reports per unit ranged from 0 to 20 (intervention group) and 0 to 7 (control group).

The number of high quality reports was higher in intervention units than in control units (37 vs. 15 reports, mean number of reports per unit ± SD: 0.5 ± 0.9 vs. 0.2 ± 0.6, P = 0.048, Table 1). Summarized, these reports (n = 52, 40% of all reports) concerned (i) serious ADRs (n = 16 [12% of all reports]), (ii) unexpected ADRs (n = 33 [25% of all reports]), and/or (iii) new drugs (n = 11 [8% of all reports]), as presented in Table 1. The high quality reports concerned 44 substances. Varenicline, acetylsalicylic acid, enalapril, citalopram, and levonorgestrel were reported more than once, and the details of the reports concerning these substances are described in Table 2.

A total of 845 physicians and 1,423 nurses worked in the primary healthcare units. A total of 1,292 questionnaires were duly filled and returned. The response rate was therefore 57% (physicians, n = 556; nurses, n = 711; other professions, n = 17 [these were not intended to receive and respond to the questionnaire, but did so anyway]). A total of 300 respondents reported having received at least one ADR information letter during 2008 (23%), and 362 (28%) had read at least one ADR information letter during the year. More persons in the intervention group than in the control group had received (29% vs. 19%, P < 0.0001) and read (31% vs. 26%, P < 0.0001) an ADR information letter during 2008. In the intervention group, more physicians than nurses had received (36% vs. 28%, P < 0.015) but not read (36% vs. 37%, P = 0.89) the ADR information letter.

**Table 1 Description of the reporting of adverse reactions from the randomized primary healthcare units in 2008**

| | Control units (n = 74) | Intervention units (n = 77) | P-value |
|---|---|---|---|
| Total number of reports | 52 | 79 | |
| Number of reporting units (% of all units) | 30 (40.5%) | 37 (48.1%) | |
| Mean number of reports per unit (± SD)** | 0.70 ± 1.21 | 1.03 ± 2.46 | 0.34 |
| Total number of high quality reports (% of all reports)* | 15 (29%) | 37 (48%) | |
| Serious | 4 | 12 | |
| Unexpected | 13 | 20 | |
| New drug and not common ADR* | 4 | 7 | |
| Mean number of high quality reports per unit (± SD) | 0.20 ± 0.57 | 0.47 ± 0.94 | 0.048 |

*A high quality report was defined as a report concerning an ADR which should be reported according to Swedish regulations, that is, an ADR which was (i) serious, (ii) unexpected, and/or (iii) related to the use of new drugs and not labelled as common in the SPC.

**Mean ± SD is presented although the non-parametric Mann Whitney test was used for comparisons between randomization groups, since median (interquartile range) would provide limited information.

ADR, adverse drug reaction; SD, standard deviation; SPC, summary of product characteristics

**Table 2 Description of high quality reports concerning substances reported more than once**

| Age (years) | Sex | Suspected substance/s | Dose | ADR diagnosis | Serious* | Unexpected* | New drug and not common ADR** | Treatment duration | Time to ADR onset | Positive dechallange | Concomitant medication | Causality assessment* |
|---|---|---|---|---|---|---|---|---|---|---|---|---|
| 55 | F | Acetylsalicylic acid/caffeine | 500/50 mg | Pruritus | N | Y | N | 1 dose | Hours | NR | NR | Probable |
| 63 | F | Acetylsalicylic acid | NR | Haemorrhagic gastric ulcer | Y | N | N | NR | NR | Y | Candesartan | Possible |
| 80 | F | Acetylsalicylic acid | NR | Gastrointestinal haemorrhage | Y | N | N | 8 weeks | 8 weeks | Died | NR | Possible |
| 56 | F | Citalopram | 60 mg | Nail disorder | N | Y | N | NR | NR | Medication continued | Folic acid Propiomazine Diazepam Levothyroxine | Possible |
| 78 | F | Citalopram Enalapril Dextropropoxyphene Omeprazole Bendroflumethiazide | 20 mg 15 mg 150 mg 20 mg 5 mg | Hyponatraemia Confusion | Y | N | N | NR | NR | Medication continued | Dipyridamole Budesonide/formoterol Tiotropium Cholecalciferol/calcium Macrogol, combinations Vitamin B-complex Paracetamol Cyanocobalamin Sodium picosulfate Ferrous sulphate Levothyroxine Antacids, salt combination Acetylcysteine | Possible |
| 38 | F | Enalapril | 5 mg | Yawning | N | Y | N | 3 weeks | Days | Y | N | Possible |
| 69 | F | Enalapril | 20 mg | Diplopia | N | Y | N | NR | NR | Medication continued | N | Possible |
| 35 | F | Levonorgestrel | NR | Fatigue Myalgia | N | Y Y | N | 15 months | Days | Y | Paracetamol Tramadol | Possible |
| 38 | F | Levonorgestrel | NR | Ectopic pregnancy | Y | N | N | 4 years | 4 years | Y | N | Possible |
| 49 | M | Varenicline | 1 mg | Thrombophlebitis | N | Y | Y | 2 months | 2 months | NR | Atenolol | Possible |
| 61 | F | Varenicline | 2 mg | Confusion | N | Y | Y | 2 weeks | NR | Y | Dipyridamole Simvastatin | Possible |
| 62 | F | Varenicline | NR | Macula-degeneration | N | Y | Y | 4 months | 5 months | NR | NR | Unclassifiable |
| 66 | F | Varenicline | NR | Oedema legs | Y | Y | Y | 5 weeks | 4 weeks | N | Naproxen Omeprazole Folic acid | Possible |

*According to the World Health Organization (WHO)[3].

**Concerning new drugs and not labelled as common in the SPC.

ADR, adverse drug reaction; F, female; M, male; N, no; NR, not reported; Y, yes.

## Discussion

In the present study, no effect of repeated one-page ADR information letters on the overall reporting rate could be detected. The results are in contrast to the findings by Castel et al., who reported an increased reporting rate after distribution of a drug safety bulletin [7]. One explanation for the divergent findings may be that the methodologies to evaluate differences in reporting rate differ between the studies; we used a randomized controlled design whereas Castel et al. used a time series methodology. Nevertheless, other interventions may be more useful when the number of ADR reports is to be increased, such as education [6,9] or detailed feedback to the reporting physician [12].

Our results show that more high quality reports were received from intervention than control units, that is, the reports more often concerned ADRs which should be reported according to Swedish regulations. Thus, repeated ADR information letters may represent a valuable means to increase the number of reports which should actually be reported. One may speculate that a combination of such letters with an educational intervention may be even more effective as regards this aspect, since the latter also has been shown beneficial [6]. Indeed, from a pharmacovigilance perspective, it is of importance that ADR reporting is focused on ADRs which are most likely to contribute to increased drug safety knowledge. ADR reports concerning well-known non-serious conditions may thus be of limited value since these contribute little to ADR signals. On the contrary, these reports constitute background noise, which may make detection of ADR signals more difficult at least as far as statistical signal detection methods within ADR databases are concerned, e.g. Proportional Reporting Ratios (PRR) [15] and Bayesian Confidence Propagation Neural Network (BCPNN) [16].

Varenicline was the most frequently reported substance in high quality reports. This substance was registered for smoking cessation in 2006 and thus the reports concerned a new drug. In addition, these reports also concerned unexpected ADRs. Indeed, the majority of high quality reports concerned unexpected ADRs. This finding may not be surprising since primary healthcare personnel probably observe serious ADRs less frequently than hospital personnel due to the definition of a serious ADR; any untoward medical occurrence that, at any dose (i) results in death; (ii) requires inpatient hospitalization or prolongation of existing hospitalization; (iii) results in persistent or significant disability/incapacity; or (iv) is life-threatening [3].

Interestingly, 84 out of 151 primary healthcare units (56%) did not report any ADR during 2008. This finding supports a high degree of under-reporting [4], and may indicate that primary healthcare personnel is an important target for interventions for improved reporting of ADRs.

Significantly more questionnaire responders had received and read the ADR information letters in the intervention group. However, the figures were generally low, indicating that ADR information letters are not prioritized reading for healthcare personnel in clinical practice. Interestingly, many questionnaire responders in the control units reported having received and read the ADR information letter. The intervention thus seems to have spilled over to the control units. Physicians and nurses may work in more than one primary healthcare unit, that is, both in the intervention group and in the control group. Furthermore, the units all belong to the same organization and information may thus easily pass from one unit to another. Another explanation for the finding that the ADR information letters were read by personnel in the control units is that ADR information from other sources, e.g. the pharmaceutical industry, may have been administered to the primary healthcare during 2008.

An important limitation of the present study is the small number of reports received from the small number of primary healthcare units. Indeed, given the available number of primary healthcare units in the region and the final results, the power of the present study to detect differences between the groups ended at 17%.

Another limitation is that our definition of quality of ADR reports was quite strict and related only to the Swedish regulations on ADR reporting. Thus, the information content of the report as regards other important aspects were not evaluated, such as factors of importance for the assessment of the strength of the relationship between the drug/s and the event/s, i.e. time to ADR onset, and response to dechallenge and rechallenge.

## Conclusions

Repeated ADR information letters to physicians and nurses was not found to increase the ADR reporting rate, However, such an intervention may still be favorable from a pharmacovigilance perspective since it resulted in an increased number of reports concerning ADRs which should be reported according to Swedish regulations.

## Additional material

**Additional file 1: ADR information letter I**. The first ADR information letter sent to physicians and nurses in the intervention units (translated to English).

**Additional file 2: ADR information letter II**. The second ADR information letter sent to physicians and nurses in the intervention units (translated to English).

**Additional file 3: ADR information letter III**. The third ADR information letter sent to physicians and nurses in the intervention units (translated to English).

**Additional file 4: Questionnaire**. Questionnaire sent to physicians and nurses in intervention and control units (translated to English).

## Acknowledgements
The authors are grateful to John Karlsson, Department of Clinical Pharmacology, for the randomization procedure. The study was funded by research grants from the Swedish Foundation for Strategic Research. The authors' work was independent of the funders.

## Author details
[1]Department of Clinical Pharmacology and Regional Pharmacovigilance Centre, Sahlgrenska University Hospital, Gothenburg, Sweden. [2]Department of Drug Research/Clinical Pharmacology, Linköping University, Linköping, Sweden.

## Authors' contributions
MLJ carried out the acquisition of data. SMW conceived the study, performed the statistical analyses and drafted the manuscript. All authors contributed to the design of the study, revised the manuscript, and read and approved the final manuscript.

## Competing interests
The authors declare that they have no competing interests.

## References

1. Wysowski DK, Swartz L: **Adverse drug event surveillance and drug withdrawals in the United States, 1969-2002: the importance of reporting suspected reactions.** *Arch Intern Med* 2005, **165**(12):1363-1369.
2. Medical Products Agency: **Code of statutes.** 2006.
3. **WHO Collaborating Centre for International Drug Monitoring.** [http://www.who-umc.org].
4. Hazell L, Shakir SA: **Under-reporting of adverse drug reactions: a systematic review.** *Drug Saf* 2006, **29**(5):385-396.
5. Lopez-Gonzalez E, Herdeiro MT, Figueiras A: **Determinants of under-reporting of adverse drug reactions: a systematic review.** *Drug Saf* 2009, **32**(1):19-31.
6. Figueiras A, Herdeiro MT, Polonia J, Gestal-Otero JJ: **An educational intervention to improve physician reporting of adverse drug reactions: a cluster-randomized controlled trial.** *Jama* 2006, **296**(9):1086-1093.
7. Castel JM, Figueras A, Pedros C, Laporte JR, Capella D: **Stimulating adverse drug reaction reporting: effect of a drug safety bulletin and of including yellow cards in prescription pads.** *Drug Saf* 2003, **26**(14):1049-1055.
8. Johansson ML, Brunlof G, Edward C, Wallerstedt SM: **Effects of e-mails containing ADR information and a current case report on ADR reporting rate and quality of reports.** *Eur J Clin Pharmacol* 2009, **65**(5):511-514.
9. Tabali M, Jeschke E, Bockelbrink A, Witt CM, Willich SN, Ostermann T, Matthes H: **Educational intervention to improve physician reporting of adverse drug reactions (ADRs) in a primary care setting in complementary and alternative medicine.** *BMC Public Health* 2009, **9**:274.
10. Gony M, Badie K, Sommet A, Jacquot J, Baudrin D, Gauthier P, Montastruc JL, Bagheri H: **Improving adverse drug reaction reporting in hospitals: results of the French Pharmacovigilance in Midi-Pyrenees region (PharmacoMIP) network 2-year pilot study.** *Drug Saf* 2010, **33**(5):409-416.
11. Backstrom M, Mjorndal T: **A small economic inducement to stimulate increased reporting of adverse drug reactions-a way of dealing with an old problem?** *Eur J Clin Pharmacol* 2006, **62**(5):381-385.
12. Wallerstedt SM, Brunlof G, Johansson ML, Tukukino C, Ny L: **Reporting of adverse drug reactions may be influenced by feedback to the reporting doctor.** *Eur J Clin Pharmacol* 2007, **63**(5):505-508.
13. Backstrom M, Ekman E, Mjorndal T: **Adverse drug reaction reporting by nurses in Sweden.** *Eur J Clin Pharmacol* 2007, **63**(6):613-618.
14. Aagaard L, Nielsen LH, Hansen EH: **Consumer reporting of adverse drug reactions: a retrospective analysis of the Danish adverse drug reaction database from 2004 to 2006.** *Drug Saf* 2009, **32**(11):1067-1074.
15. Evans SJ, Waller PC, Davis S: **Use of proportional reporting ratios (PRRs) for signal generation from spontaneous adverse drug reaction reports.** *Pharmacoepidemiol Drug Saf* 2001, **10**(6):483-486.
16. Bate A, Lindquist M, Orre R, Edwards IR, Meyboom RH: **Data-mining analyses of pharmacovigilance signals in relation to relevant comparison drugs.** *Eur J Clin Pharmacol* 2002, **58**(7):483-490.

# 12

# Pharmacokinetic and pharmacodynamic characterization of a new formulation containing synergistic proportions of interferons alpha-2b and gamma (HeberPAG®) in patients with mycosis fungoides: an open-label trial

Yanelda García-Vega[1], Idrian García-García[1], Sonia E Collazo-Caballero[2], Egla E Santely-Pravia[2], Alieski Cruz-Ramírez[1], Ángela D Tuero-Iglesias[1], Cristian Alfonso-Alvarado[2], Mileidys Cabrera-Placeres[2], Nailet Castro-Basart[2], Yaquelín Duncan-Roberts[1], Tania I Carballo-Treto[3], Josanne Soto-Matos[3], Yoandy Izquierdo-Toledo[4], Dania Vázquez-Blomquist[4], Elizeth García-Iglesias[1] and Iraldo Bello-Rivero[1]*

## Abstract

**Background:** The synergistic combination of interferon (IFN) alpha-2b and IFN gamma results in more potent *in vitro* biological effects mediated by both IFNs. The aim of this investigation was to evaluate by first time the pharmacokinetics and pharmacodynamics of this combination in patients with mycosis fungoides.

**Methods:** An exploratory, prospective, open-label clinical trial was conducted. Twelve patients, both genders, 18 to 75 years-old, with mycosis fungoides at stages IB to III, were eligible for the study. All of them received intramuscularly a single high dose ($23 \times 10^6$ IU) of a novel synergistic IFN mixture (HeberPAG®) for pharmacokinetic and pharmacodynamic studies. Serum IFN alpha-2b and IFN gamma concentrations were measured during 96 hours by commercial enzyme immunoassays (EIA) specific for each IFN. Other blood IFN-inducible markers and laboratory variables were used as pharmacodynamics and safety criteria.

**Results:** The pharmacokinetic evaluation by EIA yielded a similar pattern for both IFNs that are also in agreement with the well-known described profiles for these molecules when these are administered separately. The average values for main parameters were: Cmax: 263 and 9.3 pg/mL; Tmax: 9.5 and 6.9 h; AUC: 4483 and 87.5 pg.h/mL, half-life ($t_{1/2}$): 4.9 and 13.4 h; mean residence time (MRT): 13.9 and 13.5 h, for serum IFN alpha-2b and IFN gamma, respectively. The pharmacodynamic variables were strongly stimulated by simultaneous administration of both IFNs: serum neopterin and beta-2 microglobulin levels ($\beta_2$M), and stimulation of 2'-5' oligoadenylate synthetase (OAS1) mRNA expression. The most encouraging data was the high increment of serum neopterin, 8.0 ng/mL at 48 h, not been described before for any unmodified or pegylated IFN. Additionally, $\beta_2$M concentration doubled the pre-dose value at 24–48 hours. For both variables the values remained clearly upper baseline levels at 96 hours.

**Conclusions:** HeberPAG® possesses improved pharmacodynamic properties that may be very useful in the oncologic setting. Efficacy trials can be carried out to confirm these findings.

**Trial registration:** Registro Público Cubano de Ensayos Clínicos RPCEC00000130

* Correspondence: iraldo.bello@cigb.edu.cu
[1]Clinical Investigation Department, Center for Genetic Engineering and Biotechnology, P.O. Box 6332, Havana, Cuba
Full list of author information is available at the end of the article

## Background

Similar to other low molecular weight protein drugs, alpha or gamma interferons (IFNs) have a relatively short serum half-life. Consequently, if vascular retention is considered to be desired for enhanced efficacy, strategies that can improve a drug's pharmacokinetic (PK) and pharmacodynamic (PD) properties might improve its therapeutic benefits. Novel injectable drug delivery systems have been developed in attempts to improve PK/PD properties of therapeutic peptides and proteins. This can be achieved either by modification of the drug molecule itself (e.g. pegylation) or through a change in formulation (e.g. controlled-release formulations, liposomal preparations) [1].

Another alternative is to potentiate the pharmacodynamics of the therapeutic drug by the combination of two active principles that can act synergistically. This approach could have the same potential advantages of novel delivery mechanisms that include an increased or prolonged pharmacological activity without additional toxicity, less frequent injections, and a better patient's compliance and quality of life.

IFNs have been widely used in the treatment of human solid and hematological malignancies. However, despite antitumor activity of IFNs is well-known at present, no major advances have been achieved in the last decade. A hopeful option could be the combination of IFN alpha-2b and IFN gamma, two molecules with recognized synergistic antiproliferative effects on several tumor cell lines [2].

Takaoka *et al.* demonstrated in mouse embryonic fibroblasts that IFN gamma response is substantially augmented through autocrine IFN alpha/beta. Additionally, they observed that cross-recruitment and phosphorylation of one of the IFN alpha/beta receptor subunits (IFNAR1) occurred in response to IFN gamma [3]. Similarly, other authors showed that IFNGR1-IFNAR2 (ligand binding domains of both receptor systems) are associated in the presence of IFN alpha and IFN gamma [4]. The physical interaction between both IFN receptor complexes may be the first step for the triggering of intracellular signals that promote the synergism between both IFNs. In the clinics, the peri- and intralesional administration of a new pharmaceutical stabilized formulation containing IFNs alpha-2b and gamma (HeberPAG®), was safe and effective for the treatment of elder patients with advanced, recurrent or resistant to previous treatments basal and squamous cell skin carcinomas [5].

The main objective of this study was to characterize the PK/PD of HeberPAG® in patients with mycosis fungoides. Classical IFN-inducible biological markers, neopterin, β2-microglobulin ($\beta_2$M), and 2'-5' oligoadenylate synthetase (2'-5' OAS1), were used as indicators of their pharmacodynamic action. A secondary objective was the registration of adverse events.

## Methods

An exploratory, prospective, open-label clinical trial was carried out at the "Hermanos Ameijeiras" Hospital, Dermatology Service, Havana, Cuba. The protocol was approved by the Ethics Committee of this hospital and by the Cuban Regulatory Authority, the State Center for the Control of Drugs, Equipment & Medical Devices (CECMED, reference number: 999/16.016.09.B). The trial was in compliance with the Helsinki Declaration and its amendments. All patients prior to study enrollment provided their written informed consent.

### Subjects

Twelve patients, both genders, 18 to 75 years-old, with clinically and histologically proven mycosis fungoides, at stages IB to III, were recruited for the study. Other eligibility criteria included a measurable disease, a life expectancy of at least 24 weeks, Karnofsky's index ≥ 60%, with more than 1 month of previous disease specific treatments or more than 3 months in case of steroid use. Patients also had adequate hematological, hepatic, and renal function. Exclusion criteria were other uncompensated chronic diseases or neoplasias, pregnancy or nursing and severe psychiatric dysfunction.

### HeberPAG formulation

A stabilized formulation containing $3.5 \times 10^6$ IU of a synergistic combination of human recombinant, produced in *E. coli*, IFNs alpha-2b and gamma (HeberPAG®, Heber Biotec, Havana, Cuba), was used for all cases. Each vial also contains 18.87 mg sodium phosphates, 13 mg Dextran-40, 0.24 mg kalium phosphate, 16.59 mg sodium chloride, 0.18 mg kalium chloride, 5.0 mg manitol, 5.0 mg saccharose, and 5.5 mg human albumin. This lyophilized powder formulation was reconstituted with 2 mL bacteriostatic water for injection.

### Study design

The study was designed to calculate pharmacokinetic and pharmacodynamic parameters after a first single high dose of HeberPAG®. Each patient received, intramuscularly, in the gluteus region, a single $23 \times 10^6$ IU HeberPAG® dose, chosen to obtain detectable serum levels of both IFNs. Antipyretic medication was given orally at the same time as the HeberPAG® injection and every 4 hours thereafter, up to 12 hours or more if needed in order to mitigate the expected IFN-dependent flu-like syndrome. Patients were hospitalized during the first 96 hours after the injection under strict medical supervision. After this period the study continued to evaluate efficacy and safety of this product in the same group of patients. Then, they received $11 \times 10^6$ IU twice a week during one year.

## Laboratory evaluations

Blood samples for serum IFN alpha-2b and IFN gamma concentration determinations were collected by venipuncture before and 1, 3, 6, 12, 24, 48, 72, and 96 hours after injection. Pharmacodynamics was assessed by serum neopterin and $\beta_2M$ concentrations at the same times and by the induction of 2'-5' OAS1 mRNA expression before and at 6, 12, 24, 48, 72 and 96 hours. Routine hematological and biochemical determinations were taken as safety variables, every 24 hours during the first 96 hours. These included hemoglobin, hematocrit, leukocytes and platelets counts, transaminases, bilirubin, creatinine and urea. Patients were regularly checked for vital signs and symptoms during the whole hospitalization.

Vacutainers were used to collect blood samples to determine serum concentrations and biochemistry (8.5 mL Z Serum Sep, Greiner bio-one) and for hematology analysis (4 mL K3E K3EDTA, Greiner bio-one). Blood samples for total RNA purification were collected in PAXgene Blood RNA Tubes (2.5 mL, QIAGEN, US).

Serum IFNs, neopterin and $\beta_2M$ levels were measured using commercially available kits according to the manufacturer's instructions using sera stored at −80°C until be tested. IFN alpha-2b and IFN gamma were quantified in serum with high sensitivity enzyme immunoassay (EIA) kits specific for IFN alpha (Catalogue: BMS216CE, Bender MedSystem, GMBH) or IFN gamma (Catalogue: BMS228CE, Bender MedSystem, GMBH), respectively. Neopterin was determined by a commercial EIA kit (HENNING test, BRAHMS Diagnostica GmbH, Berlin, Germany) as well as serum $\beta_2M$ (Quantikine® IVD®, R&D System, Inc, Minneapolis).

Quantification of OAS1 mRNA levels was performed using the Real-Time Polimerase Chain Reaction (qPCR) method. Total RNAs were obtained by PAXgene purification protocol (PreAnalytiX/Qiagen, US). RNA quality was checked in a Spectrophotometer Nanodrop 1000 (ThermoScientific, US), reporting a 260/280 nm OD relation between 1.7 and 2.2. Agarose electrophoresis allowed to visualize 28S rRNA and 18S rRNA bands in a proportion higher than 1.5. Complementary DNA (cDNA) was used as template in qPCR experiments; the synthesis was carried out using Superscript II RT kit and protocol (Invitrogen, US) from total RNA samples at each time point. qPCR experiments were performed in 20 µL using ABsolute QPCR SYBR Green Mixes (ThermoScientific, ABgene, UK) and 0.3 µM of primers for amplification of OAS1 target gene (F: 5' AGCCTCATCCGCCTAGTCAA 3'; R: 5' CTCGCTCCCAAGCATAGACC 3') and reference genes GAPDH (F: 5' CCATGGGTGGAATCATATTGGA 3'; R: 5' TCAACGGATTTGGTCGTATTGG 3') and HMBS (F: 5' GGAATGTTACGAGCAGTGATGC 3'; R: 5' CCTGACTGGAGGAGTCTGGAGT 3'). All of them were designed on the basis of the GenBank database information using primer3 software [6]. All experiments were in triplicates, rendering amplifications curves between cycles 15 and 30 in RT™Cycler equipment (Capitalbio, China) with a standard program of 15 min at 95°C for enzyme activation followed by 40 cycles of 15 s at 95°C, 30s at 60°C and 30s at 72°C. Capitalbio software reports of Ct values, as the 2nd derivative maximum, and values of fluorescence per cycle, which were used for efficiency calculation by LinReg software (version 11.3, 2009), were used for calculations of relative OAS1 gene expression, at each time point respect to time 0 h, using REST-MCS (version 2, 2006) software [7], after the normalization with reference genes.

Hematological counts and blood chemistry were done according to usual clinical laboratory procedures, using advanced automated analyzers.

## Data analysis

The drug disposition data analysis was performed per patient by a non-compartmental method with a combined linear/log - linear trapezoidal rule approach. The linear trapezoidal rule was used up to peak level and the logarithmic trapezoidal rule thereafter. The first-order rate constant associated with the curve terminal (log linear) portion ($\lambda$) and terminal half-life ($t_{1/2}$) were estimated by linear regression of the included terminal data points. Time-to-peak values (Tmax) were determined directly from the experimental data as the time of maximum observed level (Cmax) considering the entire curve. Area under the serum concentration-time curve from 0 to 96 hours ($AUC_{96}$) was calculated using the linear/log linear trapezoidal rule. Mean residence time (MRT) was also calculated using the moments of the drug disposition curve. Parameters that were extrapolated to infinity, such as AUC (area under disposition curve) and AUMC (area under first moment of the disposition curve) were computed based on the last predicted value from the linear regression performed to estimate $\lambda$ and $t_{1/2}$. Some similar kinetic parameters were estimated for the pharmacodynamic markers, corrected for baseline values, neopterin and $\beta_2M$ in order to describe the kinetic behavior of the IFN-induced immunological response: Rmax (maximum response), T(Rmax) (time to reach maximum response), $\lambda$ effect (effect dissipation constant), $t_{1/2}$ effect (effect half-life), AUEC (area under the effect curve), MET (mean effect time) [8]. The WinNonlin professional software (Version 2.1, Pharsight Inc., 1997, NC, USA) was used for all these purposes. A descriptive statistic was done using SPSS for Windows version 15.0.

## Results

Twelve patients, 7 females and 5 males, with a disease stage IIA and III, were recruited. They were between 33 and 74 years-old (mean: 53.3 yrs), with a mean corporal surface of 1.79 m$^2$ (range: 1.46 – 2.28). Three clinical variants of mycosis fungoides were represented; 6 patients had plaques, 2 had erythroderma, and the rest had atypia of the epidermis. Only five patients had received prior systemic antitumor therapy, four of them IFN alpha and three methotrexate. Other previous treatments (cyclosporine, steroid cream, radiotherapy) were received by a single patient each one. Initial mean LDH was 216 U/L (range: 69 – 355). Most of the patients complied with the evaluations as previewed, except for patient No.8 whose serum samples were not available at 72 and 96 hours.

### Pharmacokinetic analysis

Except for two patients, who had 7.1 and 114 pg/mL of IFN alpha-2b, all had undetectable or very low endogenous pre-dose serum IFN concentrations (median = 0 pg/ml). The average concentration profiles obtained for both IFNs are showed in Figure 1. IFN alpha-2b concentrations started to increase notably from the first hour post-injection. At 3 hours, more than half of the patients reached 100 pg/mL. Maximum values (> 200 pg/mL) were obtained at 6–12 hours in most of the cases (Figure 1a). Patient No. 12, who had the higher baseline value, reached 440 pg/mL at 12 hours. Increments in IFN gamma levels were more

discreet with a peak at 12 hours post-injection, where 5 patients reached 15 pg/mL or more (Figure 1b). A pronounced drop of IFN concentrations was detected since 24 hours. At 48–96 hours after the injection, these values had returned near to the initial values, so the $AUC_{96}$ obtained covered more than 95% of the AUC extrapolated to infinite.

Table 1 shows the results of the pharmacokinetic parameters calculated from the above commented profiles. A high patient -dependant variability is observed, mainly with IFN gamma (see SD). Additionally, an elevated distribution volume and fast blood clearance of both IFNs was obtained (data not shown).

### Pharmacodynamic analysis

The time courses for the induction of neopterin and $\beta_2M$ are showed in Figure 2. Both variables were strongly stimulated by simultaneous administration of both IFNs with highest inductions around 24–48 hours after intramuscular administration. HeberPAG® induced an average increment of serum neopterin at 48 hours about approximately six times, until 9.6 pg/mL compared to pre-dose values (Figure 2a). Individually, five patients surpassed 10 pg/mL at this time. Figure 2b

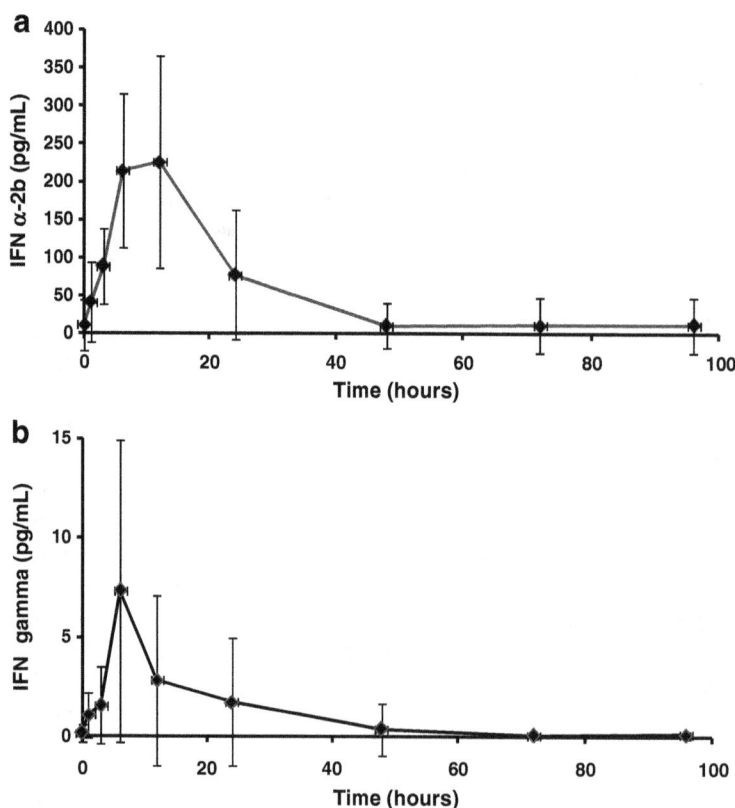

**Figure 1 Interferon concentrations in serum.** Legend: Data correspond to 12 patients with mycosis fungoides who received 23 × 10$^6$ IU of HeberPAG®. Each point represents the average and standard deviation of (**a**) IFN alpha-2b and (**b**) IFN gamma levels, both measured by EIA.

**Table 1 Pharmacokinetic parameters calculated from the IFN alpha-2b and IFN gamma concentrations in serum (N = 12)**

| Parameter | IFN alpha-2b | IFN gamma |
|---|---|---|
| Cmax (pg/mL) | 263 ± 129 | 9.3 ± 7.0 |
| Tmax (h) | 12.0 ± 6.0 | 6.0 ± 0.8 |
| $\lambda$ (h$^{-1}$) | 0.16 ± 0.06 | 0.07 ± 0.05 |
| $t_{1/2}$ (h) | 4.9 ± 1.4 | 13.4 ± 27.1 |
| AUC (pg.h/mL) | 4483 ± 4485 | 87.5 ± 89.9 |
| MRT (h) | 13.9 ± 7.9 | 13.5 ± 8.2 |

Data are reported as mean ± standard deviation, except for Tmax expressed as median ± quartile range.

shows that mean serum $\beta_2$M peaked around the double from baseline at 24–48 hours. For both variables the values remained clearly upper baseline levels until 96 hours. Notably, neopterin remained three times superior to pre-dose value at the end of the sampling period.

A pharmacokinetic-like analytical procedure was carried out with both variables (Table 2). Since patients could have pre-treatment levels of these biological markers, a more real interpretation of kinetics has to be showed as fold increases

over baseline. For neopterin Rmax was 8.0 ng/mL, with a $t_{1/2}$ effect = 40 hours and a MET around 80 hours. For $\beta_2$M, T(Rmax) was 2.7 µg/mL, and the effect dissipation phase occurred similarly slow compared to neopterin. A high intra-patient variability was again evidenced.

Since the individual induction of the enzyme 2'-5' OAS1 was measured through the relative amount of its mRNA expression using the Real-Time PCR method, an important variability could be expected. Therefore, parameters could not be rigorously calculated from the experimental data and the analysis was essentially qualitative. Figure 3 shows individual relative OAS1 mRNA levels at each time point with respect to time zero, normalized with GAPDH/HMBS levels. A single intramuscular dose of 23 x10$^6$ IU of HeberPAG® resulted in high increases of this variable with regard to their pre-dose values in all patients, in a factor between 8 and 122 times in ten patients, primarily within the first 24 hours after dosing. The expression levels return to initials by 96 hours in most of the patients.

**Safety data**

Adverse events were checked during the whole study. All the patients presented at least one event, mostly flu-like

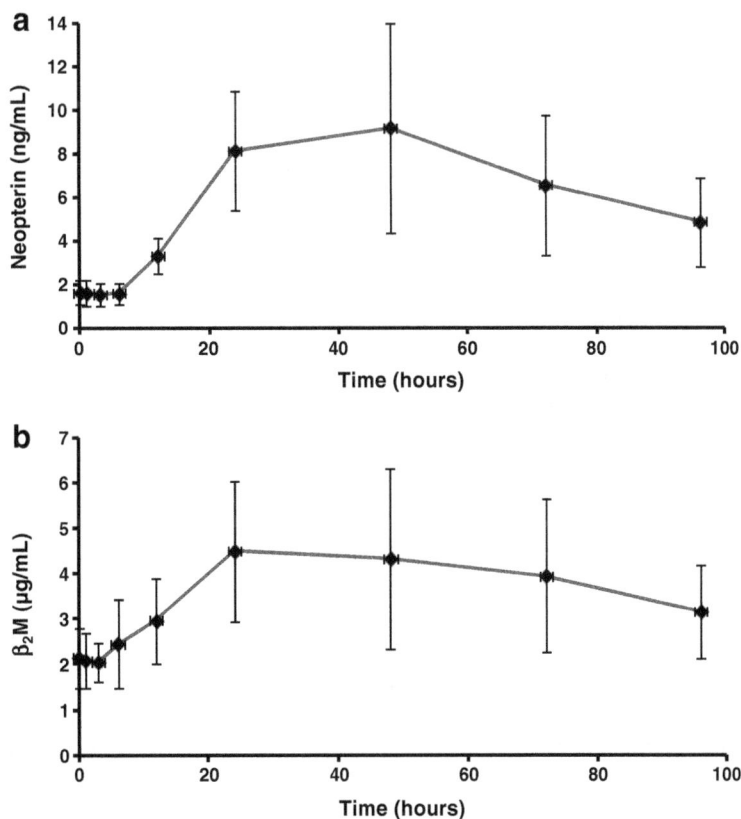

**Figure 2 Pharmacodynamic markers neopterin and β2-microglobulin in serum.** Legend: Data correspond to 12 patients with mycosis fungoides who received 23 × 10$^6$ IU of HeberPAG® at time 0. (**a**): Average neopterin concentration, measured by EIA. (**b**): Average β2M concentration, measured by EIA. Standard deviations are also showed at each time.

**Table 2 Descriptive parameters of the kinetics of serum Neopterin and serum β2-microglobulin increments (N = 12)**

| Parameter | Neopterin | β2-microglobulin |
|---|---|---|
| Rmax | 8.0 ± 4.2 ng/mL | 2.7 ± 1.4 µg/mL |
| T(Rmax) | 48 ± 24 h | 24 ± 24 h |
| λ effect | 0.02 ± 0.01 h$^{-1}$ | 0.02 ± 0.01 h$^{-1}$ |
| $t_{1/2}$ effect | 40.3 ± 12.9 h | 37.6 ± 15.9 h |
| AUEC | 661 ± 322 ng.h/mL | 195 ± 117 µg.h/mL |
| MET | 80.6 ± 17.4 h | 74.8 ± 21.9 h |

Data are reported as mean ± standard deviation, except for T(Rmax) expressed as median ± quartile range.

symptoms caused by IFN. The most frequent events were fever (100%), malaise (91.7%), headache (58.3%), tachycardia (41.6%), leucopenia (33.3%), chills (33.3%) and anemia (25%). Anorexia, arthralgias, increase of transaminases and myalgias were recorded in two patients. Most of the events (92.3%) were considered mild, none severe, being well controlled.

## Discussion

Treatment with unmodified IFNs for several malignancies and chronic viral affections requires frequent injections (e.g., daily or three times weekly) over the course of therapy due to the molecule's short circulating half-life in humans. Increase of doses and prolonged therapy could favor a better clinical response but it could also lead to magnify adverse events. Besides, patient's compliance under long-term dosing regimens is difficult to preserve. The development

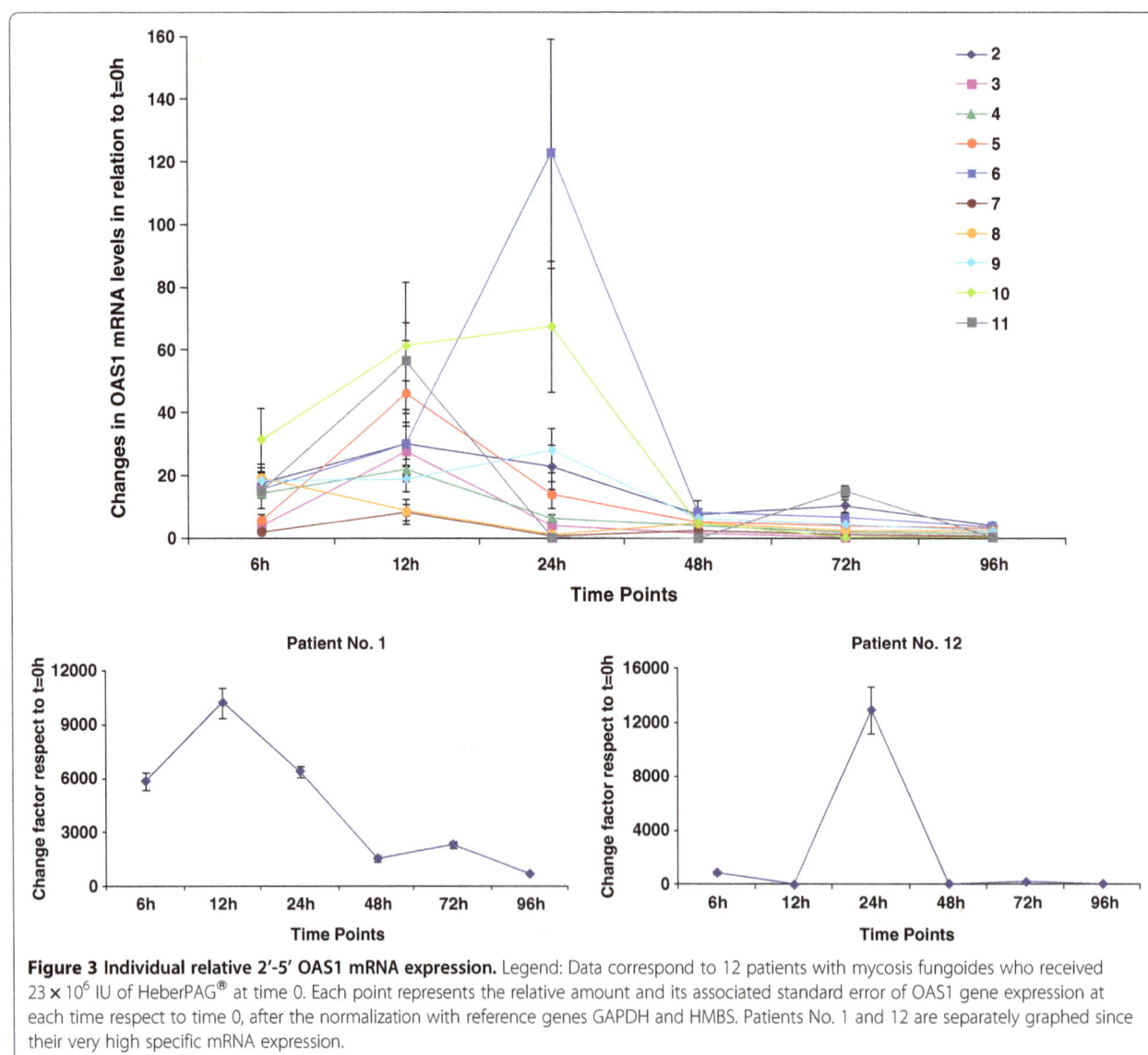

**Figure 3 Individual relative 2'-5' OAS1 mRNA expression.** Legend: Data correspond to 12 patients with mycosis fungoides who received 23 × 10$^6$ IU of HeberPAG® at time 0. Each point represents the relative amount and its associated standard error of OAS1 gene expression at each time respect to time 0, after the normalization with reference genes GAPDH and HMBS. Patients No. 1 and 12 are separately graphed since their very high specific mRNA expression.

of more slowly cleared IFNs has allowed to reduce dosing frequency and to enhance response rates in patients with chronic hepatitis C [9]. However, modified high molecular IFNs could have more difficulties to penetrate the tumor niches bearing a reduction in their antitumor effects. A significant reduction of in vitro biological activity has been demonstrated for pegylated IFNs due to non optimal interaction with IFN receptor [10].

Therefore sustained full IFN-receptor interactions with more potent antiproliferative activity are desired in the treatment of cancer. This is possible to obtain combining IFN-alpha and IFN gamma that synergize for their biological activities. HeberPAG® is a new formulation containing a mixture of recombinant IFN alpha-2b and IFN gamma at synergistic proportions. This formulation was created to improve antiproliferative and other biological effects of conventional IFNs with an adequate tolerability leading to administer fewer doses similar to others currently available therapy. This is the first PK/PD study in humans with this variety of IFN formulation.

The pharmacodynamic variables measured in this trial to characterize HeberPAG® formulation are well-known IFN-induced genes, classical surrogate markers of IFN biological actions. Neopterin is a sensitive marker of T helper 1-cell immune response, because it is primarily produced by monocytes/macrophages after activation by IFNs and augments the production of tumor necrosis factor in peripheral blood mononuclear cells [11]. Beta2-microglobulin plays an important role in the tumor growth control and metastases [12]. Progression of the cell cycle is mediated by 2'- 5'OAS levels stimulated by IFN [13]. Additionally, antiviral effects subsequent to IFNs addition are initiated by synthesis of 2'- 5'oligoadenylates that activate an endoribonuclease to cleave double-stranded viral RNA [14].

The most remarkable result was the six-fold increase of serum neopterin concentrations respect to basal value. This high increment induced by HeberPAG® has not been described before in the literature with any subtype or variant of IFN, even for pegylated forms [15-20]. The induction by pegylated IFN-alpha could only approximately tripled the neopterin basal values as maximum 48 hours after injection as reported [17,19,20]. In the case of PEG-IFN beta although half-life was greatly extended by pegylation, the neopterin response was not affected [18]. On the other hand, two times higher levels than baseline were recorded for serum $\beta_2$M 24–48 hours after injection, superior to those increments detected by other authors, which were around 60% with natural or pegylated IFN-alpha [19-21]. For both pharmacodynamic markers their more slow return to initial levels has not been observed with conventional IFN in the reports above-cited. This last result could lead to space the dosage interval for the IFN mixture formulation until twice or once a week. Recent data obtained with the same markers

but in healthy male volunteers [article in preparation] emphasize that possibility. Efficacy trials evaluating these frequencies of administration in several oncologic pathologies are under development.

After the single intramuscular injection, 2'- 5'-OAS1 mRNA levels were extensively increased which was also recently found in a group of healthy male volunteers who received $24.5 \times 10^6$ IU of a similar formulation. Although mRNA induction does not ensure the presence of active protein, it has been reported that 2'-5' OAS enzyme activity in the serum of IFN-treated patients appears to increase since the first 6 hours and maintains elevated levels for as long as 4 to 8 months after the initiation of daily IFN treatment [22].

At molecular level this beneficial pharmacodynamic effects could be explained by synergistic effects in the expression and activation of several genes regulated by both IFNs [23].

Concerning pharmacokinetics, no interferences by simultaneous administered IFNs were observed in their typical similar serum profiles. Parameters as Tmax and $t_{1/2}$ were within the reported ranges for these conventional IFNs after systemic administration either in patients or healthy volunteers even considering the expected high variability [24-27]. For IFN alpha-2b Cmax was also very similar to a previous report ours in healthy male volunteers [21].

Flu-like symptoms and other clinical and laboratory adverse events associated with HeberPAG® have been previously reported for recombinant IFN treatment [28]. Fever began 2 to 4 hours after intramuscular administration and peaked at 6 to 12 hours coincident with maximum IFN serum levels. However, the mechanisms of fever induction appear to be different between IFNs. IFN-alpha has been shown to be intrinsically pyrogenic and the body temperature rise is related to the interaction of IFN alpha to hypothalamic μ-opioid receptors [29]. Meanwhile the administration of IFN gamma stimulates the release of other lymphokines such as interleukin-1 [30], an endogenous pyrogen [31].

## Conclusion
The co-administration of IFN alpha-2b and IFN gamma with potent synergistic actions will allow us to obtain a more favorable pharmacodynamics introducing new promissory perspectives in the use of IFNs to treat several malignancies. Efficacy trials can be carried out to ratify the obtained results.

**Competing interests**
Authors YGV, IGG, ACR, ADTI, YDR, YIT, DVB, EGI and IBR are employees of the Center for Genetic Engineering and Biotechnology (CIGB), Havana network, where IFN alpha-2b and IFN gamma are produced and the new synergistic formulation (HeberPAG®) was developed. The rest of the authors have no competing interests at all. The study was financed by Heber

Biotec, Havana, Cuba (product, reagents), and the Ministry of Public Health of
Cuba (hospital facilities and general medical care of the patients).

**Authors' contributions**
YGV designed, coordinated and performed the study, analyzed the results
and revised the manuscript. IGG participated in the analyses of results and
wrote the manuscript draft. SECC (main clinical investigator), EESP and CAA
took care of patient recruitment, management, clinical examinations, and
follow-up. ACP carried out EIA determinations. EGI participated in the study
design and ADTI achieved the statistical analysis. MCP, NCB, TICT and JSM
carried out clinical laboratory determinations. YDR assisted as study monitor.
YIT and DVB did the Real time PCR method. IBR conceived the study and
took part in the design, results analysis and manuscript writing. All authors
read and approved the final manuscript.

**Acknowledgments**
The authors wish to thank the nurse Mayté Hernández for their participation
in the clinical work. They also thank the engineers Leovaldo Álvarez and
Laura Pereda for data processing and Dr. Cimara Bermúdez and the
technicians Laura Quesada, Ketty Cruz, Grettel Melo and María A Delgado for
their assistance. The authors received HeberPAG® formulation free from
Heber Biotec, Havana, Cuba.

**Author details**
[1]Clinical Investigation Department, Center for Genetic Engineering and
Biotechnology, P.O. Box 6332, Havana, Cuba. [2]"Hermanos Ameijeiras"
Hospital, Dermatology Service, Havana, Cuba. [3]"Hermanos Ameijeiras"
Hospital, Clinical Laboratory Service, Havana, Cuba. [4]Genomics Department,
Center for Genetic Engineering and Biotechnology, Havana, Cuba.

**References**
1.  Wang YS, Youngster S, Grace M, Bausch J, Bordensc R, Wyssa DF: **Structural and biological characterization of pegylated recombinant interferon alpha-2b and its therapeutic implications.** *Adv Drug Deliv Rev* 2002, **54**:547–570.
2.  Czamiecki CW, Fennie CW, Powers DB, Estell DA: **Synergistic antiviral and antiproliferative activities of E. coli derived human alpha, beta, and gamma interferons.** *J Virol* 490, **49**:496.
3.  Takaoka A, Mitani Y, Suemori H, Sato M, Yokochi T, Noguchi S, Tanaka N, Taniguchi T: **Cross talk between interferon-gamma and -alpha/beta signaling components in caveolar membrane domains.** *Science* 2000, **288**:2357–2360.
4.  Bello I, Rodes L, López-Saura P: **Antibodies against IFN gamma-binding proteins recognize a member of IFN alpha R complex.** *Biochem Biophys Res Commun* 2001, **280**:1197–1202.
5.  Anasagasti-Angulo L, Garcia-Vega Y, Barcelona-Perez S, Lopez-Saura P, Bello-Rivero I: **Treatment of advanced, recurrent, resistant to previous treatments basal and squamous cell skin carcinomas with a synergistic formulation of interferons. Open, prospective study.** *BMC Cancer* 2009, **30**:262.
6.  Rozen S, Skaletsky HJ: **Primer3 on the WWW for general users and for biologist programmers.** In *Bioinformatics methods and protocols: methods in molecular biology.* Edited by Krawetz S, Misener S. Totowa, NJ: Humana Press; 2000:365–386.
7.  Pfaffl MW, Horgan GW, Dempfle L: **Relative expression software tool REST© for group wise comparison and statistical analysis of relative expression results in real-time PCR.** *Nucleic Acids Res* 2002, **30**:E36.
8.  Krzyzanski W, Jusko WJ: **Application of moment analysis to the sigmoid effect model for drug administered intravenously.** *Pharm Res* 1997, **14**:949–952.
9.  Ferenci P: **PEG IFN alfa-2a (40KD) (Pegasys) for the treatment of patients with chronic hepatitis C.** *Int J Clin Pract* 2003, **57**:610–615.
10. Boulestin A, Kamar N, Sandres-Sauné K, Alric L, Vinel JP, Rostaing L, Izopet J: **Pegylation of IFN-alpha and antiviral activity.** *J Interferon Cytokine Res* 2006, **26**:849–853.
11. Murr C, Widner B, Wirleitner B, Fuchs D: **Neopterin as a marker for immune system activation.** *Curr Drug Metab* 2002, **3**:175–187.
12. Garcia-Lora A, Algarra I, Garrido F: **MHC class I antigens, immune surveillance, and tumor immune escape.** *J Cell Physiol* 2003, **195**:346–355.
13. Wells V, Malluci L: **Expression of the 2-5A during the cell cycle.** *Exp Cell Res* 1985, **159**:27–36.
14. Sadler AJ, Williams BR: **Interferon-inducible antiviral effectors.** *Nat Rev Immunol* 2008, **8**:559–568.
15. Alam J, McAllister A, Scaramucci J, Jones W, Rogge M: **Pharmacokinetics and pharmacodynamics of interferon beta-1a (IFN beta-1a) in healthy volunteers after intravenous, subcutaneous or intramuscular administration.** *Clin Drug Invest* 1997, **14**:35–43.
16. Xu ZX, Hoffman J, Patel I, Jonbert P: **Single-dose safety/tolerability and pharmacokinetics/pharmacodynamics (PK/PD) following administration of ascending subcutaneous doses of pegylated-interferon (PEG-INF) and interferon α-2a (INF α-2a) to healthy subjects.** *Hepatology* 1998, **28**:702A.
17. Motzer RJ, Rakhit A, Ginsberg M, Rittweger K, Vuky J, Yu R, Fettner S, Hooftman L: **Phase I trial of 40-kd branched pegylated interferon alfa-2a for patients with advanced renal cell carcinoma.** *J Clin Oncol* 2001, **19**:1312–1319.
18. Pepinsky RB, Lepage DJ, Gill A, Chakraborty A, Vaidyanathan S, Green M, Baker DP, Whalley E, Hochman PS, Martin P: **Improved pharmacokinetic properties of a polyethylene glycol-modified form of interferon-beta-1a with preserved in vitro bioactivity.** *J Pharmacol Exp Ther* 2001, **297**:1059–1066.
19. Bruno R, Sacchi P, Scagnolari C, Torriani F, Maiocchi L, Patruno S, Bellomi F, Filice G, Antonelli G: **Pharmacodynamics of PEG IFN alpha-2a and PEG IFN alpha-2b in interferon-naïve patients with chronic hepatitis C: a randomized, controlled study.** *Aliment Pharmacol Ther* 2007, **26**:369–376.
20. García-García I, González-Delgado CA, Valenzuela-Silva CM, Díaz-Machado A, Cruz-Díaz M, Nodarse-Cuní H, Pérez-Pérez O, Bermúdez-Badell CH, Ferrero-Bibilonia J, Páez-Meireles R, Bello-Rivero I, Castro-Odio FR, López-Saura PA: **Pharmacokinetic and pharmacodynamic comparison of two "pegylated" interferon alpha-2 formulations in healthy male volunteers: a randomized, crossover, double-blind study.** *BMC Pharmacol* 2010, **10**:15.
21. Garcia-Garcia I, Gonzalez-Delgado CA, Valenzuela-Silva C, Hernandez-Bernal F, Ferrero-Bibilonia J, Soto-Hernandez R, Cervantes-Llano M, Duconge J, Correa-Fernandez A, Olivera-Ruano L, Lopez-Saura P: **Bioequivalence of two recombinant interferon alpha-2b liquid formulations in healthy male volunteers.** *Drugs R D* 2004, **5**:271–280.
22. Moritz T, Weissmann B, Grunewald B, Hust H, Kummer G, Niederle N: **Induction of 2'-5' oligoadenylate synthetase during interferon treatment of chronic myelogenous leukemia.** *Mol Biother* 1992, **4**:97–102.
23. Sanda C, Weitzel P, Tsukahara T, Schaley J, Edenberg HJ, Stephens MA, McClintick JN, Blatt LM, Li L, Brodsky L, Taylor MW: **Differential gene induction by type I and type II interferons and their combination.** *J Interferon Cytokine Res* 2006, **26**:462–472.
24. Bocci V: **Pharmacokinetics of interferons and routes of administration.** In *Interferons: principles and medical applications.* Edited by Baron S, Coppenhaver DH, Dianzani F. Texas: The University of Texas Medical Branch at Galveston; 1992:417–425.
25. Zhi J, Teller SB, Satoh H, Koss-Twardy SG, Luke DR: **Influence of human serum albumin content in formulations on the bioequivalency of interferon alpha-2a given by subcutaneous injection in healthy male volunteers.** *J Clin Pharmacol* 1995, **35**:281–284.
26. Rodríguez JL, Valenzuela C, Marín N, Ferrero J, Ducongé J, Castillo R, Póntigas V, Deás M, González-Suárez R, López-Saura P: **Comparative pharmacokinetics and pharmacodynamics of Two recombinant human interferon alpha-2b formulations administered intramuscularly in healthy male volunteers.** *Biotecnol Apl* 2000, **17**:166–170.
27. Turner PK, Houghton JA, Istvan Petak David M, Tillman DM, Douglas L, Schwartzberg L, Billups CA, Panetta JC, Stewart CF: **Interferon-gamma pharmacokinetics and pharmacodynamics in patients with colorectal cancer.** *Cancer Chemother Pharmacol* 2004, **53**:253–260.
28. Vial T, Descotes J: **Clinical toxicity of the interferons.** *Drug safety* 1994, **10**:115–150.
29. Wang YX, Xu WG, Sun XJ, Chen YZ, Liu XY, Tang H, Jiang CL: **Fever of recombinant human interferon-alpha is mediated by opioid domain

interaction with opioid receptor inducing prostaglandin E2. *J Neuroimmunol* 2004, **156:**107–112.

30.  Vilcek J, Gray PW, Rinderknecht E, Sevastopoulos CG: **Interferon gamma: a lymphokine for all seasons**. In *Lymphokines*. Vol 12th edition. Edited by Pick E. Orlando: Academic Press; 1984:1–32.

31.  Duff GW, Durum SK: **The pyrogenic and mitogenic actions of interleukin-1 are related**. *Nature* 1983, **304:**449–451.

# 13

# Comparison of the anti-inflammatory effects of Cilomilast, Budesonide and a p38 Mitogen activated protein kinase inhibitor in COPD lung tissue macrophages

Marianne Jennifer Ratcliffe[1*] and Iain Gordon Dougall[2]

## Abstract

Chronic Obstructive Pulmonary Disease (COPD) is a disease characterized by a largely irreversible airflow obstruction and a persistent, excessive inflammatory response. Alveolar macrophages (AMs) are increased in the lungs of COPD patients, and act as orchestrators of the inflammatory response, releasing a range of mediators to coordinate recruitment and activation of leukocytes. Attempts to treat the inflammatory component of COPD with anti-inflammatory drugs such as steroids has met with limited success. In this study, we compared the ability of the phosphodiesterase IV (PDEIV) inhibitor Cilomilast, the steroid Budesonide, and the p38 mitogen activated protein kinase inhibitor BIRB-796 to inhibit tumour necrosis factor alpha (TNF$\alpha$) and interleukin 6 (IL-6) releases from AMs isolated from COPD lung transplant tissue. All studies were carried out with appropriate ethical approval and written, informed consent was obtained from each subject. Cilomilast had little effect on cytokine release from AMs. There was considerable variability in the responsiveness of AMs to Budesonide, with a subset of AMs responding poorly to Budesonide. BIRB-796 inhibited TNF$\alpha$ release from all AM donors, including those that responded poorly to steroids. Treatment with BIRB-796 and Budesonide together gave an additive decrease in TNFa release. These results suggest that a p38 inhibitor may provide advantages over existing anti-inflammatory treatments for COPD, either as an add-on to existing therapy, or to treat patients who respond poorly to steroids.

**Keywords:** COPD, Lung, Macrophage, TNF, Budesonide, Steroid insensitivity, p38 MAPK, PDEIV, BIRB-796

## Background

COPD is an increasingly prevalent disease, affecting up to 10% of adults aged over 40 years [1]. Current therapies include long acting $\beta_2$-receptor agonists (LABAs) and muscarinic receptor antagonists, which increase lung function by relaxing airway smooth muscle. Corticosteroids are also used, and have been shown to decrease exacerbations as well as improving other clinical parameters such as $FEV_1$[2]. However, the use of inhaled steroids in COPD is somewhat controversial due to inconsistent clinical effects and reports that these agents have limited effects on lung inflammation in COPD patients. For example, a meta-analysis of the effects of inhaled corticosteroids on inflammatory cells in the sputum of stable COPD patients showed evidence of reductions in neutrophils and lymphocytes but no effect on macrophages [3]. A similar analysis conducted recently on bronchial biopsies and bronchoalveolar lavage (BAL) fluid from stable patients showed reductions in neutrophils and lymphocytes in BAL but an increase in macrophages. The biopsy analysis indicated no effect on neutrophil and macrophage counts but a reduction in CD4[+] and CD8[+] lymphocytes [4]. In accordance with these results, macrophages from COPD patients have been reported to be insensitive to steroids [5,6]. Various mechanisms for this steroid insensitivity have been proposed, including up-regulation of NF-kB signaling and increased oxidative stress [7]. If specific mechanisms are indeed responsible for the poor efficacy of steroids in COPD, then alternative anti-inflammatory approaches may be more successful. One

* Correspondence: Marianne.ratcliffe@astrazeneca.com
[1]Personalised Healthcare and Biomarkers, AstraZeneca R&D Alderley Park, Cheshire, SK 10 4TG, UK
Full list of author information is available at the end of the article

such approach currently being considered is inhibition of PDEIV, by drugs such as Roflumilast and Cilomilast. The former drug has recently been approved as an add-on therapy for the maintenance treatment of severe COPD in the European Union and as a treatment to reduce the risk of exacerbations in the United States. These cAMP elevating agents have been shown to reduce recruitment of macrophages and CD8[+] T-cells in COPD biopsies [8] and improve $FEV_1$, alone or in combination with a bronchodilator therapy [9,10]. p38 MAP kinase is involved in transducing a number of inflammatory stimuli [11] and inhibitors of this enzyme have broad anti-inflammatory potential. Indeed, p38 inhibitors have shown evidence of anti-inflammatory effects and improvements in clinical parameters in COPD patients [12,13]. Such agents have also been shown to inhibit cytokine release from human AMs derived from patients with COPD [14,15], but the effectiveness of p38 inhibitors, steroids and PDEIV inhibitors has not been directly compared in the same donors.

In the present study we compared the ability of Cilomilast, Budesonide and BIRB-796 to inhibit cytokine release from AMs isolated from patients undergoing COPD lung transplant surgery for severe end stage disease (GOLD IV). This allowed us to directly compare the effectiveness of different mechanisms in modulating cytokine release, and assess donor to donor variability in response.

## Results
### Characterisation of LPS response
A concentration-effect curve to LPS was generated in AMs from eleven COPD transplant donors, measuring both IL-6 and TNFα release. All donors responded to LPS, with potency values of $p[A]_{50}$ = 8.2 (6 ng/ml) for TNFα and 8.3 (4 ng/ml) for IL-6. Meaned maximal response was 6.3 ± 1.6 ng/ml for TNFα and 34.1 ± 7.2 ng/ml for IL-6 (Figure 1). These cytokine levels were similar or greater to that seen in COPD macrophages used in similar published studies [14,15]. The concentration of LPS (100 ng/ml) subsequently used for testing the effects of the anti-inflammatory agents corresponded to a maximum response for both cytokine readouts.

### Response of COPD AMs to Cilomilast
The ability of Cilomilast, a PDEIV inhibitor, to inhibit LPS-induced cytokine release was tested. Cilomilast did not inhibit IL-6 release at any of the concentrations used (Figure 2B), and only inhibited TNFα release at concentrations greater than 300 nM (Figure 2A) reaching maximum levels of inhibition of 34.2 ± 6.0 at 10 μM.

### Anti-inflammatory effects of Budesonide in COPD AMs
The ability of the steroid Budesonide to inhibit TNFα or IL-6 release from COPD AMs was tested. Budesonide inhibited TNFα release by a maximum of 42.9 ± 8.0%,

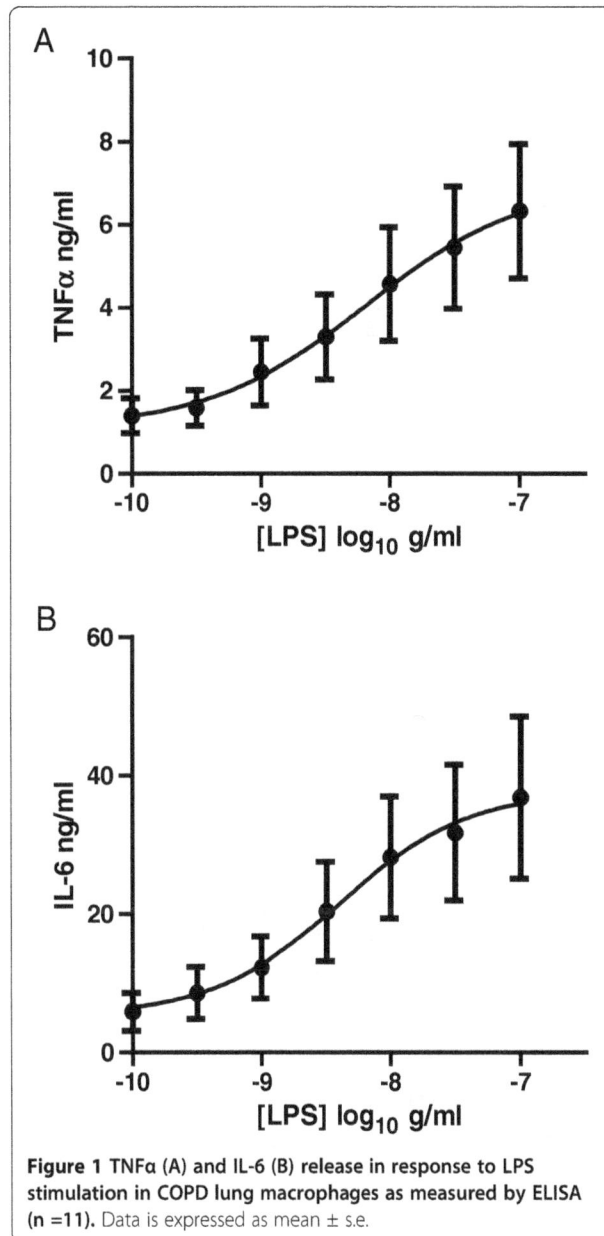

**Figure 1** TNFα (A) and IL-6 (B) release in response to LPS stimulation in COPD lung macrophages as measured by ELISA (n =11). Data is expressed as mean ± s.e.

with a $pIC_{50}$ of 8.9 (1.3 nM). A similar potency was seen against IL-6 ($pIC_{50}$ = 9.0), although the maximum effect was lower than for TNFα (30.8% ± 9.4%) (Figure 3).

### Response of COPD AMs to BIRB-796
The ability of BIRB-796, a p38 inhibitor, to inhibit macrophage cytokine release was also tested. BIRB-796 inhibited TNFα with a $pIC_{50}$ = 8.3 (5 nM) and a maximum inhibition of 63.9% ± 4.6% (Figure 4A). Effects on IL-6 release were less marked and more variable, resulting in a relatively poor fit to equation 2. The maximum inhibition achieved was 38.4% ± 8.6%, and a $pIC_{50}$ estimated as 8.2 (6.3 nM).

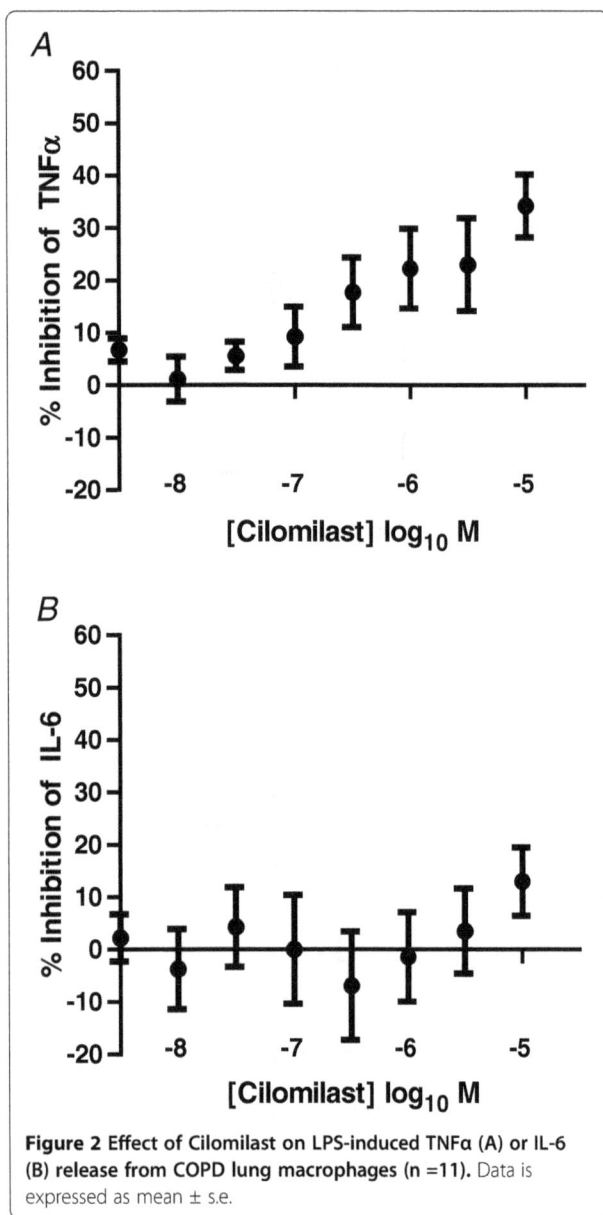

**Figure 2** Effect of Cilomilast on LPS-induced TNFα (A) or IL-6 (B) release from COPD lung macrophages (n =11). Data is expressed as mean ± s.e.

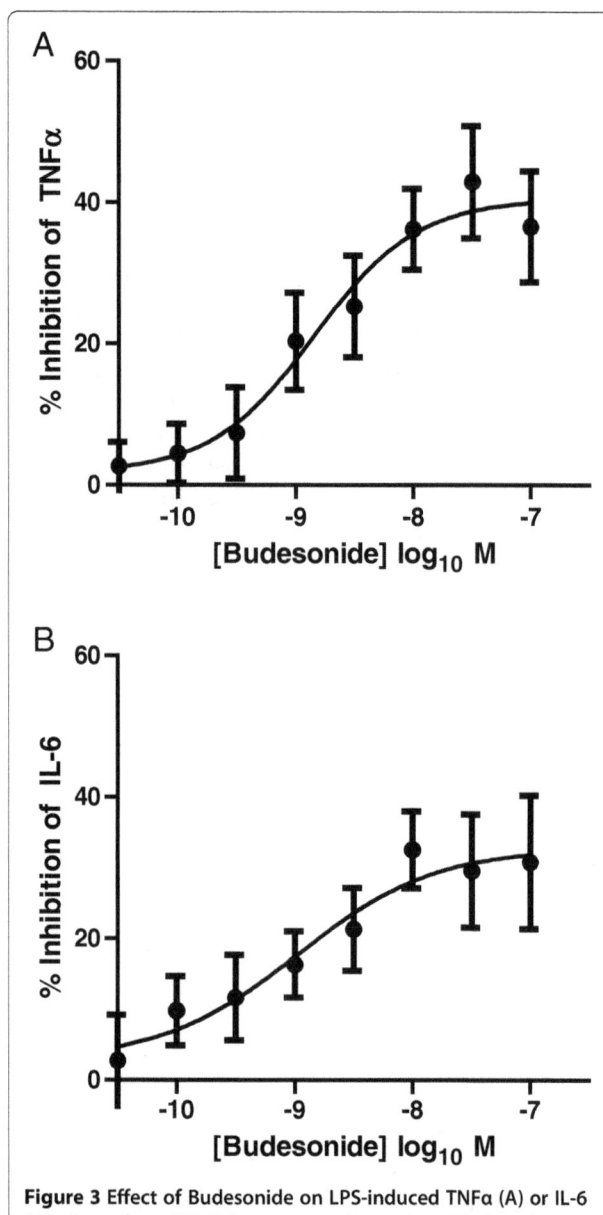

**Figure 3** Effect of Budesonide on LPS-induced TNFα (A) or IL-6 (B) release from COPD lung macrophages (n = 11). Data is expressed as mean ± s.e. and the lines drawn through the points are the result of fitting using equation 2.

**BIRB-796 responses in steroid-resistant donors**

Although the AMs from the majority of COPD donors responded to Budesonide, we observed considerable variability in the potency and maximum effect of Budesonide between different donors. For inhibition of TNFα, the average standard deviation across the concentration range in COPD donors was 21.3% for Budesonide. In comparison, the p38 response was much less variable, with an average standard deviation of 12.4%. Of note, three of the COPD donors were either unresponsive, or poorly responsive to steroid as defined by showing less than 30% inhibition of LPS-induced TNFα release at the maximal concentration of Budesonide used. The data for these three donors were separated from the remaining donors and re-plotted (Figure 5A). The inhibitory effect

of BIRB-796 in these three steroid refractory cells was similar to the steroid responsive AMs (Figure 5B). Thus the ability of BIRB-796 to inhibit TNFα release was maintained in cells with poor steroid sensitivity. We confirmed that the potency of the LPS response in the steroid resistant donors was not significantly different from that of the steroid sensitive donors, ruling out the possibility that shift in the potency of LPS could have explained the differential response to steroid (Figure 5C). The average levels of TNFα release from the steroid responsive donors appeared higher than in the non-responsive, but since the groups are small the significance of this is unclear. The

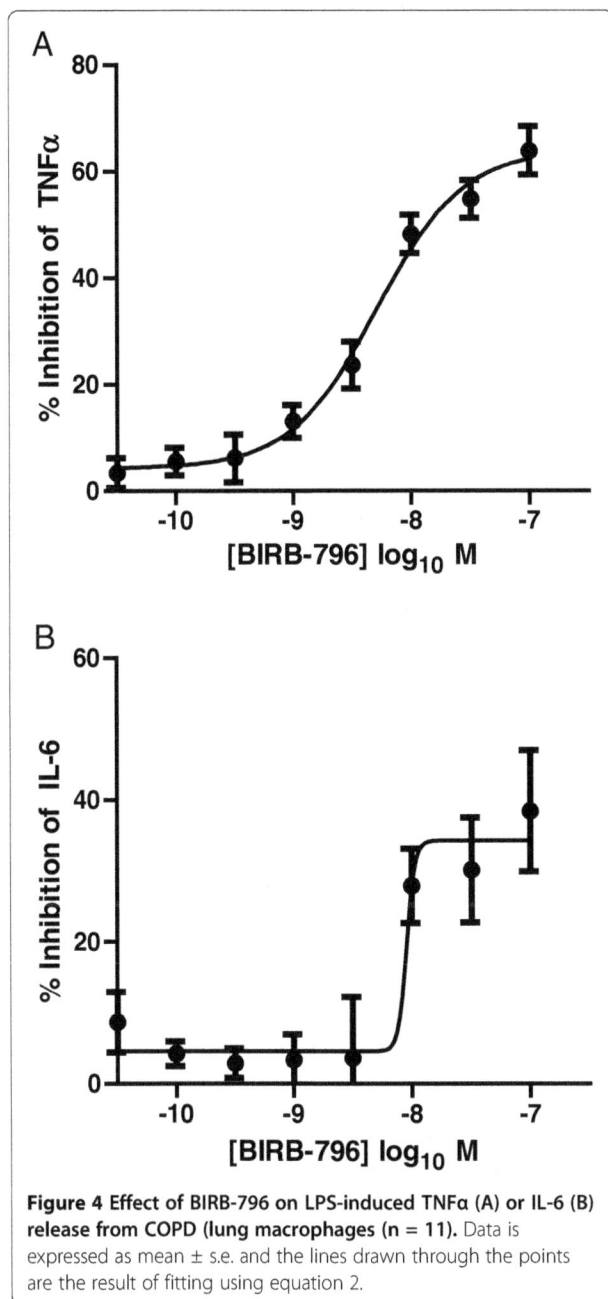

**Figure 4** Effect of BIRB-796 on LPS-induced TNFα (A) or IL-6 (B) release from COPD (lung macrophages (n = 11). Data is expressed as mean ± s.e. and the lines drawn through the points are the result of fitting using equation 2.

range of TNFα release in the steroid non-responsive group (0.6-7.6 ng/ml) lay within the range seen in the steroid responsive group (0.3-15.4 ng/ml).

## Combination of BIRB-796 and budesonide

Combination therapy is an increasing trend within the respiratory area, in an attempt to increase the therapeutic efficacy of medications. The combined effect of Budesonide and BIRB-796 was assessed in COPD AMs. Using a maximally effective concentration of Budesonide (100 nM), an additive effect of BIRB-796 on the release of TNF in response to LPS was observed (Figure 6).

## Discussion

We have investigated the pharmacological profile of three different anti-inflammatory agents in COPD lung macrophages. We used LPS as a stimulus, given the strong links between bacterial colonization and exacerbations of COPD [16]. TNF and IL-6 are both pleiotropic, pro-inflammatory cytokines which are elevated in COPD patients [17,18]. Furthermore, genetic polymorphisms in both these cytokines have been linked to development of COPD [19,20]. The response to the PDEIV inhibitor, Cilomilast, was poor, consistent with published data showing limited effects of PDEIV inhibitors in inhibiting cytokine production from human macrophages [21,22]. Such data suggests that suppression of macrophage function is not a key contributor to the observed clinical efficacy of PDEIV inhibitors in COPD, which may instead lie with anti-inflammatory effects on other cells such as neutrophils or epithelial cells. Alternatively, the modest potency of cilomilast may have limited the effects of this agent and therefore it would be interesting to evaluate the properties of other PDEIV inhibitors. The steroid Budesonide and the p38 inhibitor BIRB-796 were effective anti-inflammatory agents in alveolar macrophages although their effectiveness was dependent on the particular cytokine readout. TNFα release was significantly inhibited by both compounds, but IL-6 was more resistant to inhibition. Other studies have also demonstrated efficacy of steroids in reducing cytokine release from COPD macrophages, with the magnitude of the effect varying between readouts [15,23] . In our study, AMs exhibited a broad spectrum of sensitivities to Budesonide ranging from one donor which failed to show any inhibition of cytokine release, to donors in which the steroid gave over 75% inhibition of TNFα release. This data suggests that cellular steroid insensitivity may not be characteristic of COPD. Rather, there appears to be a significant proportion of individuals whose show a poor cellular response to steroid. Increasingly, physicians and payers are looking towards personalized healthcare approaches, so that individuals likely to respond or fail to respond to treatment can be identified. Steroid treatment is linked to a range of serious side effects, and if those patients who are steroid insensitive could be identified, an alternative treatment option could be selected, thus avoiding unnecessary exposure to steroid.

Of particular interest is our observation that BIRB-796 inhibited TNFα release from AMs equally well in COPD donors that were good or poor responders to Budesonide. This data indicates that p38 inhibitors might be effective in patients which respond poorly to steroids. p38 MAPK pathways have been shown to be active in COPD [24] and a p38 inhibitor has been shown to downregulate a different panel of mediators to steroids, which

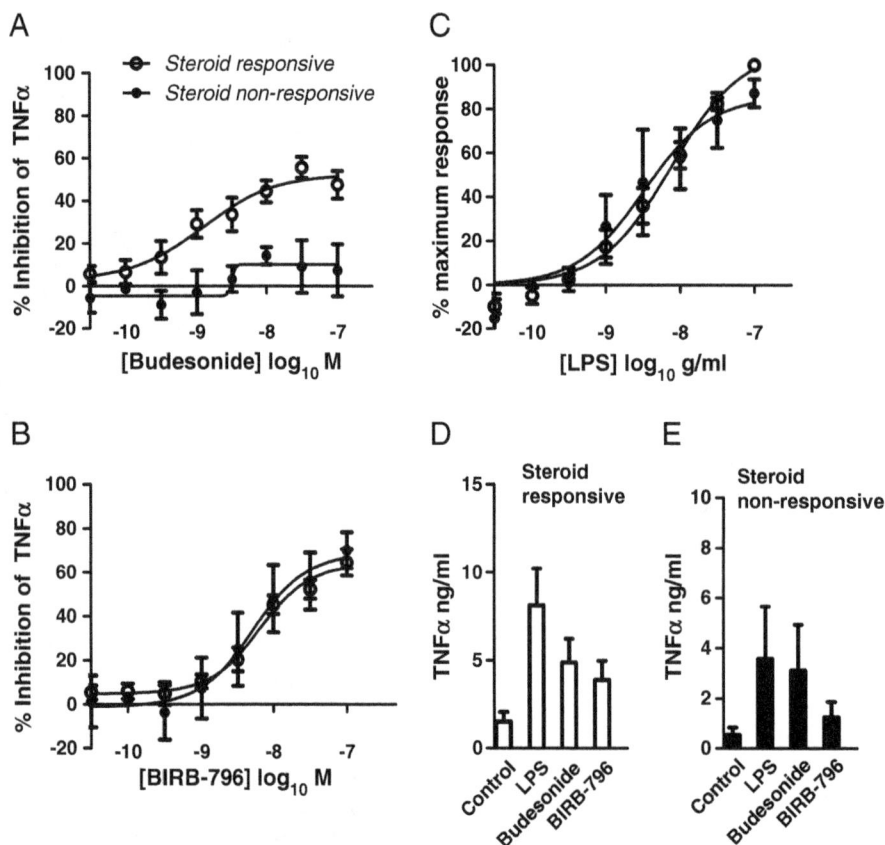

**Figure 5** The effects of Budesonide (A) and BIRB-796 (B) in COPD AMs separated into donors resistant (< 30% inhibition of LPS-induced TNFα release, n = 3), closed circles) or sensitive (> 30% inhibition, n = 8, open circles) to steroid. (C) LPS concentration-effection response curve in steroid resistant (closed circles) or steroid sensitive (open circles) COPD donors. Data is expressed as mean ± s.e. and the lines drawn through the points are the result of fitting using equations 1 (LPS data) and 2 (Budesonide and BIRB-796 data). Absolute cytokine release levels for steroid responsive (D) and steroid non-responsive (E) groups in response to LPS alone and in the presence of 100 nM Budesonide or BIRB-796.

may also provide an advantage in a disease setting [15]. Although a number of oral p38 MAPK inhibitors have ceased development due to unwanted side-effects, inhaled p38 inhibitors may have an acceptable therapeutic window and thus represent useful new anti-inflammatory agents. Indeed, PF-03715455 is being developed as an inhaled agent for the treatment of COPD [25]. Such agents could be considered as steroid replacements, or as a second-line treatment option in patients with a poor response to steroid. Recent studies have demonstrated additive effects of steroids and p38 inhibitors in reducing cytokine release from bronchoalveolar lavage (BAL) macrophages and PBMCs from asthmatics [26] and COPD patients [27]. Our data confirms and extends these results, demonstrating additive effects of BIRB-796 and Budesonide in macrophages from a different compartment (lung tissue versus BAL) and to severe (GOLD stage IV) COPD patients, as compared to mild/moderate disease. Thus, our data adds to a growing body of evidence suggesting that a combination of steroid

plus p38 inhibitor, on the background of standard bronchodilator therapy, could deliver increased clinical efficacy in severe COPD patients.

## Conclusions

In a subset of subjects with GOLD IV stage COPD, steroids are ineffective in reducing cytokine release from tissue macrophages, yet the inhibitory response to the p38 MAPK inhibitor BIRB-796 is maintained in these cells. Use of inhaled p38 MAPK inhibitors may therefore provide a more effective therapy than steroids in some COPD patients. In addition, combination of steroid with a p38 inhibitor provides additive anti-inflammatory effects in COPD lung tissue macrophages.

## Methods

### Reagents

LPS (*E. coli* 026:B6), Budesonide and Foetal Calf Serum (FCS) were from Sigma-Aldrich, Poole, Dorset UK. Cilomilast and BIRB-796 was synthesised by the Medicinal

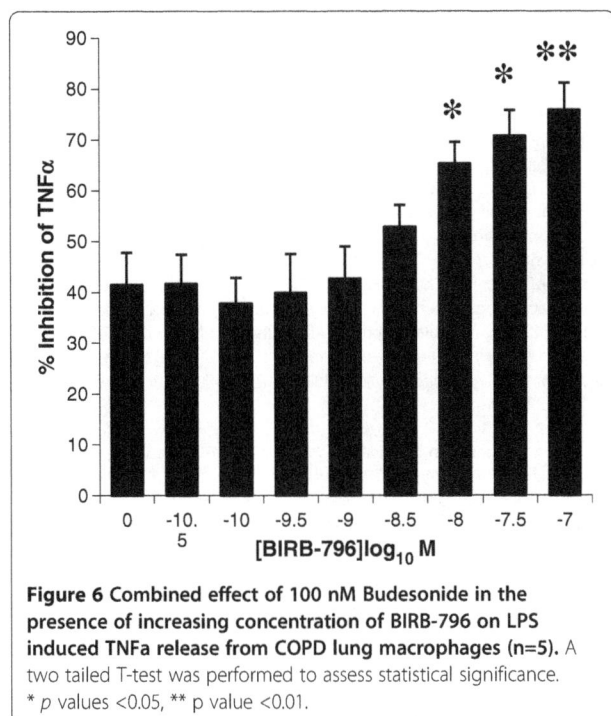

**Figure 6** Combined effect of 100 nM Budesonide in the presence of increasing concentration of BIRB-796 on LPS induced TNFa release from COPD lung macrophages (n=5). A two tailed T-test was performed to assess statistical significance. * p values <0.05, ** p value <0.01.

Chemistry Department, AstraZeneca R&D Charnwood. RPMI, DMEM, Iscoves modified Dulbecco's medium containing GlutaMAX™ (IMDM), L-glutamine and Penicillin/ Streptomycin were from Invitrogen Ltd, Paisley UK. Compounds were made up in Dimethyl Sulfoxide (DMSO) at 1000x final concentration, such that the final concentration of DMSO was 0.1%.

## Subjects

All studies were approved by the Northumberland Local Research Ethics Committee (REC reference 06/Q0902/ 57). Written, informed consent was obtained from each subject. The demographic and lung function data for the COPD transplant patients are summarised in Table 1. All patients had severe end stage disease and a diagnosis of emphysema.

## Cytokine release assays

Human AMs were obtained from COPD patients undergoing lung transplant. Macrophages were flushed from the tissue with phosphate buffered saline (PBS), then plated at 100,000 cells/well in 96 well plates in serum free RPMI for 1 hour. Contaminating cells were removed by stringent

## Table 1 Subject information. Data is average ± s.e

| | Sex (M/F) | Age (years) | FEV$_1$ (l) | FEV$_1$/FVC (%) |
|---|---|---|---|---|
| COPD transplant patients (n = 11) | 6/5 | 52.9 ± 2.4 | 0.6 ± 0.1 | 28.3 ± 6.9 |

washing in RPMI, and AMs rested in assay media for 1 hour prior to cytokine release experiments. The purity of macrophages obtained by this process was confirmed as >90% by Wright-Giemsa/May-Grünwald staining.

Cytokine release experiments were performed in IMDM containing 0.5% FCS. Compounds were added for 30 minutes, prior to addition of LPS (100 ng/ml final concentration) and cells incubated for 20 hours. Supernatants were harvested and cytokines measured using optEIA ELISA kits (BD Biosciences, Erembodegen, Belgium) according to manufacturer's instructions. The compounds had no effect on cell viability at the concentrations used as assessed by cellular morphology and/or Wst-1 viability assays.

## Data analysis

To estimate the potency of LPS, concentration-effect curve data were fitted to the following form of the Hill equation:

$$E = \frac{\alpha[A]^{nH}}{[A]^{nH} + [A]_{50}^{nH}} \quad (1)$$

in which α, $[A]_{50}$ and $n_H$ are the upper asymptote (maximum effect), location (potency) and slope parameters, respectively. $[A]_{50}$ values were assumed to be log-normally distributed and quoted as $p[A]_{50}$ ($-\log[A]_{50}$) values.

Similarly, potencies of Budesonide and BIRB-796 were estimated by fitting inhibitory concentration-effect curve data to a modified version of equation (1):

$$E = \frac{\alpha[I]^{nH}}{[I]^{nH} + [IC]_{50}^{nH}} \quad (2)$$

in which α, $[IC]_{50}$ and $n_H$ are the upper asymptote (maximum effect), location (potency) and slope parameters, respectively. $[IC]_{50}$ values were assumed to be log-normally distributed and quoted as $p[IC]_{50}$ ($-\log[IC]_{50}$) values. In all cases the individual concentration-effect curve data was averaged and this mean data fitted to equations 1 and 2. Maximum effects quoted in the results sections are the measured values rather than the values obtained from the fitting procedures. Percentage inhibition was calculated by the equation: ((LPS in presence of compound – basal) ÷ (LPS in presence of vehicle – basal)) × 100. All curve fitting was done using Graph-Pad Prism software, using a non linear regression curve fit with least squares fit. Results are expressed and plotted as mean ± s.e. Where appropriate, a two tailed T-test was performed to assess statistical significance. p values of <0.05 were considered significant.

## Abbreviations

DMSO: Dimethyl sulfoxide; TNFα: Tumor necrosis factor-alpha; IL-6: Interleukin-6; BIRB-796: 1-(5-tert-Butyl-2-p-tolyl-2H-pyrazol-3-yl)-3-[4-(2-morpholin-4-yl-ethoxy)-naphthalen-1-yl]-urea; COPD: Chronic Obstructive Pulmonary Disease; PDEIV: Phosphodiesterase IV; AM: Alveolar macrophage; FCS: Fetal calf serum; LPS: Lipopolysaccharide; BAL: Bronchoalveolar lavage.

## Competing interests

The authors are current or recent employees of AstraZeneca Plc.

## Authors' contributions

MJR conducted the experiments and performed the data analysis. IGD contributed to the data analysis. Both authors contributed to the study design and manuscript preparation. All authors read and approved the final manuscript.

## Acknowledgements

We are grateful to Professor Paul Corris, Freeman Hospital, Newcastle for supply of COPD transplant tissue. We would also like to thank Michael Dymond for statistical advice.

## Author details

[1]Personalised Healthcare and Biomarkers, AstraZeneca R&D Alderley Park, Cheshire, SK 10 4TG, UK. [2]IGD Consultancy Limited, Loughborough, LE 11 3JR, UK.

## References

1. Buist AS, McBurnie MA, Vollmer WM, Gillespie S, Burney P, Mannino DM, Menezes AM, Sullivan SD, Lee TA, Weiss KB, Jensen RL, Marks GB, Gulsvik A, Nizankowska-Mogilnicka E: International variation in the prevalence of COPD (The BOLD Study): a population-based prevalence study. *Lancet* 2007, **370**:741–750.
2. Calverley PMA, Anderson JA, Celli B, Ferguson GT, Jenkins C, Jones PW, Yates JC, Vestbo J: **Salmeterol and Fluticasone Propionate and Survival in Chronic Obstructive Pulmonary Disease.** *N Engl J Med* 2007, **356**:775–789.
3. Gan WQ, Man SP, Sin D: **Effects of inhaled corticosteroids on sputum cell counts in stable chronic obstructive pulmonary disease: a systematic review and a meta-analysis.** *BMC Pulm Med* 2005, **5**:3.
4. Jen R, Rennard SI: **Effects of inhaled corticosteroids on airway inflammation in chronic obstructive pulmonary disease: a systematic review and meta-analysis.** *International Journal of Chronic Pulmonary Obstructive Disease* 2012, **7**:587–595.
5. Barnes PJ: **New Concepts in Chronic Obstructive Pulmonary Disease.** *Annu Rev Med* 2003, **54**:113–129.
6. Culpitt SV, Rogers DF, Shah P, De Matos C, Russell REK, Donnelly LE, Barnes PJ: **Impaired Inhibition by Dexamethasone of Cytokine Release by Alveolar Macrophages from Patients with Chronic Obstructive Pulmonary Disease.** *Am J Respir Crit Care Med* 2003, **167**:24–31.
7. Adcock IM, Barnes PJ: **Molecular mechanisms of corticosteroid resistance.** *Chest* 2008, **134**:394–401.
8. Gamble E, Grootendorst DC, Brightling CE, Troy S, Qiu Y, Zhu J, Parker D, Matin D, Majumdar S, Vignola AM, Kroegel C, Morell F, Hansel TT, Rennard SI, Compton C, Amit O, Tat T, Edelson J, Pavord ID, Rabe KF, Barnes NC, Jeffery PK: **Antiinflammatory Effects of the Phosphodiesterase-4 Inhibitor Cilomilast (Ariflo) in Chronic Obstructive Pulmonary Disease.** *Am J Respir Crit Care Med* 2003, **168**:976–982.
9. Fabbri LM, Calverley PM, Izquierdo-Alonso JL, Bundschuh DS, Brose M, Martinez FJ, Rabe KF: **Roflumilast in moderate-to-severe chronic obstructive pulmonary disease treated with longacting bronchodilators: two randomised clinical trials.** *Lancet* 2009, **374**:695–703.
10. Calverley PM, Rabe KF, Goehring U, Kristiansen S, Fabbri LM, Martinez FJ: **Roflumilast in symptomatic chronic obstructive pulmonary disease: two randomised clinical trials.** *Lancet* 2009, **374**:685–694.
11. Kumar S, Boehm J, Lee JC: **p38 MAP kinases: key signalling molecules as therapeutic targets for inflammatory diseases.** *Nat Rev Drug Discov* 2003, **2**:717–726.
12. Singh D, Smyth L, Borrill Z, Sweeney L, Tal-Singer R: **A Randomized, Placebo-Controlled Study of the Effects of the p38 MAPK Inhibitor SB-681323 on Blood Biomarkers of Inflammation in COPD Patients.** *J Clin Pharmacol* 2010, **50**:94–100.
13. Lomas DA, Lipson DA, Miller BE, Willits L, Keene O, Barnacle H, Barnes NC, Tal-Singer R: **on behalf of the Losmapimod Study Investigators: An Oral Inhibitor of p38 MAP Kinase Reduces Plasma Fibrinogen in Patients With Chronic Obstructive Pulmonary Disease.** *J Clin Pharmacol* 2012, **52**:416–424.
14. Smith SJ, Fenwick PS, Nicholson AG, Kirschenbaum F, Finney-Hayward TK, Higgins LS, Giembycz MA, Barnes PJ, Donnelly LE: **Inhibitory effect of p38 mitogen-activated protein kinase inhibitors on cytokine release from human macrophages.** *Br J Pharmacol* 2006, **149**:393–404.
15. Kent LM, Smyth LJ, Plumb J, Clayton CL, Fox SM, Ray DW, Farrow SN, Singh D: **Inhibition of lipopolysaccharide-stimulated chronic obstructive pulmonary disease macrophage inflammatory gene expression by dexamethasone and the p38 mitogen-activated protein kinase inhibitor N-cyano-N'-(2-[[8-(2,6-difluorophenyl)-4-(4-fluoro-2-methylphenyl)-7-oxo-7,8-dihydropyrido [2,3-d] pyrimidin-2-yl]amino}ethyl)guanidine (SB706504).** *J Pharmacol Exp Ther* 2009, **328**:458–468.
16. Patel IS, Seemungal TAR, Wilks M, Lloyd-Owen SJ, Donaldson GC, Wedzicha JA: **Relationship between bacterial colonisation and the frequency, character, and severity of COPD exacerbations.** *Thorax* 2002, **57**:759–764.
17. Keatings V, Collins P, Scott D, Barnes P: **Differences in interleukin-8 and tumor necrosis factor-alpha in induced sputum from patients with chronic obstructive pulmonary disease or asthma.** *Am J Respir Crit Care Med* 1996, **153**:530–534.
18. Wedzicha JA, Seemungal TAR, MacCallum PK, Paul EA, Donaldson GC, Bhowmik A, Jeffries DJ, Meade TW: **Acute Exacerbations of Chronic Obstructive Pulmonary Disease Are Accompanied by Elevations of Plasma Fibrinogen and Serum IL-6 Levels.** *Thromb Haemost* 2000, **84**:210–215.
19. Gingo MR, Silveira LJ, Miller YE, Friedlander AL, Cosgrove GP, Chan ED, Maier LA, Bowler RP: **Tumour necrosis factor gene polymorphisms are associated with COPD.** *Eur Respir J* 2008, **31**:1005–1012.
20. He J, Foreman MG, Shumansky K, Zhang X, Akhabir L, Sin DD, Man SFP, DeMeo DL, Litonjua AA, Silverman EK, Connett JE, Anthonisen NR, Wise RA, Paré PD, Sandford AJ: **Associations of IL6 polymorphisms with lung function decline and COPD.** *Thorax* 2009, **64**:698–704.
21. Gantner F, Kupferschmidt R, Schudt C, Wendel A, Hatzelmann A: **In vitro differentiation of human monocytes to macrophages: change of PDE profile and its relationship to suppression of tumour necrosis factor-α release by PDE inhibitors.** *Br J Pharmacol* 1997, **121**:221–231.
22. Hatzelmann A, Schudt C: **Anti-Inflammatory and Immunomodulatory Potential of the Novel PDE4 Inhibitor Roflumilast in Vitro.** *J Pharmacol Exp Ther* 2001, **297**:267–279.
23. Armstrong J, Sargent C, Singh D: **Glucocorticoid sensitivity of lipopolysaccharide-stimulated chronic obstructive pulmonary disease alveolar macrophages.** *Clin Exp Immunol* 2009, **158**:74–83.
24. Renda T, Baraldo S, Pelaia G, Bazzan E, Turato G, Papi A, Maestrelli P, Maselli R, Vatrella A, Fabbri LM, Zuin R, Marsico SA, Saetta M: **Increased activation of p38 MAPK in COPD.** *Eur Respir J* 2008, **31**:62–69.
25. Millan DS, Bunnage ME, Burrows JL, Butcher KJ, Dodd PG, Evans TJ, Fairman DA, Hughes SJ, Kilty IC, Lemaitre A, Lewthwaite RA, Mahnke A, Mathias JP, Philip J, Smith RT, Stefaniak MH, Yeadon M, Phillips C: **Design and Synthesis of Inhaled p38 Inhibitors for the Treatment of Chronic Obstructive Pulmonary Disease.** *J Med Chem* 2011, **54**:7797–7814.
26. Bhavsar P, Khorasani N, Hew M, Johnson M, Chung KF: **Effect of p38 MAPK inhibition on corticosteroid suppression of cytokine release in severe asthma.** *Eur Respir J* 2010, **35**:750–756.
27. Armstrong J, Harbron C, Lea S, Booth G, Cadden P, Wreggett KA, Singh D: **Syngergistic effects of p38 mitogen activated protein kinase inhibition with a corticosteroid in Alveolar Macrophages from patients with Chronic Obstructive Pulmonary Disease.** *J Pharmacol Exp Ther* 2011, **338**:732.

# 14

# Efficacy of lisdexamfetamine dimesylate in adults with attention-deficit/hyperactivity disorder previously treated with amphetamines: analyses from a randomized, double-blind, multicenter, placebo-controlled titration study

Thomas Babcock[*], Bryan Dirks, Ben Adeyi and Brian Scheckner

## Abstract

**Background:** To examine the efficacy of lisdexamfetamine dimesylate (LDX) in adults with attention-deficit/hyperactivity disorder (ADHD) who remained symptomatic (ADHD Rating Scale IV [ADHD-RS-IV] total score >18) on amphetamine (AMPH) therapy (mixed AMPH salts and/or d-AMPH formulations) prior to enrollment in a 4-week placebo-controlled LDX trial vs the overall study population. In these post hoc analyses from a multicenter, randomized, double-blind, forced-dose titration study, clinical efficacy of LDX (30-70 mg/d) in adults with ADHD receiving AMPH treatment at screening vs the overall study population was evaluated. ADHD symptoms were assessed using the ADHD-RS-IV with adult prompts at screening, baseline (after prior treatment washout), and endpoint. Safety assessments included treatment-emergent adverse events (TEAEs), vital signs, laboratory findings, and electrocardiogram.

**Results:** Of 414 participants (62, placebo; 352, LDX) included in the overall study population, 41 were receiving AMPH therapy at screening (2, placebo; 39, LDX); mean AMPH dose was 35.0 and 34.1 mg/d for participants in placebo and all LDX groups, respectively. Of the 41 participants, 36 remained symptomatic (ADHD-RS-IV >18) at screening despite receiving AMPH. For the 36 participants in the placebo (n = 2) and LDX (n = 34) groups, respectively, at endpoint, mean change from screening ADHD-RS-IV total scores were -5.5 and -14.8 and from baseline scores were -13.5 and -17.8. For the overall study population, endpoint mean change from baseline ADHD-RS-IV total scores were -7.8 for placebo and -17.5 for LDX. In the prior AMPH subgroup, 2/2 (100.0%) in the placebo group and 22/39 (56.4%) participants in the LDX (all doses) group reported any TEAE. Events that occurred in ≥5% for LDX were dry mouth (5/39; 12.8%), headache (5/39; 12.8%), fatigue (3/39; 7.7%), insomnia (3/39; 7.7%), decreased appetite (2/39; 5.1%), and nausea (2/39; 5.1%). None of these events occurred in the 2 placebo patients with prior AMPH use.

**Conclusion:** In these post hoc analyses, adults with significant baseline ADHD symptoms despite adequate AMPH treatment dose showed similar improvements in ADHD symptoms with LDX treatment as the overall study population. Prospective studies are needed to confirm these findings. The safety profile of LDX in the overall study population was consistent with long-acting psychostimulant use.

**Trial registry:** Study to Assess the Safety and Efficacy of NRP104 in Adults With Attention-Deficit Hyperactivity Disorder (ADHD). Clinicaltrials.gov Identifier: NCT00334880

**Keywords:** Lisdexamfetamine dimesylate, LDX, Amphetamines, Attention-deficit hyperactivity disorder, ADHD, Adult, Switching treatment

* Correspondence: tbabcock@shire.com
Shire Development LLC, 725 Chesterbrook Blvd, Wayne, PA 19087, USA

## Background

Attention-deficit/hyperactivity disorder (ADHD) affects approximately 4.4% of adults in the United States [1]. Currently, psychostimulants, both amphetamines (AMPH) and methylphenidate (MPH), are considered first-line ADHD pharmacotherapy in adults [2-4]. Clinically non-responsive patients treated with one psychostimulant will often obtain an improved clinical response when switched to another psychostimulant class; possibly because classes may differ in mechanisms of action [5]. As reviewed by Arnold and colleagues, AMPH and MPH are reuptake inhibitors of norepinephrine and dopamine (DA) [5]. However, AMPH also stimulates neurotransmitter release from presynaptic receptors.

Moreover, it is observed in psychiatry that, when patients exhibit efficacy or tolerability concerns while on a treatment, it is not uncommon in clinical practice (e.g., depression treatment) for a patient to be switched to a different medication within the same class [6,7]. In ADHD treatment and management, this has included switching from an immediate-release or short-acting formulation to a long-acting formulation [8,9], or from a racemic mixture to a single enantiomer formulation (e.g., d-MPH) [10].

The AMPH class of psychostimulants comprises short- and long-acting formulations of mixed AMPH salts (MAS) and MAS extended release (MAS XR), respectively, and d-AMPH formulations, including short-acting d-AMPH and long-acting d-AMPH (d-AMPH-ER), and the prodrug lisdexamfetamine dimesylate (LDX). LDX is a long-acting prodrug stimulant indicated for ADHD treatment in children (6 to 12 years), adolescents (13 to 17 years), and adults [11]. The inactive prodrug is converted, primarily in the blood, to l-lysine and therapeutically active d-AMPH [12]. MAS XR is a once-daily beaded formulation, also indicated for ADHD treatment in children (6 to 12 years), adolescents (13 to 17 years), and adults [13]. Overall, studies have demonstrated the effectiveness and safety of LDX and MAS XR in adults with ADHD [14-18]. However, a qualitative comparison in a matched-group post hoc analysis suggested that LDX provided greater improvement in ADHD symptoms [16]. Unlike LDX, the pharmacokinetic profile of MAS XR is altered by gastrointestinal pH variations, as assessed by coadministration with a proton pump inhibitor that reduces stomach acid [19].

A PubMed literature search of relevant papers produced none that systematically assessed treatment response in patients switched between different formulations of the same class of stimulant (e.g., from one MPH or AMPH formulation to another). Therefore, a study assessing treatment effects of a more recent psychostimulant formulation in adults who remain symptomatic while using another psychostimulant formulation may be useful to clinicians choosing between treatment options for adults with ADHD.

The objectives of these post hoc analyses were to assess the efficacy of LDX in adults with ADHD who remained symptomatic on AMPH therapy (various formulations) prior to enrollment vs the overall study population in a 4-week, placebo-controlled, LDX trial. Comparing symptomatic recent and prior AMPH users to the overall study population of adults with ADHD treated with LDX can aid clinicians in determining if LDX may be a viable treatment option after another AMPH medication has been used with suboptimal treatment response.

## Methods

### Study design and participants

This was a multicenter, randomized, double-blind, forced-dose titration, 4-week study that evaluated efficacy of LDX (30, 50, and 70 mg/d) vs placebo in adults (18 to 55 years) with ADHD. The study was performed in accordance with the Declaration of Helsinki and the International Conference on Harmonisation Guidelines for Good Clinical Practice. All participants provided written informed consent and Institutional Review Board approval was obtained at all study sites prior to study conduct. Institutional Review Boards/Ethics Committees approving the study were Aspire IRB, 9320 Fuerte Dr, Suite 105, La Mesa, CA 91941 (multiple study sites); Duke University Medical Center IRB, Hock Plaza, 2424 Erwin Rd, Suite 405, Durham, NC 27705; Office of Institutional Review (UHC IRB) University Hospitals of Cleveland, 11100 Euclid Ave, Lakeside 1400, Cleveland, OH 44106-7061; Partners Human Research Committee, 116 Huntington Ave, Suite 1002, Boston, MA 02116; Subcommittee for Human Studies (SHS), 423 E 23rd St, 18S, New York, NY 10010; UCSF Committee on Human Research, 3333 California St, San Francisco, CA 94143-0310; University of California, Irvine, Institutional Review Board, Office of Research Administration, 300 University Tower, Irvine, CA 92697; Western Institutional Review Board (WIRB), 3535 Seventh Ave, SW, Olympia, WA 98502; and Yale University School of Medicine Human Investigation Committee (HIC), 47 College St, Suite 208, PO Box 208010, New Haven, CT 06520. The methodology and results of the primary and secondary analyses from this study have been reported elsewhere [20]. The study included participants on AMPH formulations, including MAS, MAS XR, and d-AMP (d-AMPH spansule and short-acting d-AMPH) at screening and who, at screening, remained symptomatic on their prior treatment. Post hoc analyses of these participants were conducted and are reported here. Participants may have previously been on more than one type of AMPH.

Key inclusion criteria included a primary ADHD diagnosis, by *Diagnostic and Statistical Manual of Mental Disorders, Fourth Edition, Text Revision* [21] (DSM-IV-TR) criteria and an ADHD Rating Scale IV [22] (ADHD-RS-IV) with adult prompts [23] total score of ≥28 at baseline.

### Primary efficacy assessments

The primary efficacy measure was the ADHD-RS-IV with adult prompts that assessed ADHD symptoms at screening, baseline (after washout of prior treatment), and endpoint. Endpoint was defined as the last postrandomization treatment week with a valid ADHD-RS-IV score. The primary efficacy endpoint was the mean change from baseline to endpoint in ADHD-RS-IV total score in the overall efficacy or intention-to-treat (ITT) population (all randomized and treated participants who had a baseline ADHD-RS-IV score and at least one postrandomization ADHD-RS-IV score).

### Other efficacy measures

The Clinical Global Impressions [24] (CGI) scale evaluated global ADHD symptom illness severity and improvement. CGI-Severity (CGI-S) was assessed at baseline using a 7-point scale with scores ranging from 1 (normal, not at all ill) to 7 (among the most extremely ill). The CGI-Improvement (CGI-I) scale was assessed at each postbaseline visit also on a 7-point scale with scores ranging from 1 (very much improved) to 7 (very much worse).

### Post hoc assessments

The prior AMPH subgroup was defined as all participants who took AMPH products with a stop date on or after the screening date. For purposes of this post hoc analysis, an ADHD-RS-IV total score >18 at screening in the prior AMPH subgroup was considered a suboptimal level of symptom control. ADHD symptom items are rated on a 4-point scale, which consists of scores of 0 (never or rarely), 1 (sometimes), 2 (often), and 3 (very often) [22]. An ADHD-RS-IV total score of ≤18 (an average score of 1 per item for the 18-item scale) has been used to define symptomatic remission in combined-type ADHD [25]. As reviewed by Steele and colleagues, when individuals are treated (with or without medication), symptomatic remission in ADHD should be defined as a "loss of diagnostic status, minimal or no symptoms, and optimal functioning" [26]. Moreover, on most standardized questionnaires, symptomatic remission can be "operationalized as a mean total score of ≤1" for each item or an ADHD-RS-IV total score of ≤18.

### Safety assessments

Safety assessments in the overall safety population included treatment-emergent adverse events (TEAEs), vital signs, laboratory findings, and electrocardiogram (ECG).

### Statistical analysis

Descriptive statistics were used to assess efficacy outcomes in the prior AMPH subgroup. No comparative statistical analyses were conducted between the prior AMPH-treated subgroup and the overall study population since the study was not prospectively designed to assess these comparisons. Based on established criteria [26,27], clinical response was defined as a change in ADHD-RS-IV total score of ≥30% from baseline and a CGI-I score of 1 or 2. Symptomatic remission, a measure of optimal symptom control, was defined as a postbaseline ADHD-RS-IV total score ≤18.

The overall safety population comprised all participants enrolled and randomized who received treatment. TEAEs were defined as events with onset postrandomization (i.e., first treatment date).

## Results

### Disposition

Of 420 participants randomized, 414 (62 receiving placebo, 352 LDX) were included in the efficacy population, 71 of 420 (16.9%) were discontinued, and 41 of 414 (9.9%) were receiving AMPH at screening. Of the 41 prior AMPH-treated participants, 2 were randomized to placebo and 39 were randomized to LDX (30 mg/d [n = 11], 50 mg/d [n = 16], and 70 mg/d [n = 12]). In the placebo group, 1 participant was treated with MAS and 1 with MAS XR. In the LDX (all doses) group, 11 participants were previously treated with MAS, 27 with MAS XR, and 2 with d-AMPH. Thirty-six (87.8%) of 41 participants remained symptomatic (ADHD-RS-IV >18) at screening.

### Demographics and baseline characteristics (Table 1)

The mean (standard deviation [SD]) ADHD-RS-IV total score at screening for the prior AMPH subgroup was 39.3 (7.0) for placebo and 41.0 (5.7) for LDX. Mean (SD) AMPH doses were 35.0 (7.1) mg/d for those randomized to the placebo group and 30.0 (8.9), 38.4 (17.7), and 32.2 (22.2) mg/d for those randomized to the 30-, 50-, and 70-mg/d LDX groups, respectively. Moreover, duration of prior AMPH exposure was reported in the range of approximately 2 weeks to 13 years; only 1 participant was treated for <4 weeks. Two patients reported MAS doses of <20 mg/d.

### Primary efficacy measures

At endpoint, change from baseline in mean (SD) ADHD-RS-IV total scores for LDX-treated participants was similar in AMPH groups and the overall study groups (Figure 1). Prior AMPH nonresponders (ADHD-RS-IV total score >18 at screening) in the placebo group (n = 2) had baseline mean (SD) ADHD-RS-IV total score of 41.0 (5.66) and change from baseline was -13.5 (4.95). In the placebo group of the overall efficacy population

**Table 1** Demographics and baseline characteristics of the prior AMPH subgroup (n = 41) and overall safety population (n = 420)

| Variable, n (%) | | Prior AMPH subgroup | | Overall safety population | |
| --- | --- | --- | --- | --- | --- |
| | | Placebo | LDX (all doses) | Placebo | LDX (all doses) |
| | | n = 2 | n = 39 | n = 62 | n = 358 |
| **Sex** | Male | 0 | 20 (51.3) | 32 (51.6) | 196 (54.7) |
| | Female | 2 (100.0) | 19 (48.7) | 30 (48.4) | 162 (45.3) |
| **Race** | White | 1 (50.0) | 38 (97.4) | 48 (77.4) | 301 (84.1) |
| | Non-white | 1 (50.0) | 1 (2.6) | 14 (22.6) | 57 (15.9) |
| **Ethnicity** | Hispanic/Latino | 0 | 1 (2.6) | 6 (9.7) | 34 (9.5) |
| | Non-Hispanic/Non-Latino | 2 (100.0) | 38 (97.4) | 56 (90.3) | 324 (90.5) |
| **CGI-S at baseline** | Moderately ill | 1 (50.0) | 12 (30.8) | 27 (43.5) | 115 (32.1) |
| | Markedly ill | 1 (50.0) | 17 (43.6) | 25 (40.3) | 195 (54.5) |
| | Severely/extremely ill | 0 | 10 (25.6) | 10 (16.1) | 48 (13.4) |

(n = 62), baseline mean (SD) ADHD-RS-IV total score was 39.4 (6.42) and change from baseline was -7.8 (9.28). Because of the small number of participants in the placebo-treated prior AMPH nonresponders group (n = 2), no comparisons between placebo and LDX AMPH nonresponders subgroups were warranted.

**Other efficacy measures**
The mean (SD) CGI scores were comparable between the prior AMPH subgroup and overall efficacy population in the LDX-treated groups (Table 2). At all time points assessed, the percentage of clinical responders and symptomatic remitters was comparable in both LDX groups (Figures 2a and 2b). For 2 participants in the placebo-treated prior AMPH subgroup, 1 (50.0%) achieved clinical response at week 1 through 4 and at endpoint; and 1 (50.0%)

achieved symptomatic remission at week 2 only. For participants in the overall efficacy population receiving placebo (n = 62), the proportion achieving clinical response ranged from 11.3% at week 1 to 27.4% at week 4 and 29.0% at endpoint; the proportion achieving symptomatic remission ranged from 1.6% at week 1 to 11.3% at week 3 and 11.3% at endpoint.

**Safety**
In the prior AMPH subgroup, 2 of 2 (100.0%) in the placebo group and 22 of 39 (56.4%) participants in the LDX (all doses) group reported any TEAE (Table 3). For those receiving LDX in this subgroup, TEAEs with ≥5% frequency were dry mouth (5/39; 12.8%), headache (5/39; 12.8%), fatigue (3/39; 7.7%), insomnia (3/39; 7.7%), decreased appetite (2/39; 5.1%), and nausea (2/39; 5.1%).

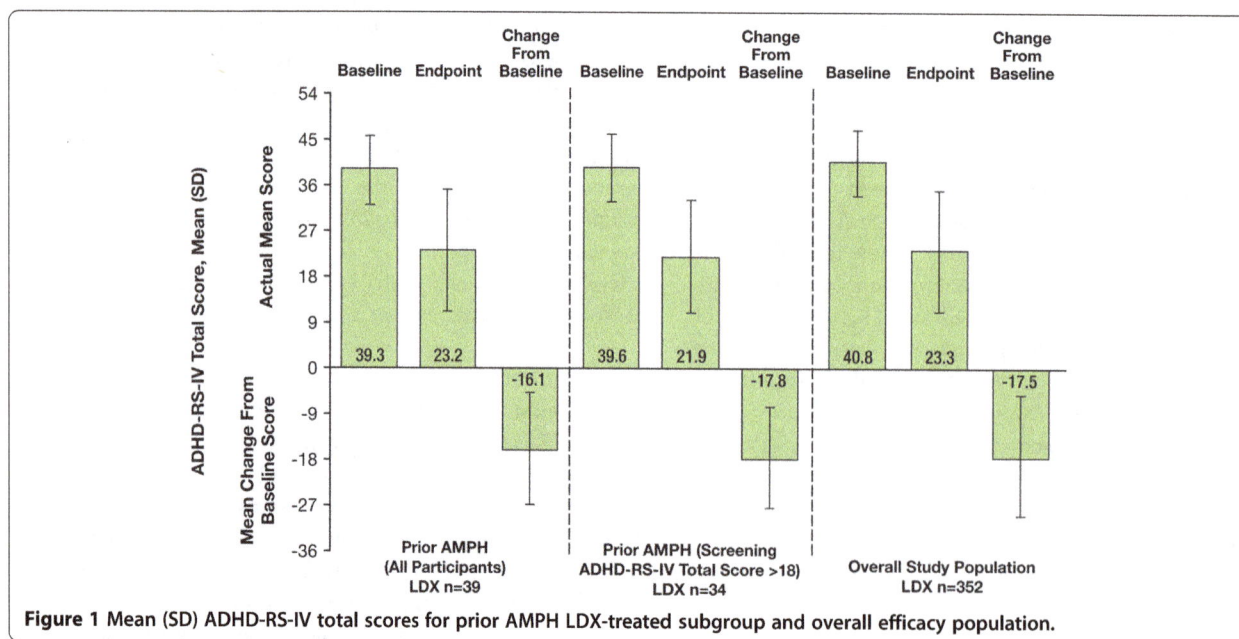

**Figure 1** Mean (SD) ADHD-RS-IV total scores for prior AMPH LDX-treated subgroup and overall efficacy population.

**Table 2 Mean (SD) CGI-S and CGI-I scores for prior AMPH subgroup and overall efficacy population**

| Variable | Mean (SD) CGI scores | | | |
| --- | --- | --- | --- | --- |
| | Prior AMPH subgroup | | Overall efficacy population | |
| | Placebo (n = 2) | LDX (n = 39) | Placebo (n = 62) | LDX (n = 352) |
| CGI-S (Baseline) | 4.5 (0.71) | 4.9 (0.76) | 4.7 (0.73) | 4.8 (0.65) |
| CGI-I (Endpoint) | 2.5 (0.71) | 2.4 (1.11) | 3.2 (1.19) | 2.4 (1.07) |

There were only 2 prior AMPH participants randomized to placebo; therefore, describing "common" TEAEs is not appropriate, but neither placebo participant experienced one of the TEAEs common in the LDX group. All TEAEs in all prior AMPH users were of mild to moderate severity and there were no serious TEAEs.

In the overall safety population, 36 of 62 (58.1%) in the placebo group and 282 of 358 (78.8%) participants in the LDX (all doses) group reported any TEAE (Table 3). The majority of TEAEs were mild to moderate in severity. Twenty-two of 420 (5.2%) participants were discontinued due to TEAEs in the overall safety population. In this population, there were no deaths, and 2 of 420 (0.5%) participants had serious AEs (leg injury due to motor vehicle accident [LDX 30 mg/d group] and postoperative knee pain [LDX 70 mg/d group]). Both reported serious

AEs were considered not treatment-related, and participants were discontinued.

At endpoint for the overall safety population, small mean increases in vital signs (systolic and diastolic blood pressure) from baseline were not statistically significant vs placebo. At endpoint for pulse, the slight mean difference vs placebo was significant ($P = .0018$). There were no significant meaningful changes in QTcF interval data from baseline between the placebo and LDX groups.

## Discussion

In these post hoc analyses, adults with significant baseline ADHD symptoms in the prior AMPH group, despite adequate mean AMPH treatment dose and duration of prior treatment (only 1 participant was treated for <4 weeks), showed improvements in symptoms with

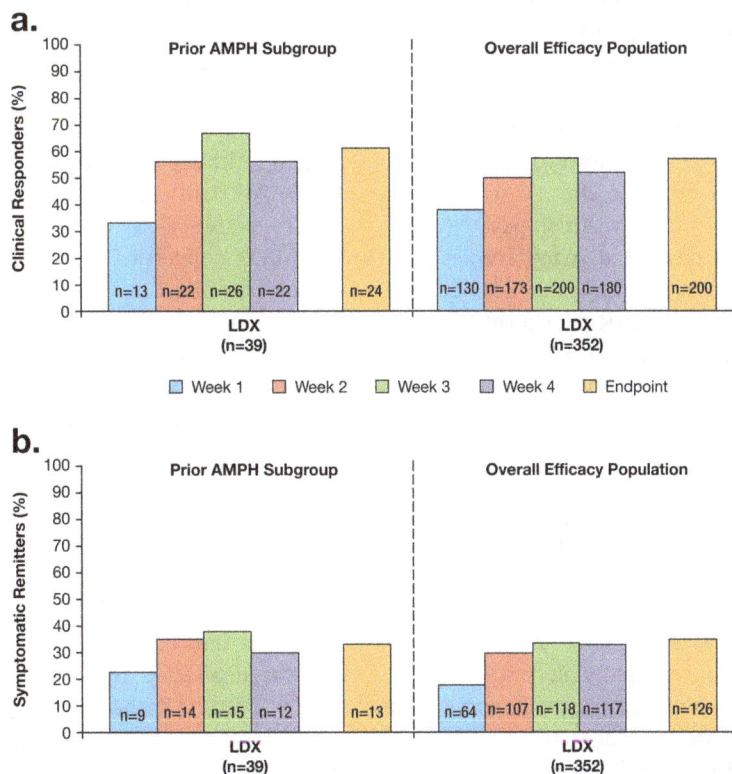

**Figure 2 Percentage of a) clinical responders and b) symptomatic remitters.** Note: Clinical response was defined as a change in ADHD-RS-IV total score of ≥30% from baseline and a CGI-I score of 1 or 2. Symptomatic Remission was defined as a post baseline ADHD-RS-IV total score of ≤18.

**Table 3 Common TEAEs with frequency ≥5% in the LDX (all doses) group and greater than placebo**

| Preferred terminology (MedDRA 9.1) | Participants, n (%) | | | |
|---|---|---|---|---|
| | Prior AMPH subgroup | | Overall safety population | |
| | Placebo n = 2 | LDX (All Doses) n = 39 | Placebo n = 62 | LDX (All Doses) n = 358 |
| All TEAEs | 2 (100) | 22 (56.4) | 36 (58.1) | 282 (78.8) |
| Anorexia | 0 | 0 | 0 | 18 (5.0) |
| Anxiety | 0 | 1 (2.6) | 0 | 21 (5.9) |
| Decreased appetite | 0 | 2 (5.1) | 1 (1.6) | 95 (26.5) |
| Diarrhea | 0 | 0 | 0 | 24 (6.7) |
| Dry mouth | 0 | 5 (12.8) | 2 (3.2) | 92 (25.7) |
| Fatigue | 0 | 3 (7.7) | 3 (4.8) | 17 (4.7) |
| Headache | 0 | 5 (12.8) | 8 (12.9) | 74 (20.7) |
| Initial insomnia | 0 | 1 (2.6) | 2 (3.2) | 18 (5.0) |
| Insomnia | 0 | 3 (7.7) | 3 (4.8) | 69 (19.3) |
| Irritability | 0 | 1 (2.6) | 4 (6.5) | 22 (6.1) |
| Nausea | 0 | 2 (5.1) | 0 | 25 (7.0) |
| Upper respiratory tract infection | 0 | 1 (2.6) | 3 (4.8) | 20 (5.6) |

LDX treatment similar to the overall study population. Improvement in ADHD symptoms in LDX-treated adults was similar in the prior AMPH subgroup and overall efficacy population. Moreover, global severity at baseline and global symptom improvement with LDX treatment were comparable across all treatment groups in the prior AMPH subgroup and overall efficacy population.

One study suggests that, although psychostimulants (both AMPH and MPH) are effective in ADHD management, some participants responded better to one type of psychostimulant than to the other [28]. However, results of studies that assess treatment response after switching between agents in the same class are few. A comparative review of psychostimulants suggests that many studies assessing differences between psychostimulants do not show comparisons at the individual participant level [5]. Thus, it is unknown if patient variability in terms of prior treatment history may affect response to current treatment.

This study suggests a differential response to various ADHD formulations within the same class of psychostimulants may occur, as indicated by the improved clinical response with LDX treatment in participants who had significant ADHD symptoms despite prior AMPH therapy. Although conducted in animals with results that may not apply to humans, a study by Joyce et al supports this contention; potential variability in response based on formulation differences among the same AMPH class of psychostimulants was suggested by differential response in AMPH-evoked DA release with MAS (racemic mixture of 76% d-AMPH and 24% l-AMPH salts), d-AMPH, and d, l-AMPH in the rat striatum [29].

Such variations in neurotransmitter release based on the differing formulations of the same class of psychostimulant may play a pivotal role in intrapatient variability to treatment response. LDX, which is a pro-drug of d-AMPH covalently bound to therapeutically inactive l-lysine, has demonstrated consistent and low inter-and intrapatient pharmacokinetic variability in d-AMPH mean observed maximum drug concentration and area under the concentration-time curve from time zero to infinity, as well as consistent delivery of d-AMPH in adults [30]. Although a small amount of LDX is hydrolyzed to d-AMPH in the gastrointestinal tract, the conversion into active d-AMPH occurs primarily in the blood. The LDX conversion to d-AMPH is unlikely to be affected by gastrointestinal pH and variations in normal gastrointestinal transit times [31,32].

Another open-label, adult study that assessed LDX and MAS XR pharmacokinetics, alone or in combination with omeprazole (proton pump inhibitor) demonstrated that MAS XR-treated participants on omeprazole experienced a shortened time to maximum drug concentration ($T_{max}$) of ≥1 hour in more than 50% of participants vs MAS-XR alone. However, LDX combination therapy with omeprazole resulted in shortened $T_{max}$ in only 25% of participants vs LDX alone [19]. Moreover, the study indicated that the distribution around the median d-AMPH $T_{max}$ for LDX was unaffected by omeprazole administration, although for MAS XR the dispersion was compressed. These aforementioned study data suggest a variable pharmacokinetic response even among the same class of psychostimulants. Data in animal models suggest that amphetamine formulations may differ in their pharmacodynamic effects as well. In rats administered equivalent doses of LDX and d-AMPH, increases in striatal dopamine release and in locomotor activity were lower in peak effect but more sustained with LDX vs d-AMPH [33].

A post hoc comparative qualitative analysis, using groups that were matched based on treatment duration, baseline ADHD symptom severity, and approximately equivalent AMPH doses of LDX and MAS XR in adults with ADHD from 2 similar short-term trials, found that both psychostimulants demonstrated efficacy vs placebo. Safety profiles were consistent with psychostimulant use [16]. However, this qualitative analysis also suggested that LDX treatment vs MAS XR demonstrated greater numerical improvements in ADHD core and global symptoms, as well as decreased frequency of percent differences (active treatment minus placebo) in AEs. Although exploratory in nature, these data suggest that there may be within-class efficacy and safety differences among psychostimulants; however, prospective and quantitative head-to-head comparison trials are needed to confirm these findings.

Findings from clinical trials have not provided clinicians with sufficient comparative data to adequately assess which psychostimulant may be optimal for individual patients, especially since large variations in response rates to drugs and doses exist, and the best sequence of dispensing the various psychostimulant treatments by the clinician is currently unknown [34]. Studies such as the present analysis may prove beneficial to clinicians in determining appropriate treatment options after nonresponse or suboptimal response to a particular psychostimulant therapy.

Overall, the safety profile of LDX was consistent with other long-acting psychostimulants. The frequency of common TEAEs ≥5% appeared to be lower in the LDX-treated prior AMPH groups compared with the overall population, perhaps because these patients were acclimated to the effects of psychostimulant medications. This effect was also seen in a pediatric study of LDX with patient groups that were previously treated with psychostimulants [35].

Limitations of this analysis include results that may not be representative of large cohorts because of the small subgroup sample sizes and the study design features discussed below. Since analyses were not designed or powered to assess group differences and were described with summary statistics, prospective studies are needed to confirm these results. The majority of participants were non-Hispanic/non-Latino, white, and moderately to markedly ill at baseline; results may not be able to be generalized to other ethnicities, races, or global illness severity levels. Due to the post hoc nature of this analysis, factors related to prior use of AMPH were not controlled or assessed in the study: despite the knowledge that adequate mean doses of prior AMPH were used, there was no information to determine if these doses were clinically optimized; data on the level of compliance with prior AMPH treatment were also lacking; and individuals with poor tolerability to AMPH would be ineligible to participate in this study, presenting another study limitation. The baseline symptom severity before AMPH treatment was unspecified. In addition, there was no apparent limitation on study enrollment that would exclude participants with sufficient clinical response to prior medication, since symptomatic non-remitters on prior AMPH were not defined by overall clinical response to AMPH, but only by the participant's screening ADHD-RS-IV total score.

## Conclusions

Overall, the analyses provide a signal suggesting that, for patients who are not optimally treated with AMPH formulations, LDX remains a potential alternative to consider for the treatment of ADHD in adults. In addition, efficacy outcomes in the prior AMPH subgroup population were consistent with those of the overall study population. The LDX safety profile was consistent with long-acting psychostimulant use. However, this study was not designed to address or compare relative advantages and disadvantages of particular pharmacotherapeutic alternatives. Prospective trials assessing this signal would be helpful in determining the utility of such options in clinical management of patients requiring treatment changes.

**Abbreviations**
ADHD: Attention-deficit/hyperactivity disorder; ADHD-RS-IV: ADHD Rating Scale IV; AEs: Adverse events; AMPH: Amphetamine; CGI: Clinical Global Impressions; CGI-I: CGI-Improvement; CGI-S: CGI-Severity; DA: Dopamine; d-AMPH: dextroamphetamine; DSM-IV-TR: Diagnostic and Statistical Manual of Mental Disorders Fourth Edition, Text Revision; ECG: Electrocardiogram; ITT: Intention to treat; LDX: Lisdexamfetamine dimesylate; l-amphetamine: levo-amphetamine; MAS: Mixed AMPH salts; MPH: Methylphenidate; SD: Standard deviation; TEAEs: Treatment-emergent AEs; T$_{max}$: Time to maximum concentration; XR: Extended release.

**Competing interests**
Dr Babcock is an employee of Shire and holds stock and/or stock options in Shire.
Dr Dirks is an employee of Shire and holds stock and/or stock options in Johnson & Johnson and Shire.
Mr Adeyi is an employee of Shire and holds stock and/or stock options in Shire.
Dr Scheckner is an employee of Shire and holds stock and/or stock options in Shire.

**Authors' contributions**
TB was the associate director, Scientific Publications, Clinical Development and Medical Affairs for this study, and made substantial contributions to the analysis and interpretation of the data. He was deeply involved in drafting the manuscript and revising the intellectual content. He has given final approval of this version. BD was the director, Clinical Development and Medical Affairs for this study, and made substantial contributions to the analysis and interpretation of the data. He was deeply involved in drafting the manuscript and revising the intellectual content. He has given final approval of this version. BA was a statistician involved in all post hoc data analysis, interpretation, and presentation. Statistician BA was fully involved in drafting and revising the intellectual content of this manuscript. Statistician

BA has given final approval to this version. **BS** was a director, Scientific Publications, Clinical Development and Medical Affairs, for this study, and made substantial contributions to the analysis and interpretation of the data. He was deeply involved in drafting the manuscript and revising the intellectual content. He has given final approval of this version.

## Authors' information
**Thomas Babcock, DO**, is currently an employee of Shire Pharmaceuticals LLC, where he has worked in the Medical Affairs Department since 2005. Dr Babcock graduated from the University of Osteopathic Medicine and Health Sciences (now Des Moines University) in Des Moines, Iowa, and earned his doctorate in anthropology working in Central America. Dr Babcock has authored 12 journal articles and 1 book as of January 2011.
**Bryan Dirks, MD**, is currently a medical director with Shire Pharmaceuticals LLC. Dr Dirks is a diplomate of the American Board of Psychiatry and Neurology in general psychiatry. He also has a master's of science degree in epidemiology from Harvard University School of Public Health in Boston, Massachusetts, and a master's of business administration degree from George Washington University in Washington, DC. His research publications include work in suicidology, schizophrenia, and ADHD.
**Ben Adeyi, MS, ACII**, is currently an employee of Shire Pharmaceuticals LLC, and has been working in the Biostatistics and Statistical Programming Department since 2008. He has worked as a senior biometrician for Merck & Co., Inc., and, prior to working in the pharmaceutical industry, he was a senior data analyst in the Nuclear Cardiology Medicine Department at Cornell University Medical College in New York, New York. Mr Adeyi was educated at Emory University in Atlanta, Georgia, and Temple University in Philadelphia, Pennsylvania. He is a charter member of the Chartered Insurance Institute of London, England, and has coauthored several abstracts and manuscripts.
**Brian Scheckner, PharmD, BCPP, CMPP**, is currently an employee of Shire Pharmaceuticals LLC, where he is a Director of Scientific Publications. He has worked for Shire since 2004 in the Clinical Development and Medical Affairs Department, serving in publication and medical communication roles. Dr Scheckner was educated at the University of the Sciences in Philadelphia (PharmD) and Rutgers University (BS, Pharmacy), and has licenses/ certifications in pharmacy, psychiatric pharmacy, and publications planning. His membership in professional associations includes the International Society for Medical Publication Professionals (ISMPP) and the College of Psychiatric and Neurologic Pharmacists (CNP). His research publications include work in ADHD and MDD.

## Acknowledgments
Clinical research was funded by the sponsor, Shire Development LLC. Under the direction of the authors, Huda Ismail Abdullah, PhD, a former employee of SCI Scientific Communications & Information (SCI), provided writing assistance for this publication. Editorial assistance in formatting, proofreading, copy editing, and fact checking was also provided by SCI. Shire Development LLC provided funding to SCI for support in writing and editing this manuscript. Although the sponsor was involved in the design, collection, analysis, interpretation, and fact checking of information, the content of this manuscript, the ultimate interpretation, and the decision to submit it for publication in *BMC Clinical Pharmacology* were made by the authors independently.

## References
1. Kessler RC, Adler L, Barkley R, Biederman J, Conners CK, Demler O, Faraone SV, Greenhill LL, Howes MJ, Secnik K, *et al*: **The prevalence and correlates of adult ADHD in the United States: results from the National Comorbidity Survey Replication.** *Am J Psychiatry* 2006, **163**(4):716.
2. Pliszka SR, Crismon ML, Hughes CW, Conners CK, Emslie GJ, Jensen PS, McCracken JT, Swanson JM, Lopez M, The Texas Consensus Conference Panel on Pharmacotherapy of Childhood Attention-Deficit/Hyperactivity Disorder: **The Texas Children's Medication Algorithm Project: revision of the algorithm for pharmacotherapy of attention-deficit/hyperactivity disorder.** *J Am Acad Child Adolesc Psychiatry* 2006, **45**(6):642.
3. Canadian ADHD Resource Alliance: **Canadian ADHD practice guidelines.** CAP-guidelines 3rd edition. http://www.caddra.ca/cms4/pdfs/ caddraGuidelines2011.pdf. Accessed September 13, 2012.
4. Nutt DJ, Fone K, Asherson P, Bramble D, Hill P, Matthews K, Morris KA, Santosh P, Sonuga-Barke E, Taylor E, *et al*: **Evidence-based guidelines for management of attention-deficit/hyperactivity disorder in adolescents in transition to adult services and in adults: recommendations from the British Association for Psychopharmacology.** *J Psychopharmacol* 2007, **21**(1):10.
5. Arnold LE: **Methylphenidate vs. amphetamine: comparative review.** *J Atten Disord* 2000, **3**(4):200.
6. Burke WJ, Bose A, Wang J, Stahl SM: **Switching depressed patients from citalopram to escitalopram is well tolerated and effective.** *Poster Presented at: American College of Neuropsychopharmacology's 42nd Annual Meeting; December 7-11, 2003.* San Juan, Puerto Rico.
7. Rush AJ, Trivedi MH, Wisniewski SR, Stewart JW, Nierenberg AA, Thase ME, Ritz L, Biggs MM, Warden D, Luther JF, *et al*: **Bupropion-SR, sertraline, or venlafaxine-XR after failure of SSRIs for depression.** *N Engl J Med* 2006, **354**(12):1231.
8. Cantwell DP: **Attention deficit disorder: a review of the past 10 years.** *J Am Acad Child Adolesc Psychiatry* 1996, **35**(8):978.
9. Pelham W Jr, Greenslade KE, Vodde-Hamilton M, Murphy DA, Greenstein JJ, Gnagy EM, Guthrie KJ, Hoover MD, Dahl RE: **Relative efficacy of long-acting stimulants on children with attention deficit-hyperactivity disorder: a comparison of standard methylphenidate, sustained-release methylphenidate, sustained-release dextroamphetamine, and pemoline.** *Pediatrics* 1990, **86**(2):226.
10. Arnold LE, Lindsay RL, Conners CK, Wigal SB, Levine AJ, Johnson DE, West SA, Sangal RB, Bohan TP, Zeldis JB: **A double-blind, placebo-controlled withdrawal trial of dexmethylphenidate hydrochloride in children with attention deficit hyperactivity disorder.** *J Child Adolesc Psychopharmacol* 2004, **14**(4):542.
11. *Vyvanse [package insert]*. Wayne, PA: Shire US Inc; 2012.
12. Pennick M: **Absorption of lisdexamfetamine dimesylate and its enzymatic conversion to d-amphetamine.** *Neuropsychiatr Dis Treat* 2010, **6**(1):317.
13. *Adderall XR [package insert]*. Wayne, PA: Shire US Inc; 2011.
14. Wigal T, Brams M, Gasior M, Gao J, Squires L, Giblin J, on behalf of the 316 Study Group: **Randomized, double-blind, placebo-controlled, crossover study of the efficacy and safety of lisdexamfetamine dimesylate in adults with attention-deficit/hyperactivity disorder: novel findings using the adult workplace environment design.** *Behav Brain Funct* 2010, **6**:34.
15. Weisler R, Young J, Mattingly G, Gao J, Squires L, Adler L, on behalf of the 304 Study Group: **Long-term safety and effectiveness of lisdexamfetamine dimesylate in adults with attention-deficit/ hyperactivity disorder.** *CNS Spectr* 2009, **14**(10):573.
16. Lasser R, Dirks B, Adeyi B, Babcock T: **Comparative efficacy and safety of lisdexamfetamine dimesylate and mixed amphetamine salts extended release in adults with attention-deficit/hyperactivity disorder.** *Prim Psychiatr* 2010, **17**(9):44.
17. Biederman J, Spencer TJ, Wilens TE, Weisler RH, Read SC, Tulloch SJ, on behalf of the SLI 381.304 Study Group: **Long-term safety and effectiveness of mixed amphetamine salts extended release in adults with ADHD.** *CNS Spectr* 2005, **10**(12 suppl 20):16.
18. Weisler RH, Biederman J, Spencer TJ, Wilens TE, Faraone SV, Chrisman AK, Read SC, Tulloch SJ, on behalf of the SLI381.303 Study Group: **Mixed amphetamine salts extended-release in the treatment of adult ADHD: a randomized, controlled trial.** *CNS Spectr* 2006, **11**(8):625.
19. Haffey MB, Buckwalter M, Zhang P, Homolka R, Martin P, Lasseter KC, Ermer JC: **Effects of omeprazole on the pharmacokinetic profiles of lisdexamfetamine dimesylate and extended-release mixed amphetamine salts in adults.** *Postgrad Med* 2009, **121**(5):11.
20. Adler LA, Goodman DW, Kollins SH, Weisler RH, Krishnan S, Zhang Y, Biederman J, on behalf of the 303 Study Group: **Double-blind, placebo-controlled study of the efficacy and safety of lisdexamfetamine dimesylate in adults with attention-deficit/hyperactivity disorder.** *J Clin Psychiatry* 2008, **69**(9):1364.
21. American Psychiatric Association: *Diagnostic and Statistical Manual of Mental Disorders DSM-IV-TR*. Washington, DC: American Psychiatric Association; 2000.

22. DuPaul GJ, Power TJ, Anastopoulos AD, Reid R: *ADHD Rating Scale-IV: Checklists, Norms, and Clinical Interpretation*. New York, NY: Guilford Press; 1998.

23. Adler L, Cohen J: **Diagnosis and evaluation of adults with attention-deficit/hyperactivity disorder.** *Psychiatr Clin North Am* 2004, **27**(2):187.

24. Guy W: **Clinical global impressions.** In *ECDEU Assessment Manual for Psychopharmacology*. Rockville, MD: US Department of Health, Education, and Welfare; Public Health Service, Alcohol, Drug Abuse and Mental Health Administration, NIMH Psychopharmacology Research Branch; 1976:218–222.

25. Stein MA, Sarampote CS, Waldman ID, Robb AS, Conlon C, Pearl PL, Black DO, Seymour KE, Newcorn JH: **A dose-response study of OROS methylphenidate in children with attention-deficit/hyperactivity disorder.** *Pediatrics* 2003, **112**(5):e404.

26. Steele M, Jensen PS, Quinn DMP: **Remission versus response as the goal of therapy in ADHD: a new standard for the field?** *Clin Ther* 2006, **28**(11):1892.

27. Swanson JM, Kraemer HC, Hinshaw SP, Arnold LE, Conners CK, Abikoff HB, Clevenger W, Davies M, Elliott GR, Greenhill LL, *et al*: **Clinical relevance of the primary findings of the MTA: success rates based on severity of ADHD and ODD symptoms at the end of treatment.** *J Am Acad Child Adolesc Psychiatry* 2001, **40**(2):168.

28. Elia J, Borcherding BG, Rapoport JL, Keysor CS: **Methylphenidate and dextroamphetamine treatments of hyperactivity: are there true nonresponders?** *Psychiatry Res* 1991, **36**(2):141.

29. Joyce BM, Glaser PE, Gerhardt GA: **Adderall produces increased striatal dopamine release and a prolonged time course compared to amphetamine isomers.** *Psychopharmacology (Berl)* 2007, **191**(3):669.

30. Ermer J, Homolka R, Martin P, Buckwalter M, Purkayastha J, Roesch B: **Lisdexamfetamine dimesylate: linear dose-proportionality, low intersubject and intrasubject variability, and safety in an open-label single-dose pharmacokinetic study in healthy adult volunteers.** *J Clin Pharmacol* 2010, **50**(9):1001.

31. Shojaei A, Ermer JC, Krishnan S: **Lisdexamfetamine dimesylate as a treatment for ADHD: dosage formulation and pH effects.** *Poster Presented at: 160th Annual Meeting of the American Psychiatric Association; May 19-24, 2007.* San Diego, CA: Poster NR; 740.

32. Krishnan S, Zhang Y: **Relative bioavailability of lisdexamfetamine 70-mg capsules in fasted and fed healthy adult volunteers and in solution: a single-dose, crossover pharmacokinetic study.** *J Clin Pharmacol* 2008, **48**(3):293.

33. Rowley H, Heal D, Hackett D: **Simultaneous measurement with hysteresis analyses of the effects of lisdexamfetamine dimesylate and d-amphetamine on striatal levels of extracellular dopamine, locomotor activity, and plasma drug concentrations in freely-moving rats.** *Poster Presented at: New Clinical Drug Evaluation Unit Annual Meeting; June 13-16, 2011.* Boca Raton, FL.

34. Greenhill LL, Pliszka S, Dulcan MK, Bernet W, Arnold V, Beitchman J, Benson RS, Bukstein O, Kinlan J, McClellan J, *et al*: **Practice parameter for the use of stimulant medications in the treatment of children, adolescents, and adults.** *J Am Acad Child Adolesc Psychiatry* 2002, **41**(2 suppl):26S.

35. Jain R, Babcock T, Burtea T, Dirks B, Adeyi B, Scheckner B, Lasser R: **Efficacy of lisdexamfetamine dimesylate in children with attention-deficit/hyperactivity disorder previously treated with methylphenidate: a post hoc analysis.** *Child Adolesc Psychiatry Ment Health* 2011, **5**(1):35.

# 15

# Experiences from consumer reports on psychiatric adverse drug reactions with antidepressant medication: a qualitative study of reports to a consumer association

Andreas Vilhelmsson[1*], Tommy Svensson[1,2], Anna Meeuwisse[3] and Anders Carlsten[4]

## Abstract

**Background:** The new European pharmacovigilance legislation has been suggested as marking the beginning of a new chapter in drug safety, making patients an important part of pharmacovigilance. In Sweden since 2008 it has been possible for consumers to report adverse drug reactions (ADRs) to the Medical Products Agency (MPA), and these reports are now understood as an increasingly valuable contribution in the monitoring of safety aspects in medicines. Already in 2002 it was possible to report experiences with medicines to the non-profit and independent organization Consumer Association for Medicines and Health (KILEN) through a web-based report form with an opportunity to describe ADR experiences in free text comments. The aim of this study was to qualitatively analyze the free text comments appended to consumer reports on antidepressant medication.

**Methods:** All reports of suspected adverse reactions regarding antidepressant medications submitted from January 2002 to April 2009 to KILEN's Internet-based reporting system in Sweden were analyzed according to reported narrative experience(s). Content analysis was used to interpret the content of 181 reports with free text comments.

**Results:** Three main categories emerged from the analyzed data material: (1) *Experiences of drug treatment* with subcategories (a) *Severe psychiatric adverse reactions*, and (b) *Discontinuation symptoms*; (2) *Lack of communication* and (3) *Trust and distrust*. A majority of the reports to KILEN were from patients experiencing symptoms of mental disturbances (sometimes severe) affecting them in many different ways, especially during discontinuation. Several report included narratives of patients not receiving information of potential ADRs from their doctor, but also that there were no follow-ups of the treatment. Trust was highlighted as especially important and some patients reported losing confidence in their doctor when they were not believed about the suspected ADRs they experienced, making them attempt to discontinue their antidepressant treatment on their own.

**Conclusions:** The present study indicates that free text comments as often contained in case reports directly submitted by patients can be of value in pharmacovigilance and provide important information on how a drug may affect the person using it and influence his or her personal life.

* Correspondence: andreas.vilhelmsson@nhv.se
[1]Nordic School of Public Health, Gothenburg, Sweden
Full list of author information is available at the end of the article

## Background

The new European pharmacovigilance legislation (Directive 2010/84/EU) (Regulation 1235/2010) [1] that came into force in July 2012 has been suggested as marking the beginning of a new chapter in drug safety [2]. Its purpose is to further accentuate patient influence, and all EU countries are now obliged to introduce patient/consumer reporting to their spontaneous reporting systems, making patients an important part of pharmacovigilance. Since under-reporting by health professionals is a well-recognized problem by the World Health Organization (WHO) [3], the Organization proclaims consumer reporting to be of great importance in safeguarding a pharmacovigilance program that will help each patient to receive optimum therapy, and on a population basis will lead to ensure the acceptance and effectiveness of public health programs [4].

Previous research has indicated that consumer reporting of adverse drug reactions (ADRs) may add value to healthcare professionals' (HCP) reports by identifying possible new reactions [5-10]. In Sweden since 2008 it has been possible for consumers to submit reports to the Medical Products Agency (MPA), and these reports are now understood as an increasingly valuable contribution in the monitoring of safety aspects in medicines [11]. The MPA also offers the opportunity for the consumer to use free text in describing the reaction(s). However, these descriptions have not previously been subjected to qualitative analysis or been published. In order to strengthen consumer rights within the health care sector, the non-profit and independent organization Consumer Association for Medicines and Health (KILEN) has provided the opportunity for consumers to report their perceptions and experiences of using medicines. KILEN had already established a consumer database in 1997 to collect consumer reports, mainly focusing on benzodiazepines and antidepressants. KILEN was created in 1992, but their co-workers had already a long history of working with pharmaceutical drug dependency when in the 1960s it became clear that the new benzodiazepines were causing dependency and harm. Since 2002 it has also been possible to report suspected ADRs to this organization through a web-based report form with the opportunity to add free text comments of the experience(s) (www.kilen.org). Previous research on the KILEN material has shown that consumer reports may contribute important information regarding more serious psychiatric adverse reactions following antidepressant treatment [9]. However, the free text comments were not scrutinized or analyzed. This study, therefore, aimed to qualitatively analyze the free text comments to consumer reports on antidepressant medication.

## Methods

All reports of suspected adverse reactions regarding antidepressant medications submitted from January 2002 to April 2009 to KILEN's Internet-based reporting system in Sweden were analyzed according to reported narrative experience(s). According to WHO, a side effect is an unintended effect of a pharmaceutical product (occurring at doses normally used by a patient) and where there is a relation to the pharmacological properties of the drug whilst an adverse drug reaction (ADR) is defined as a response to a medicine which is noxious and unintended (occurring at doses normally used in man) and where the response of the patient is of importance, in which individual factors may play an important [3]. Since the reports to KILEN contained individual responses to a drug reported as severe and noxious we decided to use the latter. The KILEN compilation and coding system is described in a previous study [9]. As Figure 1 shows, of 442 individual antidepressant reports, 393 individuals also provided a longer description of the ADR experience as free text (89%). A total of 202 antidepressant reports concerned depression as diagnosis (most reported cause for prescription) and included a narrative of the experiences (46%). A total of 21 reports were excluded since they were reported by someone other than the patient (5) or contained too little information (16). Included in the study, therefore, were 181 reports (41%) with narrative.

The project was approved by the Regional Ethics Review Board in Gothenburg, Sweden (No. 319–10).

### Data analysis

Content analysis was used to interpret the patients' accounts. Content analysis here refers to a qualitative data reduction and sense-making effort that takes a volume of qualitative material and attempts to identify core consistencies and meanings [12]. The procedure is basically as

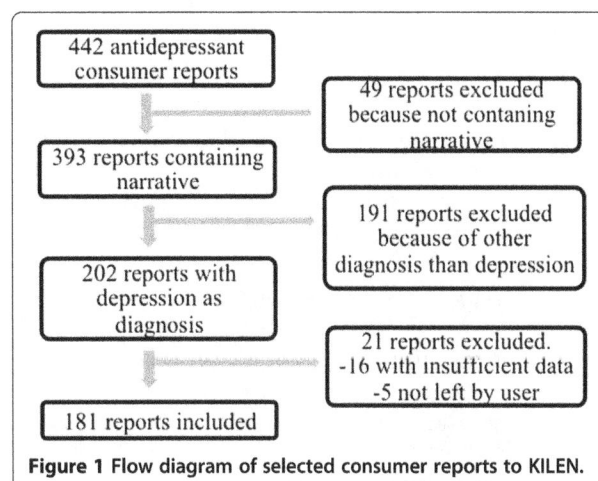

**Figure 1** Flow diagram of selected consumer reports to KILEN.

follows: data are collected and coded by theme or category; the coded data are then analyzed and presented [13]. Creating categories is the core feature of qualitative content analysis and refers to a descriptive level of content; a category often includes a number of sub-categories [14]. All 181 included consumer narratives on depression and antidepressant treatment were read thoroughly several times in order to get an understanding of their meaning. The content of these narratives was then sorted into different main categories and read again, which resulted in subcategories and sometimes new main categories [14]. As Graneheim and Lundman argue, qualitative content analysis interpretation involves a balancing act, where on one hand it is impossible and undesirable for the researcher not to add a particular perspective to the phenomena under study, but on the other hand the researcher must 'let the text talk' and not impute meaning that is not there [14]. Therefore, all authors were involved in analyzing the themes that emerged from the data and were also responsible for reading and confirming the analysis. The authors discussed the analyses – the coding, categorization and interpretation of the results – throughout the work process to gain a mutual understanding. This process was also valid for the selection of quotations describing common experiences found within certain categories. This selection was also made in order to problematize the role of the researcher and to avoid missing out on important information or exaggerate specific content.

## Results and discussion

Of the 181 consumer reports included and analyzed, women contributed 135 (75%) and men 38 (21%). The antidepressants most reported for depression as diagnosis were Sertraline (23.8%), Citalopram (23.8%), Venlafaxine (23.2%), Mirtazapine (10.5%), Paroxetine (7.7%), Escitalopram (6.1%) and Fluoxetine (5.0%). As described in Table 1, three main categories emerged from the analysis of the KILEN data: (1) *Experiences of drug treatment* with subcategories (a) *Severe psychiatric adverse reactions*, and (b) *Discontinuation symptoms*, (2) *Lack of communication* and (3) *Trust and distrust*.

## Experiences of drug treatment

A main category within the KILEN material concerned patients' experiences of suspected adverse reactions during their treatment with antidepressants. Particularly serious psychiatric adverse symptoms were perceived as something difficult during and after treatment, and especially during discontinuation.

### Severe psychiatric adverse reactions

A majority of the reports to KILEN were from patients experiencing symptoms of mental disturbances (sometimes severe) affecting them in many different ways. The level of seriousness has also been indicated in the official spontaneous reports made to the Swedish MPA in 2011 where almost half (49.7%) of a total of 597 reports from the general public were deemed serious [11]. Numerous KILEN narratives reported experiencing a kind of blunting affect of the drug, making patients perceiving feeling like 'zombies' incapable of having or sharing feelings towards others, even their own family members:

> *"I felt completely blunted, that something controlled me so I no longer had contact with my feelings anymore. I became like a zombie who was completely indifferent to everything."* Female, aged 22 years (Sertraline).

This blunting affect has been described in other research as well, where 'being-on-SSRIs' meant an increased distance between takers and their worlds and where previously emotionally close became no more important than 'anyone else' [15]. This feeling of distance was sometimes described in the KILEN narratives as a kind of depersonalization or of feeling a sensation of unreality. In a previous study on the KILEN consumer reports, feeling a sensation of unreality was a commonly reported mental disturbance, but was not listed at all as an adverse drug

**Table 1 Categorization of the analyzed components – examples of patients' statements in the KILEN consumer reports[1]**

| Meaning unit | Condensed meaning unit | Main-category | Sub-category |
|---|---|---|---|
| *"Difficulties concentrating at work, having suicidal thoughts."* | Patient experienced suicidal thoughts. | Experiences of drug treatment | Severe psychiatric adverse reactions |
| *"And when the death wish comes, I become so afraid that I start again."* | Patient experienced feelings of wanting to die when trying to end medication. | | Discontinuation symptoms |
| *"When I first started taking it I received NO [sic!] warnings of adverse drug reactions."* | Patient received no warnings of side effects from the doctor. | Lack of communication | |
| *"Decided that after three years of 'chemical terror' to discontinue, WITHOUT [sic!] doctor's approval."* | Patients decided to end drug treatment without telling the doctor. | Trust and distrust | |

[1] Categorization according to Graneheim & Lundman (2004).

reaction or side effect in the Swedish Physicians' Desk Reference FASS (building on the Summary of Product Characteristics SPC) [9].

Some of the KILEN reports contained narratives describing an increase in having suicidal thoughts or of such thoughts newly occurring. Despite its seriousness this is not something new. Already in the early 1990s Teicher and colleagues showed that some depressed patients (free of recent serious suicidal ideation) developed intense and violent suicidal preoccupation after 2–7 weeks of SSRI treatment [16], and that antidepressant medication might interfere with normal neuropsychological processes that keep suicidal thoughts from intruding into consciousness [17]. Experiencing suicidal thoughts in everyday life affected patients to a high degree, according to their narratives in the KILEN material:

*"Difficulties concentrating at work, having suicidal thoughts."* Male, aged 45 years (Venlafaxine).

Obviously it is in self-reported material often uncertain whether suicidal thoughts were evident before medication started or if they were a direct result of the use of antidepressants, but it is nevertheless important to highlight this severe psychiatric derangement, since it may have fatal consequences if ignored. One must not forget that the role of antidepressants in suicide prevention is considered a major public health question given the high prevalence of both depression and depression-related suicidality [18].

Only 16 (8.8%) consumer narratives out of the total 181 included in the study contained positive experiences of antidepressant drug treatment. This may be compared to a Swedish study of antidepressant medication in primary care where almost 67% of responding patients thought that the drug made them feel better (women 70.2% and men 58.5%) [19]. It is also important not forget that the blunting affect of the drug can sometimes be perceived as positive. Previous research has shown that the experience of younger women is that the antidepressant drug enables them to function in daily life activities [20]. The drug is perceived as working by alleviating pain and suffering [15], by suppressing sensations and stopping the person from dwelling on symptoms [21]. Patients whose narratives were positive about drug treatment in the KILEN data often emphasized that the experienced side effect of the antidepressant was a price worth paying, since the prior untreated condition had been much worse:

*"Saved me from total collapse; sure, there have been shorter episodes of depression, but without Paroxetine [Swedish antidepressant brand name – authors' note] or something like it, I would have been dead or have killed someone."* Male, aged 42 years (Paroxetine).

### Discontinuation symptoms

According to KILEN narratives, it was especially during discontinuation of antidepressant drugs that suspected psychiatric adverse reactions were experienced:

*"Discontinuation of antidepressant medication in four days on doctor's orders, from normal dosage of 50 mg to 25 mg in four days and then nothing. After three days, I experienced a fear of dying and extreme anxiety and had several panic attacks ... woke up and found myself standing with a knife towards my stomach on one occasion and on another with the bathrobe belt in my hand. I no longer tolerate any stress at all, which makes me panic and experience dizziness. Have been without antidepressant medication for nine days and experiences hell on earth."* Female, aged 35 years (Sertraline).

A previous study on the KILEN material indicated that adverse reactions in connection with discontinuation of antidepressant medication was often reported to KILEN but not always mentioned in the Swedish Physicians' Desk Reference FASS, and when it was mentioned, it was generally regarded as rare [9]. This has also been shown in an evaluation of the UK patient reporting system 'Yellow Card Scheme' which identified new 'serious' reactions not previously included in the SPC [5]. Research has shown that antidepressant discontinuation in depressed patients can be associated with worsened depression and increased suicidality [22], and that the recurrence risk for depression was much shorter after rapid than after gradual discontinuation of antidepressants [23]. Abrupt discontinuation can also cause a larger increase in the number of adverse discontinuation symptoms [24,25], and a report from the Swedish Council on Technology Assessment in Health Care (SBU) indicated that long-term use of antidepressants (particularly in high dosages) could cause these symptoms if treatment is terminated suddenly or the dosage is substantially reduced [26].

Fear of discontinuation symptoms made some patients afraid of ending their treatment; these patients often continued to take antidepressants, despite the fact that they did not want to be dependent on them. The suspected adverse reactions were not just perceived as unpleasant but also created a fear of stopping taking the antidepressant drug. A concern that the depression might return was one common feeling that was expressed:

*"And when the death wish comes, I become so afraid that I start again."* Female, aged 42 years (Citalopram).

Since the psychiatric events reported to KILEN often may also occur as a symptom of the illness for which the antidepressant had been prescribed, their (re)appearance may easily suggest that the patient is having a relapse and needs continued treatment. Distinguishing withdrawal from relapse is important but often also very difficult.

### Lack of communication

A second main category concerned the communication between patient and doctor, or rather its absence. Several KILEN narratives concerned patients experiencing a lack of information regarding adverse reactions from their doctor:

> "When I first started taking it, I received NO [sic] warning of adverse drug reactions." Female, aged 37 years (Venlafaxine).

If patients are not receiving information about potential adverse reactions, it is indeed worrying. According to treatment recommendations from the Swedish MPA, all patients with depressive symptoms should be met with understanding and empathy and have (their) opportunity to talk about their life situation, feelings and experience, as well as receive information about the disorder and its treatment options; this includes information about the effects of a drug and its potential adverse reactions [27]. However, previous studies have also provided indications that physicians rarely make reference to side effect (in only 16 of 34 consultations) [28], that patients are unaware that suspected adverse reactions may occur [29], and patients may believe that physicians are withholding information about these reactions [30]. There is also the possibility that physicians themselves are not fully aware of the side effects or adverse reactions related to the drugs they prescribe.

Such situations may lead to poor communication between physicians and patients, which may in turn increase risks [31]. Patients need, for example to be warned about, and monitored for, the possibility of increased depressive and suicidal symptoms as part of a discontinuation reaction. This is also of great importance because feelings of uncertainty regarding the safety of a drug are an important reason for nonadherence to treatment [32]. Fear of adverse effects can be a main reason for not accepting SSRI treatment [33]. Some KILEN reports included, for instance, narratives of giving up on antidepressant treatment because of difficult suspected adverse reactions:

> "Moreover, I had nightmares every night, from the moment I fell asleep, and I woke up several times every night soaked in sweat. Unable to get enough sleep, I became more strained. These adverse drug reactions were the major cause for me to give up my antidepressant treatment." Female, aged 27 years (Sertraline).

Robust and clear communications between doctor and patient if and when the patients experiences serious

adverse effects is therefore of great importance, since serious events like suicidal thoughts or attempts may continue to affect patients' lives long after the event [34]. However, it is important to acknowledge that communications about the safety of medicines are complex and generally poorly performed, and that differences in risk perception between the public and healthcare professionals exist, which may be a barrier to clear communication [35]. It is therefore vital that we challenge potential communication obstacles in order to provide a safer prescription culture. Patients need a balance of information about antidepressants so that they can decide whether or not to take (or continue to take) drugs prescribed [36]. It is however important to acknowledge that doctors alone are not to be held responsible for this lack of information. For instance, a British study indicated that the patient information leaflet (PIL), that accompanies antidepressant medication, did not always warn of discontinuation symptoms and also presented side effects in a strikingly heterogeneous way, making it difficult for patients to find the required information needed to make an informed choice [36].

In some cases in the KILEN reports patients described not just a lack of communication between doctor and patient, but also that there were no follow-ups of the treatment, and that prescriptions were renewed without a personal contact, for instance, by telephone:

> "The most appalling thing during all these years of medication was that I did not have any contact with somebody who monitored . . .either when I started, or during, or after I stopped taking my medication." Female, aged 23 years (Paroxetine).

The Swedish National Board of Health and Welfare argues that the most important measure to minimize risks is to evaluate the effect of the prescribed antidepressant drug, and on a regular basis review the treatment, so that the patient does not continue to take a drug without clear indication [19]. However, according to a study of antidepressant medication in primary care, the agency found that only 40% of Swedish patients had an appointment for follow-up, and over 60% of these had used antidepressant drugs for over a year [19]. Since antidepressants drugs are relatively often involved in the fatal adverse drug reactions (FADRs) occurring [37] (even if it is a small number of FADRs that occur in total) the extra need for surveillance is worth highlighting. Talking with patients about what influences their decisions about use of medications could affect whether these medications are used optimally [30]. Otherwise, there is risk of poor or inappropriate prescribing, wastage of drugs and unsatisfactory doctor–patient relationships if doctors' perceptions do not correspond with patients' preferences [38].

## Trust and distrust

In a third main category, some patients referred to losing trust in their doctor when they perceived that he or she did not take the patient's story and description of ADRs seriously and/or scaled down their consequences. According to several patient reports, there were sometimes problems of separating the symptoms related to the diagnosed depression from the suspected adverse reactions, where patients almost always interpreted negative experiences as belonging to the drug while the doctor construed them as evidence of the initial depression recurring.

*"She [the doctor – author's note] ignores discontinuation symptoms from the drug and wants me to start medicating again after I have been through ten days of hell. She believes that my depression has returned... It is totally wrong."* Female, aged 35 years (Sertraline).

The conflicting accounts between patients and doctors of either drug-induced reactions or initial illness symptoms were especially present during discontinuation. Some patients reported to KILEN that they perceived discontinuation symptoms over a longer period of time, which they perceived as being dismissed by their doctor. Previous research, however, has indicated that discontinuation symptoms sometimes can be severe and prolonged, and may also be mistaken for signs of physical illness or even early signs of relapse, leading to an overestimate of the true effect of the medication [39]. This is unfortunate, since studies have shown that patients can distinguish between suspected adverse reactions and other symptoms [40] and are capable of providing clear descriptions of their experiences and of balancing the benefits and burden of treatment [6]. Some patients reported losing confidence in their doctor when they were not believed about the suspected adverse reactions they experienced:

*"Decided to discontinue after three years of 'chemical terror', WITHOUT [sic] doctor's approval."* Female, aged 41 years (Paroxetine).

Patients have witnessed dismissive attitudes among health care professionals in other patient reporting systems as well (in this case, the UK 'Yellow Card Scheme') [41]. In the KILEN study, the lack of trust towards the treating doctor made some patients attempt to discontinue their antidepressant treatment on their own, sometimes abruptly leading to severe adverse symptoms as a consequence. It is important that mutual trust exists between patients and doctors in order to prevent non-adherence. Doctors with better communication and interpersonal skills are able to detect problems earlier, can prevent medical crisis and expensive intervention, and provide better support to their patients [42].

As indicated in this study, consumer reporting may be an additional way of detecting harmful effects that may have been missed in clinical trials. Patient/consumer reports (as contrasted to those reported by health professionals) come straight from the person who has experienced the drug effect(s); they describe the effect on the person's life [5,43,44]. It is hoped that the new EU-legislation on pharmacovigilance [1] will help to stimulate the systematic reporting by patients; in this way more attention can also be paid to how drug-related problems are experienced by patients themselves.

## Limitations

The study has several limitations. The KILEN data material was based on spontaneous consumer reports and thereby was selected material, which might have exaggerated a negative view and experience of antidepressant drug treatment. It is therefore unlikely that all views and experiences of antidepressants have been captured. Since it is an Internet-based reporting system, it will most likely benefit younger individuals who are used to handling a computer, but by missing out on the older age groups one risks getting a biased view of patients' experiences of treatment. A Danish study showed for instance that older female patients with depressive disorder had more negative views of the doctor–patient interaction and of antidepressants [45].

There is also the issue of gender. In a previous study, it was indicated that women reported ADRs to KILEN in a much higher degree: between three and four times more often than men, and sometimes more within certain age groups [9]. This may also be true for the use of these drugs. In this study, women accounted for 75% of the reported narratives. This may be an effect of women, possibly to a higher degree, turning to non-profit organizations for help. It may also be an effect of women tending to have a higher risk of ADRs than men, which increases with age and increased numbers of drugs prescribed [46]. This could also explain women's over-representation in ADR reporting to KILEN. Furthermore, we do not know how reporting consumers/patients were 'officially' diagnosed with depression (ICD-10, DSM IV or other), and we do not know if the reported diagnosis was a 'valid' one, since we only have the patients' own reported experiences to the KILEN website. It is also important to acknowledge that this was only the patients' perception of ADRs and doctor–patient communication, and we do not have doctors' perceptions to compare with.

Lastly, there is the question of potential problems with polypharmacy, with an unknown interaction between psychotropic drugs, for instance, different antidepressants and anxiolytics. It is therefore difficult to know if the reported suspected adverse reaction is a result of a specific medication or the combination of a number of medications. As indicated by a Swedish study, the prevalence of polypharmacy, as well as the mean number of dispensed drugs per individual increased, for instance, year-by-year in Sweden from 2005 to 2008 [47].

Despite the limitations of this study, the data are still of value since the material provides unique information of consumer reporting (in Sweden) and patients' qualitative experiences of antidepressant treatment and suspected adverse reactions.

## Conclusions

The present study indicates that free text comments as often contained in case reports directly submitted by patients can be of value in pharmacovigilance and provide important information on how a drug may affect the person using it and influence his or her personal life.

### Competing interests
The authors declare that they have no competing interests.

### Authors' contributions
AV, AM and TS were responsible for study concept and design. AV acquired the data. All authors interpreted the data. AV drafted the manuscript, to which all authors contributed. All authors read and approved the final manuscript.

### Disclaimer
The opinions or assertions contained herein are the private views of the authors and are not to be construed as official or reflecting the views of the Medical Products Agency.

### Acknowledgements
This study has received funding from Stiftelsen Kempe-Carlgrenska Fonden, Folksams Forskningsstiftelse, Stiftelsen Claes Groschinskys Minnesfond, Stiftelsen Lars Hiertas Minne and Elsa Lundberg och Greta Flerons fond för studier av läkemedelsbiverkan. The sponsors had no role in the study design; in the collection, analysis, and interpretation of data; in the writing of the manuscript; or in the decision to submit the article for publication. The researchers were independent of the funders. The authors would like to thank Lena Westin, Jan Albinsson and Kersti Andersson at KILEN for providing the research material. Kersti Andersson has also provided valuable help in organizing the data.

### Author details
[1]Nordic School of Public Health, Gothenburg, Sweden. [2]Department of Behavioural Sciences and Learning, Linkoping University, Linkoping, Sweden. [3]School of Social Work, Lund University, Lund, Sweden. [4]Medical Products Agency, Uppsala, Sweden.

### References
1. The EU Pharmacovogilance System. [http://ec.europa.eu/health/files/eudralex/vol-1/reg_2010_1235/reg_2010_1235_en.pdf]
2. Borg J-J, Aislaitner G, Pirozynski M, Mifsud S: Strengthening and rationalizing pharmacovigilance in the EU: where is Europe heading to? Drug Saf 2011, 34(3):187–197.
3. World Health Organization: Safety of Medicines-a Guide to Detecting and Reporting Adverse Drug. Reaction - Why Health Professionals Need to Take Action. Geneva: 2002.
4. World Health Organization: The Safety of Medicines in Public Health Programmes: pharmacovigilance An Essential Tool. Geneva: 2006.
5. Avery AJ, Anderson C, Bond CM, Fortnum H, Gifford A, Hannaford PC, Hazell L, Krska J, Lee AJ, McLernon DJ, Murphy E, Shakir S, Watson MC: Evaluation of the patient reporting of adverse drug reactions to the UK 'yellow card Scheme': literature review, descriptive and qualitative analyses, and questionnaire surveys. Health Technol Assess 2011, 15(20).
6. van Geffen ECG, van der Wal SW, van Hulten R, de Groot MCH, Egberts ACG, Heerdink ER: Evaluation of patients' experiences with antidepressants reported by means of a medicine reporting system. Eur J Clin Pharmacol 2007, 63:1193–1199.
7. Aagaard L, Nielsen LH, Hansen EH: Consumer reporting of adverse drug reactions. A retrospective analysis of the Danish adverse drug reaction database from 2004 to 2006. Drug Saf 2009, 32(11):1067–1074.
8. Blenkinsopp A, Wilkie P, Wang M, Routledge PA: Patient reporting of suspected adverse drug reactions: a review of published literature and international experience. Br J Clin Pharmacol 2006, 63(2):148–156.
9. Vilhelmsson A, Svensson T, Meeuwisse A, Carlsten A: What can we learn from consumer reports on psychiatric adverse drug reactions with antidepressant medication? Experiences from reports to a consumer association. BMC Clin Pharmacol 2011, 11:16.
10. Egberts TCG, Smulders M, de Koning FHP, Meyboom RHB, Leufkens HGM: Can adverse drug reactions be detected earlier? A comparison of reports by patients and professionals. BMJ 1996, 313:530–531.
11. Medical Products Agency: Inrapporterade Biverkningar 2011 från hälso- och sjukvården samt allmänheten [in Swedish]. [http://www.lakemedelsverket.se/Alla-nyheter/NYHETER-2012/Inrapporterade-biverkningar-2011/]
12. Patton MQ: Qualitative Research & Evaluation Methods. London: Sage Publications; 2002.
13. Bowling A: Research Methods in Health. Investigating Health and Health Services. Norfolk: Open University Press; 2002.
14. Graneheim UH, Lundman B: Qualitative content analysis in nursing research: concepts, procedures and measures to achieve thrustworthiness. Nurs Educ Today 2004, 24:105–112.
15. Teal J: Nothing personal: an empirical phenomenological study of the experience of "being-on-an-SSRI". J Phenomenol Psychol 2009, 40:19–50.
16. Teicher MH, Glod C, Cole JO: Emergence of intense suicidal preoccupation during fluoxetine treatment. Am J Psychiatry 1990, 147(2):207–210.
17. Teicher MH, Glod CA, Cole JO: Antidepressant drugs and the emergence of suicidal tendencies. Drug Saf 1993, 3(8):186–212.
18. Möller H-J: Is there evidence for negative effects of antidepressants on suicidality in depressive patients? Eur Arch Psychiatry Clin Neurosci 2006, 256:476–496.
19. The National Board of Health and Welfare: Antidepressiva läkemedel vid psykisk ohälsa: studier av praxis i primärvården [in Swedish]. Stockholm: 2006 [http://www.socialstyrelsen.se/Lists/Artikelkatalog/Attachments/9424/2006-103-2_20061032.pdf]
20. Knudsen P, Hansen EH, Eskildsen K: Leading ordinary lives: a qualitative study of younger women's perceived functions of antidepressants. Pharm World Sci 2003, 25(4):162–167.
21. Cornford CS, Hill A, Reilly J: How patients with depressive symptoms view their condition: a qualitative study. Fam Practi 2007, 24:358–364.
22. Tint A, Haddad PM, Anderson IM: The effect of rate of antidepressant tapering on the incidence of discontinuation symptoms: a randomised study. J Psychopharmacol 2008, 22(3):330–332.
23. Baldessarini RJ, Tondo L, Ghiani C, Lepri B: Illness risk following rapid versus gradual discontinuation of antidepressants. Am J Psychiatry 2010, 167:934–941.
24. Haddad P: Do antidepressants have any potential to cause addiction? J Psychopharmacol 1999, 3:300–307.
25. van Geffen EC, Hugtenburg JG, Heerdink ER, van Hulten RP, Egberts ACG: Discontinuation symptoms in users of selective serotonin reuptake inhibitors in clinical practice: tapering versus abrupt discontinuation. Eur J Clin Pharmacol 2005, 61:303–307.
26. The Swedish Council on Technology Assessment in Health Care: Treatment of Depression: A Systematic Review. Stockholm; 2004.
27. Läkemedelsbehandling av depression hos vuxna och äldre [in Swedish]. [http://www.sbu.se/upload/Publikationer/Content1/1/SBU_Treatment_depression.pdf]
28. Stevenson FA, Barry CA, Britten N, Barber N, Bradley CP: Doctor-patient communication about drugs: the evidence for shared decision making. Soc Sci Med 2000, 50:829–840.

29. Makoul G, Arntson P, Schofield T: **Health promotion in primary care: physician-patient communication and decision making about prescription medications.** *Soc Sci Med* 1995, **41**(9):1241–1254.

30. Dolovich L, Nair K, Sellors C, Lohfeld L, Lee A, Levine M: **Do patients' expectations influence their use of medications?** *Can Fam Physician* 2008, **54**:384–393.

31. Taylor SE: *Health Psychology.* Boston: McGraw-Hill Education; 2006.

32. Brannon L, Feist J: *Health Psychology: An Introduction to Behavior and Health.* Belmont: Wadsworth/Thomson Learning; 2004.

33. van Geffen EC, van Hulten R, Bouvry ML, Egberts AC, Heerdink ER: **Characteristics and reasons associated with nonacceptance of selective serotonin-reuptake inhibitor treatment.** *Ann Pharmacother* 2008, **42**(2):218–225.

34. Butt TF, Cox AR, Lewis H, Ferner RE: **Patient experiences of serious adverse drug reactions and their attitudes to medicines.** *Drug Saf* 2011, **34**(4):319–328.

35. Cox AR, Butt TF: **Adverse drug reactions: when the risk becomes a reality for patients.** *Drug Saf* 2012, **35**(11):977–981.

36. Haw C, Stubbs J: **Patient information leaflets for antidepressants: are patients getting the information they need?** *J Affect Disord* 2011, **128**:165–170.

37. Wester K, Jönsson AK, Spigset O, Druid H, Hägg S: **Incidence of fatal adverse drug reactions: a population based study.** *Br J Clin Pharmacol* 2008, **65**(4):573–579.

38. Britten N: **Patients' Demands for prescriptions in primary care.** *BMJ* 1995, **310**:1084–1085.

39. Reid S, Barbui C: **Long term treatment of depression with selective serotonin reuptake inhibitors and newer antidepressants.** *BMJ* 2010, **340**:752–756.

40. Krska J, Anderson C, Murphy E, Avery AJ, on behalf of the Yellow Card Study Collaboration: **How patient reporters identify adverse drug reactions: a qualitative study of reporting via the UK yellow card scheme.** *Drug Saf* 2011, **34**(5):429–436.

41. Anderson A, Krska J, Murphy E, Avery A, on behalf of the Yellow Card Study Collaboration: **The importance of direct patient reporting of suspected adverse drug reactions: a patient perspective.** *Br J Clin Pharmacol* 2011, **72**(5):806–822.

42. Ha JF, Anat DS, Longnecker N: **Doctor-patient communication: a review.** *Ochsner J* 2010, **10**:38–43.

43. Lexchin J: **Is there still a role for spontaneous reporting of adverse drug reactions?** *CMAJ* 2006, **174**(2):191–192.

44. Herxheimer A, Crombag M-R, Alves TL: *Direct Patient Reporting of Adverse Drug Reactions. A Twelve-Country Survey & Literature Review.* Amsterdam: Health Action International (HAI) (Europe); 2010.

45. Kessing LV, Hansen HV, Demyttenaere K, Bech P: **Depressive and bipolar disorders: patients' attitudes and beliefs towards depression and antidepressants.** *Psychol Med* 2005, **35**:1205–1213.

46. Zopf Y, Rabe C, Neubert A, Gaßmann KG, Rascher W, Hahn EG, Brune K, Dormann H: **Women encounter ADRs more often than do men.** *Eur J Clin Pharmacol* 2008, **64**:999–1004.

47. Hovstadius B, Hovstadius K, Astrand B, Petersson G: **Increasing polypharmacy – an individual-based study of the Swedish population 2005–2008.** *BMC Clin Pharmacol* 2010, **10**:16.

# 16

# No relevant cardiac, pharmacokinetic or safety interactions between roflumilast and inhaled formoterol in healthy subjects: an open-label, randomised, actively controlled study

Christian de Mey[1], Nassr Nassr[2] and Gezim Lahu[2*]

## Abstract

**Background:** Roflumilast is an oral, selective phosphodiesterase 4 inhibitor with anti-inflammatory effects in chronic obstructive pulmonary disease (COPD). The addition of roflumilast to long-acting bronchodilators improves lung function in patients with moderate-to-severe COPD. The present study investigated drug-drug interaction effects between inhaled formoterol and oral roflumilast.

**Methods:** This was a single-centre (investigational clinic), open, randomised, multiple-dose, parallel-group study. In Regimen A, healthy men were treated with roflumilast (500 μg tablet once daily; Day 2-18) and concomitant formoterol (24 μg twice daily; Day 12-18). In Regimen B, healthy men were treated with formoterol (24 μg twice daily; Day 2-18) and concomitant roflumilast (500 μg once daily; Day 9-18). Steady-state plasma pharmacokinetics of roflumilast, roflumilast N-oxide and/or formoterol ($C_{max}$ and $AUC_{0-\tau}$) as well as pharmacodynamics - blood pressure, transthoracic impedance cardiography (ZCG), 12-lead digital electrocardiography, peripheral blood eosinophils, and serum glucose and potassium concentrations - were evaluated through Day 1 (baseline), Day 8 (Regimen B: formoterol alone) or Day 11 (Regimen A: roflumilast alone), and Day 18 (Regimen A and B: roflumilast plus formoterol). Blood and urine samples were taken for safety assessment at screening, pharmacokinetic profiling days and Day 19. Adverse events were monitored throughout the study.

**Results:** Of the 27 subjects enrolled, 24 were evaluable (12 in each regimen). No relevant pharmacokinetic interactions occurred. Neither roflumilast nor formoterol were associated with significant changes in cardiovascular parameters as measured by ZCG, and these parameters were not affected during concomitant administration. Formoterol was associated with a slight increase in heart rate and a corresponding shortening of the QT interval, without changes in the heart rate-corrected QTc interval. There were small effects on the other pharmacodynamic assessments when roflumilast and formoterol were administered individually, but no interactions or safety concerns were seen after concomitant administration. No severe or serious adverse events were reported, and no adverse events led to premature study discontinuation.

**Conclusions:** No clinically relevant pharmacokinetic or pharmacodynamic interactions were found when oral roflumilast was administered concomitantly with inhaled formoterol, including no effect on cardiac repolarisation. Roflumilast was well tolerated.

**Trial Registration:** Clinicaltrials.gov NCT00940329

* Correspondence: gezim.lahu@nycomed.com
[2]Nycomed GmbH, Konstanz, Germany
Full list of author information is available at the end of the article

## Background

Roflumilast (3-cyclopropylmethoxy-N-(3,5-dichloropyridin-4-yl)-4-(difluoromethoxy)benzamide; CAS Registry number: 162401-32-3; molecular formula: $C_{17}H_{14}Cl_2F_2N_2O_3$) is a selective, oral, once-daily phosphodiesterase 4 (PDE4) inhibitor that has shown anti-inflammatory activity in pre-clinical studies [1-4], and in patients with chronic obstructive pulmonary disease (COPD) [5]. In large randomised clinical studies, roflumilast consistently improved lung function in patients with moderate-to-severe COPD [6], severe COPD [7], or severe airflow obstruction plus chronic bronchitis [8] compared with placebo.

Long-acting bronchodilators such as the $\beta_2$-adrenoceptor agonists formoterol and salmeterol and the anticholinergic tiotropium [9-11] are central to the treatment of COPD; however, some patients have poor symptom control with these agents, particularly patients with more severe disease [12]. Two large clinical trials have investigated whether the addition of roflumilast improves lung function in patients with moderate-to-severe COPD who are already receiving long-acting bronchodilators [13]. In these trials, patients already receiving salmeterol or tiotropium were randomised to receive either oral roflumilast 500 µg or placebo once daily for 24 weeks, in addition to continued salmeterol or tiotropium treatment [13]. Compared with placebo, the addition of roflumilast improved mean pre-bronchodilator forced expiratory volume in both trials (p < 0.0001). Further, in a separate *in vitro* study, formoterol increased the inhibitory effect of roflumilast on cytokine and tumour necrosis factor-α production from human parenchymal and bronchial explants [14].

Both PDE inhibitors and $\beta_2$-adrenoceptor agonists lead to an accumulation of intracellular cyclic adenosine monophosphate [15-17], which plays a key role in the regulation of cardiac function [18]. It is known that $\beta_2$-adrenoceptor agonists are associated with adverse cardiac events [19]. In contrast, a previous study demonstrated that roflumilast had no significant effect on cardiac repolarisation (QT/QTc interval) in healthy subjects [20].

When administered as a single, oral 500 µg dose, roflumilast is readily and almost totally absorbed in healthy individuals, with a mean bioavailability of 79% [21] and dose-proportional pharmacokinetics observed within the 250-1000 µg dose range [22]. Repeated-dose pharmacokinetic profiles of roflumilast and its active metabolite roflumilast N-oxide have been well characterised, with median time to maximum plasma concentration ($t_{max}$) values of 1 hour and 8 hours, respectively, and median effective plasma half-lives of 17 hours and 30 hours, respectively [22-24]. Roflumilast N-oxide has a

PDE selectivity profile and potency *in vivo* similar to that of roflumilast, and a substantially (10-fold) greater area under the plasma concentration-time curve (AUC) [4,22]. It is therefore estimated to account for about 90% of the overall PDE4 inhibitory activity of roflumilast. To estimate the combined PDE4 inhibition of roflumilast and roflumilast N-oxide in humans following administration of roflumilast, the parameter termed 'total PDE4 inhibitory activity' (tPDE4i) has been established [23,25]. This parameter represents the sum of the overall exposure to roflumilast and roflumilast N-oxide by accounting for differences in intrinsic activity ($IC_{50}$), free fraction (protein binding) and *in vivo* exposure (AUC values) of both compounds.

Roflumilast is metabolised to roflumilast N-oxide mainly through biotransformation via the cytochrome P450 (CYP) enzymes CYP3A4 and CYP1A2, and roflumilast N-oxide is cleared by CYP3A4. The CYP3A4 inhibitors erythromycin and ketoconazole have been shown to increase tPDE4i by 8-9% [26,27]; the CYP1A2 inhibitor fluvoxamine and the dual CYP3A4/1A2 inhibitors enoxacin and cimetidine increase tPDE4i by 59%, 25% and 47%, respectively [28-30]. Conversely, administration of the cytochrome P450 enzyme inducer rifampicin results in a reduction in tPDE4i by 58% [31].

Roflumilast and formoterol have a low potential for pharmacokinetic interaction because formoterol is eliminated mainly by direct glucuronidation and does not inhibit CYP isoenzymes at therapeutically relevant concentrations [32]. Following inhalation, formoterol is rapidly absorbed, with plasma concentrations increasing linearly with dose [32]. The kinetics of formoterol are similar after single and repeated administration, indicating no auto-induction or inhibition of metabolism [32]; however, there is a modest and self-limiting accumulation in plasma after repeated dosing in patients with COPD [32]. In a previous Phase I study, no apparent drug-drug interaction was found between roflumilast and orally co-administered formoterol (unpublished data; Nycomed GmbH, 2002). The nature and extent of a pharmacokinetic drug-drug interaction may, however, differ when formoterol is inhaled [33].

Since roflumilast is likely to be used concomitantly with a $\beta_2$-adrenoceptor agonist in some patients, it is of interest to investigate whether and to what extent concomitant administration results in relevant pharmacokinetic and pharmacodynamic drug-drug interactions with a focus on cardiovascular effects.

## Methods

The protocol (Clinicaltrials.gov registration NCT 00940329) was reviewed and approved by an independent ethics committee (Ethik-Kommission Landesärztekammer

Rheinland-Pfalz Körperschaft des öffentlichen Rechts, Mainz, Germany) and competent health authorities (Bundesinstitut für Arzneimittel und Medizinprodukte [BfArM] Fachregistratur Klinische Prüfung, Bonn, Germany). The study was planned, conducted, analysed and reported in accordance with the principles of Good Clinical Practice, the Declaration of Helsinki and the provisions for the orderly conduct of clinical trials in the country of conduct.

### Subjects

Eligibility of subjects was evaluated on the basis of an extensive screening investigation performed within 3 weeks before admission to the study clinic, which included demography, medical history, review of co-medications, physical examination, recumbent blood pressure and pulse rate, electrocardiograms (ECGs), and laboratory safety tests (haematology, clinical chemistry, urinalysis, hepatitis and HIV serology).

Eligible subjects included Caucasian males aged 18 to 45 years with a body mass index between 18 and 30 kg/m$^2$, and a body weight of > 50 kg. All subjects were willing and able to provide informed consent.

Exclusion criteria were as follows: previous participation in the study or in any other study; donation of blood or plasma within the last 30 days; presence of acute or chronic disease; presence of clinically relevant findings in the laboratory tests (including hepatitis and HIV serology and tests for alcohol and social drugs); signs or history of cardiac disease including QTc interval (Bazett's correction) ≥ 430 ms and PQ interval ≥ 220 ms; susceptibility to symptomatic orthostatic hypotension; previous gastrointestinal surgery other than appendectomy and herniotomy; use of any medication within the last 2 weeks or within less than 10 times the elimination half-life of the respective drug; history of any clinically relevant hypersensitivity (in particular to formoterol or other $\beta_2$-adrenoceptor agonists, to roflumilast or to any inactive ingredient in the trial medication); smoking more than 10 cigarettes/day or equivalent; evidence or suspicion of alcohol or social drug abuse; excessive xanthine consumption; and any concern of lack of compliance or willingness to adhere to the study directives and restrictions.

### Interventions

This was an open-label, randomised, actively controlled, multiple-dose, parallel-group study with a fixed-administration sequence. Screening took place between Day -21 and Day -1; the study period lasted from Day -1 to Day 19; and the post-study examination was conducted within 1 week of the last intake of the study medication. Subjects were admitted to the clinic from the evening of Day -1 to the morning of Day 19. Subjects were instructed to avoid strenuous physical exercise from Day -3 until the post-study examination. Smokers were required to keep their smoking habits stable, but were not allowed to smoke during the main profiling days. Alcohol- and caffeine-containing beverages, as well as grapefruit juice, were not allowed from Day -2 to Day 19. In compliance with European guidelines, both drugs were given at the maximum recommended therapeutic dosage.

For Regimen A, subjects received 500 µg oral roflumilast once daily (daily dose: one tablet of roflumilast 500 µg) from the morning of Day 2 to the morning of Day 18. From the morning of Day 12 to the evening of Day 18 subjects also received 24 µg formoterol for oral inhalation delivered by a dry powder inhaler (DPI) device (Foradil® P, Novartis Pharma GmbH, Vienna, Austria) twice daily, once in the morning and once in the evening (daily dose: 48 µg formoterol). For Regimen B, subjects received 24 µg formoterol for oral inhalation delivered by a DPI device (Foradil® P) twice daily, once in the morning and once in the evening from the morning of Day 2 to the evening of Day 18. From the morning of Day 9 to the morning of Day 18 subjects also received 500 µg roflumilast once daily. The start of the concomitant phases for each regimen was dependent on the pharmacokinetic characteristics of roflumilast and formoterol; as more time is needed to achieve steady state for roflumilast than formoterol, the timings were different between Regimen A and Regimen B.

Roflumilast was taken orally with 240 mL plain water after an overnight fast and rest; after intake, a mouth check was performed for compliance control. No fluids were allowed within 2 hours after each dose on the profile days. On days when the two medications were co-administered, formoterol was administered within 1 minute of roflumilast being administered.

The main profiling days were scheduled on Days 1, 11 and 18 for Regimen A, and on Days 1, 8 and 18 for Regimen B. On these days, subjects continued their fast from the previous evening until 8 hours after morning dosing, and standardised meals were served at 8 hours (lunch) and 12.5 hours after morning dosing (dinner).

### Pharmacokinetic methods

Blood samples for pharmacokinetic assessments were taken on Days 11 and 18 for Regimen A and Days 8 and 18 for Regimen B, 30 minutes before dosing and 0.25, 0.5, 1, 2, 4, 6, 8, 10 and 12 hours after dosing, with additional samples taken at 14 and 24 hours for roflumilast (Days 11 and 18 for Regimen A, and Day 18 for Regimen B). Pre-dose blood samples for determination of trough levels were taken on Days 9 and 10 for Regimen A (morning only), and on Days 6 and 7 (morning and evening) for Regimen B. Blood samples (4.5 mL) were collected in heparinised tubes and plasma was obtained by centrifugation at 1550 g for 15 minutes. Plasma samples were stored at -20°C or below for roflumilast, and at -70°C for formoterol. Plasma concentrations of roflumilast and roflumilast N-oxide were determined using high-performance liquid chromatography coupled with tandem mass spectrometry (HPLC-MS/MS). Before the sample analysis we determined that formoterol did not interfere with the quantification of roflumilast or roflumilast N-oxide. The lower limit of quantitation (LLOQ) was 0.1 ng/L using a sample volume of 0.4 mL for both roflumilast and roflumilast N-oxide. The inter-day precision of this assay, as determined by the analysis of quality control (QC) samples, ranged from 5.3% to 10.0% for both analytes. The inter-day accuracy of the assay, as determined by the analysis of the QC samples, ranged from -6.8% to +2.5% for both analytes. Roflumilast and roflumilast N-oxide standard curves were valid up to 20 ng/mL and 40 ng/mL, respectively. Determination of roflumilast and roflumilast N-oxide was performed at Altana Pharma AG, Konstanz, Germany (Nycomed GmbH). Plasma concentrations of formoterol were determined using HPLC-MS/MS. The LLOQ in plasma was 0.4 pg/mL using a sample volume of 1.0 mL. Formoterol standard curves were valid up to 99.9 pg/mL. The intra-day precision for QC samples ranged from 0.5% to 13.1%. The intra-day accuracy of the formoterol QC samples ranged from -10.5% to +13.6%, the inter-day precision from 6.4% to 7.6%, and the inter-day accuracy from 0.7% to 7.1%. Determination of formoterol was performed at pharm-analyt Labor GmbH, Baden, Austria, under the supervision of Altana Pharma AG(Nycomed GmbH).

For roflumilast, roflumilast N-oxide and formoterol, the maximum plasma concentration ($C_{max}$) was derived directly from the plasma concentrations. The AUC from time zero to the time of the last quantifiable concentration, which corresponded to the dosing interval of each analyte ($AUC_{0-\tau}$), was estimated using the linear trapezoidal method. Apparent clearance at steady state (CL/F; calculated by dose/$AUC_{\tau}$) was reported for roflumilast only. Pharmacokinetic variables were calculated by non-compartmental analysis using WinNonLin professional, version 4.01 (PharSight, Mountain View, California, USA). The calculation of tPDE4i was based on the equation described in Lahu et al. [27].

### Cardiovascular methods: blood pressure and transthoracic impedance cardiography

Cardiovascular effects were evaluated non-invasively by means of ECGs (cardiac rhythm, intra-cardiac conduction and ventricular repolarisation), oscillometric blood pressure and transthoracic impedance cardiography (ZCG; systolic time intervals, contractility indices and estimates of stroke volume and cardiac output). Cardiovascular assessments (oscillometric blood pressure, pulse rate, 12-lead ECG, and three-lead ZCG) were recorded before dosing and at 10, 20, 40 and 60 minutes, and at 2, 3, 4, 5, 6, 7 and 8 hours after morning dosing. Blood pressure, pulse rate and ECGs were also assessed at 12 hours after dosing, and on the morning of Day 19. All cardiovascular measurements were carried out after the subjects had been recumbent for at least 10 minutes; they generally stayed in bed from 1 hour before until 8 hours after morning dosing.

Systolic time intervals (STIs) and ZCG estimates of the systolic cardiac pump performance were derived from the simultaneous registration of a one-lead ECG, a phonocardiogram (PCG), and the rate of change of the transthoracic impedance (dZ/dt) to an AC current applied through the thoracic cage (CARDIODYNAGRAPH; Diefenbach GmbH, Wiesbaden, Germany). Tracings were captured and stored digitally during the study and subsequently analysed after the study by displaying the analogue ECG, PCG and ZCG signals on a computer screen. The relevant signal amplitudes and time intervals were delineated manually by operator-steered cursors; measurements were made for at least 10 artefact-free consecutive cardiac cycles [34,35]. From these tracings, the following variables were derived by direct measurement: RR interval (ms), total electromechanic systole (QS2 [ms]), ventricular ejection time (VET [ms]), baseline transthoracic impedance (Z0 [$\Omega$]), and maximum negative velocity of transthoracic impedance changes during the cardiac cycle (dZ/dt$_{max}$ [$\Omega$/s]). These variables were analysed for the 10 cycles and their means were used in the calculations of the following variables: heart rate (HR [bpm]), pre-ejection period (PEP [ms] = QS2 - VET), HR-corrected STIs (STI$_c$ and STI$_i$ according to Weissler et al. [36]), ZCG estimates of stroke volume (SV [mL] according to Kubicek's equation [37] using the equation of Geddes and Sadler for the specific resistance of blood [38]), cardiac output (CO [mL/min]), and total peripheral resistance (TPR [dyn.s. cm$^{-5}$]). For the latter variable, the mean blood pressure (MBP [mmHg]) was used as calculated according to Wezler and Böger [39] from the systolic blood pressure (mmHg) and the diastolic blood pressure (mmHg).

ZCG analysis was carried out by a single analyst who was blinded with regard to subject, study regimen, profiling day within regimen, and time during the day. The time courses of ZCG variables were evaluated in two main data formats: untransformed (U, all profiling days) and time-matched for control Day 1 ($\delta$, profiling days except control Day 1); the time courses of U- and $\delta$-data were characterised by their morning pre-dose baseline values (BL$_U$ and BL$_\delta$) and the observed minimum (d$_{min}$) and maximum (d$_{max}$) values over the post-dosing time. Selected variables (HR, PEP, QS2, $dZ/dt_{max}$, CO, and TPR) were compared by non-parametric estimates of the differences between the profiling days (point estimate and 95% confidence interval [CI] according to Hodges and Lehmann) [40].

### Electrocardiography

Digital 12-lead ECGs were recorded immediately after each ZCG recording. Tracings were analysed off-study by regimen-blinded qualified analysts, using previously reported methodology [20]. For each time point, three cycles were measured with regard to the RR, PQ and QT-intervals [ms]. The means of the three measurements were used for the calculation of HR and HR-corrected QTc intervals, according to Bazett's equation ($QTcB = QT/RR^{1/2}$) [41] and Fridericia's equation ($QTcF = QT/RR^{1/3}$) [41,42].

### Biological markers

During the main profiling days, blood was sampled at each ZCG time point for the determination of serum glucose and potassium concentrations. Samples were also collected 12 and 24 hours after morning dosing.

### Safety and tolerability

Blood and urine samples for conventional clinical laboratory safety tests were obtained at the screening visit, in the morning of each main profiling day, and on Day 19. Adverse events (AEs) were monitored throughout the study.

## Results

### Subjects

Twenty-seven healthy male subjects were enrolled and received the assigned investigational medication at least once (see Table 1 for demographic data). For Regimen A, 12 subjects were enrolled and all completed the study in accordance with the protocol specifications. For

**Table 1 Subject demographics for the study population (all enrolled subjects)**

| Characteristic | Regimen A (n = 12) | Regimen B (n = 15) |
|---|---|---|
| Male, n (%) | 12 (100) | 15 (100) |
| Caucasian, n (%) | 12 (100) | 15 (100) |
| Age, years (median [range]) | 33 (25-44) | 33 (21-44) |
| Body height, cm (median [range]) | 184 (169-192) | 180 (168-185) |
| Body weight, kg (median [range]) | 83 (66-95) | 75 (61-97) |
| Body mass index, kg/m² (median [range]) | 25 (23-28) | 24 (21-30) |
| Smoking status, n | | |
| Ex-smoker | 2 | 4 |
| Current | 3 | 6 |
| Never | 7 | 5 |

Regimen B, 15 subjects were enrolled: one withdrew consent on Day 11 and two were discontinued prematurely after erroneous dosing on Day 2, leaving 12 subjects who completed the study in accordance with the protocol.

### Pharmacokinetics

The time courses of geometric mean plasma concentrations of roflumilast, roflumilast N-oxide and formoterol are shown in Figures 1, 2 and 3. Geometric means and their 68% ranges of steady-state pharmacokinetics of roflumilast, roflumilast N-oxide and formoterol are shown in Tables 2 and 3. There were no relevant changes in steady-state pharmacokinetics of roflumilast and roflumilast N-oxide when formoterol was added; similarly, there were no changes in steady-state pharmacokinetics of formoterol when roflumilast was added. There were some between-group effects, since steady-state AUC and $C_{max}$ values for roflumilast and roflumilast N-oxide were about 10-15% lower when roflumilast was co-administered with formoterol (Regimen B, Day 18), compared with roflumilast alone (Regimen A, Day 11) or roflumilast after addition of formoterol (Regimen A, Day 18).

### Impedance cardiography

#### Regimen A

The treatment medians for baseline Day 1, roflumilast monotherapy alone (R; Day 11), and concomitant roflumilast plus formoterol treatment (R+F; Day 18) are shown in Table 4 for untransformed morning pre-dosing values, untransformed $d_{max}$ and $d_{min}$ post-dosing values (including contrast of R vs D1), and time-matched $d_{max}$ and $d_{min}$ post-dosing values (including contrast of R+F vs R).

Roflumilast alone had little effect on cardiovascular function and there were only small changes in the ZCG/STI variables. Concomitant administration of formoterol resulted in a protracted rise in HR compared with roflumilast alone (Figure 4), which was associated with a rise in CO (Figure 5) and a drop in TPR within 10 minutes (Figure 6). Formoterol co-administration was also associated with an increase in $dZ/dt_{max}$, particularly in the first hour after dosing, and an overall shortening of QS2 and PEP, which were mostly related to the rise in HR since they were less evident for the HR-corrected STIs (Table 4). These changes were small and within the normal physiological range.

#### Regimen B

The treatment medians for baseline Day 1, formoterol monotherapy alone (F; Day 8) and concomitant formoterol plus roflumilast (F+R; Day 18) and their contrasts are shown in Table 5. Compared with baseline, formoterol administration was associated with an increase in HR (Figure 4), a rise in CO (Figure 5) and a decrease in

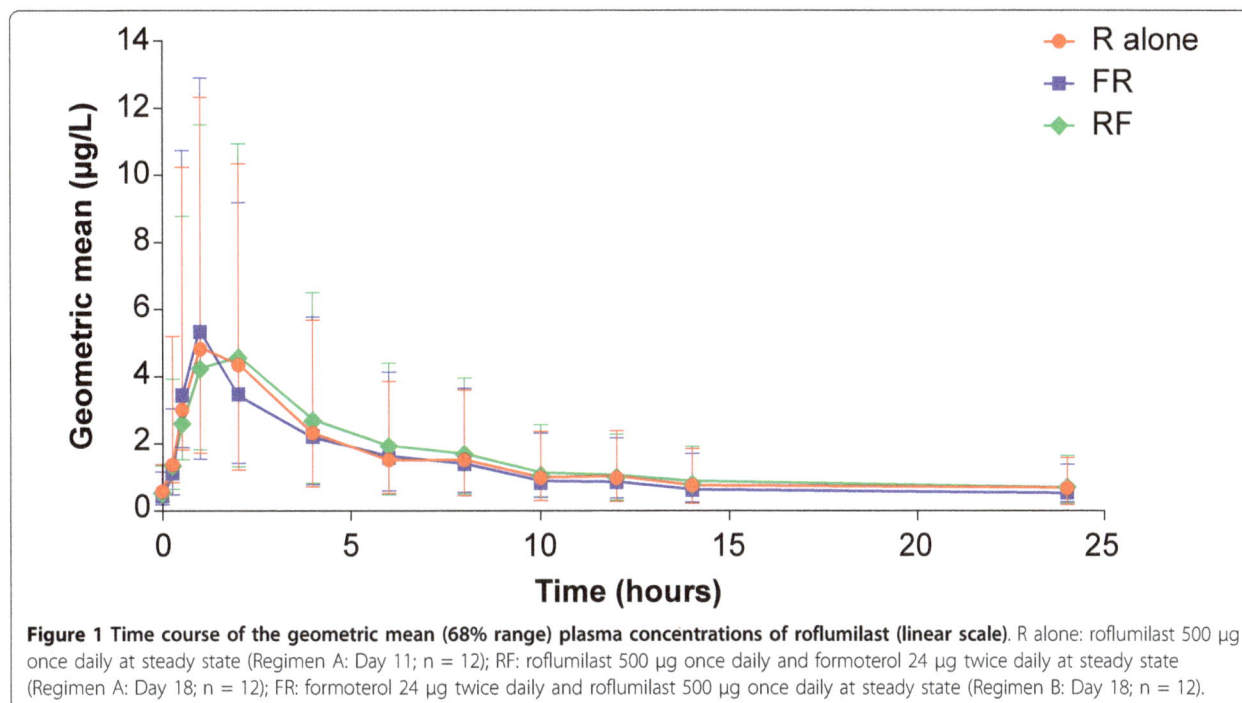

**Figure 1 Time course of the geometric mean (68% range) plasma concentrations of roflumilast (linear scale)**. R alone: roflumilast 500 μg once daily at steady state (Regimen A: Day 11; n = 12); RF: roflumilast 500 μg once daily and formoterol 24 μg twice daily at steady state (Regimen A: Day 18; n = 12); FR: formoterol 24 μg twice daily and roflumilast 500 μg once daily at steady state (Regimen B: Day 18; n = 12).

TPR (Figure 6), which were associated with an increased $dZ/dt_{max}$, and an overall shortening in QS2 and PEP. These effects were clearly apparent on Day 8 and were not amplified by the concomitant administration of roflumilast.

**Electrocardiograms**
Both roflumilast and formoterol were associated with a slight increase in HR and, correspondingly, a decrease in the duration of the QT interval. QTc values, either uncorrected or corrected using Bazett's formula or

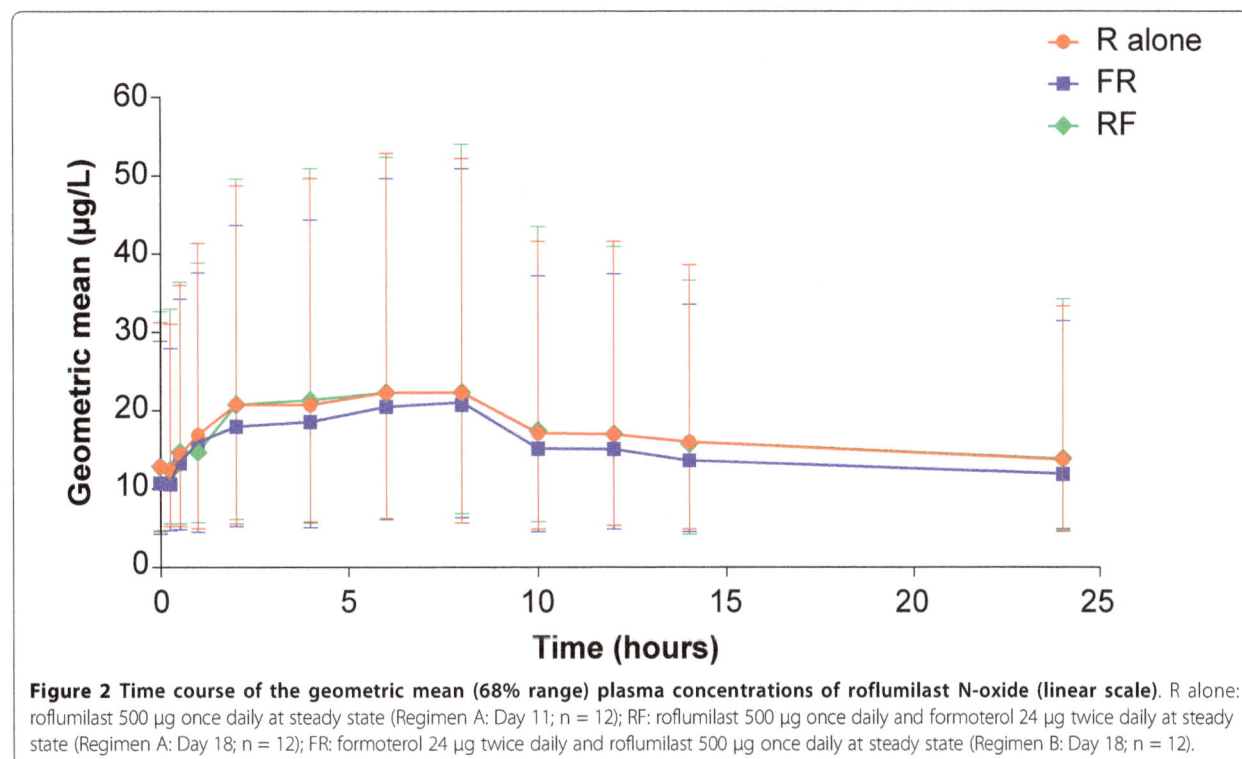

**Figure 2 Time course of the geometric mean (68% range) plasma concentrations of roflumilast N-oxide (linear scale)**. R alone: roflumilast 500 μg once daily at steady state (Regimen A: Day 11; n = 12); RF: roflumilast 500 μg once daily and formoterol 24 μg twice daily at steady state (Regimen A: Day 18; n = 12); FR: formoterol 24 μg twice daily and roflumilast 500 μg once daily at steady state (Regimen B: Day 18; n = 12).

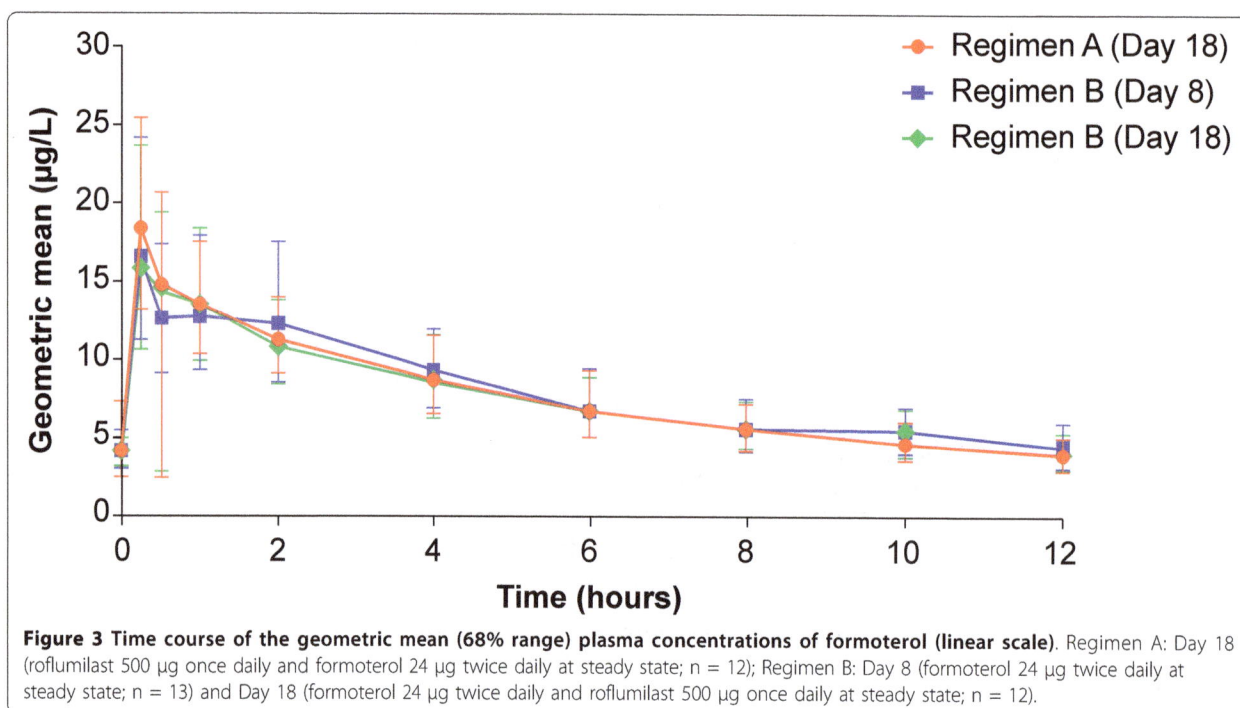

**Figure 3** Time course of the geometric mean (68% range) plasma concentrations of formoterol (linear scale). Regimen A: Day 18 (roflumilast 500 μg once daily and formoterol 24 μg twice daily at steady state; n = 12); Regimen B: Day 8 (formoterol 24 μg twice daily at steady state; n = 13) and Day 18 (formoterol 24 μg twice daily and roflumilast 500 μg once daily at steady state; n = 12).

Fridericia's formula, showed no clinically relevant changes. Categorical analyses of QT/QTc interval data did not reveal differences in the incidence of outliers between regimens, and the incidence of outliers was small. None of the subjects developed abnormal QT/QTc prolongation, and all QT/QTc intervals remained below 450 ms. No clinically relevant drug-related changes in PR or QRS intervals were observed. No clinically relevant regimen-related changes in ECG waveform morphology were detected.

### Serum glucose

With Regimen A, the median pre-dose serum glucose decreased from Day 1 (4.97 mmol/L) to Day 11 (4.75 mmol/L) and Day 18 (4.52 mmol/L). During Day 11 (roflumilast alone), glucose levels tended to remain slightly lower than pre-dose levels; in contrast, on Day 18, with concomitant formoterol plus roflumilast, there was a post-dose increase in serum glucose level that was close to the values throughout Day 1 (although the pre-dose levels had been lower).

**Table 2** Geometric means (68% inter-percentile range) of the main pharmacokinetic variables for roflumilast and roflumilast N-oxide at steady state

| | Regimen A | | Regimen B |
|---|---|---|---|
| | Day 11 (roflumilast alone) (n = 12) | Day 18 (roflumilast plus formoterol) (n = 12) | Day 18 (formoterol plus roflumilast) (n = 12) |
| **Roflumilast** | | | |
| $C_{trough}$ (μg/L) | 0.53 (0.33-0.85) | 0.50 (0.29-0.86) | 0.37 (0.18-0.77) |
| $C_{max}$ (μg/L) | 6.89 (4.94-9.62) | 6.43 (4.79-8.63) | 5.92 (4.27-8.22) |
| $AUC_{\tau}$ (μg.h/L) | 35.8 (27.8-46.1) | 36.9 (28.1-48.4) | 31.8 (21.2-47.7) |
| CL/F (L/h) | 13.9 (10.8-17.9) | 13.5 (10.3-17.7) | 15.7 (10.4-23.5) |
| **Roflumilast N-oxide** | | | |
| $C_{trough}$ (μg/L) | 12.43 (8.24-18.76) | 12.72 (8.18-19.79) | 10.66 (6.29-18.06) |
| $AUC_{\tau}$ (μg.h/L) | 417 (299-582) | 414 (293-584) | 369 (254-537) |
| $C_{max}$ (μg/L) | 23.3 (17.3-31.3) | 23.7 (17.2-32.6) | 22.04 (15.9-30.5) |

$AUC_{\tau}$, area under the plasma concentration versus time curve; $C_{max}$, maximum plasma concentration; $C_{trough}$, trough plasma concentration; CL/F, apparent clearance at steady state.

**Table 3 Geometric means (68% inter-percentile range) of the main pharmacokinetic variables for formoterol at steady state**

| | Regimen B | | Regimen A |
| --- | --- | --- | --- |
| | Day 8 (formoterol alone) (n = 13) | Day 18 (formoterol plus roflumilast) (n = 12) | Day 18 (roflumilast plus formoterol) (n = 12) |
| **Formoterol** | | | |
| $C_{trough}$ (µg/L) | 4.12 (3.05-5.57) | 3.94 (3.13-4.96) | 4.23 (2.43-7.38) |
| $C_{max}$ (µg/L) | 16.7 (11.5-24.3) | 17.2 (12.3-24.1) | 18.7 (14.3-24.6) |
| $AUC_\tau$ (µg.h/L) | 96.7 (72.8-128) | 93.1 (72.7-119) | 93.2 (72.9-119) |

$AUC_\tau$, area under the plasma concentration versus time curve; $C_{max}$, maximum plasma concentration; $C_{trough}$, trough plasma concentration.

**Table 4 Pharmacodynamic measures - Regimen A: treatment medians and treatment contrasts**

Untransformed pre-dose morning values

| | Median | | | Point estimate (95% CI) | | |
| --- | --- | --- | --- | --- | --- | --- |
| Variable | Day 1 | Day 11 (R) | Day 18 (R+F) | Day 11-Day 1 | Day 18-Day 11 | Day 18-Day 1 |
| HR (bpm) | 59 | 63 | 61 | 3 (-5 to 8) | 1 (-1 to 6) | 5 (-2 to 10) |
| PEP (ms) | 106 | 94 | 95 | -3 (-17 to 10) | -4 (-13 to 6) | -8 (-19 to 6) |
| QS2 (ms) | 435 | 423 | 430 | -10 (-21 to 2) | -1 (-14 to 12) | -12 (-23 to 4) |
| dZ/dt (Ω/s) | 1.82 | 1.67 | 1.77 | -0.06 (-0.29 to 0.16) | 0.03 (-0.08 to 0.12) | -0.05 (-0.26 to 0.15) |
| CO (L/min) | 10.4 | 9.1 | 10.4 | -0.6 (-1.7 to 0.5) | 0.1 (-1.0 to 1.7) | -0.3 (-1.0 to 0.6) |
| TPR (dyn.s.cm$^{-5}$) | 755 | 838 | 706 | 14 (-98 to 121) | -12 (-121 to 85) | -4 (-93 to 84) |

Untransformed post-dose maximum and minimum values

| | $d_{max}$ (U) | | | | $d_{min}$ (U) | | | |
| --- | --- | --- | --- | --- | --- | --- | --- | --- |
| | Median | | | Point estimate (95% CI) | Median | | | Point estimate (95% CI) |
| Variable | Day 1 | Day 11 (R) | Day 18 (R+F) | Day 11-Day 1 | Day 1 | Day 11 (R) | Day 18 (R+F) | Day 11-Day 1 |
| HR (bpm) | 62 | 64 | 70 | 3 (-4 to 6) | 52 | 54 | 61 | 4 (1 to 7) |
| PEP (ms) | 119 | 121 | 114 | 3 (-7 to 11) | 86 | 86 | 81 | 0 (-9 to 13) |
| QS2 (ms) | 457 | 454 | 432 | -1 (-11 to 11) | 416 | 410 | 399 | -9 (-21 to 8) |
| dZ/dt (Ω/s) | 2.09 | 1.93 | 2.06 | -0.05 (-0.25 to 0.15) | 1.59 | 1.56 | 1.62 | 0.03 (-0.18 to 0.20) |
| CO (L/min) | 10.3 | 10.6 | 11.7 | 0.2 (-1.1 to 1.4) | 7.6 | 8.3 | 8.8 | -0.4 (-1.2 to 0.4) |
| TPR (dyn.s.cm$^{-5}$) | 1013 | 934 | 877 | 47 (-124 to 178) | 762 | 733 | 603 | -18 (-96 to 43) |

Day 1-matched post-dose maximum and minimum values

| | $d_{max}$ (δ) | | | $d_{min}$ (δ) | | |
| --- | --- | --- | --- | --- | --- | --- |
| | Median | | Point estimate (95% CI) | Median | | Point estimate (95% CI) |
| Variable | Day 11 (R) | Day 18 (R+F) | Day 18-Day 11 | Day 11 (R) | Day 18 (R+F) | Day 18-Day 11 |
| HR (bpm) | 9 | 14 | 5 (-1 to 11) | -4 | 0 | 5 (1 to 9) |
| PEP (ms) | 25 | 19 | -8 (-19 to 4) | -27 | -30 | -2 (-11 to 10) |
| QS2 (ms) | 19 | 4 | -15 (-31 to -8) | -34 | -47 | -14 (-29 to 1) |
| dZ/dt (Ω/s) | 0.28 | 0.32 | 0.08 (-0.07 to 0.22) | -0.10 | -0.26 | 0.05 (-0.12 to 0.21) |
| CO (L/min) | 1.6 | 2.6 | 0.8 (-0.7 to 2.3) | -1.7 | -1.2 | 0.3 (-0.6 to 1.8) |
| TPR (dyn.s.cm$^{-5}$) | 126 | 108 | -42 (-179 to 77) | -128 | -168 | -42 (-131 to 43) |

CO, cardiac output; $d_{max}$, post-dose maximum values; $d_{min}$, post-dose minimum values; dZ/dt, rate of change of the transthoracic impedance; HR, heart rate; PEP, pre-ejection period; QS2, total electromechanic systole; TPR, total peripheral resistance.

Medians for baseline (Day 1), roflumilast alone (R; Day 11) and roflumilast plus formoterol (R+F; Day 18) with the corresponding point and 95% confidence interval (CI) estimates for untransformed (U) morning pre-dose values, untransformed post dose maximum and minimum values ($d_{max}$ and $d_{min}$), and Day 1 matched (δ) post-dose maximum and minimum values.

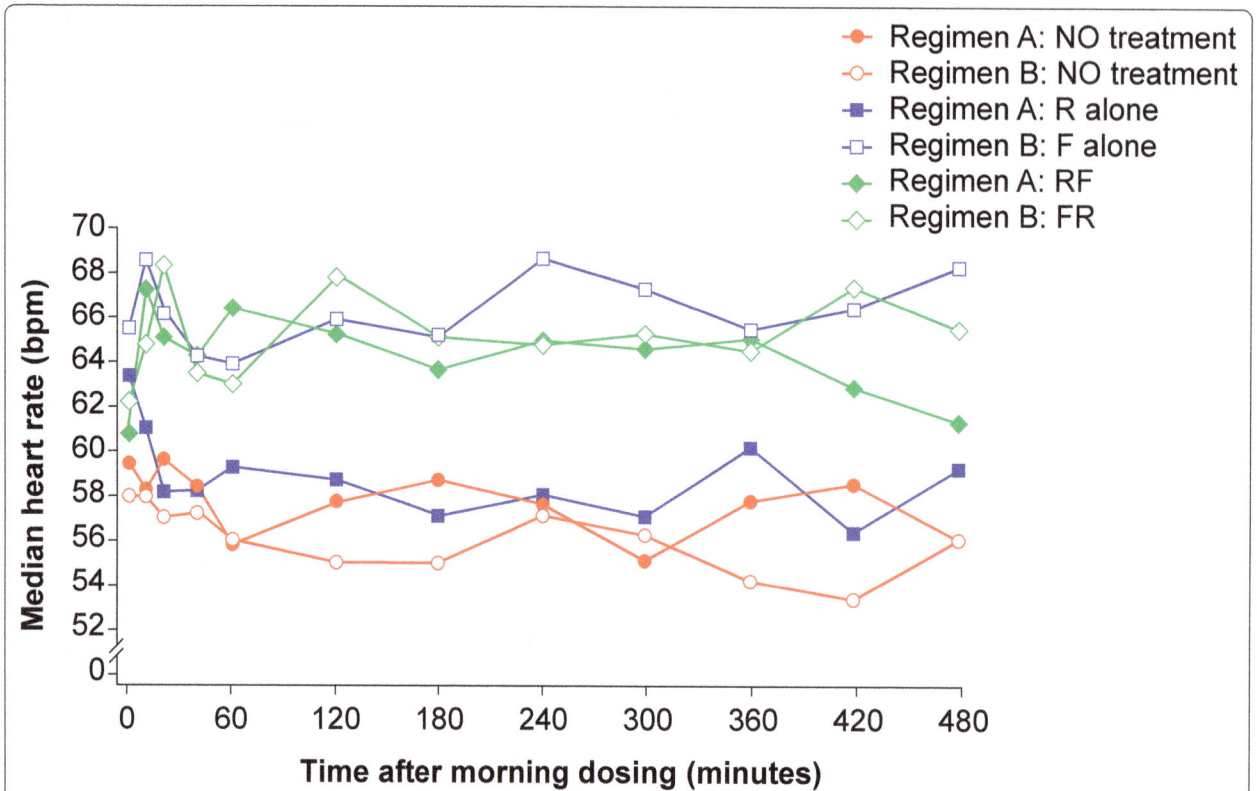

**Figure 4 Time course of the median heart rate throughout the main profiling days**. Regimen A: baseline Day 1 (NO treatment), Day 11 (R alone: roflumilast 500 µg once daily) and Day 18 (RF: roflumilast 500 µg once daily and formoterol 24 µg twice daily). Regimen B: baseline Day 1 (NO treatment), Day 8 (F alone: formoterol 24 µg twice daily) and Day 18 (FR: formoterol 24 µg twice daily and roflumilast 500 µg once daily).

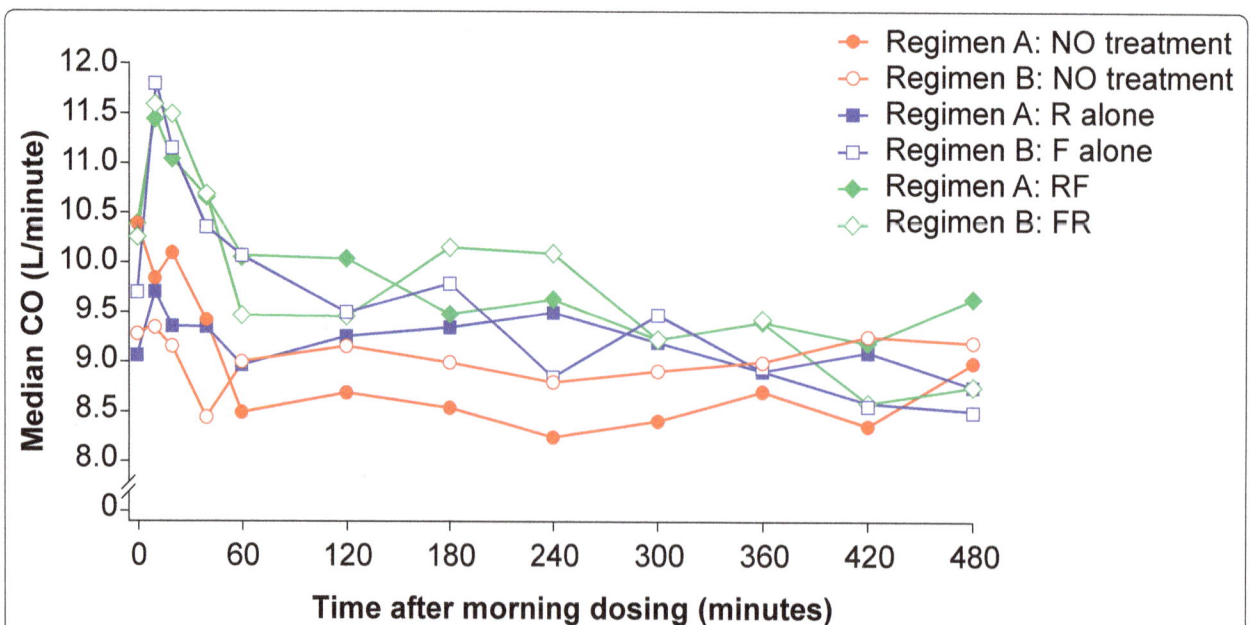

**Figure 5 Time course of the median cardiac output (CO) estimated by transthoracic impedance cardiography throughout the main profiling days**. Regimen A: baseline Day 1 (NO treatment), Day 11 (R alone: roflumilast 500 µg once daily) and Day 18 (RF: roflumilast 500 µg once daily and formoterol 24 µg twice daily). Regimen B: baseline Day 1 (NO treatment), Day 8 (F alone: formoterol 24 µg twice daily) and Day 18 (FR: formoterol 24 µg twice daily and roflumilast 500 µg once daily).

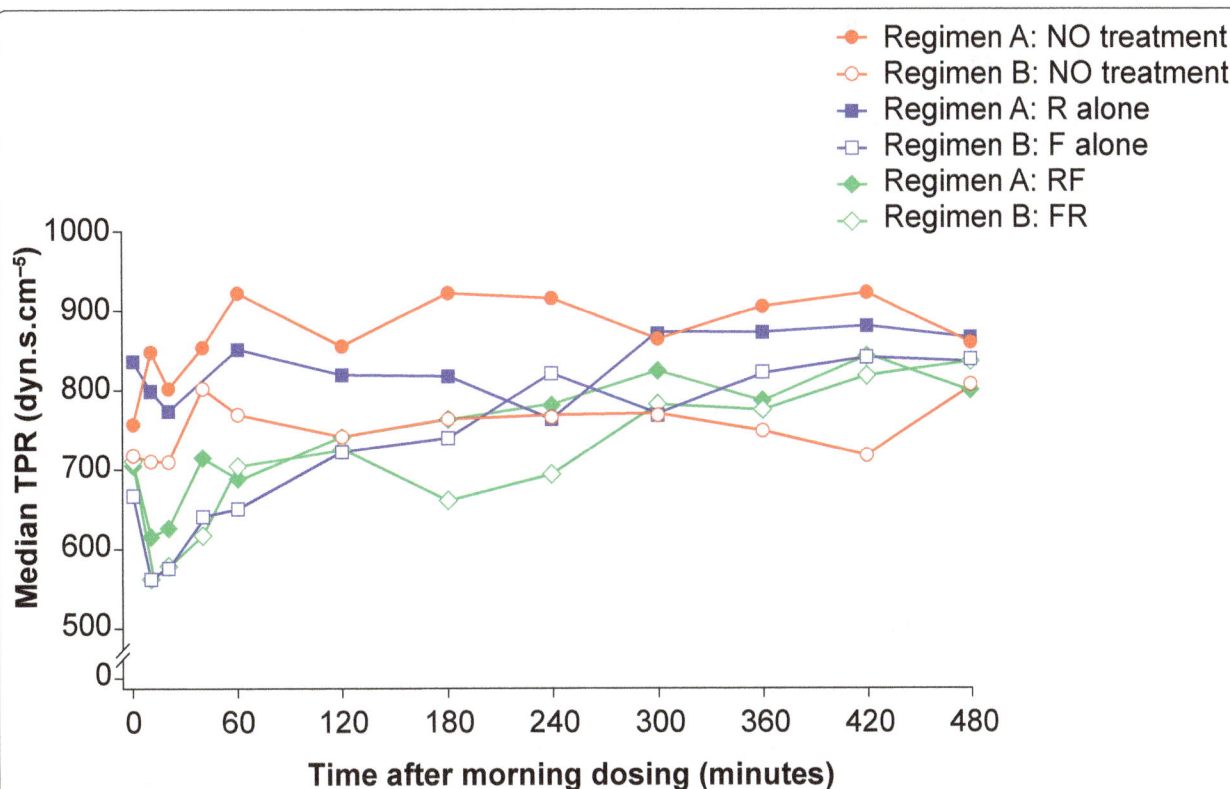

**Figure 6 Time course of the median total peripheral resistance (TPR) estimated by transthoracic impedance cardiography throughout the main profiling days.** Regimen A: baseline Day 1 (NO treatment), Day 11 (R alone: roflumilast 500 µg once daily) and Day 18 (RF: roflumilast 500 µg once daily and formoterol 24 µg twice daily). Regimen B: baseline Day 1 (NO treatment), Day 8 (F alone: formoterol 24 µg twice daily) and Day 18 (FR: formoterol 24 µg twice daily and roflumilast 500 µg once daily).

With Regimen B, there was a slight post-dose increase in serum glucose throughout Day 8 compared with Day 1; addition of roflumilast did not appear to change this formoterol effect.

### Serum potassium

With Regimen A, the median pre-dose serum potassium level was lower during roflumilast administration (4.16 mmol/L) than at Day 1 (4.34 mmol/L) or during concomitant administration of the two agents (4.35 mmol/L) on Day 18. During Day 11, when roflumilast was administered alone, serum potassium levels remained slightly lower than levels throughout Day 1. On Day 18, with concomitant formoterol plus roflumilast, serum potassium levels tended to decrease from baseline, particularly between 1 and 6 hours after morning dosing.

With Regimen B, pre-dose concentrations were similar during formoterol administration (4.38 mmol/L) on Day 8 and during concomitant administration of formoterol and roflumilast (4.32 mmol/L) on Day 18 compared with Day 1 (4.48 mmol/L). On both Day 8 (formoterol) and Day 18 (concomitant administration), serum potassium levels tended to decrease from baseline throughout the course of the day.

### Safety

For Regimen A, during administration of roflumilast alone (Day 2 to Day 11), 7 subjects experienced 17 AEs; during subsequent concomitant administration of roflumilast and formoterol (Day 12 to Day 18), 8 subjects experienced 22 AEs. The most common AE was tremor, which was seen exclusively after addition of formoterol to roflumilast (11 of 22 AEs). Dizziness and myalgia were each reported on four occasions when roflumilast was administered alone; myalgia was also reported on four occasions when formoterol was added.

For Regimen B, during administration of formoterol alone (Day 2 to Day 8), no AEs were reported. Subsequently, during concomitant administration of formoterol and roflumilast (Day 9 to Day 18), 17 AEs were reported for 6 subjects; dizziness and headache were each reported on five occasions and tremor on two occasions.

All AEs were considered to be of mild (35/39 and 16/17 AEs reported with Regimens A and B, respectively) or moderate (4/39 and 1/17 AEs reported with Regimens A and B, respectively) intensity, and most were considered likely related to the investigational medication (35/39 and 14/17 AEs reported with Regimens A

**Table 5 Pharmacodynamic measures - Regimen B: treatment medians and treatment contrasts**

Untransformed pre-dose morning values

| Variable | Median | | | Point estimate (95% CI) | | |
|---|---|---|---|---|---|---|
| | Day 1 | Day 8 (F) | Day 18 (F+R) | Day 8-Day 1 | Day 18-Day 8 | Day 18-Day 1 |
| HR (bpm) | 58 | 66 | 62 | 5 (2 to 9) | -1 (-4 to 3) | 4 (2 to 7) |
| PEP (ms) | 105 | 97 | 98 | -7 (-22 to 7) | 3 (-9 to 17) | -5 (-19 to 20) |
| QS2 (ms) | 434 | 431 | 445 | -4 (-18 to 9) | 4 (-7 to 13) | 2 (-13 to 16) |
| dZ/dt (Ω/s) | 1.81 | 1.94 | 1.82 | 0.06 (-0.07 to 0.19) | -0.08 (-0.37 to 0.07) | -0.03 (-0.30 to 0.16) |
| CO (L/min) | 9.7 | 9.7 | 10.3 | 0.7 (-0.9 to 2.0) | -0.5 (-1.7 to 0.6) | 0.3 (-1.7 to 2.1) |
| TPR (dyn.s.cm$^{-5}$) | 657 | 668 | 709 | -18 (-198 to 70) | 28 (-80 to 100) | -36 (-186 to 105) |

Untransformed post-dose maximum and minimum values

| Variable | $d_{max}$ (U) | | | | | $d_{min}$ (U) | | | |
|---|---|---|---|---|---|---|---|---|---|
| | Median | | | Point estimate (95% CI) | | Median | | | Point estimate (95% CI) |
| | Day 1 | Day 8 (F) | Day 18 (F+R) | Day 8-Day 1 | | Day 1 | Day 8 (F) | Day 18 (F+R) | Day 8-Day 1 |
| HR (bpm) | 62 | 72 | 72 | 9 (5 to 11) | | 51 | 62 | 60 | 7 (3 to 10) |
| PEP (ms) | 122 | 117 | 116 | -4 (-14 to 2) | | 87 | 84 | 85 | 0 (-7 to 6) |
| QS2 (ms) | 459 | 440 | 445 | -14 (-27 to 4) | | 424 | 408 | 410 | -13 (-22 to -3) |
| dZ/dt (Ω/s) | 2.05 | 2.10 | 2.20 | 0.01 (-0.15 to 0.21) | | 1.53 | 1.64 | 1.60 | 0.03 (-0.13 to 0.17) |
| CO (L/min) | 9.8 | 11.8 | 11.8 | 1.7 (0.6 to 2.6) | | 8.4 | 8.2 | 8.0 | 0.5 (-0.5 to 1.4) |
| TPR (dyn.s.cm$^{-5}$) | 870 | 882 | 865 | -49 (-160 to 80) | | 655 | 561 | 556 | -96 (-188 to -24) |

Day 1-matched post-dose maximum and minimum values

| Variable | $d_{max}$ (δ) | | | | $d_{min}$ (δ) | | |
|---|---|---|---|---|---|---|---|
| | Median | | Point estimate (95% CI) | | Median | | Point estimate (95% CI) |
| | Day 8 (F) | Day 18 (F+R) | Day 18-Day 8 | | Day 8 (F) | Day 18 (F+R) | Day 18-Day 8 |
| HR (bpm) | 16 | 14 | -2 (-6 to 2) | | -2 | -3 | -1 (-2 to 1) |
| PEP (ms) | 25 | 21 | 3 (-19 to 4) | | -26 | -25 | 0 (-4 to 4) |
| QS2 (ms) | 13 | 15 | 4 (-7 to 13) | | -47 | -37 | 8 (-1 to 15) |
| dZ/dt (Ω/s) | 0.32 | 0.28 | 0.05 (-0.16 to 0.17) | | -0.29 | -0.37 | -0.05 (-0.27 to 0.15) |
| CO (L/min) | 2.9 | 3.3 | 0.0 (-1.0 to 1.5) | | -0.6 | -0.6 | -0.4 (-1.3 to 0.6) |
| TPR (dyn.s.cm$^{-5}$) | 61 | 66 | -18 (-95 to 73) | | -221 | -224 | -42 (-107 to 35) |

CO, cardiac output; $d_{max}$, post-dose maximum values; $d_{min}$, post-dose minimum values; dZ/dt, rate of change of the transthoracic impedance; HR, heart rate; PEP, pre-ejection period; QS2, total electromechanic systole; TPR, total peripheral resistance.

Medians for baseline (Day 1), formoterol alone (F; Day 8) and formoterol plus roflumilast (F+R; Day 18) with the corresponding point and 95% confidence interval (CI) estimates for untransformed (U) morning pre-dose values, untransformed post-dose maximum and minimum values ($d_{max}$ and $d_{min}$), and Day 1-matched (δ) post-dose maximum and minimum values.

and B, respectively). There were no severe or serious AEs and no AEs led to premature discontinuation from the trial.

## Discussion

Roflumilast improves lung function in patients with COPD who are also treated with a long-acting broncho-dilator [13]; accordingly, the concomitant administration of roflumilast and a $\beta_2$-adrenoceptor agonist in patients with COPD is of interest. The present study investigated whether relevant drug-drug interactions might occur with the combination of oral roflumilast and inhaled formoterol. The steady-state plasma pharmacokinetics of roflumilast and its active metabolite roflumilast N-oxide were not altered by the addition of formoterol; similarly, the steady-state pharmacokinetics of formoterol were unaffected by the addition of roflumilast. Concomitant

administration of inhaled formoterol resulted in changes that were less than 1% in peak concentration and expo-sure compared with roflumilast alone treatment There-fore, this co-administration is unlikely to result in clinically relevant interactions.

Cardiovascular effects were investigated by ZCG, which enabled measurement of STIs and allowed deriva-tion of method-specific non-invasive estimates of systo-lic pump function [35,43]. These ZCG/STI methods are particularly sensitive to within-subject positive inotropic and vasodilatory cardiovascular changes, especially when chronotropic and inotropic reflexes are triggered by vasodilatation ('chrono-inodilatory' responses) [34,44]. Such measures are affected by changes in posture and food intake [45-47]. In all these measures the detectable effects were small. With formoterol alone there was a discrete trend towards a slightly higher HR, shorter PEP, increased CO and decreased TPR; these changes are likely to reflect a vasodilatory effect of formoterol [48,49]. Roflumilast had no effect on the ZCG/STI criteria and did not appear to potentiate the effects of formoterol.

Electrocardiographic investigations confirmed a slight increase in HR for formoterol, which was associated with an HR-dependent shortening of the QT interval with no change in HR-corrected QTc. Accordingly, there was no indication of a safety-relevant cardiovascular drug-drug interaction.

There was a slight decrease in fasting serum glucose level with roflumilast, which did not induce any hypoglycaemia. This effect was blunted when formoterol was administered concomitantly. Formoterol is known to increase serum glucose concentrations at supra-therapeutic levels [50]; however, at the 24 µg dose used in this study, there was only a slight increase in serum glucose level when formoterol was administered both alone and in combination with roflumilast. Supra-therapeutic doses of $\beta_2$-agonists are also associated with decreased serum potassium concentrations [50,51]; in this study, a mild but consistent decrease was seen with formoterol, which was unaffected by concomitant roflumilast. A mild decrease in serum potassium level was also seen with roflumilast.

None of the other parameters examined (blood pressure, body temperature, clinical laboratory tests) showed safety-relevant changes that might be attributable to roflumilast, formoterol or their combination. The reported AEs were generally mild, with no severe or serious AEs, and mostly reflected the known properties of the investigated medications. There were some differences between the two regimens with regard to the incidence of tremor: tremor was reported 13 times when formoterol was added to roflumilast (11 times in Regimen A and twice in Regimen B), but was not observed when roflumilast or formoterol were administered alone (Regimens A and B respectively).

Although this study was performed in healthy men, results from clinical trials conducted in the roflumilast target population - patients with severe COPD, chronic bronchitis and a history of exacerbations - also support the absence of any relevant interaction between roflumilast and long-acting $\beta_2$-adrenoreceptor agonists. The two 1-year roflumilast pivotal studies (M2-124 and M2-125) were conducted in 3091 patients, approximately half of whom were receiving concomitant $\beta_2$-adrenoreceptor agonists [8]. In a pooled analysis of the two studies, roflumilast proved effective irrespective of $\beta_2$-adrenoreceptor agonist use, and the overall pattern of AEs with or without concomitant $\beta_2$-adrenoreceptor agonists was similar to that reported across all patients; there was no indication that roflumilast increased AEs

associated with $\beta_2$-adrenoreceptor agonists (such as tachycardia or cardiovascular events), and the co-administration of the two drugs did not increase the frequency of events associated with roflumilast alone [52]. Similar results were observed in a 6-month study (M2-127) conducted in patients with moderate to severe COPD receiving concomitant salmeterol [13]. Furthermore, a population pharmacokinetic analysis of roflumilast and roflumilast N-oxide [53] indicated that only a slight increase (12.6%) in tPDE4i is expected in patients with COPD compared with healthy individuals. The fact that during the clinical development of roflumilast the co-administration with long-acting $\beta_2$-adrenoreceptor agonists was evaluated in patients with COPD for periods of up to 1 year also suggests that safety issues can be excluded, not only in the short term considered in this crossover study, but also in chronic use.

Given that $\beta_2$-adrenoreceptor agonists can be used in combination with inhaled corticosteroids in the symptomatic treatment of severe COPD, concerns may arise regarding the addition of roflumilast to this therapeutic combination. Results from two 1-year randomised clinical trials (M2-111 and M2-112) in patients with severe and very severe COPD showed that the co-administration of inhaled corticosteroids does not affect the AE profile of roflumilast [55]. Furthermore, a drug-drug interaction study evaluating the effects of the co-administration of roflumilast and budesonide, a commonly used inhaled corticosteroid metabolised by CYP3A enzymes [54], revealed no relevant pharmacokinetic interactions and no alteration of the safety and tolerability profiles of either drug in healthy volunteers [24]. As mentioned earlier, roflumilast is metabolised by parallel CYP pathways, which suggests that specific CYP inducers or inhibitors are unlikely to alter its pharmacokinetic profile significantly. Although the combination of roflumilast, formoterol and inhaled corticosteroids has not been specifically investigated, based on these observations it is unlikely that the concomitant administration of the three drugs will cause relevant drug-drug interactions.

## Conclusions

In summary, the study results demonstrate that concomitant administration of oral roflumilast and inhaled formoterol under steady-state conditions does not affect the pharmacodynamics or pharmacokinetics of either drug. In particular, there was no evidence of a relevant pharmacodynamic interaction with regard to myocardial repolarisation or cardiac function in general. Moreover, the concomitant administration of roflumilast and formoterol did not negatively influence the safety profile of either drug.

## Acknowledgements and Funding
The authors thank Polly Field, DPhil, of Caudex Medical Ltd, Oxford, UK (supported by Nycomed GmbH, Konstanz, Germany [formerly ALTANA Pharma AG]) for editorial assistance with the preparation of the manuscript; Dr Robert Hermann (CR Appliance, Radolfzell, Germany) for his contribution to conceptual study design and data interpretation; and Dr Andreas Huennemeyer and Dr Markus Hinder of Nycomed GmbH for their contribution to the preparation of the manuscript and critical evaluation of the data. Nycomed GmbH provided funding for the design and conduct of the study; collection, management, analysis, and interpretation of the data; and preparation, review, and approval of the manuscript.

## Author details
[1]ACPS - Applied Clinical Pharmacology Services, Mainz-Kastel, Germany. [2]Nycomed GmbH, Konstanz, Germany.

## Authors' contributions
CdM served as a study investigator and was responsible for the acquisition of trial data. In addition he was involved in the study conception and design, in collaboration with GL. All three authors (CdM, GL and NN) contributed significantly to the analysis and interpretation of data; were involved in drafting the manuscript or revising it critically for important intellectual content; and gave final approval of the version to be published.

## Competing interests
This study was sponsored by Nycomed GmbH (formerly ALTANA Pharma AG), Konstanz, Germany. CdM has received financial support for research and consulting services from Nycomed GmbH. NN and GL are employees of Nycomed GmbH, Konstanz, Germany.

## References
1. Hatzelmann A, Morcillo EJ, Lungarella G, Adnot S, Sanjar S, Beume R, Schudt C, Tenor H: The preclinical pharmacology of roflumilast - a selective, oral phosphodiesterase 4 inhibitor in development for chronic obstructive pulmonary disease. Pulm Pharmacol Ther 2010, 23:235-256.
2. Bundschuh DS, Eltze M, Barsig J, Wollin L, Hatzelmann A, Beume R: In vivo efficacy in airway disease models of roflumilast, a novel orally active PDE4 inhibitor. J Pharmacol Exp Ther 2001, 297:280-290.
3. Jones NA, Boswell-Smith V, Lever R, Page CP: The effect of selective phosphodiesterase isoenzyme inhibition on neutrophil function in vitro. Pulm Pharmacol Ther 2005, 18:93-101.
4. Hatzelmann A, Schudt C: Anti-inflammatory and immunomodulatory potential of the novel PDE4 inhibitor roflumilast in vitro. J Pharmacol Exp Ther 2001, 297:267-279.
5. Grootendorst DC, Gauw SA, Verhoosel RM, Sterk PJ, Hospers JJ, Bredenbroker D, Bethke TD, Hiemstra PS, Rabe KF: Reduction in sputum neutrophil and eosinophil numbers by the PDE4 inhibitor roflumilast in patients with COPD. Thorax 2007, 62:1081-1087.
6. Rabe KF, Bateman ED, O'Donnell D, Witte S, Bredenbroker D, Bethke TD: Roflumilast - an oral anti-inflammatory treatment for chronic obstructive pulmonary disease: a randomised controlled trial. Lancet 2005, 366:563-571.
7. Calverley PM, Sanchez-Toril F, McIvor A, Teichmann P, Bredenbroeker D, Fabbri LM: Effect of 1-year treatment with roflumilast in severe chronic obstructive pulmonary disease. Am J Respir Crit Care Med 2007, 176:154-161.
8. Calverley PM, Rabe KF, Goehring UM, Kristiansen S, Fabbri LM, Martinez FJ: Roflumilast in symptomatic chronic obstructive pulmonary disease: two randomised clinical trials. Lancet 2009, 374:685-694.
9. Global Initiative for Chronic Obstructive Lung Disease: Global Strategy for the Diagnosis, Management and Prevention of Chronic Obstructive Pulmonary Disease (Updated 2009) Bethesda: National Heart, Lung and Blood Institute; 2009.
10. O'Donnell DE, Hernandez P, Kaplan A, Aaron S, Bourbeau J, Marciniuk D, Balter M, Ford G, Gervais A, Lacasse Y, Maltais F, Road J, Rocker G, Sin D, Sinuff T, Voduc N: Canadian Thoracic Society recommendations for management of chronic obstructive pulmonary disease - 2008 update - highlights for primary care. Can Respir J 2008, 15(Suppl A):1A-8A.
11. Celli BR, MacNee W: Standards for the diagnosis and treatment of patients with COPD: a summary of the ATS/ERS position paper. Eur Respir J 2004, 23:932-946.
12. Calverley PM: COPD: what is the unmet need? Br J Pharmacol 2008, 155:487-493.
13. Fabbri LM, Calverley PM, Izquierdo-Alonso JL, Bundschuh DS, Brose M, Martinez FJ, Rabe KF: Roflumilast in moderate-to-severe chronic obstructive pulmonary disease treated with longacting bronchodilators: two randomised clinical trials. Lancet 2009, 374:695-703.
14. Buenestado A, Naline EN, Chapelier AC, Bellamy JFB, Devillier PD: Roflumilast and its active metabolite inhibit LPS-induced cytokines production from human parenchymal and bronchial explants: interaction with formoterol [abstract]. Eur Respir J 2009, 34:581s.
15. Spina D: Phosphodiesterase-4 inhibitors in the treatment of inflammatory lung disease. Drugs 2003, 63:2575-2594.
16. Spina D: PDE4 inhibitors: current status. Br J Pharmacol 2008, 155:308-315.
17. Anderson GP: Current issues with beta2-adrenoceptor agonists: pharmacology and molecular and cellular mechanisms. Clin Rev Allergy Immunol 2006, 31:119-130.
18. Zaccolo M, Movsesian MA: cAMP and cGMP signaling cross-talk: role of phosphodiesterases and implications for cardiac pathophysiology. Circ Res 2007, 100:1569-1578.
19. Cazzola M, Matera MG, Donner CF: Inhaled beta2-adrenoceptor agonists: cardiovascular safety in patients with obstructive lung disease. Drugs 2005, 65:1595-1610.
20. Hermann R, Lahu G, Huennemyer A, Knoerzer D, Bethke TD, Haverkamp W: No effect of roflumilast on cardiac repolarization in healthy subjects [abstract]. Eur Respir J 2006, 28(Suppl 50):660s.
21. David M, Zech K, Seiberling M, Weimar C, Bethke TD: Roflumilast, a novel, oral, selective PDE4 inhibitor, shows high oral bioavailability. J Allergy Clin Immunol 2004, 113:S220-S221.
22. Bethke TD, Böhmer GM, Hermann R, Hauns B, Fux R, Morike K, David M, Knoerzer D, Wurst W, Gleiter CH: Dose-proportional intraindividual single- and repeated-dose pharmacokinetics of roflumilast, an oral, once-daily phosphodiesterase 4 inhibitor. J Clin Pharmacol 2007, 47:26-36.
23. Hermann R, Nassr N, Lahu G, Peterfai E, Knoerzer D, Herzog R, Zech K, de Mey C: Steady-state pharmacokinetics of roflumilast and roflumilast N-oxide in patients with mild and moderate liver cirrhosis. Clin Pharmacokinet 2007, 46:403-416.
24. Hermann R, Siegmund W, Giessmann T, Westphal K, Weinbrenner A, Hauns B, Reutter F, Lahu G, Zech K, Bethke TD: The oral, once-daily phosphodiesterase 4 inhibitor roflumilast lacks relevant pharmacokinetic interactions with inhaled budesonide. J Clin Pharmacol 2007, 47:1005-1013.
25. Hermann R, Lahu G, Hauns B, Bethke T, Zech K: Total PDE4 inhibitory activity: a concept for evaluating pharmacokinetic alterations of roflumilast and roflumilast N-oxide in special populations and drug-drug interactions [abstract]. Eur Respir J 2006, 28:436s.
26. Lahu G, Hünnemeyer A, Herzog R, McCracken N, Hermann R, Elmlinger M, Zech K: Effect of repeated dose of erythromycin on the pharmacokinetics of roflumilast and roflumilast N-oxide. Int J Clin Pharmacol Ther 2009, 47:236-245.
27. Lahu G, Hünnemeyer A, von Richter O, Hermann R, Herzog R, McCracken N, Zech K: Effect of single and repeated doses of ketoconazole on the pharmacokinetics of roflumilast and roflumilast N-oxide. J Clin Pharmacol 2008, 48:1339-1349.
28. von Richter O, Lahu G, Hünnemeyer A, Herzog R, Zech K, Hermann R: Effect of fluvoxamine on the pharmacokinetics of roflumilast and roflumilast N-oxide. Clin Pharmacokinet 2007, 46:613-622.
29. Lahu G, Nassr N, Herzog R, Elmlinger M, Ruth P, Hinder M, Huennemeyer A: Effect of steady-state enoxacin on single-dose pharmacokinetics of roflumilast and roflumilast N-Oxide. J Clin Pharmacol 2011, 51:586-593.
30. Bohmer GM, Gleiter CH, Morike K, Nassr N, Walz A, Lahu G: No Dose Adjustment on Coadministration of the PDE4 Inhibitor Roflumilast With a Weak CYP3A, CYP1A2, and CYP2C19 Inhibitor: An Investigation Using Cimetidine. J Clin Pharmacol 2011, 51:594-602.
31. Nassr N, Huennemeyer A, Herzog R, von RO, Hermann R, Koch M, Duffy K, Zech K, Lahu G: Effects of rifampicin on the pharmacokinetics of roflumilast and roflumilast N-oxide in healthy subjects. Br J Clin Pharmacol 2009, 68:580-587.

32.  Electronic Medicines Compendium: **Formoterol summary of product characteristics.** 1950 [http://www.medicines.org.uk/EMC/medicine/19503/SPC/Formoterol+Easyhaler+12+micrograms+per+actuation+inhalation+powder/].

33.  Lecaillon JB, Kaiser G, Palmisano M, Morgan J, Della CG: **Pharmacokinetics and tolerability of formoterol in healthy volunteers after a single high dose of Foradil dry powder inhalation via Aerolizer.** *Eur J Clin Pharmacol* 1999, **55**:131-138.

34.  de Mey C, Erb K, Schroeter V, Belz GG: **Differentiation of inodilatory responses by non-invasive measures of cardiovascular performance in healthy man.** *Int J Clin Pharmacol Ther* 1996, **34**:525-532.

35.  de Mey C, Erb KA: **Usefulness, usability, and quality criteria for noninvasive methods in cardiovascular clinical pharmacology.** *J Clin Pharmacol* 1997, **37**:11S-20S.

36.  Weissler AM, Harris WS, Schoenfeld CD: **Systolic time intervals in heart failure in man.** *Circulation* 1968, **37**:149-159.

37.  Kubicek WG, Karnegis JN, Patterson RP, Witsoe DA, Mattson RH: **Development and evaluation of an impedance cardiac output system.** *Aerosp Med* 1966, **37**:1208-1212.

38.  Geddes LA, Sadler C: **The specific resistance of blood at body temperature.** *Med Biol Eng* 1973, **11**:336-339.

39.  Wezler K, Boeger A: **Die dynamik des arteriellen. Systems.** *Ergebn Physiol* 1939, **41**:292-606.

40.  Hodges JL, Lehmann EL: **The efficiency of some nonparametric competitors of the t-test.** *Ann Math Statist* 1956, **27**:324-335.

41.  Bazett HC: **An analysis of the time-relations of electrocardiograms.** *Heart* 1920, **7**:353-370.

42.  Fridericia LS: **Die Systolendauer im Elektrokardiogramm bei normalen Menschen und bei Herzkranken.** *Acta Med Scand* 1920, **53**:469-486.

43.  de Mey C, Belz GG, Nixdorf U, Butzer R, Schroeter V, Meyer J, Erbel R: **Relative sensitivity of four noninvasive methods in assessing systolic cardiovascular effects of isoproterenol in healthy volunteers.** *Clin Pharmacol Ther* 1992, **52**:609-619.

44.  de Mey C, Enterling D, Hanft G: **Noninvasive assessment of the inodilator action of amrinone in healthy man.** *Eur J Clin Pharmacol* 1991, **40**:373-378.

45.  de Mey C, Enterling D: **Non-invasive estimates of cardiac performance during and immediately after single and repeated passive upright tilt in normal man: volume dependency of systolic time intervals and maximum velocity of transthoracic impedance changes.** *Am J Noninvasive Cardiol* 1987, **1**:188-196.

46.  de Mey C, Hansen-Schmidt S, Enterling D: **Food intake as a source of methodological bias in cardiovascular clinical pharmacology.** *Pharmaceut Med* 1987, **2**:251-257.

47.  de Mey C, Hansen-Schmidt S, Enterling D: **Postprandial haemodynamic changes: a source of bias in cardiovascular research affected by its own methodological bias.** *Cardiovasc Res* 1988, **22**:703-707.

48.  Kirby DA, Vatner SF: **Enhanced responsiveness to carotid baroreceptor unloading in conscious dogs during development of perinephritic hypertension.** *Circ Res* 1987, **61**:678-686.

49.  Carlsson E, Dahlof CG, Hedberg A, Persson H, Tangstrand B: **Differentiation of cardiac chronotropic and inotropic effects of beta-adrenoceptor agonists.** *Naunyn Schmiedebergs Arch Pharmacol* 1977, **300**:101-105.

50.  Bennett JA, Tattersfield AE: **Time course and relative dose potency of systemic effects from salmeterol and salbutamol in healthy subjects.** *Thorax* 1997, **52**:458-464.

51.  Palmqvist M, Ibsen T, Mellen A, Lotvall J: **Comparison of the relative efficacy of formoterol and salmeterol in asthmatic patients.** *Am J Respir Crit Care Med* 1999, **160**:244-249.

52.  Bateman ED, Rabe K, Calverley PMA, Goehring UM, Brose M, Bredenbrocker D, Fabbri LM: **Roflumilast with long-acting $\beta_2$ agonists for COPD: influence of exacerbation history.** *Eur Respir J* 2011.

53.  Lahu G, Hünnemeyer A, Diletti E, Elmlinger M, Ruth P, Zech K, McCracken N, Facius A: **Population Pharmacokinetic Modelling of Roflumilast and Roflumilast N-Oxide by Total Phosphodiesterase 4 Inhibitory Activity and Development of a Population Pharmacodynamic-Adverse Event Model.** *Clin Pharmacokinet* 2010, **49**:589-606.

54.  Jonsson G, Astrom A, Andersson P: **Budesonide is metabolized by cytochrome P450 3A (CYP3A) enzymes in human liver.** *Drug Metab Dispos* 1995, **23**:137-142.

55.  Rennard SI, Calverley PM, Goehring UM, Bredenbroker D, Martinez FJ: **Reduction of exacerbations by the PDE4 inhibitor roflumilast–the**

importance of defining different subsets of patients with COPD. *Respir Res* 2011, **12**:18.

# 17

# An open prospective study of amikacin pharmacokinetics in critically ill patients during treatment with continuous venovenous haemodiafiltration

Deirdre M D'Arcy[2], Eoin Casey[1], Caitriona M Gowing[3], Maria B Donnelly[1*] and Owen I Corrigan[2]

## Abstract

**Background:** The objectives of the current study were to determine amikacin pharmacokinetics in patients undergoing treatment with continuous venovenous haemodiafiltration (CVVHDF) in an Intensive Care Unit (ICU), and to determine whether peak and trough concentration data could be used to predict pharmacokinetic parameters. An open prospective study was undertaken, comprising five critically ill patients with sepsis requiring CVVHDF.

**Methods:** Peak and trough plasma concentrations and multiple serum levels in a dosage interval were measured and the latter fitted to both a one- and two-compartment model. Blood and ultrafiltrate samples were collected and assayed for amikacin to calculate the pharmacokinetic parameters; total body clearance (TBC), elimination rate constant (k) and volume of distribution ($V_d$). The concentration of amikacin in ultrafiltrate was used to determine the clearance via CVVHDF. CVVHDF was performed at prescribed dialysate rates of 1-2l h$^{-1}$ and ultrafiltration rate of 2l h$^{-1}$. Blood was pumped at 200ml/min using a Gambro blood pump and Hospal AN69HF haemofilter. Amikacin dosing was according to routine clinical practice in the Intensive Care Unit.

**Results:** The multi serum level study indicated that the one compartment model was adequate to characterize the pharmacokinetics in these patients suggesting that peak and trough plasma level data may be used to estimate individual patient pharmacokinetic parameters and to optimise individual patient dosing during treatment with CVVHDF. CVVHDF resulted in an amikacin k of 0.109+/−0.025 h, $t_{1/2}$ of 6.74 +/− 1.69h, TBC of 3.39+/−0.817 h$^{-1}$, and $V_d$ of 31.4 +/− 3.27. The mean clearance due to CVVHDF of 2.86 l h$^{-1}$ is similar to the creatinine clearance of 2.74 +/−0.4 lh$^{-1}$. Amikacin was significantly cleared by CVVHDF, and its half life in patients on CVVHDF was approximately 2–3 times that reported in subjects without renal impairment and not undergoing haemodiafiltration for any reason.

**Conclusions:** CVVHDF contributes significantly to total clearance of amikacin. The use of pharmacokinetic parameter estimates obtained from two steady state serum-drug concentrations (peak and trough) can be used to guide individualised dosing of critically ill patients treated with CVVHDF. This is considered a useful strategy in this patient cohort, particularly in avoiding the risk of underdosing.

**Keywords:** Amikacin, Pharmacokinetics, Haemodiafiltration

* Correspondence: maria.donnelly@amnch.ie
[1]Intensive Care Medicine, Tallaght Hospital, Dublin 24, Ireland
Full list of author information is available at the end of the article

## Background

Aminoglycoside antibiotics are used to treat serious infections caused by gram negative microorganisms in intensive care unit (ICU) patients. They are an increasingly popular choice for both empiric and directed therapy as they are less likely to engender resistance than quinolones [1] and have a lesser incidence of promoting Clostridium difficile infection than other antibiotics [2]. The intersection of aminoglycoside and continuous veno-venous haemodiafiltration (CVVHDF) use is an ever increasing likelihood in the ICU setting. The use of amikacin in particular is increasing as it may offer a more extensive spectrum of cover than gentamicin [3], especially with the advent of Extended Spectrum Beta-Lactamase (ESBL) producing organisms.

Elimination of amikacin is mainly via the renal route. Its dosage regimens must therefore be adjusted in severe renal insufficiency to prevent accumulation of the drug to toxic levels and the associated risk of oto- and nephrotoxicity. However, this drug's hydrophilicity and low molecular weight also make it likely to be cleared by CVVHDF and consequently pharmacokinetic studies during CVVHDF are required to optimise dosing regimens and obtain therapeutic concentrations.

In general, data relating toxicity with aminoglycoside concentrations refer to trough plasma concentrations [4]. Low serum peak aminoglycoside concentrations are associated with an increased risk of clinical failure [5,6] and the emergence of resistant strains [7]. A marked variability in aminoglycoside pharmacokinetic parameters has been reported in critically ill patients [8,9]. For example an increased volume of distribution for aminoglycoside antibiotics has been found in critically ill patients with sepsis [10] and ascites [11]. Additionally, augmented renal clearance has been described in certain patient cohorts, e.g. burns patients.

There are some studies investigating the effects of CVVH on clearance of amikacin [12-14] but there is little published evidence describing the effect of CVVHDF. CVVH depends predominantly on convection alone while CVVHDF involves a combination of solute clearance by diffusion and convection, and is generally expected to have increased removal efficiency over CVVH [15]. One study has suggested that 40% of an amikacin dose could be removed by CVVHDF based on a study of six renal failure patients [16]. Another study recently published investigated pharmacokinetics of amikacin in patients on CVVHDF suffering from sepsis or septic shock following administration of a 25 mg/kg loading dose [17]. This study illustrated that the half life (~6.5 h) of amikacin in these patients on CVVHDF was much lower than reported for patients with renal impairment not receiving dialysis [18] (> 30 hours in anuric patients during the interhemofiltration period). However it did not determine specifically the contribution of CVVHDF to amikacin clearance. Furthermore, it was suggested that accumulation following high loading dose

may be an issue in subsequent doses if the dosage interval is not adequately extended. A further recent case report of two patients demonstrated the value of clearance via CVVHDF when administering high doses of amikacin to patients with sepsis due to panresistant *Pseudomonas aeruginosa*. As this combination was used as a therapeutic option to enable higher dosing, no pharmacokinetic analysis was presented in that study [19]. CVVHDF is the preferred modality of continuous renal replacement therapy in the hospital setting of the current work.

A 1-compartment model is considered adequate to describe amikacin pharmacokinetics in most clinical settings to facilitate aminoglycoside dosage adjustments/calculations [4], once peak concentrations are measured after a short distribution phase e.g. 30 minutes after a 30 minute infusion. In the study by Taccone et al. a 2-compartment model was used for the pharmacokinetics analysis of amikacin plasma concentrations following the high loading dose in patients on CVVHDF [17]. Due to the unknown pharmacokinetic behaviour of amikacin in patients on CVVHDF, it was desirable to establish whether a 1-compartment model rather than a 2-compartment model would still be a suitable model selection in these patients. Collection and analysis of multiple serum concentration data is not routine in the clinical setting, therefore assessment of the suitability of the use of peak and trough data only, to calculate pharmacokinetic parameters is mandated. This type of data would be routine in a standard therapeutic drug monitoring (TDM) scenario.

The practice in the hospital setting of the current study prior to the commencement of this study was for the dosage of aminoglycosides to be modified during CVVHDF, on the basis of the best prescribing recommendations of the time. The levels (peak and trough values) obtained indicated potential underdosing and suggested significant CVVHDF induced clearance.

The deficit of data on amikacin pharmacokinetics during treatment with CVVHDF, and the evident potential for underdosing due to clearance via CVVHDF in these patients prompted this study.

The objectives of the study were:

a) to carry out a prospective study of patients treated with amikacin and CVVHDF, and to determine amikacin pharmacokinetic parameters including an estimate of clearance due to CVVHDF

b) to determine whether a 1-compartment model or a 2-compartment model better fitted multiple serum concentration data over the course of one dosage interval in patients on CVVHDF.

c) to determine whether peak and trough data alone would be adequate to calculate pharmacokinetic parameters and subsequent dose recommendations, as this data is obtained during routine therapeutic drug monitoring (TDM) practice.

## Methods

### Patient Selection

The decision to treat with CVVHDF and amikacin was determined prior to the inclusion of the patients in the study. It was an open, prospective, non-interventional study. Demographic data and clinical characteristics are given in Table 1. Estimates of creatinine clearance (CrCl) were obtained using the method of Jelliffe and Jelliffe [20].

Ethical approval was obtained from the Joint Hospitals Ethics Committees (St James Hospital/Adelaide and Meath Hospital Dublin, Incorporating the National Children's Hospital Ref No. 041007/7704). Approval was obtained from the Irish Medicines Board. Written informed consent to participate and publish (predominantly consent by proxy) was obtained in compliance with Helsinki declaration.

### CVVHDF procedure

A 0.6 m$^2$ polyacrilonitrile cylinder haemofilter (Prisma M100, Preset AN69HF, Hospal, Lyon, France) was utilised. Blood was pumped through the membrane at a rate of 200 ml min$^{-1}$. The dialysate fluid passed once across the membrane into the dialysate compartment of the filter at a rate of 1–2 l h$^{-1}$. The ultrafiltration rate and predilution replacement solution infusion rates were both 2 l h$^{-1}$.

### Administration of amikacin

Multiple doses of amikacin were administered to each patient. Each dose of amikacin was infused intravenously over a period of 30 minutes. Blood samples (7 ml) were taken immediately prior to the administration of a subsequent dose (trough) and 30 minutes after the infusion was complete (peak).

Additionally, multiple serum concentrations (minimum of seven; at the end of the infusion, and at 1, 2, 5, 8, 12, 18 hours) in a dosage interval were obtained for at least one dosage interval for each patient.

In the hospital setting of this study, current target peak and trough plasma concentrations using once-daily dosing (extended interval dosing) are 50–60 mg/L and <5

mg/L respectively and these criteria are consistent with literature ranges of approximately 40 - 60 mg/L and <5 mg/L [4,21,22]. It should be noted that the study time period straddled the hospital's transition from multiple daily dosing (7.5 mg kg$^{-1}$ twice daily, trough <2.5 mg l$^{-1}$, peak not greater than 30 mg l$^{-1}$) to once daily/extended interval dosing.

### Analytical Procedures

Concentrations of amikacin in serum and dialysis effluent fluid were measured using a TDx analyser (Abbott) using a fluorescence polarization immunoassay. An amikacin standard concentration curve was constructed using calibrators (0, 5.0, 10, 20, 30 and 50 mg l$^{-1}$). Blood samples were stored at 4°C prior to prompt analysis.

Amikacin clearance by CVVHDF was investigated for a single dosage interval. The amount of amikacin in each effluent collection during the dosage interval was calculated by multiplying the measured effluent concentration in each effluent sample by the volume of effluent collected over the corresponding time period. Effluent samples were stored at 4°C pending assay.

### Pharmacokinetic analysis

*Multiple concentration data over a dosage interval – 1 compartment model*

Multiple serum concentrations during one dose interval were used to determine k, $V_d$, $t_{1/2}$ and total body clearance (TBC). k was calculated through fitting of the concentration time data to a 1-compartment infusion model using WinNonlin pharmacokinetic software version 5.2, (Pharsight Corporation, North Carolina, USA).

*Multiple concentration data over a dosage interval - 2 compartment model*

It was attempted to fit the concentration-time data from multiple samples taken over a dosage interval to a 2-compartment infusion model using WinNonlin version 5.2, (Pharsight Corporation, North Carolina, USA).

**Table 1 Summary of patients' clinical and demographic data**

| ID | Sex | Age | Diagnosis | Infective diagnosis | APACHE II Score[1] | CrCl[2] | Duration CVVHDF (days) |
|----|-----|-----|-----------|---------------------|-----------------|------|------------------------|
| P1 | M | 57 | Cirrhosis of liver, sepsis, ARF | Pseudomonas aeruginosa | 39 | 10 | 7 |
| P2 | F | 68 | Colonic obstruction, post-op ARF, sepsis | Pseudomonas aeruginosa | 28 | 8 | 14 |
| P3 | M | 59 | ALL with neutropenic sepsis and ARF | Empiric cover for sepsis | 24 | 5 | 10 |
| P4 | M | 63 | Ruptured abdominal aortic aneurysm repair with post-op ARF and sepsis | Acinetobacter baumanni | 18 | 5 | 13 |
| P5 | F | 70 | Pneumonia, ARDS | Klebsiella pneumoniae | 24 | 2 | 11 |
| **Mean** | | **63.4** | | - | **26.6** | **6** | **11** |

[1] Initial/ICU admission value.
[2] Creatinine clearance value on day 1 of CVVHDF, prior to commencing CVVHDF therapy. Units = ml/min; estimated using the method of Jelliffe and Jelliffe.
ARF = Acute renal failure.
ALL = Acute lymphocytic leukaemia.
ARDS = Acute Respiratory Distress Syndrome.

Fitting multiple serum concentration data to a 2-compartment model facilitated the calculation of TBC, $V_1$, k, $t_{1/2 (el)}$, $t_{1/2\alpha}$, $t_{1/2\beta}$ and Vss. Vss is the estimated volume of distribution at steady state. In this case, $t_{1/2(el)}$ is the elimination half life, comparable to $t_{1/2}$ for the one compartment model. In order to calculate initial estimates, the post-infusion concentration data was fitted to a bi-exponential curve of the form $C_{pt}=A_1e^{-\alpha t}+B_1e^{-\beta t}$, where $C_{pt}$ is the plasma concentration at time, t. The parameters $A_1$ and $B_1$ were then transformed to A and B using equation 1, where T is the duration of the infusion, $C_i = A$ or B, $Y_i = A_1$ or $B_1$ and $\lambda_i = \alpha$ or $\beta$ [23].

$$C_i = \frac{\lambda_i T Y_i}{e^{\lambda_i T} - 1} \qquad (1)$$

The relevant pharmacokinetic parameters were then calculated using the following standard equations:

$$\frac{A\beta + B\alpha}{A + B} = k_{21} \qquad (2)$$

$$k_{10} = \frac{\alpha\beta}{k_{21}} \qquad (3)$$

$$V_1 = \frac{Dose}{A + B} \qquad (4)$$

where $V_1$ is the volume of the central compartment.

### Peak and trough values

In order to evaluate serum concentration data which would be available under routine therapeutic drug monitoring conditions, individualized pharmacokinetic parameters were determined from each patient's peak and trough serum concentration data using the method of Sawchuk and Zaske [24]. The half life ($t_{1/2}$), elimination rate constant (k), TBC and volume of distribution ($V_d$) were calculated as follows:

$$k = \frac{\left(\ln C_{p\,max} - \ln C_{p\,min}\right)}{\tau - t^1} \qquad (5)$$

where $\tau$ is the dosage interval and $t^1$ is time of the peak sample.

$$t_{\frac{1}{2}} = \frac{0.693}{k} \qquad (6)$$

$$V_d = \frac{\frac{D}{T}\left(1 - e^{-kT}\right)}{k\left(C_{p\,max} - \left(C_{p\,min^1}e^{-kT}\right)\right)} \qquad (7)$$

where D is the dose, T is the duration of the infusion and $C_{p\,min^1}$ is the trough concentration from the previous dose [24]. In the case of the first dose, the term $C_{p\,min^1}e^{-kT}$ was omitted from Equation 7.

$$TBC = k \times V_d \qquad (8)$$

## Results

### Patient demographics

Three men and two women treated with amikacin during CVVHDF therapy, ages 57–70 (mean +/– SD: 63.4 +/– 5.6 years) were enrolled in the study. Demographic data and clinical characteristics are given in Table 1. All five patients enrolled in the prospective study had severe renal impairment. Three were anuric throughout treatment (patients 1, 2, 3) and two patients were anuric on commencing CVVHDF but became oliguric during treatment (day 11 and day 10), at which time treatment with amikacin had stopped. The average measured effluent flow rate was 3.5 +/–0.6 l $h^{-1}$.

The mean APACHE II (Acute Physiology and Chronic Health Evaluation II) score was 26.6 +/– 7.8. The mean duration of CVVHDF therapy was 11.0 +/– 2.7 days. Patients 1–4 were diagnosed with sepsis and two patients (1 and 4) had concomitant liver and renal impairment.

### Pharmacokinetic results

In total 68 amikacin concentrations were determined, ranging from 1.8 mg $l^{-1}$ to 68.3 mg $l^{-1}$. All samples were quantifiable.

### *Measuring multiple serum concentrations over a dosage interval and fitting to 1- and 2-compartment models*

The multiple amikacin serum concentrations sampled in a dosage interval for each of the five patients are presented graphically in Figure 1. This post infusion data was analysed in terms of the 1- and, where possible, 2-

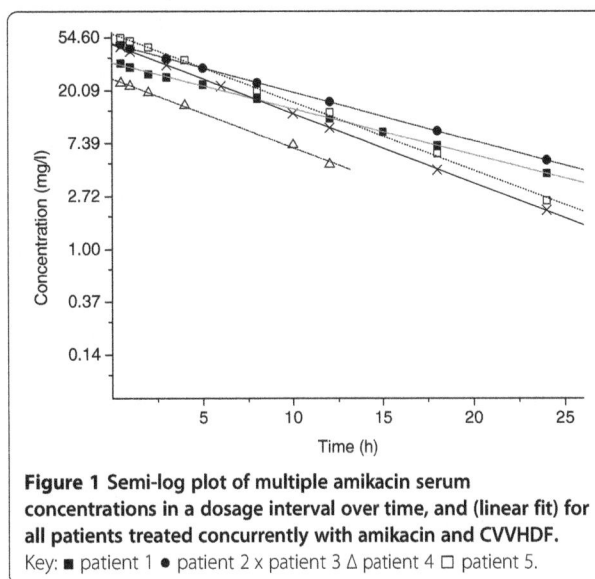

**Figure 1** Semi-log plot of multiple amikacin serum concentrations in a dosage interval over time, and (linear fit) for all patients treated concurrently with amikacin and CVVHDF.
Key: ■ patient 1 ● patient 2 x patient 3 Δ patient 4 □ patient 5.

compartment open models, and the parameters obtained are summarized in Tables 2 and 3 respectively.

Estimates of the pharmacokinetic parameters, k, $t_{1/2}$, TBC and $V_d$, were initially obtained for each patient on the basis of a 1-compartment model. The results are presented in Table 2.

The same amikacin serum concentration time data, fitted to a 2-compartment model gave estimates of the pharmacokinetic parameters, k, $t_{1/2(el)}$, $t_{1/2\alpha}$, $t_{1/2\beta}$, $V_1$, TBC and $V_{ss}$ shown in Table 3. It was not possible to reasonably fit the data for patients 4 and 5 to a 2-compartment model. The best fit to a 2-compartment model was with the data from patient 1 where a short but clear distribution phase was evident. Nevertheless, the highest CV% values were associated with the estimates for k21, $t_{1/2\alpha}$ and $V_2$, illustrating the variability surrounding the fitting of data to the distribution phase, when it is not very distinct and only captured by 1–2 points. Although the data was fitted to a 2-compartment model for patients 2 and 3, the standard residual and CV% values were much higher for all parameters, and more so those associated with the distribution phase and the second compartment. Overall the relevant pharmacokinetic parameters were similar in Tables 2–3, when considering the values from the same patient. Therefore, the current data suggest that, although it was possible to fit the data to a 2-compartment model in some cases, parameter estimates were similar to those obtained with a 1-compartment model. Most importantly, as can be seen from Figure 1, there was little or no distribution phase evident from the concentration-time profiles, further supporting the use of a 1-compartment model for pharmacokinetic analysis of this data. A short distribution phase is anticipated with aminoglycoside antibiotics, which is generally expected to be complete by 30 minutes after the end of the 30 minute infusion [4]. Therefore, in the case of these patients the distribution phase was evidently very rapid and of a small magnitude in comparison with the magnitude and time scale of the rest of the concentration-time profile.

### Estimates of pharmacokinetic parameters and dosage recommendations using peak and trough data only

Individual patient estimates of amikacin pharmacokinetic parameters during treatment with CVVHDF were obtained from amikacin serum concentration data. Estimates of $t_{1/2}$, k, $V_d$, and TBC obtained from peak and trough values are presented for each patient in Table 4.

Initial doses in patients 1, 2 and 4 were commenced prior to pharmacokinetic recommendations being available, according to the then current dosing practice on the ICU (pre-dating the change in dosing strategy). Subsequently pharmacokinetic parameters calculated for patients 1 and 2 were similar, and a dosing regime of 1500 mg at intervals of 31–32 hours was recommended. The initial results from these two patients illustrate the confusion which can surround "once daily" vs. "extended interval" dosing. The initial dose (900 mg) in patient 1 was subsequently increased to 1100 mg every 24 hours. Possibly due to the high $V_d$ observed in this patient, this dose was not adequate to achieve recommended peak levels, however the interval of 24 hours contributed to a degree of accumulation. This dosing schedule did not achieve target $C_{pmax}$ concentrations in this patient during CVVHDF therapy.

Subsequently, in patient 2, the recommended dose of 1500 mg was prescribed, achieving recommended peak concentrations. However the interval was not increased immediately and accumulation was noted. The interval was increased on day 5 and the rate of accumulation decreased.

In the case of patient 2, stopping CVVHDF therapy resulted in a three-fold increase in the amikacin half-life. Figure 2 shows amikacin serum concentrations over time for Patient 2. The arrow indicates the point at which CVVHDF therapy was stopped and a subsequent

**Table 2** Individual patient estimates of amikacin pharmacokinetic parameters during treatment with CVVHDF, obtained from multiple amikacin serum concentrations in a dosage interval fitted to a one-compartment model

| ID | k (h$^{-1}$) | CV%_k | $t_{1/2}$ (h) | $V_d$ (l) | TBC (l h$^{-1}$) |
|---|---|---|---|---|---|
| P1B | 0.088 | 2.8 | 7.91 | 28.47 | 2.49 |
| P2C | 0.094 | 2.31 | 7.37 | 31.97 | 3.01 |
| P3C | 0.130 | 1.27 | 5.33 | 32.48 | 4.22 |
| P4B | 0.141 | 5.99 | 4.91 | 29.45 | 4.15 |
| P5C | 0.126 | 1.98 | 5.49 | 27.88 | 3.51 |
| Mean +/– | 0.116 +/– | | 6.21 | 30.05 | 3.48 |
| s.d. | 0.024 | | +/– | +/– | +/– |
| | | | 1.34 | 2.07 | 0.74 |
| Median | 0.126 | | 5.5 | 29.45 | 3.51 |

$t_{1/2}$: half life. $V_d$: volume of distribution. TBC: Total body clearance. k: elimination rate constant. CV%: coefficient of variation. PX (1–5) patients 1–5.

**Table 3 Individual patient estimates of amikacin pharmacokinetic parameters during CVVHDF therapy assuming a two compartment model**

| ID | k ($h^{-1}$) | $V_1$ (l) | TBC (l $h^{-1}$) | $T_{1/2\alpha}$ (h) | $T_{1/2\beta}$ (h) | $T_{1/2el}$ (h) | $V_{ss}$ (l) |
|---|---|---|---|---|---|---|---|
| P1B | 0.093 | 25.0 | 2.32 | 0.25 | 8.18 | 7.45 | 27.33 |
| P2C | 0.131 | 21.95 | 2.88 | 0.035 | 7.61 | 5.29 | 31.5 |
| P3C | 0.172 | 24.31 | 4.19 | 0.028 | 5.29 | 4.02 | 31.94 |

$t_{1/2\alpha}$: half life of the alpha phase. $t_{1/2\beta}$: half life of the beta phase. $t_{1/2el}$: elimination half life. $V_{ss}$: volume of distribution at steady state. $V_1$: volume of distribution of the central compartment. TBC: Total body clearance. k: elimination rate constant. CV%: coefficient of variation. PX (1–5) patients 1–5.

increase in serum concentrations was observed. Despite the significant increase in interval between peak and trough sampling (53.5 h), the need for a further extension in dosage interval and decrease in dose due to the decrease in clearance after CVVHDF was discontinued is evident from the high trough level.

For patient 3, a 1500 mg dose achieved adequate $C_{pmax}$ concentrations, while the $C_{pmin}$ concentrations were also below the target threshold with a dosage interval of 24 hours. The mean clearance estimate, 4.4 +/- 0.51 l $h^{-1}$, was high and this value was close to the mean observed effluent flow rate during CVVHDF (4.1 l $h^{-1}$).

**Table 4 Peak and trough concentration data and estimates of amikacin pharmacokinetic parameters**

| Patient profile | Dose (mg) | Dosage interval (h) | Cpmax (mg $l^{-1}$) | Cpmin (mg $l^{-1}$) | $t_{1/2}$ (h) | k ($h^{-1}$) | TBC (l $h^{-1}$) | $V_d$ (l) |
|---|---|---|---|---|---|---|---|---|
| P1A | 900 | 24 | 31.3 | 3 | 6.80 | 0.102 | 2.858 | 28.03 |
| P1B | 900 | 24 | 33.8 | 4 | 7.63 | 0.091 | 2.583 | 28.44 |
| P1C | 1100 | 24 | 35.7 | 6.2 | 9.10 | 0.076 | 2.579 | 33.89 |
| **Mean** | | | | | **7.84** | **0.090** | **2.674** | **30.12** |
| P2A | 300 | 19 | 7.6 | 1.8 | 8.66 | 0.080 | 3.096 | 38.69 |
| P2B | 1500 | 24 | 50.2 | 2.8 | 5.52 | 0.125 | 3.761 | 29.97 |
| P2C | 1500 | 24 | 48.5 | 5.4 | 7.42 | 0.093 | 2.987 | 31.98 |
| P2D | 1500 | 29 | 49.4 | 5 | 8.47 | 0.082 | 2.719 | 33.24 |
| P2E | 1500 | 32 | 55.9 | 6.1 | 9.70 | 0.071 | 2.062 | 28.85 |
| P2F | 1500 | 29 | 53.8 | 7 | 9.51 | 0.073 | 2.239 | 30.74 |
| **Mean** | | | | | **8.21** | **0.088** | **2.811** | **32.25** |
| CVVHDF Stopped P2G | 1500 | 53.5 | 68.3 | 16.1 | 25.18 | 0.028 | 0.668 | 24.26 |
| P3A | 1500 | 24 | 44.9 | 2.8 | 5.74 | 0.121 | 3.911 | 32.42 |
| P3B | 1500 | 24 | 42.4 | 1.9 | 5.13 | 0.135 | 4.923 | 36.46 |
| P3C | 1500 | 24 | 46.5 | 2.1 | 5.26 | 0.132 | 4.278 | 32.46 |
| **Mean** | | | | | **5.38** | **0.129** | **4.371** | **33.78** |
| P4A | 600 | 12 | 16.2 | 4 | 5.45 | 0.127 | 4.563 | 35.88 |
| P4B | 600 | 12 | 23.4 | 5 | 5.16 | 0.134 | 3.961 | 29.52 |
| **Mean** | | | | | **5.31** | **0.131** | **4.262** | **32.70** |
| P5A | 1500 | 24 | 48.2 | 2.1 | 5.09 | 0.136 | 4.099 | 30.08 |
| P5B | 1500 | 25 | 52.4 | 2.4 | 5.39 | 0.128 | 3.701 | 28.81 |
| P5C | 1500 | 28 | 54.4 | 2.5 | 5.29 | 0.131 | 3.649 | 27.84 |
| P5D | 1500 | 28 | 55.8 | 2.5 | 6.03 | 0.115 | 3.137 | 27.28 |
| **Mean** | | | | | **5.45** | **0.128** | **3.646** | **28.50** |
| **Overall mean\*** | | | | | **6.74** | **0.109** | **3.39** | **31.4** |
| **Standard deviation** | | | | | **1.69** | **0.025** | **0.82** | **3.27** |
| **Median** | | | | | **5.88** | **0.118** | **3.39** | **30.4** |

\* Excluding profile P2G.
Cpmax: maximum serum concentration Cpmin: minimum serum concentration.
$t_{1/2}$: half life. $V_d$: volume of distribution. TBC: Total body clearance. k: elimination rate constant.
PX (1–5): patients 1–5. PXA-PXE: first (A) to fifth (E) dosing interval during which serum concentration data was collected for patient PX.

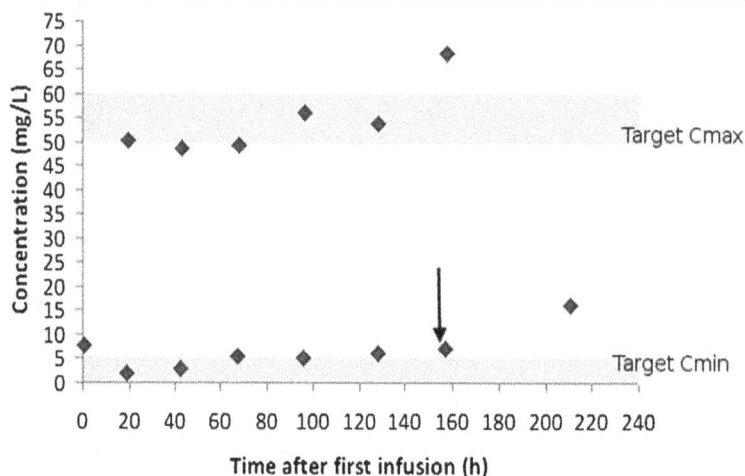

**Figure 2 Amikacin serum concentration-time data for Patient P2.** The arrow indicates the point at which CVVHDF was ceased. The shaded areas indicate the target therapeutic peak and trough ranges.

As mentioned in the methods section, this study straddled the period of transition from multiple daily dosing to extended interval dosing of aminoglycosides. In the case of patient 4, Acetinobacter baumanni was isolated from sputum samples and amikacin therapy was initiated. Instead of administering a high dose at extended interval, 600mg amikacin was administered twice daily. The $C_{pmax}$ concentration achieved by the 600 mg dose was 16.2 mg/L and the $C_{pmin}$ concentration was 4 mg $l^{-1}$, which is above the recommended trough level. If the patient had continued on amikacin following the second dose, an extended interval should have been considered due to the decrease in clearance and higher than recommended trough values.

For patient 5, a dosing schedule of 1500 mg once daily achieved effective $C_{pmax}$ concentrations, based on a target $C_{pmax}$/MIC ratio of 10. The MIC for the sensitive microorganism was 5ug $ml^{-1}$ amikacin. For profiles C and D, the dosage interval was extended somewhat to avoid excessively high $C_{pmin}$ concentrations. Serum concentration-time data for this patient, illustrating the dosing regime accomplishing target concentrations, is depicted in Figure 3.

The estimates of pharmacokinetic parameters from the 1-compartment model, obtained from the multiple amikacin serum concentration versus time data, can also be compared with pharmacokinetic parameters estimates (TBC, $V_d$, k) obtained from typical TDM data (Sawchuk and Zaske method) from the same patient profiles. It is clear that values calculated using both methods for each patient are similar (Tables 2 and 4). The data from this study therefore supports the usefulness of the Sawchuk and Zaske method to obtain appropriate amikacin PK parameters for patients on CVVHDF. These parameters are suitable for dosage regimen calculation/adjustment,

thereby supporting a practical approach of individualising amikacin dosing based on routinely available troughs and peaks in patients on CVVHDF.

### Amikacin Clearance due to CVVHDF

Details of amikacin and creatinine clearances obtained during CVVHDF, together with the CVVHDF conditions employed are given in Table 5. The mean clearance of amikacin by CVVHDF was 2.86 +/− 0.41 l $h^{-1}$, ~89% of the mean total body clearance for these patient profiles. The sieving coefficient for amikacin was 0.83 +/− 0.05, which was consistent with that previously reported in the literature (0.93 +/− 0.16), although different filters and CRRT conditions were in use [13]. The observed sieving coefficient was similar to the unbound fraction of amikacin, assuming a fraction unbound of 0.8 based on the fact that 20% or less of amikacin is bound to

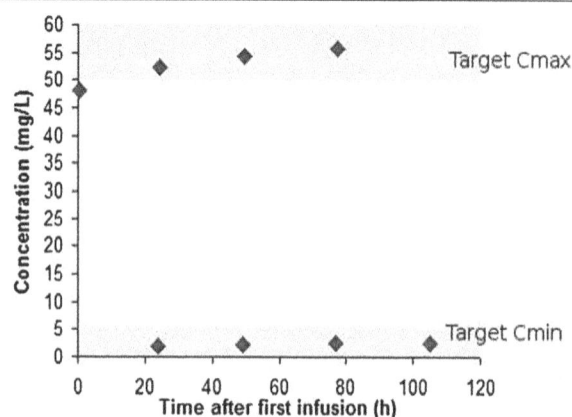

**Figure 3 Amikacin serum concentration time data for Patient P5.** The shaded areas indicate the target therapeutic peak and trough ranges.

**Table 5 Clearance of amikacin and creatinine by CVVHDF and summary of CVVHDF conditions**

| Patient profile | $Cl_{CVVHDF}$ (l h$^{-1}$) | $F_{CVVHDF}$ | CrCl (l h$^{-1}$) | Actual effluent flow rate (l h$^{-1}$) | Number. of filters ^ | Age of filter* (h) |
|---|---|---|---|---|---|---|
| P1C | 2.53 | 0.98 | 2.19 | 3.16 | 1 | 16 |
| P2D | 2.55 | 0.94 | 2.70 | 2.91 | 1 | 27 |
| P3A | 3.40 | 0.87 | 3.20 | 4.10 | 1 | 1 |
| P5B | 2.97 | 0.80 | 2.86 | 3.95 | 1 | 26 |
| **Mean** | **2.86** | **0.90** | **2.74** | **3.53** | **1** | - |
| +/- | +/- | +/- | +/- | +/- | | |
| **s.d.** | **0.412** | **0.08** | **0.42** | **0.584** | | |

*At start of dosage interval.
^ During dosage interval.
PX (1–5) patients 1–5. $Cl_{CVVHDF}$: clearance via CVVHDF $F_{CVVHDF}$: Fraction of total body clearance via CVVHDF. CrCl: Creatinine clearance.

serum protein [3]. The amikacin clearance due to CVVHDF estimated using the sieving coefficient, 2.93 l h$^{-1}$, was similar to the actual measured clearance (2.86 l h$^{-1}$). Creatinine clearance (2.74 +/– 0.42 l h$^{-1}$) by the filter was similar to amikacin clearance. The sieving coefficient for creatinine was 0.80 +/– 0.1. This value was very close to the sieving coefficient for amikacin, but was slightly lower and more variable.

## Discussion

CVVHDF was observed to increase amikacin clearance, with a mean TBC value of 3.39 l h$^{-1}$. The results demonstrate that CVVHDF is capable of significant amikacin clearance, accounting for most of the measured TBC in all patients. As such, the CVVHDF status of a patient, i. e. whether CVVHDF is commenced, temporarily interrupted or discontinued, is of primary importance when estimating the dose regimen.

The mean half-life during CVVHDF therapy was 6.74 hours, and the median half-life estimate of 5.88 h comparing well with that of 6.5 h reported by Taccone et al. [17] Additionally, the mean elimination rate constant was 0.109 h$^{-1}$ indicating that elimination is ~ one third that observed in subjects with normal renal function. In patients with normal renal function, the half-life is 2–3 hours but in anephric patients, the half-life increases to 30–60 hours [4]. A wide range of values for the $V_d$ of aminoglycosides (0.1 to 0.5 l kg$^{-1}$ ~ 7–35 l)) has been reported and the observed mean value from the current study (31.4 +/– 3.27 l) lies at the higher end of this range (based on Ideal Body Weight (IBW)). Assuming a 70 kg patient weight, this corresponds to a value of 0.45 l kg$^{-1}$, which is comparable to the estimate of $V_{ss}$ of 0.5 l kg$^{-1}$ determined by Taccone et al. [17]. Interestingly, the value for $V_1$ reported in that study was lower (median 0.29 l kg$^{-1}$) than estimated in the current work; however it ranged from 0.21-0.62 l kg.

A large volume of distribution in critically ill patients is not unexpected as sepsis [10], total parenteral

nutrition and factors associated with critical illness such as aggressive fluid therapy and hypoalbuminemia have been associated with an increased volume of distribution for aminoglycoside antibiotics [25]. As a result of this increased volume of distribution and the fact that aminoglycosides demonstrate concentration dependent killing, higher loading doses may be required to obtain clinically relevant peak concentration values, as is occurring in practice [17].

'Once-daily' aminoglycoside dosing is more correctly described as extended-interval dosing and extension of the dosage far beyond 24 hours will be required in some patients with renal dysfunction. The importance of acknowledging this concept, rather than attempting to maintain a rigid 'once-daily' dosage interval, is illustrated in the cases of patients 1 and 2. In the treatment of the first patient, where strict 'once-daily' dosing was applied, lower doses at 24-hour intervals failed to achieve target peak concentrations. The high $V_d$ combined with a lower dose in patient 1 contributed to the peak concentration failing to reach the recommended target value. The risk of accumulation following higher doses to achieve appropriate peak concentrations has also been highlighted by Taccone et al. [17], and evidence is provided in the current work to support this concern, where accumulation was evident in patients 1 and 2. However, in contrast to patient 1, in the case of patient 2, use of the recommended dose and extension of the dosage interval beyond 24 hours, allowed target peak serum concentrations to be achieved, while limiting accumulation. Estimates of amikacin pharmacokinetic parameters were similar for both patients and the dosage recommendation for patient 2 was 1500 mg every 32 hours. It is imperative that clinicians be aware of the significant impact of CVVHDF on amikacin clearance and thus the effect of stopping, interrupting or changing dialysis modality on amikacin serum concentrations. The observed effect of stopping CVVHDF was evident in patient 2 (Figure 2).

This study supports the approach of using routinely measured (both peak and trough) amikacin serum levels in estimating pharmacokinetic parameters and thus guiding dosage regimens. For each patient the values of the pharmacokinetic parameters calculated from peak and trough data were similar to those calculated from multiple serum concentration data within a dosing interval fitted to a 1-compartment model. As obtaining multiple serum concentrations within a dosing interval would not be practical in the routine clinical setting, a standard TDM approach of using peak and trough data only is shown to be suitable for obtaining ongoing meaningful individual pharmacokinetic data. Use of regularly obtained peak and trough data to assess individual pharmacokinetic parameters is likely to be particularly valuable in the context of critically ill patients receiving CRRT. This is due to the complex interaction between the patient, drug factors and CRRT factors in influencing drug pharmacokinetics.

Careful consideration should be given to the importance of the timing of the peak and trough sampling. Although several of the profiles in the current work had no discernible distribution phase, the peak sample should be taken approximately 30 minutes after the end of the infusion [4]. It has been suggested that in some cases a longer distribution phase may be present [4]. In any case, consideration should always be given to the timing of the peak sample data used to generate the target peak range used. Furthermore, trough samples should be taken 2–4 half lives after the peak sample [4]. In addition, caution must be applied in the interpretation of drug serum levels when interruptions in CVVHDF therapy have occurred, for example due to filter clotting or medical interventions.

It has been suggested that the reduced amikacin half life observed in the study by Robert et al. [12], of patients receiving CVVH, compared to that reported by Armendariz et al. [13] arose because of the higher haemofiltration rate contributing to the higher observed clearance of amikacin. Furthermore, the longer observed half life during CVVH compared with CVVHDF is consistent with an increased dialysis efficiency from CVVHDF in comparison with CVVH [15]. Therefore it would be anticipated that shorter half lives would be observed in patients undergoing CVVHDF in comparison with those observed in patients undergoing CVVH, as demonstrated by the current study. These differences in observed half lives underline the relevance of continuous renal replacement therapy mode employed and conditions used (e.g. flow rate) when considering potential for drug clearance during dialysis. In addition to the study by Taccone et al. [17], at present, the authors are aware of only one other prospective analysis of amikacin pharmacokinetics in patients undergoing CVVHDF. That study reported a mean half life of 11.3 h (+/− 1.5) [16] which is longer than that determined in the current study. This is likely explained by higher blood flow

rates (100 ml min$^{-1}$ vs. 200 ml min$^{-1}$ in the current study), dialysate flow rates and pre-dilution replacement flow rates (1 l h$^{-1}$ vs lh$^{-1}$ to 2 lh$^{-1}$ in the current study). Although both the current study and that by Moon et al. [16] found evidence of significant amikacin clearance via CVVHDF, the differences in calculated pharmacokinetic parameters further illustrate the effect of CVVHDF conditions employed on amikacin clearance. On the other hand, no correlation was found by Taccone et al. between CVVHDF conditions employed and calculated clearance or trough levels within the range of conditions employed. The observed clearance values [17] were thought to be affected by residual renal function and/or potential filter absorbance. Due to this lack of clarity, a more comprehensive study of CVVHDF parameters employed and amikacin levels is warranted to ascertain the effect of CVVHDF conditions employed on amikacin clearance.

It has been recommended recently that more aggressive dosing practices need to be employed for patients undergoing dialysis who are treated with aminoglycosides, as poorer outcomes were observed retrospectively among dialysis patients receiving aminoglycosides, with one of the risk factors for mortality being lower peak concentrations relative to MIC [26]. Recently CVVHDF was employed to enable use of high amikacin doses to achieve appropriate peak levels while avoiding nephrotoxicity [19]. This approach should contribute to prevention of treatment failure and minimisation of the emergence of resistance. This illustrates that there is a growing acceptance of both the high peak levels of aminoglycosides required in many cases along with the potential for significant clearance via CVVHDF. However, to date data have been lacking to support initial dosage regimen estimates and the expected range of individual pharmacokinetic parameters for amikacin in critically ill patients on CVVHDF.

### Limitations of the current study

The limited patient number (5) in this study, together with their heterogeneity, limits in-depth statistical analysis of the data. The results are presented as the ranges and absolute values which might be expected from 5 critically ill patients undergoing CVVHDF.

### Conclusions

CVVHDF contributes significantly to total clearance of amikacin. The use of pharmacokinetic parameter estimates obtained from two appropriately timed steady state serum-drug concentrations (peak and trough) can be used to guide individualised dosing of critically ill patients treated with CVVHDF. This is considered a useful monitoring strategy particularly in avoiding the risk of underdosing. The potential for underdosing coupled with the notable decrease in clearance when

CVVHDF is discontinued indicates that individualised dosing of patients treated with CVVHDF using estimates of pharmacokinetic parameters is required.

## Abbreviations

Cl: Clearance; $C_{pmax}$: Maximum plasma concentration; $C_{pmin}$: Minimum plasma concentration; CrCl: Creatinine clearance; CV%: Coefficient of variation; CVVH: Continuous venovenous haemofiltration; CVVHDF: Continuous veno-venous haemodiafiltration; ESBL: Extended spectrum beta lactamases; $F_{CVVHDF}$: Cl via CVVHDF as fraction of TBC; ICU: Intensive care unit; k: Elimination rate constant; MIC: Minimum inhibitory concentration; T: Duration of infusion; $t_{1/2}$: Half life; TBC: Total body clearance; TDM: Therapeutic drug monitoring; $V_1$: Volume of central compartment; $V_2$: Volume of peripheral compartment; $V_d$: Volume of distribution; Vss: Volume of distribution at steady state.

## Competing interests

The authors declare that they have no competing interests.

## Authors' contributions

OC, CG, and MD initiated and supervised the study from its inception. EC co-ordinated sample and consent acquisition. DD completed the pharmacokinetic analysis and modelling. OC authored the first draft, with review and additions by DD, MD and CG. OC, CG, MD, EC and DD read and approved the final manuscript.

## Acknowledgements

The authors acknowledge the tireless commitment of the ICU nursing staff to data collection, ongoing research and patient care.

## Author details

[1]Intensive Care Medicine, Tallaght Hospital, Dublin 24, Ireland. [2]School of Pharmacy and Pharmaceutical Sciences, Trinity College Dublin, Dublin 2, Ireland. [3]Pharmacy Department, Tallaght Hospital, Dublin 24, Ireland.

## References

1. Leone M, Martin C: **Antibiotics in the ICU.** In *25 years of progress and innovation in intensive care medicine*. Edited by Kuhlen R, Moreno R, Ranierie M, Rhodes A. Berlin: Medizinisch Wissenschaftliche Verlagsgesellschaft; 2007.
2. Kelly CP, LaMont T: *Antibiotic-associated diarrhea caused by Clostridium difficile (Beyond the basics)*.; www.uptodate.com Accessed 20/04/2012.
3. Bristol-Myers Squibb HL: *Amikacin Injection 100mg/2ml Summary of Product Characteristics*. Dublin: Irish Pharmaceutical Healthcare Association - medicines information online; 2012.
4. Winters M: *Basic Clinical Pharmacokinetics*. 5th edition. New York: Lippincott Williams and Wilkins; 2010.
5. Moore R, Smith C, Lietman P: **Association of aminoglycoside plasma levels with therapeutic outcome in gram-negative pneumonia.** *Am J Med* 1984, **77**:657–662.
6. Moore R, Lietman P, Smith C: **Clinical Response to aminoglycoside therapy: importance of the ratio of peak concentration to minimal inhibitory concentration.** *J Infect Dis* 1987, **155**(1):93–99.
7. Roberts J, Kruger P, Paterson D, Lipman J: **Antibiotic resistance- What's dosing got to do with it?** *Crit Care Med* 2008, **36**(8):2433–2440.
8. Barletta J, Johnson S, Nix D, Nix L, Erstad B: **Population pharmacokinetics in critically ill trauma patients on once-daily regimens.** *J Trauma* 2000, **49**(5):869–872.
9. Zaske D, Strate R, Kohls P: **Amikacin pharmacokinetics: wide interpatient variation in 98 patients.** *J Clin Pharmacol* 1991, **31**(2):158–163.
10. Lugo G, Castaneda-Hernandez G: **Relationship between hemodynamic and vital support measures and pharmacokinetic variability of amikacin in critically ill patients with sepsis.** *Crit Care Med* 1997, **255**:806–811.
11. Udy A, Roberts J, Lipman J: **Implications of augmented renal clearance in critically ill patients.** *Nat Rev Nephrol* 2011, **7**(9):539–543.
12. Robert R, Rochard E, Malin F, Bouquet S: **Amikacin pharmacokinetics during continuous veno-venous hemofiltration.** *Crit Care Med* 1991, **19**(4):588–589.
13. Armendariz E, Chelluri L, Ptachcinski R: **Pharmacokinetics of amikacin during continuous venovenous hemofiltration.** *Crit Care Med* 1990, **18**(6):675–676.
14. Akers K, Cota J, Frei C, Chung K, Mende K, Murray C: **Once-daily amikacin dosing in burns patients treated with continuous venovenous hemofiltration.** *Antimicrob Agents Chemother* 2011, **55**(10):4639–4642.
15. Pea F, Pierluigi V, Pavan F, Furlanut M: **Pharmacokinetic considerations for Antimicrobial Therapy in Patients Receiving Renal Replacement Therapy.** *Clin Pharmacokinet* 2007, **46**(12):997–1038.
16. Moon S-Y, Oh K-H, Oh Y, Curie A, Joo K, Kim Y, Han J, Kim S, Lee J, Kim J-R, et al: **Removal of amikacin in patients undergoing continuous veno-venous hemodiafiltration.** *The Korean J Nephrology* 2006, **25**(4):595–601.
17. Taccone FS, de Backer D, Laterre P-F, Spapen H, Dugernier T, Delattre I, Wallemacq P, Vincent J-L, Jacobs F: **Pharmacokinetics of a loading dose of amikacin in septic patients undergoing continuous renal replacement therapy.** *Int J Antimicrob Agents* 2011, **37**(6):531–535.
18. Kinowski J, Coussaye JD, Bressole F, Fabre D, Saissi G, Bouvet O, Galtier M, Eledjam J: **Muliple-dose pharmacokinetics of amikacin and ceftaizidime in critically ill patients with septic multiple-organ failure during intermittent haemofiltration.** *Antimicrob Agents Chemother* 1993, **37**(3):464–473.
19. Layeux B, Taccone F, Fagnoul D, Vincent J-L, Jacobs F: **Amikacin monotherapy for sepsis caused by panresistant Pseudomonas aeruginosa.** *Antimicrob Agents Chemother* 2010, **54**:4939–4941.
20. Jelliffe R, Jelliffe S: **A computer program for estimation of creatinine clearance from unstable serum creatinine levels, age, sex and weight.** *Math Biosci* 1972, **14**(1–2):17–24.
21. Bressolle F, Gouby A, Martinez J-M, Joubert P, Saissi G, Guillaud R, Goment R: **Population pharmacokinetics of amikacin in critically ill patients.** *Antimicrob Agents Chemother* 1996, **40**(7):1682–1689.
22. Marik P, Lipman J, Kobilski S, Scribante J: **A prospective randomized study comparing once- versus twice-daily amikacin dosing in critically ill adult and paediatric patients.** *J Antimicrob Chemother* 1991, **28**:753–764.
23. Gabrielsson J, Weiner D: *Pharmacokinetic and pharmacodynamic data analysis:concepts and applications*. 4th edition. Stockholm: Swedish Pharmaceutical Press; 2000.
24. Sawchuk R, Zaske D: **Pharmacokinetics of dosage regimens which utilize multiple intravenous infusions: gentamicin in burn patients.** *J Pharmackinet Biopharm* 1976, **4**(2):183–195.
25. Ronchera-Oms C, Tormo C, Ordovas J, Abad J, Jimenez N: **Expanded gentamicin volume of distribution in critically ill adult patients receiving total parenteral nutrition.** *J Clin Pharm Ther* 1995, **20**(5):253–258.
26. Heintz B, Matzke G, Dager W: **Antimicrobial dosing concepts and reccomendations for critically ill adult patients receiving continuous renal replacement therapy or intermittent hemodialysis.** *Pharmacotherapy* 2009, **29**(5):662–577.

# 18

# Cognitive functioning in opioid-dependent patients treated with buprenorphine, methadone, and other psychoactive medications: stability and correlates

Pekka Rapeli[1,2,3*], Carola Fabritius[2], Hely Kalska[3] and Hannu Alho[2,4]

## Abstract

**Background:** In many but not in all neuropsychological studies buprenorphine-treated opioid-dependent patients have shown fewer cognitive deficits than patients treated with methadone. In order to examine if hypothesized cognitive advantage of buprenorphine in relation to methadone is seen in clinical patients we did a neuropsychological follow-up study in unselected sample of buprenorphine- vs. methadone-treated patients.

**Methods:** In part I of the study fourteen buprenorphine-treated and 12 methadone-treated patients were tested by cognitive tests within two months (T1), 6-9 months (T2), and 12 - 17 months (T3) from the start of opioid substitution treatment. Fourteen healthy controls were examined at similar intervals. Benzodiazepine and other psychoactive comedications were common among the patients. Test results were analyzed with repeated measures analysis of variance and planned contrasts. In part II of the study the patient sample was extended to include 36 patients at T2 and T3. Correlations between cognitive functioning and medication, substance abuse, or demographic variables were then analyzed.

**Results:** In part I methadone patients were inferior to healthy controls tests in all tests measuring attention, working memory, or verbal memory. Buprenorphine patients were inferior to healthy controls in the first working memory task, the Paced Auditory Serial Addition Task and verbal memory. In the second working memory task, the Letter-Number Sequencing, their performance improved between T2 and T3. In part II only group membership (buprenorphine vs. methadone) correlated significantly with attention performance and improvement in the Letter-Number Sequencing. High frequency of substance abuse in the past month was associated with poor performance in the Letter-Number Sequencing.

**Conclusions:** The results underline the differences between non-randomized and randomized studies comparing cognitive performance in opioid substitution treated patients (fewer deficits in buprenorphine patients vs. no difference between buprenorphine and methadone patients, respectively). Possible reasons for this are discussed.

## Background

Opioid agonists buprenorphine and methadone prevent opioid withdrawal symptoms and reduce craving for opioids [1,2]. Both drugs are used in opioid substitution treatment (OST), also known as opioid maintenance treatment. OST has proven effective in reducing illicit drug use, somatic diseases, mortality, and social or mental health problems in opioid-dependent patients [3,4]. Cognitive effects of OST drugs have been examined in clinical and experimental studies, but the results have been mixed. Studies comparing OST patients against healthy controls have, in general, shown cognitive impairment among patients [5-8]. Yet, it has not been proven that the impairment would be specifically related to opioid substitution drugs [5,9,10]. In non-randomized studies, however, buprenorphine-treated

* Correspondence: pekka.rapeli@hus.fi
[1]Department of Psychiatry. Helsinki University Central Hospital, Finland
Full list of author information is available at the end of the article

opioid-dependent patients have performed better than methadone patients in several cognitive tests [7,11-13].

It is important to know if the possible cognitive differences between unselected buprenorphine vs. methadone patients are stabile during the treatment and what are the correlates of cognitive performance. Therefore, we compared cognitive performance of buprenorphine and methadone patients against healthy controls thrice (T1 - T3) during the first year in the OST by (part I of the study). In part II we analyzed correlates of cognitive performance in patients after six (T2) and twelve (T3) months in treatment by using extended patient pool. The present study is an extension to our previous studies [7,14].

### Part I: Stability

Opioid and dopamine systems in the brain have important interactions, and current opioid drug use may negatively affect cognitive functioning, especially working memory [15-17]. However, Pirastu et al. have presented evidence that buprenorphine as being a partial mu opioid agonist and kappa opioid receptor antagonist may improve cognitive performance after long-term opioid abuse. According to them methadone as being a full mu opioid agonist may lack properties for supporting normal cognitive function [18]. Also, there is evidence that adverse interactive effects benzodiazepines (BZD) and opioid substitution drugs on cognitive performance are greater for methadone than buprenorphine [19,20]. Therefore, we hypothesized that patients treated with buprenorphine combined in most cases with BZD and other comedications would show greater cognitive improvement in long-term treatment in comparison to methadone-treated ones.

### Part II: correlates

In the part II of the study the patient sample was extended to include additional patients examined at all test points, but whose data were excluded at T1. After this, data from 36 patients could be analyzed at T2 and T3. We hypothesized that there would be negative correlations between medication variables (opioid agonist dose, BZD dose, and the number of psychoactive drugs) and cognitive performance in opioid-dependent patients treated either with buprenorphine or methadone. In addition, we hypothesized that those with the highest opioid dose would have higher BZD doses, because BZDs have been associated with craving for higher opioid dose [21]. The negative effects of methadone and buprenorphine on cognition are dose-dependent in healthy volunteers, although little is known about the development of tolerance [22,23]. It is known that BZDs have negative effects on memory performance in opioid substitution treated patients, and these effects are

stronger for methadone than for buprenorphine [24]. Little is known about possible effects of polypharmacy on cognition in opioid-agonist treated patients. However, in other patient populations, those patients treated with several drugs perform worse in cognitive tests than patients treated with single drug [25-27].

Negative correlations were also hypothesized between cognitive performance and frequency of substance abuse in the past month, benzodiazepine dosage, the number of other psychoactive drugs, early onset of substance abuse, early-onset mental health or behavioral problems, opioid-related overdoses, and duration of lifetime alcohol abuse. In our sample recent alcohol and/or cannabis abuse were common, and these negatively affect cognitive function [28-31]. Early onset substance abuse and childhood mental health or behavioral problems have been associated with poor adult cognitive functioning among individuals with substance abuse problems [32-35]. High number of opioid-related overdoses, lifetime alcohol abuse, and low level of education have all been associated with poor cognitive performance among opioid-dependent patients [5,36,37]. Verbal intelligence (IQ) and years of education were hypothesized to correlate positively with memory performance.

### Methods

All participants included in the study were between 18 - 50 years of age and participated voluntarily. Inclusion criteria for patients were opioid dependence and BZD dependence or abuse according to Diagnostic and Statistical Manual of Mental Disorders (DSM-IV), treatment of opioid dependence with methadone, buprenorphine, or buprenorphine/naloxone. We excluded participants with uncontrolled polysubstance abuse, acute alcohol abuse, or acute axis I psychiatric morbidity according to DSM-IV other than substance abuse disorders. Full description of our inclusion and exclusion criteria is given in our previous report [7].

In order to screen for substance abuse an urine sample was collected from each patient on each day of testing and at least once in the preceding week. Each healthy control participant was screened for substance abuse once during the study period. In addition, we interviewed all participants about their past month and lifetime substance use by using the European Addiction Severity Index as a basis for further inquiry [38]. If any indication of intoxication was observed, we excluded them. Breath alcohol testing was used when considered necessary. Participants who had used within 24 h alcohol more than four/five drinks (females/males, respectively) or significant as-needed benzodiazepine dose (5 mg or more as diazepam equivalent dose) were excluded as well. The study protocol was accepted by the Ethics Committee of Helsinki University Central Hospital. We obtained a written informed consent according to the Declaration of Helsinki from all participants, and paid them € 60 if they attended all study visits.

## Part I participants

Participants who were eligible for T1-T3 follow-up (sample I) represent 42% (14/35) of the all buprenorphine patients tested at T1, 55% (12/22) of the methadone patients and 78% (14/18) of the healthy controls, respectively. To test whether the follow-up completers of either group were significantly different from the non-completers of that group, we compared these groups by independent samples $t$-tests, chi-square tests, or Mann-Whitney $U$-tests ($p$-value = 0.05). No statistically significant differences emerged in demographic, medication or cognitive variables. Because there were few follow-up non-completers (n = 4) among the potential healthy controls, these comparisons were not made in healthy controls.

When the groups were compared on demographic variables with analysis of variance (ANOVA) or chi-square-test (Table 1) there were no statistically significant differences in age, sex, or estimated premorbid intelligence. Healthy controls had completed more years in education than either one of the patient groups. Because BZD use on prescription was very common, their doses were converted to diazepam equivalent doses according to the conversion tables given by Nelson and Chouinard [39]. Temazepam doses were halved in order to account for their use as hypnotics on the night before testing. Substance abuse in the past month was estimated as frequency of use. Because accurate number of the days of abuse was hard to obtain we dichotomized the frequency of the past month substance abuse into two categories. The first category was labeled as low to moderate use, and it included abstinence or substance abuse up to two days a week. The second category was labeled as high frequency group and included all the participants with substance use of three days a week or more. This classification was based on the findings showing that mean three days of substance use a week is one of the threshold values for getting into serious substance abuse problems [40,41]. In the buprenorphine group, 79% of the patients were given buprenorphine/ naloxone at all test points. Thus, they were also given sublingual naloxone in the ratio 1:4 combined with their buprenorphine dose. When the tablet is taken sublingually the absorption of naloxone is low and eliminates within first hours [42]. It has been concluded that naloxone has minimal, if any effect, on the bioavailability or pharmacokinetics of buprenorphine [43,44]. Also, buprenorphine and buprenorphine/naloxone have similar physiological effects [43]. On the basis of these findings, we combined patients using either one of the buprenorphine compounds. Table 2 shows medication

characteristics of the sample I within the last 24 h before testing. Both patient groups used more psychoactive medications than healthy controls.

## Part II participants

Sample II (n = 36) included 51% of all the buprenorphine-treated and 59% of methadone-treated patients who entered the follow-up at T1. The methadone group included also five patients who were tested without opioid medication at T1, but who then started methadone treatment within few days after the testing. Thus, all patients were tested after minimum 6 (T2) and 12 months (T3) of OST. They had been tested at start of their treatment, but were excluded from the part I sample. Substance abuse history variables included in the analyses were onset ages of any substance and opioid abuse, years of heavy alcohol use, and the number of self-reported opioid-related overdoses. Whenever possible, the data was checked using medical reports. It turned out that no reliable information about the number of opioid-related overdoses could be obtained. Therefore this variable was excluded from the analyses. Current substance abuse variables were frequency of substance abuse in the past month (low vs. high) and drug screen result (positive vs. negative). Medication drug use variables that were examined included opioid substitution drug (buprenorphine vs. methadone), benzodiazepine dose (diazepam equivalent), and the number of other psychoactive drugs other than opioid substitution drug. Demographic variables included in the analyses were age, sex, years of education, early neurobehavioral problems, and verbal IQ. Data about childhood mental health or behavioral problems was gathered using the Childhood Behavioral Checklist as a basis for interview, and medical reports were used, whenever possible [45]. Those participants who had had treatment or referral to special services due to mental health or behavioral problems before the onset of substance abuse were rated as early-onset neurobehavioral problem group (31%). If significant change was seen in cognitive performance then change (T3 - T2) in that that variable, as well in medication, and substance use changes were analyzed. Medication and substance abuse change variables were made more reliable by dichotomizing the data. Change in opioid drug dose between T2 and T3 was dichotomized as steady or reduced dose group (58%) or higher dose group (42%). Change in BZD dose between T2 and T2 was grouped respectively. The majority of the patients belonged to steady or reduced BZD dose group (83%), and the rest (17%) had higher BZD dose at T3. All those who reduced their frequency of substance abuse as indicated by the shift from the high frequency group to low to moderate frequency group were put into group of reduced substance abuse.

**Table 1 Group demographics in sample I**

| | Buprenorphine (n = 14) | Methadone (n = 12) | Healthy control (n = 14) | Group comparison p-values |
|---|---|---|---|---|
| Age (M ± SD) | 30 ± 7 | 31 ± 8 | 29 ± 10 | ns |
| Sex (female/male) | 36%/64% | 50%/50% | 50%/50% | ns |
| Intelligence[a] (M ± SD) | 101 ± 11 | 98 ± 9 | 105 ± 8 | ns |
| Education, years | 10 ± 2 | 10 ± 1 | 13 ± 1 | BN & M < HC *** |
| Main opioid of abuse used within last month at T1 (%) | | | | |
|     Buprenorphine | 93% | 83%? | - | ns[b] |
|     Heroin | 7% | 17% | - | ns[b] |
| Days in opioid substitution treatment at test (M ± SD) | | | | |
|     T1 | 21 ± 15 | 20 ± 14 | - | ns[b] |
|     T2 | 210 ± 20 | 200 ± 28 | - | ns[b] |
|     T3 | 414 ± 46 | 405 ± 31 | - | ns[b] |
| Examined in inpatient settings % | | | | |
|     T1 | 21% | 25% | - | ns[b] |
|     T2 | 7% | 0% | - | ns[b] |
|     T3 | 7% | 8% | - | ns[b] |
| Participants with high frequency of use of any substance of abuse [c] % | | | | |
|     T1 | 86% | 67% | 14% | BN > HC ***; M > HC * |
|     T2 | 29% | 42% | 7% | ns ; ns |
|     T3 | 36% | 33% | 7% | ns ; ns |
| | T2 < T1** | T3 < T1* | | |
| | T3 < T1* | | | |
| Participants with the past month extra doses of any opioid [d], % | | | | |
|     T1 | 86% | 92% | - | ns[b] |
|     T2 | 29% | 33% | - | ns[b] |
|     T3 | 36% | 33% | - | ns[b] |
| | T2 < T1** | T2 < T1** | | |
| | T3 < T1* | T3 < T1** | | |
| Participants with the past month nicotine use (daily) | | | | |
|     T1 | 100% | 100% | 36% | BN & M > HC *** |
|     T2 | 100% | 100% | 36% | BN & M > HC *** |
|     T3 | 100% | 93% | 29% | BN > HC **; M > HC *** |

Note. BN = buprenorphine patients, HC = healthy control group, and M = methadone patients.

[a] Estimation based on the vocabulary and picture completion subtests of the Wechsler Adult Intelligence Scale - Revised (WAIS-R) [67].

[b] Tested only between patient groups.

[c] High frequency = three or more days a week. Alcohol use was taken into account if it was at least mean weekly 16 portions (12 g) for females and 24 portions for males or binge drinking occurred on any day.

[d] Extra doses of any non-prescribed opioid use during the recent month seen in drugs screens or admitted by the patients.

> = superior than, *** = statistically significant at level $p < 0.001$. ** = statistically significant at level $p < 0.01$. * = statistically significant at level $p < 0.05$.

This group included also the patients who belonged to the low to moderate frequency group at both time points, totaling 58% of the patients. The rest were put into group of non-reduced substance abuse (42%). Change in the number of psychoactive drugs was dichotomized similarly. All those with less psychoactive drugs at T3 in comparison to T2 or no other psychoactive prescribed drugs than opioid drug at both time points were put in the group of reduced use of psychoactive drugs (42%). The rest were put into group of non-reduced use of psychoactive drugs (58%). Table 3 presents the demographic characteristics of the sample II. In the buprenorphine group, 78% of the patients were given buprenorphine/naloxone at all test points. Table 4 shows other medication characteristics of the sample II within the last 24 h before testing.

## Procedure

Cognitive tests were administered between three to six hours after opioid substitution drug had been given.

**Table 2 Medications given to participants within the last 24 h before testing in sample I**

| | Buprenorphine (n = 14) | Methadone (n = 12) | Healthy control (n = 14) | Group or time point comparison p-values |
|---|---|---|---|---|
| Opioid agonist drug, dose | | | | |
| Buprenorphine (M ± SD; (range) ) | | | | |
| T1 | 16 ± 3 mg (12 - 24 mg) | - | - | - |
| T2 | 20 ± 5 mg (14 - 28 mg) | - | - | T2 > T1** |
| T3 | 21 ± 6 mg (6 - 28 mg) | - | - | T3 > T1** |
| Methadone (M ± SD;(range) ) | | | | |
| T1 | - | 71 ± 39 mg (30 - 135 mg) | - | - |
| T2 | - | 127 ± 36 mg (80 - 180 mg) | - | T2 > T1 *** |
| T3 | - | 135 ± 34 mg (75 - 180 mg) | - | T3 > T1 *** |
| Participants treated with BZD medication | | | ' | |
| T1 | 79% | 100% | 0% | BN & M > HC *** |
| BZD dose at T1 (M ± SD) | 20 ± 17 mg | 21 ± 11 mg | - | ns [a] |
| T2 | 71% | 100% | 0% | BN & M > HC *** |
| BZD dose at T2 (M ± SD) | 16 ± 11 mg | 22 ± 11 mg | - | ns [a] |
| T3 | 64% | 100% | 0% | BN & M > HC *** |
| BZD dose at T3 (M ± SD) | 13 ± 12 mg | 22 ± 9. mg | - | BN < M * |
| Number of other medications with possible cognitive effects [b] (M ± SD (range)) | | | | |
| T1 | 1.9 ± 1.1 (0 - 4) | 3.0 ± 1.3 (0 - 5) | 0.2 ± 0.4 (0 - 1) | BN & M > HC ***; M > BN * |
| T2 | 1.9 ± 1.2 (0 - 3) | 2.3 ± 0.8 (1 - 4) | 0.2 ± 0.4 (0 -1) | BN & M > HC *** |
| T3 | 1.8 ± 1.3 (0 -4) | 2.2 ± 1.0 (1 -4) | 0.2 ± 0.4 (0 -1) | BN & M > HC *** |

[a] Tested only between patient groups.

[b] These included antidepressants, neuroleptics (used with anxiolytic indications), non-benzodiazepine hypnotics, and substance abuse withdrawal symptom or (non-opioid) pain relievers. There were no significant differences between time points within the groups in medication variables.

> = superior than, *** = statistically significant at level $p < 0.001$. ** = statistically significant at level $p < 0.01$. * = statistically significant at level $p < 0.05$.

**Attention** was assessed by two tests from the Test for Attentional Performance (TAP) [46]. In the Alertness test, the participant was instructed to respond to visual stimuli by pressing a response key as quickly as possible. The stimuli were presented without or with auditory warning signal. The condition without warning signal is a simple reaction time task reflecting tonic alertness. The condition with auditory warning signal reflects both tonic and phasic alertness. In the Go/NoGo test, the participant was instructed to respond only to two out of five alternative stimuli. Thus, selective attention and executive control of action was assessed.

**Working memory** was assessed by two tests. In the Letter-Number Sequencing task from the Wechsler Memory Scale - III the participant was instructed to repeat letters and numbers in specific order [47]. In the Paced Auditory Serial Addition Task ( PASAT) the participant was instructed to add two consecutive numbers from an auditory series of digit [48]. A new digit was presented after every 1.6 seconds. Both tests are thought to tap complex working memory because simultaneous storage and manipulation of the material is needed.

**Verbal memory** was assessed by the Logical Memory from the Wechsler Memory Scale - III. However, only

**Table 3 Group demographics in sample II**

| | Buprenorphine or Buprenorphine/ Naloxone (n = 18) | Methadone (n = 18) | Group or time point comparison p-values |
|---|---|---|---|
| Age, years at T1 (M ± SD) | 30 ± 8 | 32 ± 8 | ns |
| Sex: females/males, % | 28/72% | 33/67% | ns |
| Verbal IQ [a] (M ± SD) | 101 ± 8 | 100 ± 11 | ns |
| Education, years (M ± SD) | 10 ± 2 | 11 ± 1 | ns |
| Participants with early neurobehavioral problems % | 33% | 28% | ns |
| Examined in inpatient settings % | | | |
| T2 | 6% | 6% | ns |
| T3 | 11% | 11% | ns |
| Participants with high frequency use of any substance of abuse % [b] | | | |
| T2 | 44% | 39% | ns |
| T3 | 44% | 44% | ns |
| Participants with recent month extra doses of any opioid % [c] | | | |
| T2 | 36% | 36% | ns |
| T3 | 36% | 43% | ns |
| Nicotine, participants using daily, % | | | |
| T2 | 100% | 100% | ns |
| T3 | 100% | 100% | ns |
| Days in opioid substitution treatment at test (M ± SD) | | | |
| T2 | 211 ± 19 | 196 ± 27 | ns |
| T3 | 411 ± 43 | 405 ± 29 | ns |
| Age of onset, any substance abuse (M ± SD) | 16 ± 4 | 15 ± 3 | ns |
| Age of onset, opioid abuse (M ± SD) | 19 ± 5 | 19 ± 4 | ns |
| Participants with lifetime alcohol abuse | 72% | 83% | ns |
| Years of any substance abuse at T1 (M ± SD) | 15 ± 7 | 17 ± 7 | ns |
| Years of alcohol abuse at T1 (M ± SD) | 3 ± 4 | 3 ± 3 | ns[b] |
| Years of opioid abuse at T1, years (M ± SD) | 10 ± 7 | 12 ± 7 | ns |

[a] Estimation based on the WAIS-R Vocabulary score.

[b] High frequency = three or more days a week Alcohol use was considered heavy if it was at least mean weekly 16 portions for females and 24 portions for males. One portion was defined as 12 g of alcohol.

[c] Non-prescribed doses of opioids during the recent month seen in drugs screens or admitted by the patient.

one story was presented. A full description of the tasks is given in our previous report [7].

## Statistical analyses: stability of function

Longitudinal changes in cognitive function were examined by repeated-measures analysis of variance (ANOVA) using general linear model approach. Group was used as between-subjects factor and time as within-subjects factor. Before the analyses normality assumptions of cognitive variables were examined by Shapiro-Wilk's test and homogeneity of variance by Levene's test. The data were also screened for outlying values.

On the basis of these procedures, reaction time and the PASAT scores were subjected to log transformations before further analyses, and the Go/NoGo errors were examined by non-parametric Kruskal-Wallis ANOVA. Sphericity assumption was tested by Mauchly's test, and when appropriate, analyses of effects were interpreted using Huynh-Feldt correction. The effects of demographic variables on cognitive performance were tested as covariates. Only significant covariates were retained in the model. Statistically significant between groups effects were followed by planned contrast using healthy controls as a reference group. Significant time effects we

**Table 4 Medications given to participants within the last 24 h before testing in sample II**

| | Buprenorphine or Buprenorphine/ Naloxone (n = 18) | Methadone (n = 18) | Group or time point comparison p-values |
|---|---|---|---|
| Opioid drug, dose (M ± SD (range) ) | | | |
| T2 | 22 ± 5 mg ( 10 - 28 mg) | - | T2 vs. T3, ns |
| T3 | 21 ± 6 mg ( 6 - 30 mg) | - | |
| T2 | - | 119. ± 33 mg (80 - 180 mg) | T2 vs. T3, ns |
| T3 | - | 129 ± 33 mg (75 - 180 mg) | |
| Participants using BZD medication | | | |
| T2/T3 | 78%/67% | 89%/94% | ns/ns |
| BZD dose at T2 (M ± SD (range)) | 20 ± 16 mg (0 - 60 mg) | 21 ± 16 mg (0 - 70 mg) | T2 vs. T3, ns ns |
| BZD dose at T3 (M ± SD (range)) | 16 ± 14 mg (0 - 40 mg) | 20 ± 10 mg (0 - 40 mg) | ns T2 vs. T3, ns |
| Number of other medications with possible cognitive effects [a] | | | |
| T2/T3 (M ± SD ; (range)) | 1.8 ± 1.1 (0 - 3) | 2.2 ± 0.7 (1 -4) | ns |
| | 1.9 ± 1.4 (0 - 4) | 2.0 ± 1.0 (1 - 4) | ns |
| | | | T2 vs. T3, ns |

These included antidepressants, neuroleptics (used with anxiolytic indications), non-benzodiazepine hypnotics, and substance abuse withdrawal symptom or (non-opioid) pain relievers.

C = controls, M = methadone, BN = buprenorphine or buprenorphine/naloxone

> = superior than, *** = statistically significant at level $p < 0.001$. ** = statistically significant at level $p < 0.01$. * = statistically significant at level $p < 0.05$.

examined using repeated contrast (T2 vs. T1 and T3 vs. T2). When a significant group by time interaction effect was noted, it was examined further by combining previous contrasts (healthy control vs. buprenorphine group * T2 vs. T1, healthy control vs. buprenorphine group * T3 vs. T2; and healthy control vs. methadone group, respectively). All statistical analyses were done by SPSS statistical software, version 15.0, with an exception of the effect size calculations. These were done by an effect size calculator provided by Durham University, UK [49]. For the effect size estimation we pooled the samples and corrected the values by Hedge's correction for small sample bias.

**Statistical analyses: correlates of cognitive functioning**
Cognitive tests selected for the analyses were the same as in the part I, except that the PASAT was excluded from the second set of analyses. Improvement in the PASAT is shown to be related to practice effect [50]. This makes it problematic to analyze the correlates of this measure in repeated testing. In order to reduce the number of cognitive variables correlations between the variables analyzed, and whenever justified, domain-wise cognitive sum scores for T2 and T3 performances were

formed. T2 performance was used as a reference point in T3 summed scores. Analysis of correlation is sensitive for the effects of outliers. Therefore, visual inspections of scatter plots were used to check the linearity of the relationship between variables and the role of possible outliers. Then correlations between cognitive variables we analyzed by the Pearson product moment method. As expected there were high positive correlations between all reaction time measures at both test points (range .52 - .86); whereas correlations between reaction time measures and other cognitive measures ranged from zero to moderate (-.38 as highest). Therefore, a mean composite score called attention performance was calculated after converting the test scores into z-scores. The working memory measure, the Letter-Number Sequencing task, showed only low to moderate correlations with other measures (.38 as highest) and therefore it was not combined with other measures. The verbal memory measures, immediate and delayed recall of the Logical Memory, correlated strongly at both test points (.80 at T2 and .91 at T3). Therefore, a mean sum score called verbal memory was formed after z-score conversion. Then group differences in cognitive function were examined by repeated-measures analysis of variance

(ANOVA) using general linear model approach. Group was used as between-subjects factor and time as within-subjects factor. After this all significant or three highest correlates of each cognitive variable were further examined by checking for intercorrelations between these variables and other variables of interest. Also, medication variables were checked for significant intercorrelations. The sample size did not allow for multiple regression analysis. Instead three highest correlations for each cognitive domain were investigated with analyses of semipartial correlations. Correlations between .10 - .19 were considered to show low association and .20 - 29 mild association. Only some of these are reported. Correlations between, .30 - .49 were considered to show moderate association, .50 - 69 substantial and those .70 or above a strong association [51].

## Results

### Stability of cognitive functioning in sample I

The pattern of means in Table 5 identifies change over time in cognitive performance in each group. There were statistically significant overall group differences in all attention and memory measures. As apparent from the Table 5, the methadone-treated patient group constantly lagged behind the healthy control group in the TAP reaction time tests measuring alertness and selective attention. Planned contrasts confirmed that the healthy controls outperformed the methadone group in these measures ($p = 0.002$ for the TAP tonic alertness/ simple reaction time; $p = 0.002$ for the TAP phasic alertness/reaction time with-auditory-warning-signal; and $p = 0.001$ for the TAP Go/NoGo reaction time/ selective attention). There were neither significant time nor group by time interaction effects in these measures. Errors in the Go/NoGo task were rare in all groups, and no significant between groups differences were observed. In both working memory measures there was an overall group effect. In the PASAT the planned contrast revealed that both patient groups performed *overall* worse than the healthy controls at the level of $p = 0.001$. In the Letter-Number Sequencing the values were $p = 0.016$, for healthy controls vs. buprenorphine patients and $p = 0.008$ for healthy controls vs. methadone patients. However, because there was also time effect (the PASAT), or a group by time interaction effect (the Letter-Number Sequencing) in these measures, further analyses are needed before the final interpretation. In the PASAT the improvement in overall performance between T1 and T2 turned out to be non-significant, but the overall improvement between T2 and T3 was significant, $p = 0.01$. As apparent from Figure 1, the source of group by time interaction in the Letter-Number Sequencing was due to differences

between the groups between T2 and T3. This was confirmed by a planned contrast which showed improved performance in the buprenorphine patients between T2 and T3 relative to healthy control group, $p = 0.017$. Effect size of the T2 - T3 improvement in the buprenorphine group, as measured by Cohen's **d**, was 0.77. In verbal memory, there was a significant overall group effect both in immediate and delayed condition of the Logical Memory. Both patient groups performed worse than the healthy controls in the immediate Logical Memory, $p = 0.029$ for the buprenorphine group; and $p = 0.007$ for the methadone group. In the delayed Logical Memory the values were $p = 0.005$, and $p = 0.028$, respectively.

### Cognitive functioning in sample II

The cognitive group comparisons in the part II (T2 - T3) sample brought results that were in line with the part I sample analyses. Buprenorphine patients outperformed methadone patients in the combined attention performance ($p = 0.004$), and no significant time or group by time effect were seen. In working memory as measured by the Letter-Number Sequencing there was a main effect of time ($p = 0.01$) and a significant group by time interaction, ($p = 0.04$) indicating again that improvement in this measure was due to enhanced performance in the buprenorphine patients between T2 and T3. In the combined verbal memory measure there were no significant differences between groups, time effect, or group by time interaction.

### Correlations between medication variables and non-cognitive variables in sample II

At T2, buprenorphine dose correlated substantially with BZD dose (.62, $p = 0.006$) and moderately with the number of psychoactive drugs (.40, *ns*). In the methadone group, respective values were (.47, *ns;* and .58, $p = 0.013$). At T3, buprenorphine dose correlated at moderate level with BZD dose (.33, *ns*) and at very low level with the number of psychoactive drugs (.10, *ns*). In the methadone group respective values were mild (.25, ns; and .20, ns). In general, buprenorphine or methadone doses did not show significant correlations with substance abuse or demographic variables. As an exception buprenorphine dose correlated negatively with years of alcohol abuse, at T2 the value was -.56 ($p = 0.016$) and at T3 -.64 ($p = 0.004$). In the methadone group, no significant correlations emerged. Other significant correlations between medication variables and other non-cognitive variables of interest are presented in Table 6. It can be noted that high BZD dose was associated with high frequency of substance abuse in the past month and younger age at both time points.

**Table 5 Group comparisons of cognitive performances using repeated measures ANOVA in sample I**

| | | | | | |
|---|---|---|---|---|---|
| TAP Tonic Alertness/simple reaction time (ms) | | | | | |
| | T1 | 232 ± 25 | 261 ± 21 | 238 ± 22 | **Group, *p* = 0.002** |
| | T2 | 236 ± 18 | 263 ± 21 | 233 ± 21[a] | Time, *ns* |
| | T3 | 242 ± 25 | 267 ± 36 | 241 ± 25 | Group × Time, *ns* |
| TAP Phasic Alertness/ reaction time with warning signal (ms) | | | | | |
| | T1 | 227 ± 24 | 244 ± 20 | 226 ± 21 | **Group, *p* = 0.005** |
| | T2 | 229 ± 21 | 255 ± 28 | 224 ± 21[a] | Time, *ns* |
| | T3 | 229 ± 19 | 254 ± 45 | 225 ± 22 | Group × Time, *ns* |
| TAP Go-NoGo reaction time (ms) | | | | | |
| | T1 | 490 ± 50 | 548 ± 74 | 460 ± 41 | **Group, *p* = 0.001** |
| | T2 | 480 ± 42 | 548 ± 104 | 443 ± 72[a] | **Group, *p* = 0.002** |
| | T3 | 493 ± 43 | 529 ± 63 | 462 ± 47 | **Age, *p* = 0.022** |
| | | | | | Time, *ns* |
| | | | | | Group × Time, *ns* |
| TAP Go-NoGo errors | | | | | |
| | T1 | 1.1 ± 1.3 | 0.7 ± 0.6 | 0.5 ± 0.5 | *ns* |
| | T2 | 0.5 ± 0.7 | 1.0 ± 0.9 | 0.5 ± 0.8[a] | *ns* |
| | T3 | 0.6 ± 0.8 | 0.5 ± 1.0 | 0.2 ± 0.4 | *ns* |
| The Letter-Number Sequencing | | | | | |
| | T1 | 8.4 ± 2.2 | 9.3 ± 2.4 | 11.8 ± 3.4 | **Group, *p* = 0.009** |
| | T2 | 8.8 ± 2.2 | 8.5 ± 2.3 | 11.6 ± 3.0 | Time, *ns* |
| | T3 | 10.6 ± 2.2 | 8.8 ± 2.4 | 11.2 ± 3.2 | **Group × Time, *p* = 0.007** |
| The PASAT | | | | | |
| | T1 | 32.4 ± 10.5 | 31.0 ± 8.5 | 46.3 ± 9.7 | **Group, *p* = 0.001** |
| | T2 | 35.0 ± 6.8 | 33.4 ± 10.1 | 45.8 ± 9.0[a] | **Time, *p* = 0.013** |
| | T3 | 35.8 ± 10.0 | 34.9 ± 11.0 | 49.8 ± 8.4 | Group × Time, *ns* |
| Logical memory, immediate | | | | | |
| | T1 | 12.8 ± 2.6 | 14.9 ± 4.5 | 15.9 ± 3.3 | **Group, *p* = 0.016** |
| | T2 | 13.8 ± 3.1 | 14.8 ± 3.7 | 16.3 ± 3.2 | Time, *ns* |
| | T3 | 15.5 ± 4.1 | 14.3 ± 4.3 | 17.9 ± 2.9 | Group × Time, *ns* |
| Logical memory, delayed | | | | | |
| | T1 | 11.8 ± 3.0 | 13.1 ± 4.0 | 13.9 ± 4.0 | **Group, *p* = 0.013** |
| | T2 | 12.0 ± 4.0 | 13.7 ± 4.0 | 15.6 ± 3.1 | Time, *ns* |
| | T3 | 12.4 ± 4.1 | 11.8 ± 4.7 | 15.9 ± 3.6 | Group × Time, *ns* |

Bold indicates statistically significant effects.

[a] One missing value was replaced by the carry-over value from the preceding testing point.

### Correlates of cognitive performances in sample II

As shown in Table 7, the only significant correlate for attention performance at both test points was the opioid substitution drug group. High frequency of substance abuse correlated negatively with the Letter-Number Sequencing performance at both time points. Figures 2 and 3 depict this association. It can be noted from these Figures that the association between working memory performance and frequency of substance abuse in the past month is similar in both groups. The T2 negative correlation remained significant after controlling for two next highest correlates. The T3 correlation dropped to non-significant level after controlling for two next highest correlates (-.18). At T3, high benzodiazepine dose correlated negatively with the Letter-Number

Sequencing performance. After controlling for the two other highest correlates, this association was no longer significant (-.22). In further analysis no evidence in support of high association between BZD dose and the Letter-Number Sequencing performance was seen, because T2 correlation between these variables was at zero level (.02). Belonging to the buprenorphine group was the only variable that correlated significantly (.34) with change of the Letter-Number Sequencing performance. After controlling for two other highest correlates, this association was no longer significant.

The number of psychoactive drugs correlated positively with verbal memory performances at both testing points. At T3, the positive association with the number of psychoactive drugs reached significant level after two other

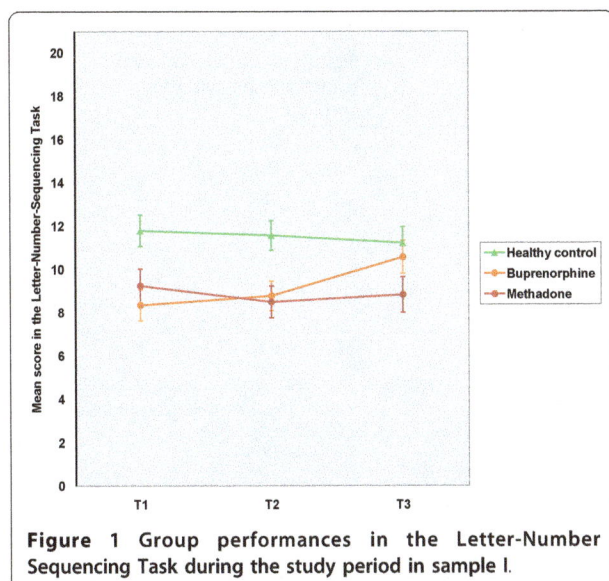

**Figure 1** Group performances in the Letter-Number Sequencing Task during the study period in sample I.

correlates were taken into account. At T2, there was a negative association with the highly frequent past month substance abuse and verbal memory performance. After controlling for two other highest this correlation dropped to non-significant level (.28). Furthermore, at T3 the correlation between highly frequent substance abuse in the past month and verbal memory was very low and to the opposite direction (-.08).

Correlations between opioid substitution drug dose and cognitive performances opioid drug doses could be examined only group-wise (n = 18 in both groups). None of the correlations reached statistical significance. Because there was a significant group by time interaction in the Letter-Number Sequencing indicating specific improvement in this task in the buprenorphine group, correlates for the improvement in the buprenorphine group were examined. No significant correlates for the change score emerged.

## Discussion

This study was designed to evaluate stability and correlates of cognitive functioning in unselected buprenorphine- vs. methadone treated opioid-dependent patients during the first year in OST. The main findings are the following. Buprenorphine-treated opioid-dependent patients do not show deficits in attention, improve in one of the working memory tests, the Letter-Number Sequencing, but they show stable deficits in the other working memory test, the PASAT, and verbal memory. Methadone-treated opioid-dependent patients show stabile cognitive deficits in attention, working memory, and verbal memory. When correlates of cognitive performances are analyzed 6 and 12 after the start of the OST drug type (buprenorphine vs. methadone) is moderately associated with attention performance. Highly frequent substance abuse in the past month is negatively associated with performance in the Letter-Number Sequencing. The number of other psychoactive drugs and verbal IQ both show mild positive correlation with verbal memory.

### Stability of buprenorphine patients' cognitive function during the first year in treatment

Our observation of no reaction time deficits in buprenorphine-treated opioid-dependent patients in relation to healthy controls is in accordance with the idea that some of the negative effects of buprenorphine on cognition disappear after the development of tolerance. Most patients had abused buprenorphine before the treatment (Table 1). Further studies are needed to examine if buprenorphine patients' normal performance in attention tests is related to the development of tolerance only, or if a population selection process is affecting performance in patient samples.

Our finding of partial recovery of working memory function in buprenorphine-treated patients during the OST is in line with the idea of Spiga et al. [52]. The idea is supported by observations by Pirastu et al. showing that buprenorphine patients outperform methadone patients in spatial working memory [18]. They suggest that buprenorphine could preserve working memory function better than methadone because of its antagonism on kappa opioid receptor, which then affects prefrontal dopamine tone known to be important for working memory. This reasoning, however, does not explain why the improvement in working memory in our study took place between 6 and 12 months in the treatment.

**Table 6 Significant correlations between medication variables and other non-cognitive variables in sample II**

| Medication variables | Substance abuse variables | Demographic variables |
|---|---|---|
| Benzodiazepine dose (T2) | Frequency of substance abuse in the past month **.36 ( $p$ = 0.033)** | Age **-.34 ($p$ = 0.040)** |
| Benzodiazepine dose (T3) | Frequency of substance abuse in the past month **.50 ($p$ = 0.002)** | Age **-.33 ($p$ = 0.048)** |
| Number of other psychoactive drugs (T2) | | |
| Number of other psychoactive drugs (T3) | Years of opioid abuse **-.37 ($p$ = 0.028)** | |

**Table 7 Highest correlations between cognitive and non-cognitive variables in sample II**

| Domain or test | Medication variables | Substance abuse variables | Demographic variables | Significant correlations after controlling for two other correlates |
|---|---|---|---|---|
| Attention (T2) | Opioid substitution drug **.48 (p = 0.003)** Number of other psychoactive drugs (T2) .24 | Opioid abuse onset age .25 | | Opioid substitution drug **.46, (p = 0.004)** |
| Attention (T3) | Opioid substitution drug **.37 (p = .024)** | Opioid abuse onset age .28 | Age .26 | Opioid substitution drug **.37, (p = 0.021)** |
| The Letter-Number Sequencing Task (T2) | Number of other psychoactive drugs .25 | Frequency of substance abuse in the past month **-49 (p= .002)** | Verbal IQ .29 | Frequency of substance abuse in the past month **-44 (p = .005)** |
| The Letter-Number Sequencing Task (T3) | Benzodiazepine dose **.-38** | Frequency of substance abuse in the past month **.-34 (p = .044)** Years of opioid abuse .28 | | |
| Change score in the Letter-Number Sequencing Task (T3 - T2) | Opioid substitution drug **.34 (p = .039)** | | Change in the opioid agonist dose -.33 Change in the number of psychoactive drugs -.24 | |
| Verbal memory (T2) | Number of other psychoactive drugs (T2) .25 | Frequency of substance abuse in the past month **-. 34 (p = .044)** | Verbal IQ .28 | |
| Verbal memory (T3) | Number of other psychoactive drugs (T3) .31 | | Verbal IQ .32 Years of education .27 | Number of other psychoactive drugs **.34 (p = .035)** |

Bold indicates statistically significant correlation.

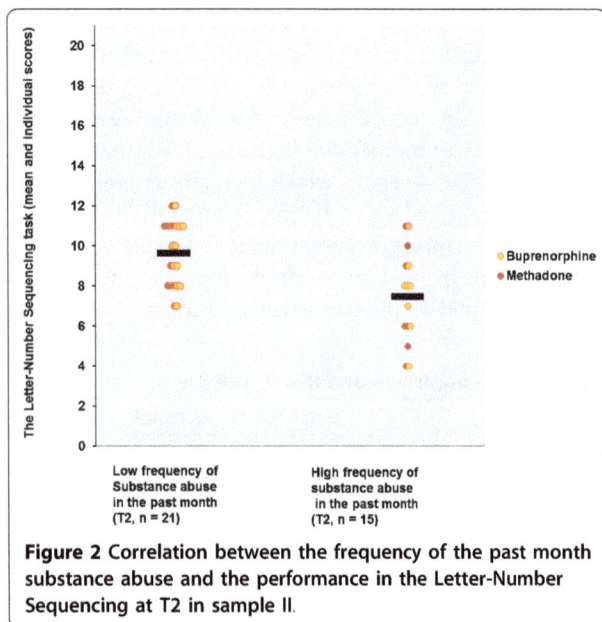

**Figure 2** Correlation between the frequency of the past month substance abuse and the performance in the Letter-Number Sequencing at T2 in sample II.

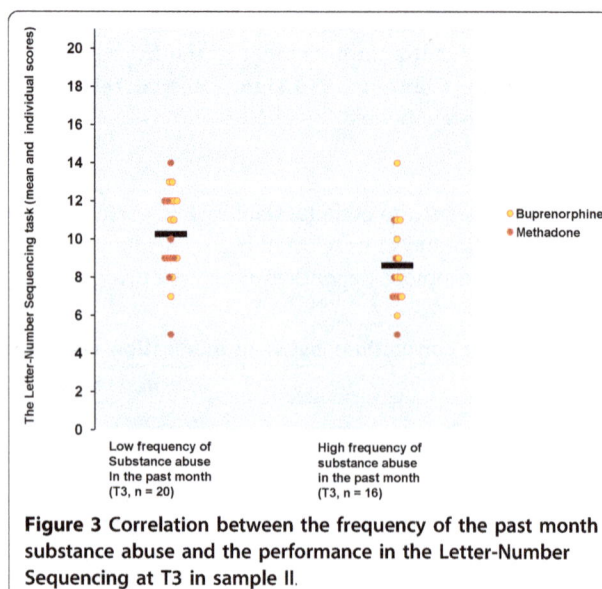

**Figure 3** Correlation between the frequency of the past month substance abuse and the performance in the Letter-Number Sequencing at T3 in sample II.

In the other working memory measure, the PASAT, both patient groups are inferior to healthy controls while all groups show improvement during the study period. Improvement that is seen in all groups is a normal finding when the PASAT is administered, and most likely reflects practice effect [50]. The result of no specific improvement in the buprenorphine patients in this measure may be related to the finding that also several other cognitive processes than working memory are needed for good performance in the PASAT [53].

In verbal memory buprenorphine-treated patients perform worse than healthy controls during the whole follow-up. Buprenorphine dose given to our patients was relative high (range mean 16 mg (T1) - 21 mg (T3)). High dose of buprenorphine (32 mg) have been associated with verbal memory impairment [54]. In addition, in recent study by Messinis et al. buprenorphine-treated opioid-dependent patients with a fairly low mean dose of buprenorphine (7 mg) performed worse than healthy controls in verbal memory. Abstinent opioid-dependent patients treated with mu opioid antagonist naltrexone showed no significant difference relative to healthy controls. In sum, buprenorphine may negatively affect verbal memory, although evidence is still insufficient.

### Stability of methadone patients' cognitive function during the first year in treatment

In this study, methadone patients show cognitive deficits in all domains studied: attention, working memory and verbal memory. Not all studies, however, have shown attention deficits among them. Gordon found that methadone-treated opioid-dependent patients outperformed controls in simple visual and visual multiple choice reaction times [55]. Curran et al. found that 3 h after methadone dose opioid-dependent patients in methadone-aided opioid withdrawal actually had faster simple reaction times than before the dose [56]. On the other hand, in the Lintzeris et al study high dose of methadone (150% of normal dose) was associated with slower reaction times in OST patients [20]. Thus, the issue whether methadone dose prolongs reaction times in opioid-dependent patients is not fully resolved.

We found a stabile working memory deficit in both complex working memory measures, the Letter-Number Sequencing and the PASAT, in methadone patients. In early study Gritz et al. found no deficit in methadone patients in "simple" working memory test, the Digit Span from the Wechsler scales, in which the items needs to repeated without organizing them [57]. However, in a more recent study Darke et al. found medium effect size difference between methadone patients and healthy controls in the same test [5]. Interestingly, in abstinent opioid-dependent patients "simple" working memory seems to be spared while complex working

memory performance is impaired [58,59]. Thus, it would be informative to compare methadone patients against abstinent opioid-dependent patients using both simple and complex working memory measures.

Methadone patients were inferior to healthy controls in verbal memory. Also, in the Darke et al. study opioid-dependent patients treated with methadone for a minimum 5 months were impaired relative to healthy controls in verbal memory [5]. However, in the Curran et al. study opioid-dependent patients treated with methadone for a minimum 6 months were given their normal dose, 33% increased dose, or placebo linctus; and then tested 3-4 after the dose. No significant treatment effect was seen, and the authors conclude that single doses of methadone are devoid of verbal memory effects among long-term methadone users. Thus, negative effect of methadone on verbal memory is not well-confirmed.

### Correlates of cognitive functioning in opioid substitution treated patients

The most consistent finding of analyses of correlates of cognitive functioning after 6 (T2) or 12 months (T3) in treatment is that belonging to the methadone group negatively associates with attention performance. However, as stated earlier in randomized or well-controlled studies methadone patients, in general, have performed at equal level than buprenorphine ones in tests measuring attention. Thus, it is possible that patient selection or other medication or substance abuse factor is affecting the results in non-randomized studies, in which methadone patients perform worse than buprenorphine patients.

We hypothesized that the number of prescribed psychoactive drugs given to the patients would show negative correlations with performance in cognitive tests. Our results, however, show three mild to moderate *positive* correlations between the number of psychoactive drugs and verbal memory. Thus, the results do not confirm the hypothesis that the number of psychoactive drugs as such would correlate negatively with cognitive performance in OST patients. We hypothesized that those with the high opioid substitution drug dose would have higher BZD doses. The results were in line with this hypothesis. Benzodiazepine use was very common in both patient groups, and experimental studies have shown that benzodiazepines, when given in combination with opioid substitution drug may affect negatively attention or verbal memory functioning [24]. Therefore, we hypothesized that a negative correlation between the BZD dose and cognitive measures would be seen. Although one moderate negative correlation between working memory measures and BZD dose is seen in our clinical sample, this does not remain significant when two other correlates are taken into account. In sum, substantial differences between test points and many significant intercorrelations show that relationships between medication variables and cognitive performance are not easily discovered in clinical sample studies.

High frequency of substance abuse in the past month was negatively associated with the working memory measure with executive function component, the Letter-Number Sequencing, at both test points. This finding is line with studies reporting negative association between working memory and recent substance abuse, possibly affecting fluid intelligence in general [31,58,60]. In addition, frequency of substance abuse in the past month correlates positively with BZD dose at both test points (.36 - .50), and BZD dose correlated negatively with the T2 Letter-Number Sequencing performance. Furthermore, the opioid substitution drug doses show moderate or substantial correlations with the BZD doses. There is temptation to suggest an association between the past month frequent substance abuse, high opioid agonist dose, high BZD dose, and impaired working memory performance. Yet, our data do not allow controlling for all these intercorrelations.

The hypothesis of negative effect of lifetime substance abuse on cognitive performance was examined using substance abuse onset ages and durations of abuse as correlates for cognitive performance. Some negative correlations emerged, but these were moderate at best.

Demographic variables have been shown to be important correlates for cognitive performance in opioid-dependent patients [10,36,37]. In our study, the only consistent finding is the positive correlation between Verbal IQ measured by the vocabulary test and verbal memory. This relationship is not surprising because vocabulary and verbal memory correlate moderately in normal and clinical populations [61,62].

### Limitations

The main limitation of part I of this study is the fact that, while the opioid-dependent patient groups were comparable to each other in variables of interest, our healthy comparison group had hardly any medication or substance abuse. Although these differences relate to the 'dark side' of addiction [63] they limit the specificity of our results. Some of the cognitive deficits seen in patients may be premorbid or related to early-onset substance abuse [64,65]. In order to examine these questions analyses of correlations were done in extended population in part II of our study.

Because of high drop-out rate in our study we could not use statistical methods to test causal relationships in part II. On the other hand, comparison of correlations from two testing points gives possibility to evaluate their reliability and consistency. In case of

prescription opioid drug, drug screen do not show extra doses. Thus, it is possible that opioid doses are not fully accurate. While much is known about the pharmacological comparisons between different BZDs, the values of BZD equivalent doses are approximations instead of precise values [39]. Alcohol use estimates may not be fully accurate. These estimates were based on information given by the participants. Breath alcohol analyzer or other objective test was used only when considered necessary. Finally, our results do not imply that functional capacity of an opioid-dependent patient could be determined on the basis of his/her drug group. Instead, validation of cognitive test battery to a functional task, for instance driving a car, as well as exploration of non-cognitive factors is needed [66]. Only then individual assessment of the functional capacity can be made.

### Conclusions

In conclusion, our results show again that in non-randomized clinical studies buprenorphine patients tend to perform better than methadone patients. The results do not support the idea that there would be substantial negative associations with medication variables and cognitive performance among patients in OST. A longitudinal study of opioid substitution treated patients who switch from buprenorphine to methadone or vice versa would be ideal in detecting cognitive effects of these drugs and the roles of other clinical variables.

### Acknowledgements

This work was funded by the National Institute of Health and Welfare, Finland (THL), the Yrjö Jahnsson Foundation, the Rauha and Jalmari Ahokas Foundation, the Emil Aaltonen Foundation, The Finnish Cultural Foundation, and the Psychiatry Department of Helsinki University Central Hospital. We thank Mikko Salaspuro, Veijo Virsu, and Kristian Wahlbeck for helpful comments during the study, and Pertti Keskivaaara and Jari Lipsanen for statistical advice. We are grateful to the patients and personnel of the clinics who participated in the study.

### Author details

[1]Department of Psychiatry. Helsinki University Central Hospital, Finland. [2]Department of Mental Health and Substance Abuse Services, National Institute for Health and Welfare (THL), Finland. [3]Institute of Behavioural Sciences, University of Helsinki, Finland. [4]Research Unit of Substance Abuse Medicine, University of Helsinki, Finland.

### Authors' contributions

PR planned and performed cognitive testing and statistical analysis. He wrote the first version of the manuscript and prepared the final manuscript. HA conceived the idea of the study and advised in manuscript preparation. HK participated in the design of the study and in manuscript preparation. CF carried out psychiatric investigations. All authors prepared, read and accepted the final manuscript.

### Competing interests

Pekka Rapeli has given a paid lecture in training organized by Schering-Plough, the former manufacturer of buprenorphine.

## References

1. Walsh SL, Eissenberg T: The clinical pharmacology of buprenorphine: extrapolating from the laboratory to the clinic. *Drug Alcohol Depend* 2003, 70:S13-S27.
2. Dole VP, Nyswander ME: Use of Methadone for Narcotic Blockade. *Br J Addict* 1968, 63(1-2):55-57.
3. Degenhardt L, Randall D, Hall W, Law M, Butler T, Burns L: Mortality among clients of a state-wide opioid pharmacotherapy program over 20 years: Risk factors and lives saved. *Drug Alcohol Depend* 2009, 105(1-2):9-15.
4. Wittchen HU, Apelt SM, Soyka M, Gastpar M, Backmund M, Golz J, Kraus MR, Tretter F, Schafer M, Siegert J, *et al*: Feasibility and outcome of substitution treatment of heroin-dependent patients in specialized substitution centers and primary care facilities in Germany: A naturalistic study in 2694 patients. *Drug Alcohol Depend* 2008, 95(3):245-257.
5. Darke S, Sims J, McDonald S, Wickes W: Cognitive impairment among methadone maintenance patients. *Addiction* 2000, 95(5):687-695.
6. Mintzer MZ, Stitzer ML: Cognitive impairment in methadone maintenance patients. *Drug Alcohol Depend* 2002, 67(1):41-51.
7. Rapeli P, Fabritius C, Alho H, Salaspuro M, Wahlbeck K, Kalska H: Methadone vs. buprenorphine/naloxone during early opioid substitution treatment: a naturalistic comparison of cognitive performance relative to healthy controls. *BMC clinical pharmacology* 2007, 7:5.
8. Messinis L, Lyros E, Andrian V, Katsakiori P, Panagis G, Georgiou V, Papathanasopoulos P: Neuropsychological functioning in buprenorphine maintained patients versus abstinent heroin abusers on naltrexone hydrochloride therapy. *Human Psychopharmacology-Clinical and Experimental* 2009, 24(7):524-531.
9. Prosser J, Cohen LJ, Steinfeld M, Eisenberg D, London ED, Galynker II: Neuropsychological functioning in opiate-dependent subjects receiving and following methadone maintenance treatment. *Drug Alcohol Depend* 2006, 84(3):240-247.
10. Specka M, Finkbeiner T, Lodemann E, Leifert K, Kluwig J, Gastpar M: Cognitive-motor performance of methadone-maintained patients. *European addiction research* 2000, 6(1):8-19.
11. Baewert A, Gombas W, Schindler SD, Peternell-Moelzer A, Eder H, Jagsch R, Fischer G: Influence of peak and trough levels of opioid maintenance therapy on driving aptitude. *European addiction research* 2007, 13(3):127-135.
12. Giacomuzzi SM, Thill C, Riemer Y, Garber K, Ertl M: Buprenorphine-and Methadone Maintenance Treatment: Influence on Aspects of Cognitive and Memory Performance. *The Open Addiction Journal* 2008, 1(1):5-6.
13. Loeber S, Kniest A, Diehl A, Mann K, Croissant B: Neuropsychological functioning of opiate-dependent patients: a nonrandomized comparison of patients preferring either buprenorphine or methadone maintenance treatment. *The American journal of drug and alcohol abuse* 2008, 34(5):584-593.
14. Rapeli P, Fabritius C, Kalska H, Alho H: Memory function in opioid-dependent patients treated with methadone or buprenorphine along with benzodiazepine: longitudinal change in comparison to healthy individuals. *Substance abuse treatment, prevention, and policy* 2009, 4:6.
15. Aalto S, Bruck A, Laine M, Nagren K, Rinne JO: Frontal and temporal dopamine release during working memory and attention tasks in healthy humans: a positron emission tomography study using the high-affinity dopamine D2 receptor ligand [11C]FLB 457. *The Journal of neuroscience: the official journal of the Society for Neuroscience* 2005, 25(10):2471-2477.
16. Hagelberg N, Aalto S, Kajander J, Oikonen V, Hinkka S, Nagren K, Hietala J, Scheinin H: Alfentanil increases cortical dopamine D2/D3 receptor binding in healthy subjects. *Pain* 2004, 109(1-2):86-93.
17. Melis M, Spiga S, Diana M: The dopamine hypothesis of drug addiction: hypodopaminergic state. *International review of neurobiology* 2005, 63:101-154.
18. Pirastu R, Fais R, Messina M, Bini V, Spiga S, Falconieri D, Diana M: Impaired decision-making in opiate-dependent subjects: effect of pharmacological therapies. *Drug Alcohol Depend* 2006, 83(2):163-168.
19. Lintzeris N, Mitchell TB, Bond A, Nestor L, Strang J: Interactions on mixing diazepam with methadone or buprenorphine in maintenance patients. *Journal of clinical psychopharmacology* 2006, 26(3):274-283.
20. Lintzeris N, Mitchell TB, Bond AJ, Nestor L, Strang J: Pharmacodynamics of diazepam co-administered with methadone or buprenorphine under

high dose conditions in opioid dependent patients. *Drug Alcohol Depend* 2007, 91(2-3):187-194.
21. Heikman PK, Ojanperä IA: Inadequate Dose of Opioid-agonist Medication is Related to Misuse of Benzodiazepines. *Addictive Disorders & Their Treatment* 2009, 8(3):145-153.
22. Zacny JP: A Review of the Effects of Opioids on Psychomotor and Cognitive Functioning in Humans. *Experimental and Clinical Psychopharmacology* 1995, 3(4):432-466.
23. Zacny JP, Conley K, Galinkin J: Comparing the subjective, psychomotor and physiological effects of intravenous buprenorphine and morphine in healthy volunteers. *The Journal of pharmacology and experimental therapeutics* 1997, 282(3):1187-1197.
24. Lintzeris N, Nielsen S: Benzodiazepines, methadone and buprenorphine: interactions and clinical management. *The American journal on addictions/ American Academy of Psychiatrists in Alcoholism and Addictions* 2010, 19(1):59-72.
25. Meador KJ: Cognitive side effects of medications. *Neurologic clinics* 1998, 16(1):141-155.
26. Starr JM, McGurn B, Whiteman M, Pattie A, Whalley LJ, Deary IJ: Life long changes in cognitive ability are associated with prescribed medications in old age. *International journal of geriatric psychiatry* 2004, 19(4):327-332.
27. Oken BS, Flegal K, Zajdel D, Kishiyama SS, Lovera J, Bagert B, Bourdette DN: Cognition and fatigue in multiple sclerosis: Potential effects of medications with central nervous system activity. *Journal of rehabilitation research and development* 2006, 43(1):83-90.
28. Horner MD, Waid LR, Johnson DE, Latham PK, Anton RF: The relationship of cognitive functioning to amount of recent and lifetime alcohol consumption in outpatient alcoholics. *Addictive behaviors* 1999, 24(3):449-453.
29. Mann K, Gunther A, Stetter F, Ackermann K: Rapid recovery from cognitive deficits in abstinent alcoholics: A controlled test-retes study. *Alcohol Alcohol* 1999, 34(4):567-574.
30. Pope HG Jr, Gruber AJ, Hudson JI, Huestis MA, Yurgelun-Todd D: Neuropsychological performance in long-term cannabis users. *Arch Gen Psychiatry* 2001, 58(10):909-915.
31. Hanson KL, Winward JL, Schweinsburg AD, Medina KL, Brown SA, Tapert SF: Longitudinal study of cognition among adolescent marijuana users over three weeks of abstinence. *Addictive behaviors* 2010, 35(11):970-976.
32. Ferrett HL, Carey PD, Thomas KG, Tapert SF, Fein G: Neuropsychological performance of South African treatment-naive adolescents with alcohol dependence. *Drug Alcohol Depend* 2010, 110(1-2):8-14.
33. Tapert SF, Granholm E, Leedy NG, Brown SA: Substance use and withdrawal: Neuropsychological functioning over 8 years in youth. *Journal of the International Neuropsychological Society* 2002, 8(07):873-883.
34. Bates ME, Labouvie EW, Voelbel GT: Individual differences in latent neuropsychological abilities at addictions treatment entry. *Psychology of Addictive Behaviors* 2002, 16(1):35-46.
35. Tessner KD, Hill SY: Neural circuitry associated with risk for alcohol use disorders. *Neuropsychology review* 2010, 20(1):1-20.
36. Guerra D, Sole A, Cami J, Tobena A: Neuropsychological performance in opiate addicts after rapid detoxification. *Drug Alcohol Depend* 1987, 20(3):261-270.
37. Rounsaville BJ, Novelly RA, Kleber HD, Jones C: Neuropsychological impairment in opiate addicts: risk factors. *Annals of the New York Academy of Sciences* 1981, 362:79-80.
38. Kokkevi A, Hartgers C: EuropASI: European adaptation of a multidimensional assessment instrument for drug and alcohol dependence. *European addiction research* 1995, 1(4):208-210.
39. Nelson J, Chouinard G: Guidelines for the clinical use of benzodiazepines: pharmacokinetics, dependency, rebound and withdrawal. Canadian Society for Clinical Pharmacology. *The Canadian journal of clinical pharmacology* 1999, 6(2):69-83.
40. Nocon A, Wittchen HU, Pfister H, Zimmermann P, Lieb R: Dependence symptoms in young cannabis users? A prospective epidemiological study. *Journal of psychiatric research* 2006, 40(5):394-403.
41. Shakeshaft AP, Bowman JA, Sanson-Fisher RW: A comparison of two retrospective measures of weekly alcohol consumption: diary and quantity/frequency index. *Alcohol Alcohol* 1999, 34(4):636-645.
42. Chiang CN, Hawks RL: Pharmacokinetics of the combination tablet of buprenorphine and naloxone. *Drug Alcohol Depend* 2003, 70(2 Suppl):S39-47.

43. Harris DS, Mendelson JE, Lin ET, Upton RA, Jones RT: **Pharmacokinetics and subjective effects of sublingual buprenorphine, alone or in combination with naloxone: lack of dose proportionality.** *Clinical pharmacokinetics* 2004, **43(5)**:329-340.

44. Orman JS, Keating GM: **Buprenorphine/Naloxone A Review of its Use in the Treatment of Opioid Dependence.** *Drugs* 2009, **69(5)**:577-607.

45. Tarter RE, McBride H, Buonpane N, Schneider DU: **Differentation of alcoholics.** *Arch Gen Psych* 1977, **34(7)**:761-768.

46. Zimmermann P, Fimm B: *Test for Attentional Performance (TAP)* Herzogenrath: PsyTest; 1995.

47. Wechsler D: *Wechler Memory Scale.* Third edition. San Antonio, TX: The Psychological Corporation; 1997.

48. Gronwall DM: **Paced auditory serial-addition task: a measure of recovery from concussion.** *Perceptual and motor skills* 1977, **44(2)**:367-373.

49. **Effect Size Calculator.** [http://www.cemcentre.org/evidence-based-education/effect-size-calculator].

50. Tombaugh TN: **A comprehensive review of the Paced Auditory Serial Addition Test (PASAT).** *Archives of clinical neuropsychology: the official journal of the National Academy of Neuropsychologists* 2006, **21(1)**:53-76.

51. Kotrlik JW, Williams HA: **The incorporation of effect size in information technology, learning, and performance research.** *Information Technology, Learning, and Performance Journal* 2003, **21(1)**:1-7.

52. Spiga S, Lintas A, Diana M: **Addiction and Cognitive Functions.** In *Drug Addiction: Research Frontiers and Treatment Advances. Volume 1139.* Edited by: Kuhar MJ. Oxford: Blackwell Publishing; 2008:299-306.

53. Lockwood AH, Linn RT, Szymanski H, Coad ML, Wack DS: **Mapping the neural systems that mediate the Paced Auditory Serial Addition Task (PASAT).** *J Int Neuropsychol Soc* 2004, **10(1)**:26-34.

54. Mintzer MZ, Correia CJ, Strain EC: **A dose-effect study of repeated administration of buprenorphine/naloxone on performance in opioid-dependent volunteers.** *Drug Alcohol Depend* 2004, **74(2)**:205-209.

55. Gordon NB: **Reaction-times of methadone treated ex-heroin addicts.** *Psychopharmacologia* 1970, **16(4)**:337-344.

56. Curran HV, Kleckham J, Bearn J, Strang J, Wanigaratne S: **Effects of methadone on cognition, mood and craving in detoxifying opiate addicts: a dose-response study.** *Psychopharmacology (Berl)* 2001, **154(2)**:153-160.

57. Gritz ER, Shiffman SM, Jarvik ME, Haber J, Dymond AM, Coger R, Charuvastra V, Schlesinger J: **Physiological and psychological effects of methadone in man.** *Arch Gen Psychiatry* 1975, **32(2)**:237-242.

58. Rapeli P, Kivisaari R, Autti T, Kahkonen S, Puuskari V, Jokela O, Kalska H: **Cognitive function during early abstinence from opioid dependence: a comparison to age, gender, and verbal intelligence matched controls.** *BMC Psychiatry* 2006, **6(1)**:9.

59. Wang Z-X, Xiao Z-W, Zhang D-R, Liang C-Y, Zhang JX: **Verbal working memory deficits in abstinent heroin abusers.** *Acta Neuropsychiatrica* 2008, **20(5)**:265-268.

60. Shelton JT, Elliott EM, Hill BD, Calamia MR, Gouvier WD: **A Comparison of Laboratory and Clinical Working Memory Tests and Their Prediction of Fluid Intelligence.** *Intelligence* 2009, **37(3)**:283..

61. Bowden SC, Ritter AJ, Carstairs JR, Shores EA, Pead J, Greeley JD, Whelan G, Long CM, Clifford CC: **Factorial invariance for combined Wechsler Adult Intelligence Scale-revised and Wechsler Memory Scale-revised scores in a sample of clients with alcohol dependency.** *Clinical Neuropsychologist* 2001, **15(1)**:69-80.

62. Alexander JRM, Smales S: **Intelligence, learning and long-term memory.** *Personality and Individual Differences* 1997, **23(5)**:815-825.

63. Koob GF, Le Moal M: **Plasticity of reward neurocircuitry and the 'dark side' of drug addiction.** *Nature neuroscience* 2005, **8(11)**:1442-1444.

64. Block RI, Erwin WJ, Ghoneim MM: **Chronic drug use and cognitive impairments.** *Pharmacology, Biochemistry and Behavior* 2002, **73(3)**:491-504.

65. Brown SA, Tapert SF, Granholm E, Delis DC: **Neurocognitive functioning of adolescents: Effects of protracted alcohol use.** *Alcohol Clin Exp Res* 2000, **24(2)**:164-171.

66. Shmygalev S, Damm M, Weckbecker K, Berghaus G, Petzke F, Sabatowski R: **The impact of long-term maintenance treatment with buprenorphine on complex psychomotor and cognitive function.** *Drug Alcohol Depend* 2011, **117(2-3)**:190-197.

67. Wechsler D: *Wechsler Adult Intelligence Scale - Revised (WAIS-R) Finnish version* Helsinki: Psykologien Kustannus; 1993.

# 19

# Quality and safety of medication use in primary care: consensus validation of a new set of explicit medication assessment criteria and prioritisation of topics for improvement

Tobias Dreischulte[1*], Aileen M Grant[2], Colin McCowan[2], John J McAnaw[3] and Bruce Guthrie[2]

## Abstract

**Background:** Addressing the problem of preventable drug related morbidity (PDRM) in primary care is a challenge for health care systems internationally. The increasing implementation of clinical information systems in the UK and internationally provide new opportunities to systematically identify patients at risk of PDRM for targeted medication review. The objectives of this study were (1) to develop a set of explicit medication assessment criteria to identify patients with sub-optimally effective or high-risk medication use from electronic medical records and (2) to identify medication use topics that are perceived by UK primary care clinicians to be priorities for quality and safety improvement initiatives.

**Methods:** For objective (1), a 2-round consensus process based on the RAND/UCLA Appropriateness Method (RAM) was conducted, in which candidate criteria were identified from the literature and scored by a panel of 10 experts for 'appropriateness' and 'necessity'. A set of final criteria was generated from candidates accepted at each level. For objective (2), thematically related final criteria were clustered into 'topics', from which a panel of 26 UK primary care clinicians identified priorities for quality improvement in a 2-round Delphi exercise.

**Results:** (1) The RAM process yielded a final set of 176 medication assessment criteria organised under the domains 'quality' and 'safety', each classified as targeting 'appropriate/necessary to do' (quality) or 'inappropriate/necessary to avoid' (safety) medication use. Fifty-two final 'quality' assessment criteria target patients with unmet indications, sub-optimal selection or intensity of beneficial drug treatments. A total of 124 'safety' assessment criteria target patients with unmet needs for risk-mitigating agents, high-risk drug selection, excessive dose or duration, inconsistent monitoring or dosing instructions. (2) The UK Delphi panel identified 11 (23%) of 47 scored topics as 'high priority' for quality improvement initiatives in primary care.

**Conclusions:** The developed criteria set complements existing medication assessment instruments in that it is not limited to the elderly, can be implemented in electronic data sets and focuses on drug groups and conditions implicated in common and/or severe PDRM in primary care. Identified priorities for quality and safety improvement can guide the selection of targets for initiatives to address the PDRM problem in primary care.

**Keywords:** Medication error, quality indicator, primary health care, adverse drug events, preventable drug related morbidity

* Correspondence: T.Dreischulte@dundee.ac.uk
[1]Tayside Medicines Unit, NHS Tayside, Mackenzie Building, Kirsty Semple Way, Dundee, Scotland, DD2 4BF, UK
Full list of author information is available at the end of the article

## Background

Systematic reviews have demonstrated deficits in the quality and safety of medication use in primary care to an extent sufficient to constitute a public health threat. Three to four percent of all unplanned hospital admissions are due to preventable drug related morbidity (PDRM), with the majority attributed to high-risk prescribing and inconsistent monitoring [1-4]. Antiplatelets, diuretics, non-steroidal anti-inflammatory drugs (NSAIDs) and anticoagulants account for almost half of preventable drug-related admissions to hospital, with opioid analgesics, beta-blockers, drugs affecting the renin angiotensin system and anti-diabetic agents also frequently implicated [1]. In addition, safety alerts have been issued for drugs less commonly implicated in PDRM but associated with preventable deaths, such as prescribing and monitoring of methotrexate [5] and use of antipsychotics in older people with dementia [6]. These figures are likely to underestimate PDRM caused in primary care, since the negative consequences of under-use of effective guideline recommended drugs have not consistently been considered by the hospitalisation studies included in systematic reviews [1-4].

The 'Data-driven Quality Improvement in Primary care (DQIP)' research programme is designing and testing a complex intervention to improve the quality and safety of medication use in UK primary care. It is based on encouraging and facilitating primary care medical practices to systematically and continuously identify, correct or otherwise manage drug therapy risks that are potential pre-cursors to PDRM [7]. The DQIP approach requires explicit medication assessment criteria which can (1) be operationalised in existing UK electronic data sources in order to (2) identify patients at risk of common or severe PDRM in primary care.

A number of explicit medication assessment tools have been developed in recent years. The Beers criteria set [8] lists potentially inappropriate drugs in the elderly and can be relatively easily implemented in electronic data sets. However, a large proportion of listed items are not licensed or rarely used in the UK and many of the drug groups frequently associated with preventable harm are not considered. More recently published tools that also focus on the elderly, such as 'Assessing care of vulnerable elders' (ACOVE) [9], 'Screening Tool of Older Person's Prescriptions (STOPP)' and 'Screening Tool to Alert doctors to Right Treatment' (START) [10] have a broader scope, but many of the included criteria require manual record review and/or clinical judgement, which are barriers to routine or large scale applications. Other instruments that have been implemented in electronic records and target the primary care population at large [11-13] cover a limited spectrum of medication use issues, especially with respect to medication safety.

The study had two aims. First, we aimed to develop and classify by clinical importance a set of up-to-date medication assessment criteria that can be implemented in routine primary care clinical datasets to identify instances of (a) sub-optimally effective medication use for conditions commonly encountered in primary care and (b) high-risk use of drugs that have been shown to either commonly cause harm and/or cause severe harm in primary care. Second, we aimed to elicit the extent to which thematically-related medication assessment criteria, subsequently referred to as *topics*, are perceived to be priorities for quality improvement by professionals working in UK primary care.

## Methods

### Study design

The study was conducted in three stages. First, an extensive list of candidate medication assessment criteria was generated based on a structured literature review. Second, an expert panel participating in a modified RAND/UCLA (University College of Los Angeles) Appropriateness Method (RAM) study scored these items by clinical importance based on a summary of research evidence and their clinical judgement. Candidate criteria with high importance scores were translated into a final criteria set by removing redundancies (see below). Final criteria were characterised by the type of medication use targeted, informed by available taxonomies [13-15]. Third, thematically related final criteria were clustered into medication improvement topics and those derived from candidates with high importance scores were presented to a larger Delphi panel of clinicians working in UK primary care for prioritisation. The study was approved by the Tayside Committee on Medical Research Ethics A (reference no. 09/S1401/54).

### Literature review

Prescribing is a ubiquitous feature of medical care which makes a systematic evaluation of the literature on prescribing quality or safety unfeasible in a single research project. We therefore focussed on medication use for conditions commonly encountered in primary care and drugs with clear evidence of significant benefit or harm. The literature review drew initially on UK national clinical guidelines, prescribing advice, and safety alerts, supplemented by European or other clinical guidelines and targeted primary literature review in selected areas as detailed below.

Candidate medication assessment criteria either described potentially beneficial medication use ('quality') or the use of potentially harmful treatments ('safety'). Candidate 'quality' criteria targeted common conditions where there are compelling indications for drug therapy based on UK and European guidelines [16-25]. Common conditions that may or may not require drug treatment for adequate management (depression, anxiety, dyspepsia, acute infections) or where we anticipated that undertreated patients would not be reliably identifiable from UK electronic data sets (chronic pain, chronic obstructive pulmonary disease, rheumatoid arthritis, thyroid disorders, epilepsy) were not considered. The following conditions were selected: primary and secondary prevention of vascular disease [26,27], management of diabetes [28], heart failure [29], atrial fibrillation [30], asthma [31] and osteoporosis [32,33].

In order to identify candidate safety criteria, the drug groups reported to be most frequently implicated in PDRM hospital admissions were identified from systematic reviews and large scale studies [1-4,34]. For each drug or drug group identified, a more extensive literature search was conducted in order to identify patient and/or treatment related risk factors that make patients particularly vulnerable to drug-related toxicity by virtue of age, medical history, co-prescription, treatment duration and/or dose. Standard medicines information resources [35-39] and the primary research literature were considered in addition to selected previously published medication assessment instruments [8-10,40]. Safety alerts in the British National Formulary [36], the UK National Prescribing Centre [38] and the Medicines and Healthcare products Regulatory Agency [39] were examined to identify prescribing that was less commonly reported to be implicated in drug-related hospital admissions but associated with severe harm. Candidate safety criteria targeting potentially harmful prescribing in vulnerable groups were identified drawing on the above literature sources (children and young adults, the elderly) as well as current clinical practice guidelines (heart failure [22]). Potentially important aspects of high-risk prescribing that relied on data items which are not consistently recorded in UK primary care electronic data sets (monitoring or achievement of international normalised ratio targets, monitoring of blood glucose in patients co-prescribed drugs known to enhance sensitivity to insulin or oral anti-diabetics, medication use in pregnancy/lactation) were excluded.

### RAND/UCLA Appropriateness Method (RAM) study
The RAND/University of California Los Angeles (UCLA) appropriateness method is a rigorous way of combining research evidence with expert opinion [41], and has previously been applied to develop explicit criteria for the assessment of a range of health care procedures including medication use [42]. A panel of ten members was selected with clinical, public health or academic expertise in medication use in UK primary care. The panel was composed of four general medical practitioners (of whom two had National Health Service

prescribing improvement roles) and six pharmacists (including two academics with a special interest in primary care, two working in medicines governance at health board level, and two working directly with general practices). All ten participants completed two rounds of scoring.

The questionnaire aimed to classify candidate medication assessment criteria derived from the literature as either 'necessary' or 'appropriate' care (table 1). 'Necessary' is a more stringent rating standard than 'appropriate', because it represents care that would be *improper* not to be offered or avoided, whereas 'appropriate' is a more neutral balancing of net benefit or harm [43-45]. Following the RAM recommendations, ordinal scales of 1 to 9 were used for all ratings [43,46].

All candidate quality and safety assessment criteria were scored for 'appropriateness'. Candidate criteria with a median rating of 4 to 6 ('uncertain') or disagreement (three or more ratings of 7 to 9 *and* three or more ratings of 1 to 3) on the appropriateness scale were rejected. Those items with median ratings of 7 to 9 were accepted as 'appropriate' and those with median ratings of 1 to 3 as 'inappropriate'.

Candidate quality assessment criteria were additionally scored on a 'necessary to do' scale, where items with a median rating of 7 to 9 (= clearly necessary to do) were accepted. Candidate safety assessment criteria were additionally scored on a 'necessary to avoid' scale, where items with a median rating of 1 to 3 (= clearly necessary to avoid) were accepted. Candidate criteria with median ratings of < 7 on the 'necessary to do' and > 3 on the necessary to avoid scale and those showing disagreement (defined as above) were rejected. The concept of 'necessary to avoid' was an extension to the original RAM method to differentiate between prescribing that is 'generally not worthwhile' from 'improper' in safety terms (see box 2).

The ten RAM panel members were emailed the first round questionnaire and a summary of the supporting evidence base. Panellists were asked to rate each item with reference to an 'average' patient consulting an 'average' primary care clinician in 2009 based on both the evidence summary and their clinical judgement [44]. Panellists subsequently met for a full day, where a summary of the first round ratings was fed back to panellists anonymously. This formed the basis for a moderated discussion of each item before the second round ratings were placed. All findings reported in this paper are based on second round ratings.

### Delphi study
A random sample of general medical practitioners (GPs) and eligible pharmacists in Scotland and England was invited to participate by e-mail. In order to be eligible,

**Table 1 Definitions of rating categories used in the modified RAM study [55]**

| Rating category | Definition |
| --- | --- |
| 'Appropriate' | In an average patient, the expected health benefit usually exceeds the expected negative consequences by a sufficiently wide margin that prescribing is worthwhile, irrespective of cost |
| 'Inappropriate' | In an average patient, the expected negative consequences usually exceed the expected health benefits by a sufficiently wide margin that prescribing is not worthwhile, irrespective of cost |
| 'Necessary to do' | In an average patient, it would be considered improper care NOT to prescribe as stated, because<br>(1) there is sufficient evidence, that the patient is likely to benefit AND<br>(2) the likely benefit to the patient is large enough to be clinically significant |
| 'Necessary to avoid' | In an average patient, it would be considered improper care to prescribe as stated, because<br>(1) there is sufficient evidence, that the patient is likely to be harmed AND<br>(2) the likely harm to the patient is large enough to be clinically significant |

pharmacists had to have experience of working in medicines governance, as a prescribing advisor or as a practice pharmacist. Twenty three (64%) GPs and 13 (36%) pharmacists agreed to participate.

The Delphi questionnaire listed the medication improvement topics to be scored together with a short summary of the scientific rationale for each topic. For each item, panellists were asked to state their level of agreement with the statement *'The described topic is a priority for collaborative quality improvement in primary care'*. The term 'collaborative' was used in order to emphasise that the intended purpose of this study was to identify priority topics for quality improvement rather than measures for judging practitioners or practices as part of performance management.

As in the RAM study, all ratings used an ordinal scale of 1 to 9 (1 = strongly disagree and 9 = strongly agree). Panellists were instructed to rate topics in relation to primary care in general, rather than their own practice. The first round ratings were summarised and returned to participants by email for a second round of scoring. Topics with second round median ratings of 7 to 9 without disagreement (30% or more ratings of 1 to 3 *and* 30% or more ratings of 7 to 9) were accepted as 'priority', with median ratings of 8 or 9 defined as 'high priority'. All findings reported in this paper refer to second round ratings.

## Results

### Literature review and RAM study

The questionnaire listed 389 (100 quality and 289 safety) candidate assessment criteria. Upon completion of the second rating round, 318 (82%) candidates (93 quality and 225 safety) were accepted at the 'appropriate' and 275 (71%) items (73 quality and 202 safety) at the 'necessary' level. A number of candidate criteria were duplicates, in the sense that they were designed to determine thresholds beyond which care was judged appropriate and necessary. For example, 18 candidate quality assessment criteria related to glycated haemoglobin (HbA1c) levels beyond which treatment intensification was appropriate or necessary. Removing redundant

candidate criteria yielded 52 quality and 124 safety assessment criteria to be included in the final set. Forty (77%) final quality assessment criteria and 107 (86%) final safety assessment criteria were derived from candidates accepted at the 'necessary' level. The results of the RAM study are summarised in tables 2 and 3 and the final list of quality and safety assessment criteria is presented in tables 4 and 5.

Table 2 shows the number of accepted quality assessment criteria categorised (1) by medical condition and (2) by four medication quality categories (MQ 1 to 4) referring to 'need (indication)', 'selection' or 'intensity' of drug treatment that were informed by available taxonomies [13-15]. The majority (87%) of the final 52 quality assessment criteria focus on the prevention (including diabetes mellitus) or management of vascular disease with lower proportions addressing asthma (8%) and osteoporosis (6%). Over half (52%) of final quality criteria target patients with unmet indications for drug therapy (MQ1) and 43% focus on treatment intensity (MQ3 and MQ4) for effective disease management with the remainder (8%) targeting selection of first line agents within a therapeutic class (MQ2).

Similarly, table 3 categorises the number of accepted safety assessment criteria generated (1) by high-risk drug or patient group targeted and (2) by eight medication safety categories (MS 1 to 8), referring to 'need (indication)', 'selection', treatment 'intensity', 'compliance' issues and 'monitoring'.

The majority of safety assessment criteria are drug-focussed (74%), either targeting drugs reported to be frequently implicated in PDRM hospital admissions (54% - section A) or others implicated in severe preventable harm (20% - section B). The remainder (26% - section C) target medication use in particularly vulnerable groups, namely the elderly (15%), patients with heart failure (8%) and children (4%). Over a third (36%) of final safety assessment criteria focus on potentially harmful use of NSAIDs, antiplatelets, anticoagulants and diuretics, the drug groups most frequently implicated in PDRM hospital admissions [1].

**Table 2 Summary of final quality assessment criteria designed from candidates accepted in the modified RAM study as appropriate (App) or necessary to do (NecDo)**

| Condition targeted | Final quality assessment criteria | | | | |
|---|---|---|---|---|---|
| | Medication quality category (MQ): Targeted prescribing | Associated PDRM event | Count | | |
| | | | App | NecDo | Total |
| HYPERTENSION | MQ2: Selection of first line antihypertensives | CV events | - | 1 | 13 (25%) |
| | MQ3: Blood pressure control | CV events | 5 | 7 | |
| DIABETES | MQ1: Use of ACEI/ARB if micro-albuminuria | DM complications | - | 1 | 6 (12%) |
| | MQ2: Selection of metformin if overweight | DM complications | - | 1 | |
| | MQ3: HbA1c control | DM complications | 2 | 2 | |
| AT RISK OF PRIMARY/SECONDARY VASCULAR EVENTS | MQ1: Use of antiplatelet or anticoagulant | CV events | 1 | 4 | 17 (33%) |
| | Use of statin | CV events | 1 | 3 | |
| | Use of ACEI or ARB in CHD | CV events | 1 | 1 | |
| | Use of beta blockers in CHD | CV events | - | 2 | |
| | MQ4: Achievement of target statin dose | CV events | - | 4 | |
| CHRONIC HEART FAILURE | MQ1: Use of ACEI or ARB | CHF progression | - | 1 | 5(10%) |
| | Use of beta blocker | CHF progression | - | 1 | |
| | MQ2: Selection of beta blocker licensed for CHF | CHF progression | 1 | - | |
| | MQ4: Achievement of target ACEI/ARB dose | CHF progression | - | 1 | |
| | Achievement of target BB dose | CHF progression | - | 1 | |
| ATRIAL FIBRILLATION | MQ1: Use of antiplatelet or anticoagulant | Stroke/Embolism | - | 3 | 4(8%) |
| | MQ2: Selection of warfarin in high risk of stroke | Stroke/Embolism | - | 1 | |
| ASTHMA | MQ1: Use of inhaled corticosteroid | Asthma exacerbation | 1 | 3 | 4 (8%) |
| OSTEOPOROSIS | MQ1: Use of bone protecting agent | Fractures | - | 1 | 3(6%) |
| | Use of calcium/vitamin D supplement | Fractures | - | 2 | |
| **Total** | | | **12** | **40** | **52 (100%)** |
| **Medication Quality categories** | | | | | |
| 1. INDICATION | MQ1: Need for treatment to control condition | | 4 | 22 | 26 (52%) |
| 2. SELECTION | MQ2: Selection of first line option within drug class | | 1 | 3 | 4 (8%) |
| 3. INTENSITY | MQ3: Achievement of intermediate outcome target | | 7 | 9 | 16 (31%) |
| | MQ4: Achievement of target dose | | - | 6 | 6 (12%) |
| **Criteria restricted to the elderly** | | | | | |
| Aged ≥ 75 | | | 4 | 4 | 8 (15%) |
| Aged ≥ 80 | | | - | 2 | 2 (4%) |

MQ1 to 4 refer to medication quality categories as specified in the bottom half of the table.

Over half (52%) of safety criteria target the selection of high-risk drugs (MS2 to 4), either for indications where safer (and equally effective) alternatives exist (MS2) or in patients particularly susceptible to adverse reactions because of age/co-morbidity (MS3) or co-prescription (MS4). A further 15 (12%) criteria target omissions of drugs indicated to mitigate the risk of adverse events from high-risk treatments (MS1), while twenty (16%) criteria target inconsistent laboratory monitoring (MS8). Two (2%) criteria focus on prescribing that may jeopardise patient compliance with methotrexate dosing schedules (MS7).

The majority of quality (81%) and safety (71%) assessment criteria are not restricted to the elderly (patients aged 65 years or older).

### Delphi study

Grouping of thematically related assessment criteria that were derived from candidates accepted at the 'necessary' level yielded a total of 47 (18 quality and 29 safety) medication improvement topics to be rated by the Delphi panel. Thirty-six Delphi study participants completed a first round and 26 (73%) a second round questionnaire (table 6). Fifteen (83%) quality and 23 (79%) safety topics were accepted as 'priorities for quality improvement in primary care'. Eleven (7 quality and 4 safety) topics were classified as 'high priorities' and nine (3 quality and 6 safety) topics were rejected because of lower than stipulated median ratings (table 7). There were no differences between pharmacists and GPs with respect to the

**Table 3 Summary of final safety assessment criteria designed from candidates accepted in the modified RAM study as inappropriate (InApp) or necessary to avoid (NecAv)**

| High-risk drug/patient group | Final safety assessment criteria | | | | |
|---|---|---|---|---|---|
| | Medication safety category (MS): Targeted prescribing/monitoring | Associated PDRM event | InApp | NecAv | Total |
| **Drugs frequently implicated in PDRM hospital admissions** | | | | | |
| ANTIPLATELET | MS1: Use without gastroprotection | GI toxicity/bleeding | 1 | 4 | 5 (4%) |
| DIURETIC | MS1: Unmet need for allopurinol in thiazide users | Gout | - | 1 | 11 (9%) |
| | MS3: Use of thiazides in CKD | Renal toxicity | - | 1 | |
| | Use of aldosterone antagonist in CKD | Hyperkalaemia | - | 1 | |
| | MS6: Excess duration of potassium supplement | Hyperkalaemia | - | 1 | |
| | MS8: Inconsistent monitoring of U&E's | Electrolyte disturbances | 2 | 5 | |
| NSAID | MS1: Unmet need for gastroprotection | GI toxicity/bleeding | 1 | 4 | 18 (15%) |
| | MS2: Use of COX II selective agents in aspirin users | CV events | - | 1 | |
| | Paracetamol not tried first | General NSAID toxicity | 1 | 2 | |
| | MS3: Use in CKD | Renal toxicity | - | 2 | |
| | Use of COX II selective agents in high CV risk | CV events | - | 2 | |
| | MS4: Co-prescription with diuretic and/or ACEI or ARB | Renal toxicity | 2 | 3 | |
| ANTICOAGULANT | MS2: Use of warfarin in AF and low risk of stroke | Bleeding | - | 1 | 11 (9%) |
| | MS4: Co-prescription of high-risk anti-infectives | Bleeding | 1 | 9 | |
| OPIOID | MS1: No laxative co-prescribed in strong opioid users | Constipation | 1 | 1 | 2 (2% |
| BETA BLOCKER | MS3: Use in asthma | Asthma exacerbation | 1 | 2 | 4 (3%) |
| | MS4: Co-prescription with verapamil/diltiazem | Bradycardia | - | 1 | |
| ACEI/ARB | MS8: Inconsistent monitoring of U&E's | Hyperkalaemia | - | 2 | 2 (2%) |
| ANTIDIABETIC | MS3: Use of long acting sulphonylureas in CKD | Hypoglycaemia | - | 1 | 2 (2%) |
| | Use of metformin in CKD | Lactic acidosis | - | 1 | |
| DIGOXIN | MS5: Excessive dose in CKD or the elderly | Digoxin toxicity | - | 2 | 10 (8%) |
| | Excessive dose in patients on interacting drugs | | - | 6 | |
| | MS8: Inconsistent monitoring of U&E's | | - | 2 | |
| ORAL STEROID | MS1: Unmet need for bone protecting agents | Bone fracture | - | 2 | 2 (2%) |
| **Other drugs implicated in severe adverse drug events** | | | | | |
| DMARD | MS7: Lack of dose instructions/Use of 2 strengths | Miscellaneous | - | 2 | 10 (8%) |
| | MS8: Inconsistent monitoring of FBC | Blood dyscrasias | 2 | 6 | |
| FEMALE | MS3: Use of estrogens in women w/o hysterectomy | Gynaecological cancer | - | 1 | 7 (6%) |
| STEROIDS | MS3: Use in women with CVD or CVD risk > 20% | Vascular events | 2 | 2 | |
| | MS6: Excess duration in postmenopausal women | | 1 | 1 | |
| AMIODARONE | MS8: Inconsistent monitoring of thyroid function | Thyroid disturbances | - | 1 | 1 (1%) |
| THEOPHYLLIN | MS2: Use without inhaled anticholinergics/steroids | Theophylline toxicity | - | 1 | 1 (1%) |
| STATIN | MS5: Excessive dose in patients on interacting drugs | Rhabdomyolysis | - | 5 | 5 (4%) |
| **Particularly vulnerable patient groups** | | | | | |
| ELDERLY | MS3: Miscellaneous drugs to be avoided | Miscellaneous | 1 | 10 | 18 (15%) |
| | MS6: Miscellaneous drugs for excessive duration | Miscellaneous | - | 7 | |
| HEART FAILURE | MS3: Miscellaneous drugs to be generally avoided | HF exacerbation | - | 10 | 10 (8%) |
| CHILDREN | MS3: Miscellaneous drugs to be generally avoided | Miscellaneous | 1 | 4 | 5 (4%) |
| **Total** | | | 17 | 107 | 124 (100%) |
| **Medication Safety (MS) categories** | | | | | |
| 1. INDICATION | MS1: Unmet need for risk mitigating drug | | 3 | 12 | 15 (12%) |
| 2. SELECTION | MS2: High risk drug without compelling indication | | 1 | 5 | 64 (52%) |
| | MS3: Drug-disease or Drug-age interaction | | 5 | 37 | |
| | MS4: Drug-Drug interaction (DDI) | | 3 | 13 | |
| 3. INTENSITY | MS5: Excessive dose | | - | 13 | 23 (19%) |

**Table 3 Summary of final safety assessment criteria designed from candidates accepted in the modified RAM study as inappropriate (InApp) or necessary to avoid (NecAv)** *(Continued)*

|  |  |  |  |  |
|---|---|---|---|---|
|  | MS6: Excessive duration | 1 | 9 |  |
| 4. COMPLIANCE | MS7: Issues related to patient compliance | - | 2 | 2 (2%) |
| 5. MONITORING | MS8: Inconsistent laboratory monitoring | 4 | 16 | 20 (16%) |
| **Criteria restricted to the elderly** |  |  |  |  |
| Aged ≥ 65 |  | 3 | 21 | 24 (19%) |
| Aged ≥ 75 |  | 2 | 9 | 11 (9%) |
| Aged ≥ 85 |  | 1 | - | 1 (1%) |

MS 1 to 8 refer to medication quality categories as specified in the bottom half of the table.

**Table 4 Quality assessment criteria generated from candidates that the RAM panel classified as 'appropriate but not necessary to do' (A) and 'appropriate and necessary to do' (N)**

| Topic No. | Treatment targeted - Associated PDRM event (Medication quality category) |
|---|---|
| HYPERTENSION |  |

**Q1** **Selection of first line antihypertensives - Hypertension complications (MQ2)**

1. (N) Patient with HTN and without CHD - is started on antihypertensive treatment with a first-line antihypertensive

**Q2** **Treatment to blood pressure (BP) target - Hypertension complications (MQ3)**

Patient aged < 75 years, who has a history of hypertension WITHOUT complications

2. (N) and BP is > 150/90 mmHg on < 3 antihypertensive drugs - has antihypertensive treatment intensified

3. (N) and BP is > 140/85 mmHg on < 2 antihypertensive drugs - has antihypertensive treatment intensified

4. (A) and BP is > 140/85 mmHg on < 3 antihypertensive drugs - has antihypertensive treatment intensified

Patient aged ≥ 75 years, who has a history of hypertension WITHOUT complications

5. (N) and BP is > 150/90 mmHg on < 2 antihypertensive drugs - has antihypertensive treatment intensified

6. (N) and BP is > 140/85 mmHg without antihypertensive treatment - has antihypertensive treatment started

7. (A) and BP is > 150/90 mmHg on < 3 antihypertensive drugs - has antihypertensive treatment intensified

8. (A) and BP is > 140/85 mmHg on < 2 antihypertensive drugs - has antihypertensive treatment intensified

Patient aged < 75 years, who has a history of hypertension WITH complications

9. (N) and BP is > 130/80 mmHg on < 2 antihypertensive drugs - has antihypertensive treatment intensified

Patient aged ≥ 75 years, who has a history of hypertension WITH complications

10. (N) and BP is > 140/85 mmHg on < 2 antihypertensive drugs - has antihypertensive treatment intensified

11. (N) and BP is > 130/80 mmHg without antihypertensive treatment - has antihypertensive treatment intensified

12. (A) and BP is > 140/85 mmHg on < 3 antihypertensive drugs - has antihypertensive treatment intensified

13. (A) and BP is > 130/80 mmHg on < 2 antihypertensive drugs - has antihypertensive treatment intensified

DIABETES MELLITUS

**Q3** **Treatment to HbA1c target - Diabetes complications (MQ3)**

Patient with diabetes mellitus type 2,

14. (N) who has HbA1c of > 7% on < 2 oral antidiabetic drugs - has antidiabetic treatment intensified

15. (N) who has HbA1c of > 9% on < 3 oral antidiabetic drugs - has antidiabetic treatment intensified

16. (A) who has HbA1c of 6.6 to 7% without antidiabetic treatment - has antidiabetic treatment intensified

17. (A) who has HbA1c of 7.6 to 9% on < 3 oral antidiabetic drugs - has antidiabetic treatment intensified

**Q4** **Selection of first line oral antidiabetic - Diabetes complications (MQ2)**

18. (N) Patient with diabetes mellitus type 2, who is overweight - is started on metformin

**Q5** **Indication for ACEI or ARB in patients with renal complications - Diabetes complications (MQ1)**

19. (N) Patient with diabetes mellitus and micro-albuminuria - is prescribed an ACEI or ARB

AT RISK OF/MANIFEST VASCULAR DISEASE

**Q6** **Indication for statin in patients with manifest vascular disease or risk factors - Vascular events (MQ1)**

20. (N) Patient with previous vascular events (MI, stroke or TIA) - is prescribed a statin

21. (N) Patient with peripheral vascular disease - is prescribed a statin

22. (N) Patient aged > 40 with DM without established vascular disease - is prescribed a statin

23. (A) Patient with 10 year CVD risk > 20% without diabetes - is prescribed a statin

**Table 4 Quality assessment criteria generated from candidates that the RAM panel classified as 'appropriate but not necessary to do' (A) and 'appropriate and necessary to do' (N)** *(Continued)*

| | |
|---|---|
| Q7 | **Treatment to target statin dose in patients with manifest vascular disease or risk factors - Vascular events (MQ4)** |
| | 24. (N) Patient with previous vascular events (MI, stroke or TIA) - is prescribed simvastatin ≥ 40 mg/d (or equivalent) |
| | 25. (N) Patient with peripheral vascular disease - is prescribed simvastatin ≥ 40 mg/d (or equivalent) |
| | 26. (N) Patient aged > 40 with DM without established vascular disease - is prescribed simvastatin ≥ 40 mg/d (or equiv.) |
| | 27. (N) Patient with 10 year CVD risk > 20% without diabetes - is prescribed simvastatin ≥ 40 mg/d (or equivalent) |
| Q8 | **Indication for thrombo-embolic prophylaxis in patients with CHD - Vascular events (MQ1)** |
| | 28. (N) Patient with previous vascular events (MI, stroke or TIA) - is prescribed any thrombo-embolic prophylaxis |
| | 29. (N) Patient with a history of peripheral vascular disease - is prescribed any thrombo-embolic prophylaxis |
| | Indication for dual antiplatelets in CHD with a history of ACS - Vascular events (MQ1) |
| | 30. (N) Patient with previous stroke/TIA - is co-prescribed aspirin and dipyridamole (unless on warfarin or clopidogrel) |
| | 31. (N) Patient with ACS 0 to 3 months ago - is co-prescribed aspirin and clopidogrel (unless on warfarin) |
| | 32. (A) Patient with ACS 4 to 9 months ago - is co-prescribed aspirin and clopidogrel (unless on warfarin) |
| Q9 | **Indication for beta blockers in CHD - Vascular events (MQ1)** |
| | 33. (N) Patient with a history of acute coronary syndrome - is prescribed a beta blocker |
| | 34. (N) Patient with stable angina without a history of acute coronary syndrome - is prescribed a beta blocker |
| Q10 | **Indication for ACEI or ARB in CHD - Vascular events (MQ1)** |
| | 35. (N) Patient with a history of acute coronary syndrome - is prescribed an ACEI or ARB |
| | 36. (A) Patient with stable angina without a history of acute coronary syndrome - is prescribed an ACEI or ARB |

**CHRONIC HEART FAILURE**

| | |
|---|---|
| Q11 | **Indication for ACEI or ARB in CHF - Heart failure progression (MQ1)** |
| | 37. (N) Patient with CHF - is prescribed an ACE or ARB |
| Q12 | **Indication for Beta blocker in CHF - Heart failure progression (MQ1)** |
| | 38. (N) Patient with CHF - is prescribed a beta blocker |
| | **Selection of licensed beta blocker in CHF - Heart failure progression (MQ2)** |
| | 39. (A) Patient with CHF and treated with a BB - is prescribed a BB licensed for CHF |
| Q13 | **Treatment to target dose (ACEI and ARB) in CHF - Heart failure progression (MQ4)** |
| | 40. (N) Patient with CHF and treated with an ACEI or ARB - has achieved the recommended target dose |
| Q13 | **Treatment to target dose (beta blocker) - CHF- Prevention of heart failure progression (MQ4)** |
| | 41. (N) Patient with CHF and treated with a beta blocker - has achieved the recommended target dose |

**ATRIAL FIBRILLATION**

| | |
|---|---|
| Q14 | **Indication for thrombo-embolic prophylaxis in AF - Thrombo-embolism (MQ1)** |
| | 42. (N) Patient with atrial fibrillation and a CHADS2 score of 0 or 1 - is prescribed thrombo-embolic prophylaxis |
| | 43. (N) Patient with atrial fibrillation and a CHADS2 score of 2 - is prescribed thrombo-embolic prophylaxis |
| | 44. (N) Patient with atrial fibrillation and a CHADS2 score ≥ 3 - is prescribed thrombo-embolic prophylaxis |
| Q15 | **Selection of thrombo-embolic prophylaxis in AF - Thrombo-embolism (MQ2)** |
| | 45. (N) Patient with AF and a CHADS$_2$ score ≥ 3 treated with an antithrombotic - is prescribed an oral anticoagulant |

**ASTHMA**

| | |
|---|---|
| Q16 | **Indication for inhaled corticosteroids in asthma - Asthma exacerbation (MQ1)** |
| | Patient aged > 4 with asthma but without COPD and |
| | 46. (N) is treated with a step 3 drug* - is also prescribed an inhaled corticosteroid |
| | 47. (N) has received oral prednisolone in last 12 weeks - is also prescribed an inhaled corticosteroid |
| | 48. (N) has received ≥ 3 prescriptions of SABAs in last 12 weeks - is also prescribed an inhaled corticosteroid |
| | 49. (A) has received 2 prescriptions of SABAs in last 12 weeks - is also prescribed an inhaled corticosteroid |
| | * long acting beta agonist, leukotriene receptor antagonist or theophylline |

**OSTEOPOROSIS**

| | |
|---|---|
| Q17 | **Indication for bone protecting agents in patients with osteoporosis - Fractures (MQ1)** |
| | 50. (N) Female patient with osteoporosis who had a vertebral fracture - is prescribed a bone protecting agent* |
| | * a bisphosphonate, strontium ranelate, raloxifene or teriparatide |
| Q18 | **Indication for Calcium/vitamin D in patients at risk of osteoporosis - Fractures (MQ1)** |
| | 51. (N) Female patient aged ≥ 80 who is housebound - is prescribed calcium and vitamin D |

**Table 4 Quality assessment criteria generated from candidates that the RAM panel classified as 'appropriate but not necessary to do' (A) and 'appropriate and necessary to do' (N)** *(Continued)*

| |
|---|
| 52. (N) Female patient aged ≥ 80 who lives in a nursing home/residential care - is prescribed calcium and vitamin D |

The criteria are organised hierarchically by medical condition, followed by the drug group targeted, quality topic scored in the Delphi study (Q) and by medication use quality category (MQ). MQ1 = indication for beneficial treatment, MQ2 = Selection of most effective option within drug class, MQ3 = Achievement of intermediate outcome target, MQ4 = Achievement of target dose

**Table 5 Safety assessment criteria generated from candidates that the RAM panel classified as 'inappropriate' (I) or 'necessary to avoid' (N)**

| Topic No. | Treatment targeted - Associated PDRM event (Medication safety category) |
|---|---|
| **A. DRUGS FREQUENTLY IMPLICATED IN PDRM HOSPITAL ADMISSIONS** | |
| ANTIPLATELETS | |
| S1 | **High-risk use without gastro-intestinal protection (GIP) - GI toxicity/bleeding (MS1)** |
| | 1. (N) Patient with previous peptic ulcer (PU) treated with low dose aspirin - is not prescribed GIP |
| | 2. (N) Patient aged ≥ 65 treated with warfarin AND low dose aspirin - is not prescribed GIP |
| | 3. (N) Patient aged ≥ 65 treated with warfarin AND clopidogrel - is not prescribed GIP |
| | 4. (N) Patient aged ≥ 65 treated with low dose aspirin AND clopidogrel - is not prescribed GIP |
| | 5. (I) Patient aged ≥ 75 years treated with low dose aspirin - is not prescribed GIP |
| NSAIDS | |
| S1 | **High-risk use without gastroprotection (GIP) - GI toxicity/bleeding (MS1)** |
| | 6. (N) Patient with previous PU treated with an oral NS NSAID for > 12 weeks - is not prescribed GIP |
| | 7. (N) Patient is aged ≥ 75 years treated with an oral NS NSAID for > 12 weeks - is not prescribed GIP |
| | 8. (I) Patient is aged 65 to 74 treated with an oral NS NSAID for > 12 weeks - is not prescribed GIP |
| S1 | **High-risk use without gastroprotection - GI toxicity/bleeding (MS1)** |
| | 9. (N) Patient aged ≥ 65 treated with warfarin AND an oral NS NSAID - is not prescribed GIP |
| | 10. (N) Patient aged ≥ 65 treated with low dose aspirin AND an oral NS NSAID for > 12 weeks - is not prescribed GIP |
| S2 | **High risk drug without compelling indication - General drug specific toxicity (MS2)** |
| | 11. (N) Patient aged ≥ 65 - is prescribed an oral NSAID for osteoarthritis without previous trial of full dose paracetamol |
| | 12. (N) Patient aged ≥ 75 - is prescribed an oral NSAID for minor trauma without previous trial of full dose paracetamol |
| | 13. (I) Patient aged 65 to 74 - is prescribed an oral NSAID for minor trauma without previous trial of full dose paracetamol |
| S3 | **High-risk selection in renal impairment - Renal toxicity (MS3)** |
| | 14. (N) Patient with CKD stage 3 - is prescribed an oral NSAID |
| | 15. (N) Patient with CKD stage 4 or 5 - is prescribed an oral NSAID |
| S3 | **Drug-Drug interaction (additive toxicity) - Renal toxicity (MS4)** |
| | 16. (N) Patient aged ≥ 65 treated with an ACEI or ARB but no diuretic - is co-prescribed an oral NSAID |
| | 17. (N) Patient aged ≥ 75 treated with a diuretic but no ACEI or ARB - is co-prescribed an oral NSAID |
| | 18. (N) Patient treated with an ACEI or ARB AND a diuretic - is co-prescribed an oral NSAID |
| | 19. (I) Patient aged ≤ 65 treated with an ACEI or ARB but no diuretic - is co-prescribed an oral NSAID |
| | 20. (I) Patient aged 65 to 74 treated with a diuretic but no ACEI or ARB - is co-prescribed an oral NSAID |
| S4 | **High-risk drug without compelling indication - CV events (MS2)** |
| | 21. (N) Patient treated with low-dose aspirin - is prescribed an oral COX II selective NSAID |
| S5 | **High-risk selection in patients at high vascular risk- Vascular events (MS3)** |
| | 22. (N) Patient aged > 40 and CVD risk > 20% - is prescribed a COX II selective NSAID |
| | 23. (N) Patient with a history of vascular events - is prescribed a COX II selective NSAID |
| DIURETICS | |
| S6 | **Monitoring of U&E's - Electrolyte imbalance (MS8)** |
| | 24. (N) Patient treated with a potassium sparing diuretic -had no U&Es check before treatment start |
| | 25. (N) Patient treated with a potassium sparing diuretic - had no U&Es check in the last 48 weeks |
| | 26. (N) Patient treated with a loop diuretic - had no U&Es check before treatment start |
| | 27. (N) Patient treated with a loop AND a thiazide diuretic or metolazone - had no U&Es check in the last 24 weeks |
| | 28. (N) Patient treated with a potassium sparing diuretic AND an ACEI or ARB - had no U&Es check in the last 48 weeks |
| | 29. (I) Patient treated with a potassium wasting diuretic - had no U&Es check in the last 48 weeks |

**Table 5 Safety assessment criteria generated from candidates that the RAM panel classified as 'inappropriate' (I) or 'necessary to avoid' (N)** *(Continued)*

|     |     |
| --- | --- |
|     | 30. (I) Patient treated with a potassium sparing diuretic AND an ACEI or ARB - had no U&Es check in the last 24 weeks |
| S7  | **High-risk selection in renal impairment - Renal toxicity/Treatment failure (MS3)** |
|     | 31. (N) Patient with chronic kidney disease stage 4 or 5 - is prescribed a thiazide diuretic |
| S8  | **High-risk use without allopurinol - Gout (MS1)** |
|     | 32. (N) Patient with a history of gout and treated with a thiazide diuretic - is not prescribed allopurinol |
| S9  | **High-risk selection in renal impairment - Electrolyte imbalance (MS3)** |
|     | 33. (N) Patient with CKD stage 4 or 5 - is prescribed an aldosterone antagonist |
| S10 | **Excess duration - Electrolyte imbalance (MS6)** |
|     | 34. (N) Patient treated with a potassium (KI) sparing diuretic - is prescribed a K+ supplement for ≥ 4 weeks |
| ANTICOAGULANTS | |
| S11 | **Drug-Drug interaction (pharmacokinetic) - Bleeding (MS4)** |
|     | 35. (N) Patient treated with warfarin - is co-presribed a macrolide |
|     | 36. (N) Patient treated with warfarin - is co-prescribed a sulfonamide |
|     | 37. (N) Patient treated with warfarin - is co-prescribed an azole antifungal |
|     | 38. (N) Patient treated with warfarin - is co-prescribed metronidazole |
|     | 39. (N) Patient treated with warfarin - is co-prescribed chloramphenicol |
|     | 40. (N) Patient treated with warfarin- is co-prescribed isoniazid |
|     | 41. (N) Patient treated with warfarin - is co-prescribed rifampin |
|     | 42. (N) Patient treated with warfarin - is co-prescribed griseofulvin |
|     | 43. (N) Patient treated with warfarin - is co-prescribed ribavirin |
|     | 44. (I) Patient treated with warfarin - is co-prescribed tetracyclines |
| S12 | **High risk drug without compelling indication- Bleeding (MS2)** |
|     | 45. (N) Patient with atrial fibrillation - is prescribed warfarin despite CHADS2 score = 0 |
| OPIOIDS - CONSTIPATION | |
| S13 | **High-risk use without laxative - Constipation (MS1)** |
|     | 46. (N) Patient treated with a strong opioid (morphine > 10 mg or equivalent) for > 4 weeks - is not prescribed a laxative |
|     | 47. (I) Patient aged ≥ 65 treated with a strong opioid (morphine > 10 mg or equivalent) - is not prescribed a laxative |
| BETA BLOCKERS | |
| S14 | **Drug-drug interaction (additive toxicity) - Bradycardia (MS4)** |
|     | 48. (N) Patient treated with a beta-blocker - is co-prescribed verapamil or diltiazem |
| S15 | **High-risk selection in asthma - Asthma exacerbation (MS3)** |
|     | 49. (N) Patient with active asthma (prescribed beta agonist inhaler in last year) without COPD - is prescribed any oral BB |
|     | 50. (N) Patient with active asthma without COPD - is prescribed a non-cardio-selective oral BB |
|     | 51. (I) Patient with active asthma without COPD - is prescribed beta-blocker eye drops |
| ACE INHIBITORS (ACEIs) AND ANGIOTENSIN RECEPTOR BLOCKERS (ARBs) | |
| S6  | **Monitoring of U&E's - Electrolyte imbalance (MS8)** |
|     | 52. (N) Patient co-prescribed an ACEI AND ARB - has not had a U&Es check > 24 weeks ago |
|     | Monitoring of U&E's - Electrolyte imbalance (MS8) |
|     | 53. (N) Patient prescribed an ACEI or ARB - has not had a U&Es check before treatment start |
| ANTIDIABETICS | |
| S16 | **High-risk selection in renal impairment- Lactic acidosis (MS3)** |
|     | 54. (N) Patient with chronic kidney disease (CKD) stage 4 or 5 - is prescribed metformin |
| S17 | **High-risk selection in renal impairment - Hypoglycaemia (MS3)** |
|     | 55. (N) Patient with CKD stage 4 or 5 - is prescribed a sulphonylurea other than gliclazide or tolbutamide |
| DIGOXIN | |
| S18 | **Excessive dose (Elderly) - General digoxin toxicity (MS5)** |
|     | 56. (N) Patient aged ≥ 65 years - is prescribed digoxin ≥ 250 mcg/day |
|     | 57. (N) Patient with CKD stage 3, 4 or 5 (eGFR < 60) - is prescribed digoxin ≥ 250 mcg/day |
| S18 | **Excessive dose (DDI without dose adjustment) - General digoxin toxicity (MS5)** |
|     | 58. (N) Patient treated with digoxin and amiodarone - is prescribed digoxin ≥ 250 mcg/day |

## Table 5 Safety assessment criteria generated from candidates that the RAM panel classified as 'inappropriate' (I) or 'necessary to avoid' (N) (Continued)

|  |  |
|---|---|
|  | 59. (N) Patient treated with digoxin and propafenone - is prescribed digoxin ≥ 250 mcg/day |
|  | 60. (N) Patient treated with digoxin and chloroquine or hydroxychloroquine - is prescribed digoxin ≥ 250 mcg/day |
|  | 61. (N) Patient treated with digoxin and quinine - is prescribed digoxin ≥ 250 mcg/day |
|  | 62. (N) Patient treated with digoxin and a calcium channel blocker * - is prescribed digoxin ≥ 250 mcg/day |
|  | 63. (N) Patient treated with digoxin and ciclosporin - is prescribed digoxin ≥ 250 mcg/day |
|  | * lercanidipine, nicardipine, nifedipine, diltiazem, verapamil) |
| S8 | **Monitoring of U&E's - General digoxin toxicity (MS8)** |
|  | 64. (N) Patient is co-prescribed a potassium wasting diuretic AND digoxin with last U&Es check before treatment start |
|  | 65. (N) Patient is co-prescribed a potassium wasting diuretic AND digoxin with last U&Es check > 48 weeks ago |

CORTICOSTEROIDS

| S19 | **High-risk use without bone protecting agent - Bone fracture (MS1)** |
|---|---|
|  | 66. (N) Patient aged ≥ 65 years treated with an oral corticosteroid for ≥ 12 weeks - is not prescribed bone protection * |
|  | 67. (N) Patient with low trauma fracture and treated with an oral corticosteroid for ≥ 12 weeks - is not prescribed bone protection* |
|  | *a bisphosphonate, calcitriol or hormone replacement therapy |

## B. OTHER HIGH RISK DRUGS

DMARDS

| S20 | **High-risk drug without taking action to ensure patient compliance - General toxicity (MS7)** |
|---|---|
|  | 68. (N) Patient treated with methotrexate - has not been given explicit dose instructions of weekly dosing |
|  | 69. (N) Patient treated with methotrexate - is prescribed > 1 strength of methotrexate tablets |
| S21 | **Monitoring of full blood count (FBC) - Blood dyscrasias (MS8)** |
|  | 70. (N) Patient treated with auranofin - had no FBC check in the last 8 weeks |
|  | 71. (N) Patient treated with aurothiomalate - had no FBC check in the last 8 weeks |
|  | 72. (N) Patient treated with penicillamine - had no FBC check in the last 8 weeks |
|  | 73. (N) Patient treated with leflunomide - had no FBC check in the last 12 weeks |
|  | 74. (N) Patient treated with methotrexate - had no FBC check in the last 12 weeks |
|  | 75. (N) Patient treated with azathioprine - had no FBC check in the last 12 weeks |
|  | 76. (I) Patient treated with cyclophosphamide - had no FBC check in the last 24 weeks |
|  | 77. (I) Patient treated with sulfasalazine - had no FBC check in the last 24 weeks |

FEMALE HORMONES

| S22 | **Selection in patients at high vascular risk - Vascular events (MS3)** |
|---|---|
|  | 78. (N) Patient with previous vascular disease/events - is prescribed any hormone replacement therapy (HRT) |
|  | 79. (N) Patient with an estimated 10 year CVD risk ≥ 20% - is prescribed combined contraceptives |
|  | 80. (I) Patient with an estimated 10 year CVD risk ≥ 20% and aged 50 to 59 - is prescribed combined HRT |
|  | 81. (I) Patient with an estimated 10 year CVD risk ≥ 20% and aged ≥ 60 - is prescribed (any) HRT |
| S23 | **Excess duration - Gynaecological cancer (MS6)** |
|  | 82. (N) Patient aged ≥ 50 - is prescribed combined HRT for ≥ 5 years |
|  | 83. (N) Patient aged ≥ 50 without hysterectomy - is prescribed estrogens without cyclical progestogen |
|  | 84. (I) Patient aged ≥ 50 - is prescribed estrogens only HRT for ≥ 5 years |

AMIODARONE

| S24 | **Monitoring of thyroid function - Hypo-/Hyperthyroidism (MS8)** |
|---|---|
|  | 85. (N) Patient prescribed amiodarone - had no thyroid function test in last 9 months |

THEOPHYLLINE

| S25 | **High-risk drug without compelling indication - General theophylline toxicity (MS2)** |
|---|---|
|  | 86. (N) Patient aged ≥ 65 with COPD - is prescribed theophylline without use of a long acting beta2 - agonist or antimuscarinic |

STATINS

| S26 | **Excessive dose (DDI without dose adjustment) - Rhabdomyolysis (MS5)** |
|---|---|
|  | 87. (N) Patient treated with simvastatin and an HIV protease inhibitor - is prescribed simvastatin > 10 mg/day |
|  | 88. (N) Patient treated with simvastatin and ciclosporin - is prescribed simvastatin > 10 mg/day |
|  | 89. (N) Patient treated with simvastatin and verapamil - is prescribed simvastatin > 10 mg/day |
|  | 90. (N) Patient treated with simvastatin and a fibrate (except fenofibrate) - is prescribed simvastatin > 10 mg/day |

**Table 5 Safety assessment criteria generated from candidates that the RAM panel classified as 'inappropriate' (I) or 'necessary to avoid' (N)** *(Continued)*

|  |  |
|---|---|
|  | 91. (N) Patient treated with simvastatin and amiodarone - is prescribed simvastatin > 20 mg/day |

**C. PATIENT GROUPS PARTICULARLY VULNERABLE TO ADVERSE DRUG EVENTS**

ELDERLY PATIENTS

| S27 | **High-risk drug selection in the elderly - Miscellaneous (MS3)** |
|---|---|
|  | 92. (N) Patient aged ≥ 65 with dementia - is prescribed a TCA |
|  | 93. (N) Patient aged ≥ 65 with dementia but no psychosis - is prescribed an antipsychotic |
|  | 94. (N) Patient aged ≥ 65 with dementia and psychosis - is prescribed antipsychotic other than risperidone |
|  | 95. (N) Patient aged ≥ 65 - is prescribed a long acting benzodiazepine |
|  | 96. (N) Patient aged ≥ 65 with Parkinson's disease - is prescribed an antipsychotic other than quetiapine or clozapine |
|  | 97. (N) Patient aged ≥ 65 with Parkinson's disease - is prescribed a phenothiazine antiemetic |
|  | 98. (N) Patient aged ≥ 75 - is prescribed a TCA |
|  | 99. (N) Patient aged ≥ 75 - is prescribed a short acting benzodiazepine |
|  | 100. (N) Patient aged ≥ 75 - is prescribed a Z-drug |
|  | 101. (N) Patient aged ≥ 75 - is prescribed an antihistamine with antimuscarinic properties |
|  | 102. (A) Patient aged > 85 - is prescribed an antispasmodic with antimuscarinic properties |
| S27 | **Excess duration - Miscellaneous (MS6)** |
|  | 103. (N) Patient aged ≥ 65 - is prescribed a TCA for ≥ 4 weeks |
|  | 104. (N) Patient aged ≥ 65 - is prescribed a short acting benzodiazepine for ≥ 4 weeks |
|  | 105. (N) Patient aged ≥ 65 - is prescribed a Z-drug for ≥ 4 weeks |
|  | 106. (N) Patient aged ≥ 65 - is prescribed an antispasmodic with antimuscarinic properties for ≥ 4 weeks |
|  | 107. (N) Patient aged ≥ 65 with dementia and psychosis - is prescribed risperidone for ≥ 12 weeks |
|  | 108. (N) Patient aged 66 to 75 - is prescribed an antihistamine with antimuscarinic properties for ≥ 4 weeks |
|  | 109. (N) Patient aged ≥ 75 - is prescribed urologicals with antimuscarinic properties for ≥ 4 weeks |

PATIENTS WITH HEART FAILURE

| S28 | **Use in heart failure - Heart failure exacerbation (MS3)** |
|---|---|
|  | 110. (N) Patient with chronic heart failure - is prescribed a class 1 or 3 antiarrhythmics except amiodarone |
|  | 111. (N) Patient with chronic heart failure - is prescribed verapamil or diltiazem |
|  | 112. (N) Patient with chronic heart failure - is prescribed minoxidil |
|  | 113. (N) Patient with chronic heart failure - is prescribed any oral NSAID |
|  | 114. (N) Patient with chronic heart failure - is prescribed a glitazone |
|  | 115. (N) Patient with chronic heart failure - is prescribed a tricyclic antidepressant |
|  | 116. (N) Patient with chronic heart failure - is prescribed itraconazole |
|  | 117. (N) Patient with chronic heart failure - is prescribed other antifungals (e.g. ketoconazole, fluconazole) |
|  | 118. (N) Patient with chronic heart failure - is prescribed tadalafil |
|  | 119. (N) Patient with chronic heart failure - is prescribed disulfiram |

CHILDREN AND YOUNG ADULTS

| S29 | **Use in children - Miscellaneous (MS3)** |
|---|---|
|  | 120. (N) Patient aged ≤ 20 - is prescribed a phenothiazine anti-emetic |
|  | 121. (N) Patient aged ≤ 16 who has no record of Kawasaki disease - is prescribed aspirin |
|  | 122. (N) Patient aged ≤ 12 - is prescribed a tetracycline |
|  | 123. (N) Patient aged ≤ 18 - is prescribed an antidepressant other than fluoxetine |
|  | 124. (I) Patient aged ≤ 18 - is prescribed fluoxetine |

The criteria target high-risk use of (A) drugs frequently implicated in PDRM hospital admissions, (B) other drugs implicated in severe PDRM events and (C) medication use in vulnerable groups. Within each domain A to C, the criteria are organised hierarchically by the high-risk drug (group) that is the focus of each criterion, followed by safety topic scored in the Delphi study (S) and medication use safety category (MS). MS1 = Indication for risk mitigating drug; MS2 = High risk drug without compelling indication; MS3 = Drug-disease or Drug-age interaction; MS4 = Drug-Drug interaction (DDI); MS5 = Excessive dose; MS6 = Excessive duration; MS7 = Prescribing issues linked to patient compliance; MS8 = Inconsistent monitoring

assignment of priority levels, and no panel disagreement on any topic (defined in terms of variation in scoring as detailed in the methods section above).

## Discussion

This paper reports the development of a set of 176 explicit assessment criteria to identify patients at risk of

**Table 6 Delphi study: Demographics of the 26 panellists, who completed both rounds of ratings**

| | Pharmacists n = 9 (35%) | | General practitioners n = 17 (65%) | | Total |
|---|---|---|---|---|---|
| | Currently | Previously | Currently | Previously | |
| Works in primary care | 7 | 2 | 17 | - | 26 (100%) |
| Has a prescribing role | 2 | 1 | 17 | - | 20 (77%) |
| Has a strategic role | 2 | - | 1 | 1 | 4 (15%) |
| Mean age in years (SD) | 47 (9) | | 47 (9) | | 47 (9) |
| Mean years since training completed (SD) | 22 (11) | | 22 (9) | | 23 (10) |
| Mean years of experience of working in primary care (SD) | 11 (11) | | 19 (8) | | 15 (8) |

**Table 7 Delphi study priority ratings by the 26 panellists**

| Topic | | Median | Mean | Priority |
|---|---|---|---|---|
| | **Accepted as priorities** | | | |
| | ***Quality*** | | | |
| Q 16 | Not using inhaled corticosteroids in patients with uncontrolled asthma | 8 | 8.0 | ++ |
| Q 15 | Not using oral anticoagulants in patients with AF and high risk of stroke | 8 | 7.9 | ++ |
| Q 11 | Not using ACEIs or ARBs in patients with a history of chronic heart failure | 8 | 7.9 | ++ |
| Q 14 | Not using thrombo-embolic prophylaxis in AF patients at low/moderate risk of stroke | 8 | 7.7 | ++ |
| Q 5 | Not using ACEIs or ARBs in patients with DM and renal complications | 8 | 7.7 | ++ |
| Q 12 | Not using beta blockers in patients with a history of chronic heart failure | 8 | 7.7 | ++ |
| Q 4 | Not using metformin as first line antidiabetic in overweight type 2 diabetics | 8 | 7.6 | ++ |
| Q 8 | Not using antiplatelets in patients at risk of vascular events | 7 | 7.5 | + |
| Q 6 | Not using statins in patients at high risk of cardiovascular events | 7 | 7.4 | + |
| Q 17 | Not using bone sparing agents in female patients at high risk of fractures | 7 | 7.3 | + |
| Q 3 | Low intensity antidiabetic treatment despite suboptimal HbA1c control | 7 | 7.2 | + |
| Q 10 | Not using ACEIs or ARBs in patients with a history of ACS | 7 | 7.0 | + |
| Q 2 | Low intensity antihypertensive treatment despite suboptimal BP control | 7 | 6.9 | + |
| Q 9 | Not using beta blockers in coronary heart disease | 7 | 6.8 | + |
| Q 7 | Underdosing of statins in patients at high risk of cardiovascular events | 7 | 6.7 | + |
| | ***Safety*** | | | |
| S 20 | Using MTX without taking precautionary action to prevent patient overdosing | 9 | 8.4 | ++ |
| S 1 | Not using gastro-protection in oral NSAIDs/antiplatelets users at high risk of bleeding | 8 | 8.2 | ++ |
| S 3 | Using oral NSAIDs in patients at increased risk of renal failure | 8 | 7.9 | ++ |
| S 21 | Inconsistent monitoring of FBC in patients on DMARDs | 8 | 7.8 | ++ |
| S 27 | Using sedatives, antipsychotics, anticholinergics in elderly patients | 7 | 7.3 | + |
| S 19 | Using bone protection in users of long term oral corticosteroids | 7 | 7.3 | + |
| S 23 | Excess duration of female hormones in patients at risk of gynaecological cancer | 7 | 7.3 | + |
| S 10 | Excess duration of potassium supplements *and* potassium sparing diuretics | 7 | 7.2 | + |
| S 28 | Using drugs to avoid in patients with heart failure | 7 | 7.1 | + |
| S 18 | Excessive dosing of digoxin in patients susceptible to digoxin toxicity | 7 | 7.1 | + |
| S 24 | Inconsistent monitoring of thyroid function in patients prescribed amiodarone | 7 | 7.0 | + |
| S 6 | Inconsistent monitoring of U&Es in patients at risk of electrolyte imbalance | 7 | 7.0 | + |
| S 14 | Co-prescribing beta blockers and rate-limiting calcium channel blockers | 7 | 6.9 | + |
| S 25 | Using theophylline in elderly COPD patients without a compelling indication | 7 | 6.9 | + |
| S 15 | Using beta blockers in patients with active asthma | 7 | 6.8 | + |
| S 13 | Not using of laxatives in strong opioid users | 7 | 6.8 | + |
| S 29 | Using drugs to avoid in children and young adults | 7 | 6.7 | + |
| S 5 | Using COX II inhibitors in patients at high risk of cardiovascular events | 7 | 6.6 | + |
| S 7 | Using thiazide diuretics in patients with a history of CKD | 7 | 6.6 | + |
| S 17 | Using long acting sulphonylureas in patients at risk of hypoglycaemia | 7 | 6.6 | + |

**Table 7 Delphi study priority ratings by the 26 panellists** (Continued)

| | | | | |
|------|-------------------------------------------------------------------------------------------------------------------|---|-----|---|
| S 4 | Using COX II inhibitors without compelling indication (low dose aspirin users) | 7 | 6.4 | + |
| S 16 | Using metformin in patients with CKD | 7 | 6.4 | + |
| S 26 | Excessive dosing of statins in patients on interacting drugs | 7 | 6.3 | + |
| | **Not scored as priorities for medication improvement** | | | |
| | *Quality* | | | |
| Q 13 | Inadequate dose titration of ACEI, ARBs and BBs in chronic heart failure | 6 | 6.2 | |
| Q 1 | Not using first line antihypertensives when initiating treatment for high blood pressure | 6 | 6.4 | |
| Q 18 | Not using calcium/vitamin D supplementation in female elderly patients | 6 | 6.4 | |
| | *Safety* | | | |
| S 2 | Using oral NSAIDs in the elderly without compelling indication (no previous trial of full dose paracetamol) | 6 | 6.6 | |
| S 9 | Using of aldosterone antagonists in patients with a history of CKD | 6 | 6.5 | |
| S 11 | Co-prescribing anti-infectives with high risk of affecting INR in patients on warfarin | 6 | 6.4 | |
| S 12 | Using warfarin without a compelling indication in AF with low risk of stroke | 6 | 6.3 | |
| S 22 | Using HRT in female patients at high risk of cardiovascular events | 6 | 6.2 | |
| S 8 | Not using allopurinol in thiazide users with a history of gout | 6 | 5.8 | |

Topics are ranked by median scores. Clusters of topics with the same median are ranked in descending order of mean score. Topics with a median of 8 or higher ('high priority') are coded '++' and those with a median of 7 ('priority') '+'.

PDRM from electronic data sources routinely held in UK primary care. The criteria set targets suboptimal selection, intensity or omissions of beneficial drug treatments (medication use quality) and high-risk use, inconsistent monitoring or patient instructions for drugs implicated in preventable harm (medication use safety) in primary care. All items are classified by clinical importance (appropriateness and necessity) as the output of an extended RAM process. Key professionals in UK primary care identified eleven clusters of thematically related medication assessment criteria (topics) as 'high priority' for quality improvement initiatives. The three highest rated topics related to methotrexate dosing instructions, high-risk prescribing of NSAIDs and antiplatelets and underuse of corticosteroids in asthma.

### Development process of the DQIP criteria set

The RAM approach had advantages over the Delphi technique as an initial step in the criteria development process, because the face-to-face meeting ensured the necessary commitment of panellists to place ratings on an extensive and thematically broad list of candidate criteria that were grounded in the evidence base. The original RAM approach was extended in this study by introducing the concept of 'necessary to avoid', in order to distinguish between inappropriate ('not worthwhile') and 'improper' medication use in safety terms (see table 1). As for the distinction between 'appropriate' and 'necessary', panellists required examples to apply and reason the concepts, but the absence of paradoxical 'appropriateness' and 'necessity' ratings is consistent with a reliable rating process.

A limitation of consensus methods such the RAM is that ratings may depend on panel composition [42]. The chosen panel combined clinical, public health and academic expertise in primary care medication use in general, rather than specialist expertise in the management of each medical condition covered. It is possible that generalists underestimate the implications of suboptimal medication use because they do not individually see relatively rare PDRM events that have significant impact at population level. Conversely, specialists tend to overestimate the importance of practices that fall within their own specialty [47,48]. However, since relatively few candidate criteria (22%) were rejected, it seems unlikely that including specialists would have substantially altered the results.

### Scope and focus of the DQIP criteria set

Consistent with the intended use of the DQIP criteria set, our literature search targeted commonly encountered medical conditions and drug groups implicated in PDRM events in primary care rather than exclusively focussing on the elderly. As a consequence, only 27% of all developed criteria are restricted to patients over 65 years with the majority of generated assessment criteria covering aspects of medication use which are not or not exclusively relevant to the elderly [8-10,49], such as primary prevention of vascular events, use of anti-diabetics in renal impairment [36] and treatments that are potentially harmful in children [36]. The fact that all topics identified as 'high priority' by the Delphi panel are age independent additionally underlines the relevance of not restricting a criteria set to be used in primary care to the elderly as is the case with many existing criteria sets [8-10,49].

A limitation of the medication assessment criteria developed for this study is that several established and potentially important criteria were not considered because the study focused on those that could be applied routinely to existing UK electronic clinical data. For example, international normalised ratio (INR) results in the UK are often held in bespoke systems which hinder the implementation of meaningful measures for monitoring anticoagulant use [1-4]. Similarly, although a broad spectrum of medication use categories are covered, the criteria set is mainly focussed on the prescribing and monitoring stages of the medication use process with minimal coverage of patient education and compliance. In the future, the increasing sophistication of clinical information systems and the ability to link clinical datasets with laboratory systems and dispensing data would make an even broader set of assessment criteria feasible.

Although the DQIP criteria set has been developed for application in UK primary care, the drug groups reported to be implicated in PDRM events in primary care are similar internationally [50-52], and we would expect the areas focused on to be relevant in other countries and health care settings. Nevertheless, some local adaptation may be required in order to account for differences in drug licensing, available resources, and clinical guidelines.

## Implications for quality improvement initiatives

The Delphi approach allowed stakeholders in primary care to prioritise the chosen medication use topics for improvement initiatives in UK primary care. The Delphi panel was deliberately chosen to include both day to day prescribers (GPs do almost all primary care prescribing, especially of the more complex kind being assessed in this study, but pharmacists prescribe for some patients and conditions) and those involved in prescribing governance and improvement (predominately pharmacists but including GPs with a more strategic role). A limitation is that our focus on professionals involved in primary care prescribing meant that we did not seek to include either specialist or patient/public perspectives in the Delphi panel. Since there is evidence that practitioners' perceptions of a targeted behaviour as meaningful is a pre-requisite to changing behaviour [53] we aimed to identify medication improvement topics which met this condition to inform the design of an intervention targeting primary care professionals.

It is important to note that even those topics that were not considered to be priorities (3 quality - and 6 safety topics) contain individual criteria that were agreed to be 'necessary' to do or avoid by the RAM panel. Examples are 'inadequate dose titration of ACEI, ARBs and beta blockers in chronic heart failure', and the 'using of warfarin without a compelling indication in atrial fibrillation

with low risk of stroke'. These should therefore not be neglected. Lower priority ratings nevertheless indicate that changing and improving the corresponding medication use aspects may require targeted effort (or resources) in order to influence prescribing behaviour.

## Conclusions

The DQIP medication assessment criteria set presented here has been developed using established consensus methods and complements existing medication assessment instruments by not being limited to the elderly and by targeting a wide spectrum of medication use practices implicated in common and/or severe PDRM events in primary care. As all previously published explicit medication assessment tools, the criteria set presented here does not, however, provide comprehensive coverage of all situations that put patients at risk of PDRM, reflecting the large scope and high complexity of medication use in primary care and the limitations of current UK clinical information systems. The best choice of criteria set will therefore depend on the main purpose to be addressed and will be guided by local priorities. Informed by the priority ratings of a panel of UK primary care professionals, we have selected a subset of the DQIP criteria to serve as outcome measures in a cluster randomised trial evaluating the effectiveness of a complex intervention to improve prescribing safety (Trial registration number NCT01425502).

The DQIP criteria were primarily developed to facilitate the identification of patients at risk of PDRM from routine electronic data sets for a targeted review of their medication. However, we anticipate that they could also serve a range of other purposes, for example by informing the design of clinical decision support systems, where the classification of criteria by 'appropriateness' and 'necessity' may guide the selection of alerts that should or should not be interruptive to clinicians' workflow. Performance feedback is a further potential application, but in order not to overwhelm practitioners, the developed criteria are likely to require further prioritisation and/or the design of meaningful composites, for example by aggregating items that address the same topic [54] or medication use category [13].

An inherent limitation of explicit assessment criteria is that they cannot fully account for clinical factors that may justify deviations from what is considered to be best practice in an 'average' patient. The extent to which patients identified to be at risk of PDRM are judged by practitioners to represent actual opportunities for improvement (concurrent validity) and the extent to which any improvements in prescribing or monitoring translate into improved patient outcomes (predictive validity) therefore deserve further study.

## List of abbreviations

**ACEI:** Angiotensin converting enzyme inhibitor; **ACOVE:** Assessing care of vulnerable elders; **ACS:** Acute coronary syndrome; **ADE:** Adverse drug event; **AF:** Atrial fibrillation; **ARB:** Angiotensin receptor blocker; **BB:** Beta blocker; **BP:** Blood pressure; **CCB:** Calcium channel blocker; **CHADS$_2$:** Score for stroke risk assessment in atrial fibrillation based on the following risk factors: cardiac failure, hypertension, age > 75, diabetes and stroke; **CHD:** Coronary heart disease; **CHD:** Coronary Heart Disease; **CHF:** Chronic heart failure; **CKD:** Chronic kidney disease; **CKD:** Chronic kidney disease; **COPD:** Chronic obstructive pulmonary disease; **COX:** Cyclo-oxygenase; **CVD:** Cardiovascular disease; **DM:** Diabetes mellitus; **DMARD:** Disease modifying antirheumatic drug; **DQIP:** Data driven quality improvement in primary care; **eGFR:** Estimated glomerular filtration rate; **FBC:** Full blood count; **GIP:** Gastro-intestinal protective agents; **GP:** General practitioner; **HbA1c:** Glycated haemoglobin; **HIV:** Human immunodeficiency virus; **HRT:** Hormone replacement therapy; **HTN:** Hypertension; **INR:** International normalised ratio; **IT:** Information technology; **MI:** Myocardial infarction; **MTX:** Methotrexate; **NSAID:** Non-steroidal anti-inflammatory drug (includes non-selective and COXII selective agents unless stated otherwise); **NS NSAID:** Non-selective NSAID **NYHA:** New York Heart Association; **PDRM:** Preventable drug related morbidity; **RAM:** RAND appropriateness method; **SABA:** Short acting beta 2 receptor agonist; **SD:** Standard deviation; **START:** Screening tool to alert doctors to right treatment; **STOPP:** Screening tool of older person's prescriptions; **TCA:** Tricyclic antidepressant; **TIA:** Transient ischaemic attack; **U&E:** Urea and electrolytes; **UCLA:** University College of Los Angeles; **UK:** United Kingdom; **Z-drug:** zopiclone, zolpidem or zaleplone.

## Acknowledgements

The study was funded by the Chief Scientist Office of Scottish Government Health Directorates programme grant ARPG/07/02. The authors would like to thank all participants in the RAM and Delphi panels and Debby O'Farrell for administrative support for both consensus studies.

## Author details

[1]Tayside Medicines Unit, NHS Tayside, Mackenzie Building, Kirsty Semple Way, Dundee, Scotland, DD2 4BF, UK. [2]Population Health Sciences, University of Dundee, Mackenzie Building, Kirsty Semple Way, Dundee, Scotland, DD2 4BF, UK. [3]NHS 24 East Contact Centre, 2 Ferrymuir, South Queensferry, Scotland, EH3 0 9QZ, UK.

## Authors' contributions

The study is part of the Data-driven Quality Improvement in Primary Care (DQIP) research programme, which is led by BG. TD led the literature review, conduct of RAM and Delphi studies, data analysis and wrote the first draft of the manuscript. All co-authors contributed to subsequent drafts. All authors have read and approved the final manuscript.

## Competing interests

The authors declare that they have no competing interests.

## References

1. Howard RL, Avery AJ, Slavenburg S, Royal S, Pipe G, Lucassen P, Pirmohamed M: **Which drugs cause preventable admissions to hospital? A systematic review.** *British Journal of Clinical Pharmacology* 2006, **63**(2):136-147.

2. Pirmohamed MJ, Meakin S, Green C, Scott AK, Walley TJ, Farrar K, Park BK, Breckenridge AM: **Adverse drug reactions as a cause of admission to hospital: prospective analysis of 18 820 patients.** *BMJ* 2004, **329**:15-19.

3. Thomsen LA, Winterstein AG, Søndergaard B, Haugbølle LS, Melander A: **Systematic Review of the Incidence and Characteristics of Preventable Adverse Drug Events in Ambulatory Care.** *The Annals of Pharmacotherapy* 2007, **41**:1411-1426.

4. Winterstein AG SB, Hepler CD, Poole C: **Preventable drug related hospital admissions.** *Ann Pharmacother* 2002, **36**:1238-1248.

5. National Patient Safety Agency (2006): **Improving compliance with oral methotrexate guideline.**, Available at http://www.nrls.npsa.nhs.uk/resources/?entryid45=59800.

6. Medicines and Healthcare Products Regulatory Agency CoHM: **Antipsychotics: use in elderly people with dementia.** *Drug Saf Update* 2009, **2**(8).

7. Howard R, Avery A, Bissell P: **Causes of preventable drug-related hospital admissions: a qualitative study.** *Qual Saf Health Care* 2007, **17**:109-116.

8. Fick DM, Cooper JW, Wade WE, Waller JL, Maclean JR, Beers MH: **Updating the Beers Criteria for Potentially Inappropriate Medication Use in Older Adults: Results of a US Consensus Panel of Experts.** *Arch Intern Med* 2003, **163**(22):2716-2724.

9. Shekelle PG, MacLean CH, Morton SC, Wenger NS: **Acove quality indicators.** *Annals of Internal Medicine* 2001, **135**(8 Pt 2):653-667.

10. Gallagher P, Ryan C, Byrne S, Kennedy J, O'Mahony D: **STOPP (Screening Tool of Older Person's Prescriptions) and START (Screening Tool to Alert doctors to Right Treatment). Consensus validation.** *International Journal of Clinical Pharmacology & Therapeutics* 2008, **46**(2):72-83.

11. Instituut vor Verantwoord Medicijngebruik (IVM): **Rapport. Benchmark Voorschrijven 2010 (in Dutch).**, Available at http://www.medicijngebruik.nl/projecten/benchmark-voorschrijven.html.

12. National Prescribing Service Limited: **Indicators of Quality Prescribing in Australian General Practice (2006). A manual for users.**, Available at http://www.nps.org.au/health_professionals/tools/quality_prescribing_indicators_in_australian_general_practice.

13. Wessell AM, Litvin C, Jenkins RG, Nietert PJ, Nemeth LS, Ornstein SM: **Medication prescribing and monitoring errors in primary care: a report from the Practice Partner Research Network.** *Quality & Safety in Health Care* 2010, **19**(5):e21.

14. Strand LM, Cipolle RJ, Morley PC, Frakes MJ: **The impact of Pharmaceutical care Practice on the practitioner and the patient in the ambulatory care setting: 25 years of experience.** *Current Pharmaceutical Design* 2004, 3987-4001.

15. Martirosyan L, Voorham J, Haaijer-Ruskamp FM, Braspenning J, Wolffenbuttel BH: **A systematic literature review: prescribing indicators related to type 2 diabetes mellitus and cardiovascular risk management.** *Pharmacoepidemiol Drug Saf* 2010, **19**(4):319-334.

16. The American College of Cardiology and American Heart Association Task Force on practice guidelines and the European Society of Cardiology Committee for Practice Guidelines (Writing Committee to Revise the 2001 guidelines for the management of patients with atrial fibrillation): **ACC/AHA/ESC 2006 guidelines for the management of patients with atrial fibrillation. Developed in collaboration with the European Heart Rhythm Association and the Heart Rhythm Society.** *Europace* 2006, **8**(9):651-745.

17. National Collaborating Centre for Chronic Conditions: **Atrial fibrillation: National clinical guideline for management in primary and secondary care (update).** *National Institute for Clinical Excellence, London* 2006, Available at http://www.nice.org.uk/nicemedia/live/10982/30055/30055.pdf.

18. National Collaborating Centre for Chronic Conditions: **Type 2 Diabetes: National clinical guideline for management in primary and secondary care (update).** *National Institute for Clinical Excellence, London* 2008, Available at http://www.nice.org.uk/nicemedia/live/11983/40803/40803.pdf.

19. National Institute for Health and Clinical Excellence: **Alendronate, etidronate, risedronate, raloxifene, strontium ranelate and teriparatide for the secondary prevention of osteoporotic fragility fractures in postmenopausal women. NICE Technology appraisal guidance number 161.** *National Institute for Health and Clinical Excellence, London* 2008, Available at http://www.nice.org.uk/nicemedia/pdf/TA160guidance.pdf.

20. Scottish Intercollegiate Guidelines Network: **Acute coronary syndromes.** *SIGN publication number 93, Edinburgh* 2007, Available at http://www.sign.ac.uk/guidelines/fulltext/93-97/index.html.

21. Scottish Intercollegiate Guidelines Network: **Management of stable angina.** *SIGN publication number 96, Edinburgh* 2007, Available at http://www.sign.ac.uk/guidelines/fulltext/93-97/index.html.

22. Scottish Intercollegiate Guidelines Network: **Management of chronic heart failure.** *SIGN publication number 95, Edinburgh* 2007, Available at http://www.sign.ac.uk/guidelines/fulltext/93-97/index.html.

23. Scottish Intercollegiate Guidelines Network: **Risk estimation and the prevention of cardiovascular disease.** *SIGN publication number 97, Edinburgh* 2007, Available at http://www.sign.ac.uk/guidelines/fulltext/93-97/index.html.

24. Scottish Intercollegiate Guidelines Network: **British guideline on the management of asthma.** *SIGN publication number 101. Edinburgh* 2008, Available at http://www.sign.ac.uk/guidelines/fulltext/101/index.html.

25. The Task Force for the diagnosis and treatment of acute and chronic heart failure of the European Society of Cardiology (ESC): ESC guidelines for the diagnosis and treatment of acute and chronic heart failure 2008. Developed in collaboration with the Heart Failure Association of the ESC (HFA) and endorsed by the European Society of Intensive Care Medicine (ESICM). *European Journal of Heart Failure* 2008, **10(10)**:933-989.

26. Komajda M, Drexler H: Lessons from the European heart survey. *Circulation* 2006, **113(7)**:f25-26.

27. Anselmino M, Bartnik M, Malmberg K, Ryden L: Euro Heart Survey I: Management of coronary artery disease in patients with and without diabetes mellitus. Acute management reasonable but secondary prevention unacceptably poor: a report from the Euro Heart Survey on Diabetes and the Heart. *European Journal of Cardiovascular Prevention & Rehabilitation* 2007, **14(1)**:28-36.

28. Leiter LA, Betteridge DJ, Chacra AR, Chait A, Ferrannini E, Haffner SM, Kadowaki T, Tuomilehto J, Zimmet P, Newman CB, Hey-Hadavi J, Walkinshaw C: AUDIT study. Evidence of global undertreatment of dyslipidaemia in patients with type 2 diabetes mellitus. *The British Journal of Diabetes & Vascular Disease* 2006, **6(1)**:31-40.

29. Cleland JGF, Swedberg K, Follath F, Komajda M, Cohen-Solal A, Aguilar JC, Dietz R, Gavazzi A, Hobbs R, Korewicki J, Madeira HC, Moiseyev VS, Preda I, van Gilst WH, Widimsky J, Freemantle N, Eastaugh J, Mason J: The EuroHeart Failure survey programme–a survey on the quality of care among patients with heart failure in Europe. *European Heart Journal* 2003, **24(5)**:442-463.

30. Nieuwlaat R, Capucci A, Camm AJ, Olsson SB, Andresen D, Davies DW, Cobbe S, Breithardt G, Le Heuzey J-Y, Prins MH, Levy S, Crijns H: Atrial fibrillation management: a prospective survey in ESC member countries: The Euro Heart Survey on Atrial Fibrillation. *European Heart Journal* 2005, **26(22)**:2422-2434.

31. Turner S, Thomas M, von Ziegenweidt J, Price D: Prescribing trends in asthma: a longitudinal observational study. *Archives of Disease in Childhood* 2009, **94(1)**:16-22.

32. Feldstein AC, Elmer PJ, Nichols GA, Herson M: Practice patterns in patients at risk for glucocorticoid-induced osteoporosis. *Osteoporosis International* 2005, **16(12)**:2168-2174.

33. Elliot-Gibson V, Bogoch ER, Jamal SA, Beaton DE: Practice patterns in the diagnosis and treatment of osteoporosis after a fragility fracture: a systematic review. *Osteoporosis International* 2004, **15(10)**:767-778.

34. Gurwitz JH, Field TS, Harrold LR, Rothschild J, Debellis K, Seger AC, Cadoret C, Fish LS, Garber L, Kelleher M, Bates DW, Gurwitz JH, Field TS, Harrold LR, Rothschild J, Debellis K, Seger AC, Cadoret C, Fish LS, Garber L, Kelleher M, Bates DW: Incidence and preventability of adverse drug events among older persons in the ambulatory setting. *JAMA* 2003, **289(9)**:1107-1116.

35. Stockley's drug interactions. [online]. Edited by: Baxter K. Pharmaceutical Press, London; 2009:.

36. Joint Formulary Committee (British Medical Association and The Royal Pharmaceutical Society of Great Britain): British National Formulary. London; 2009**57**.

37. BMJ Clinical evidence [online]. In *BMJ Publishing Group Limited, London* Edited by: Minhas R 2009, Available at http://clinicalevidence.bmj.com/ceweb/index.jsp.

38. National Prescribing Centre: Evidence based therapeutics. *MeRec monthly* 2009, Available at http://www.npc.nhs.uk/merec/.

39. Medicines and Healthcare products Regulatory Agency (MHRA) and Commission on Human Medicines: *Drug Safety Update* , Available at http://www.mhra.gov.uk/Publications/Safetyguidance/DrugSafetyUpdate/index.htm.

40. Morris CJ, Cantrill JA: Preventing drug-related morbidity-the development of quality indicators. *Journal of Clinical Pharmacy & Therapeutics* 2003, **28(4)**:295-305.

41. Campbell SM, Braspenning J, Hutchinson A, Marshall MN: Research methods used in developing and applying quality indicators in primary care. *BMJ* 2003, **326(7393)**:816-819.

42. Shekelle PG, MacLean CH, Morton SC, Wenger NS: Assessing Care of Vulnerable Elders: Methods for Developing Quality Indicators. *Annals of Internal Medicine* 2001, **135(8 Part 2)**:647-652.

43. Kahan JP BS, Leape LL: Measuring the necessity of medical procedures. *Med Care* 1994, **32(357)**-365.

44. Naylor CD: What is appropriate care? *N Engl J Med* 1998, **338**:1918-1920.

45. Shekelle PG: Are appropriateness criteria ready for use in clinical practice? *NEngl JMed* 2001, **344(9)**:677-678.

46. Brook RH CM, Fink A: A method for the detailed assessment of the appropriateness of medical technologies. *Int J Technol Assess Health Care* 1986, **2**:53-63.

47. Leape LL, Park RE, Kahan JP, Brook RH: Group judgements of appropriateness: the effect of panel composition. *Quality Assurance Health Care* 1992, **4**:151-159.

48. Campbell SM, Cantrill JA: Consensus methods in prescribing research. *Journal of Clinical Pharmacy & Therapeutics* 2001, **26(1)**:5-14.

49. Morris CJ, Cantrill JA, Hepler CD, Noyce PR: Preventing drug-related morbidity-determining valid indicators. *International Journal for Quality in Health Care* 2002, **14(3)**:183-198.

50. Bigby J, Dunn J, Goldman L, Adams JB, Jen P LC, Komaroff AL: Assessing the preventability of emergency hospital admissions. A method for evaluating the quality of medical care in a primary care facility. *Am J Med* 1987, **83**:1031-1036.

51. Chan M, Nicklason F, Vial JH: Adverse drug events as a cause of hospital admission in the elderly. *Intern Med* 2001, **31**:199-205.

52. Courtman BJ, Stallings SB: Characterisation of drug-related problems in elderly patients on admissions to a medical ward. *Can J Hosp Pharm* 1995, **48**:161-166.

53. Ajzen I: The theory of planned behaviour. *Organizational behaviour and human decision processes* 1991, **50**:170-211.

54. Guthrie B, McCowan C, Davey P, Simpson CR, Dreischulte T, Barnett K: High risk prescribing in primary care patients particularly vulnerable to adverse drug events: cross sectional population database analysis in Scottish general practice. *BMJ* 2011, **342**:d3514.

55. Fitch K, Bernstein S, Aguilar M, Burnand B, LaCalle J, Lazaro P: The RAND/UCLA appropriateness method user's manual. *RAND Corporation* 2003.

# 20

# Association between statin therapy and outcomes in critically ill patients: a nested cohort study

Shmeylan A Al Harbi[1], Hani M Tamim[2] and Yaseen M Arabi[3*]

## Abstract

**Background:** The effect of statin therapy on mortality in critically ill patients is controversial, with some studies suggesting a benefit and others suggesting no benefit or even potential harm. The objective of this study was to evaluate the association between statin therapy during intensive care unit (ICU) admission and all-cause mortality in critically ill patients.

**Methods:** This was a nested cohort study within two randomised controlled trials conducted in a tertiary care ICU. All 763 patients who participated in the two trials were included in this study. Of these, 107 patients (14%) received statins during their ICU stay. The primary endpoint was all-cause ICU and hospital mortality. Secondary endpoints included the development of sepsis and severe sepsis during the ICU stay, the ICU length of stay, the hospital length of stay, and the duration of mechanical ventilation. Multivariate logistic regression was used to adjust for clinically and statistically relevant variables.

**Results:** Statin therapy was associated with a reduction in hospital mortality (adjusted odds ratio [aOR] = 0.60, 95% confidence interval [CI] 0.36-0.99). Statin therapy was associated with lower hospital mortality in the following groups: patients >58 years of age (aOR = 0.58, 95% CI 0.35-0.97), those with an acute physiology and chronic health evaluation (APACHE II) score >22 (aOR = 0.54, 95% CI 0.31-0.96), diabetic patients (aOR = 0.52, 95% CI 0.30-0.90), patients on vasopressor therapy (aOR = 0.53, 95% CI 0.29-0.97), those admitted with severe sepsis (aOR = 0.22, 95% CI 0.07-0.66), patients with creatinine ≤100 µmol/L (aOR = 0.14, 95% CI 0.04-0.51), and patients with GCS ≤9 (aOR = 0.34, 95% CI 0.17-0.71). When stratified by statin dose, the mortality reduction was mainly observed with statin equipotent doses ≥40 mg of simvastatin (aOR = 0.53, 95% CI 0.28-1.00). Mortality reduction was observed with simvastatin (aOR = 0.37, 95% CI 0.17-0.81) but not with atorvastatin (aOR = 0.80, 95% CI 0.84-1.46). Statin therapy was not associated with a difference in any of the secondary outcomes.

**Conclusion:** Statin therapy during ICU stay was associated with a reduction in all-cause hospital mortality. This association was especially noted in high-risk subgroups. This potential benefit needs to be validated in a randomised, controlled trial.

## Background

Statins, also known as 3-hydroxy-3-methylglutaryl coenzyme A reductase inhibitors, were first introduced in the late 1980s as cholesterol-lowering drugs for the prevention of cardiovascular events. However, recent studies have demonstrated a wide variety of statin properties independent of their lipid-lowering ability. These properties, known as pleiotropic effects [1-4], include multiple anti-inflammatory actions, the direct activation of heme oxygenase, direct interference in leucocyte-endothelial interactions, and direct inhibition of major histocompatibility complex class II (MHC II) [5-10].

The effect of statin therapy on mortality in critically ill patients is controversial, with some studies suggesting a benefit and others no benefit or even potential harm [11-17]. These divergent results are probably related to

---

* Correspondence: yaseenarabi@yahoo.com
[3]Intensive Care Department, Medical Director, Respiratory Services, and Associate Professor, College of Medicine, King Saud bin Abdulaziz University for Health Sciences, King Abdulaziz Medical City, Riyadh, Saudi Arabia
Full list of author information is available at the end of the article

differences in study designs, patient populations [4,11-14,18,19], statin types, and doses [4,15,17,20]. Therefore, we sought to evaluate the association of statin therapy during the intensive care unit (ICU) stay with all-cause mortality in critically ill medical surgical patients.

## Methods

### Setting

This study was conducted in a 900-bed tertiary academic medical centre. The adult ICU admits medical, surgical, and trauma patients, and it operates as a closed unit with 24-hr, 7-day onsite coverage by a critical care board of certified intensivists. The nurse-to-patient ratio at the unit is approximately 1:1.2 [21].

### Study design

This was a nested cohort study within two randomised, controlled trials.

The first trial, conducted between January 2004 and March 2006 included 532 patients, compared intensive insulin therapy (IIT) (for patients with a blood glucose level of 4.4-6.1 mmol/L or 80-110 mg/dl) to conventional insulin therapy (CIT) (for patients with a blood glucose level of 10-11.1 mmol/L or 180-200 mg/dl) [22]. This trial showed no significant difference in ICU mortality between the IIT and CIT groups (13.5% vs. 17.1%, p = 0.3). Hypoglycemia occurred more frequently in the IIT than in the CIT group (28.6% vs. 3.1% of patients; p < 0.0001) [22].

The second trial, conducted between February 2006 and January 2008, included 240 patients and assessed the effects on outcomes of permissive underfeeding (a caloric goal of 60-70% of the calculated requirement) versus target feeding (caloric goal of 90-100% of the calculated requirement) with either IIT or CIT in critically ill patients [23]. The study found no difference between the two groups in 28-day mortality (18% vs. 23%, p = 0.34). However, hospital mortality was lower in the permissive underfeeding compared with the target-feeding group (30% vs. 43%, p = 0.04) [23]. All patients enrolled in the original two trials were included in this study.

### Statin therapy

Statins for critically ill patients were prescribed as part of the medication reconciliation process if they had been prescribed in the pre-ICU period. Occasionally, statin therapy was initiated in the ICU for patients admitted with acute coronary syndrome or stroke. The prescribed dose was at the discretion of the treating physician. Data regarding the use, type (simvastatin or atorvastatin) and dose of statin were collected from the hospital information system. Doses of atorvastatin were converted into the equivalent dose of simvastatin at a atorvastatin: simvastatin ratio of 1:2.

### Data Collection

Patient outcomes and the following data were retrieved from the two original studies: age, gender, acute physiology and chronic health evaluation (APACHE II) score [24], sequential organ failure assessment (SOFA) score [25], creatinine, platelet count, bilirubin, international normalised ratio (INR), Glasgow coma scale (GCS) score [26], admission category, history of diabetes, need for mechanical ventilation, vasopressor therapy, sepsis, severe sepsis and septic shock and the presence of chronic cardiac, respiratory, renal, hepatic, or immunocompromising diseases, as defined by the APACHE II system [24].

### Outcomes

The primary outcomes were all-cause ICU and hospital mortality. Secondary outcomes included the development of sepsis and severe sepsis during the ICU stay, ICU and hospital length of stay, and the duration of mechanical ventilation. Sepsis and severe sepsis were defined according to the 2001 International Sepsis Definitions Conference [27]. The two trials were approved by the research committee and institutional review board of King Abdulaziz Medical City.

### Statistical analysis

Statistical analyses were performed using Statistical Analysis Software (SAS, release 8, SAS Institute, Cary, NC, 1999). We compared patients who received statins during their ICU admission (statin group) with those who did not (non-statin group). Baseline characteristics and outcome variables were compared using $t$-test for continuous data and Chi-square test for nominal data. To control for any potential confounding effects of baseline characteristics, we used multivariate logistic regression to calculate adjusted odds ratios (aOR) and 95% confidence intervals (CI) for the association between statin use and outcome. Adjustments were made for clinically relevant variables and for those that showed a statistically significant difference between the two groups at baseline. These variables included age, gender, admission category, APACHE II score, history of diabetes, creatinine, platelets, GCS, and the presence of chronic cardiac, renal, or respiratory diseases. We further examined the dose effects of statins on the primary and secondary outcomes by stratifying patients on the basis of doses equivalent to <40 mg and ≥ 40 mg of simvastatin. Additionally, we conducted stratified analyses by age, gender, admission category, APACHE II score, history of diabetes, the presence of chronic cardiac problems, vasopressor therapy, sepsis, severe sepsis and septic shock, creatinine, platelet count, bilirubin, INR, GCS, ICU length of stay, mechanical ventilation and type of statin, to detect any change in the association between intervention and outcome measures on the basis of any of these factors. Statistical significance was defined as a p value ≤ 0.05.

## Results

Of the 763 patients enrolled in the study, 107 (14%) received statins during their ICU stay, and 656 (86%) did not. Atorvastatin was prescribed to 63 patients (58.9%), with doses ranging between 10 and 80 mg/day. Simvastatin was prescribed to 44 patients (41.1%), with doses ranging between 10 and 40 mg/day. Table 1 compares the baseline characteristics of the statin and non-statin groups. Patients who received statins were older; more likely to be females; diabetic; more likely to have chronic cardiac, renal or respiratory illness; and had higher APACHE II scores.

Table 2 summarises the association between statin therapy and mortality using multivariate analysis adjusting for the selected confounders. Statin therapy was associated with lower all-cause hospital mortality (aOR = 0.60, 95% CI 0.36-0.99). The association between statins and ICU mortality was not statistically significant

(aOR = 0.84, 95% CI 0.47-1.51). When stratified by statin dose, a significant reduction in hospital mortality was observed with doses of ≥40 mg (aOR = 0.53, 95% CI 0.28-1.00).

Table 3 shows the association between statin therapy and all-cause hospital mortality stratified by different characteristics using multivariate analysis. Statin therapy was associated with lower hospital mortality in patients older than 58 years (aOR = 0.58, 95% CI 0.35-0.97), those with an APACHE II score >22 (aOR = 0.54, 95% CI 0.31-0.96), diabetic patients (aOR = 0.52, 95% CI 0.30-0.90), patients on vasopressor therapy (aOR = 0.53, 95% CI 0.29-0.97), those with creatinine ≤100 μmol/L (aOR = 0.14, 95% CI 0.04-0.51), patients with severe sepsis (aOR = 0.22, 95% CI 0.07-0.66), and patients with a GCS ≤ 9 (aOR = 0.34, 95% CI 0.17-0.71). When stratified by statin type, statistically significant association with lower mortality was observed by simvastatin (aOR = 0.37, 95% CI 0.17-0.81), but not with atorvastatin.

There was no significant association between statin use and the development of sepsis or severe sepsis and septic shock, ICU and hospital length of stay, or the duration of mechanical ventilation (Table 4).

## Discussion

Our study demonstrates that statin therapy in critically ill patients is associated with lower hospital mortality. This effect was observed predominantly in elderly patients, diabetics, patients with higher severity of illness, with a low GCS, patients on vasopressors, with severe sepsis, and those on simvastatin.

Several studies have shown favourable effects of statin therapy on outcomes in critically ill patients. Liappies et al. retrospectively reviewed patients with documented bacteraemia and found that statin therapy was associated with a significant reduction in overall hospital mortality and infection rates (11). Almog et al. found that prior statin therapy was associated with a reduction in severe sepsis and the incidence of ICU admission [12]. Kruger et al. studied a cohort of bacteraemia patients and found a significantly lower incidence of mortality and bacteraemia-related mortality with statin therapy [13]. Mortensen et al. found that statin therapy before ICU admission was associated with a decreased 30-day mortality [20]. A recent systematic review examined the effect of statins on mortality in patients with infection and/or sepsis. The review included a total of 20 studies, with 18 cohort studies (12 retrospective and 6 prospective), 1 matched cohort study with 2 case-controlled studies, and 1 randomised, controlled trial. The review demonstrated a protective effect of statin therapy for various infection-related outcomes compared with placebo in patients with sepsis and/or other infections [28]. These studies are in concordance with ours, which

## Table 1 Baseline characteristics of patients on statin therapy and non-statin therapy

|  | Statin (n = 107) | Non-Statin (n = 656) | P-value |
|---|---|---|---|
| Age, mean ± SD (yrs) | 68.8 ± 11.0 | 49.3 ± 21.7 | < 0.0001 |
| Female gender, no. (%) | 44 (41.1) | 164 (25) | 0.0005 |
| APACHE II, mean ± SD | 27.2 ± 6.9 | 23.0 ± 8.1 | < 0.0001 |
| SOFA day 1, mean ± SD | 9.3 ± 3.2 | 9.2 ± 3.5 | 0.92 |
| Creatinine, mean ± SD, μmol/L* | 200.8 ± 152.6 | 152.3 ± 152.1 | 0.002 |
| Platelets, mean ± SD, x10⁹/L | 270.7 ± 117.8 | 193.3 ± 123.3 | 0.0001 |
| Bilirubin, mean ± SD, μmol/l | 26.4 ± 63.6 | 31.6 ± 55.2 | 0.50 |
| INR, mean ± SD | 1.5 ± 0.7 | 1.5 ± 0.9 | 0.72 |
| GCS, mean ± SD | 9.4 ± 4.5 | 8.5 ± 4.0 | 0.05 |
| ICU admission category, no. (%) |  |  |  |
| Postoperative | 4 (3.7) | 119 (18.1) | 0.0002 |
| Nonoperative | 103 (96.3) | 537 (81.9) |  |
| History of diabetes, no. (%) | 84 (78.5) | 219 (33.4) | < 0.0001 |
| Mechanically ventilated, no. (%) | 92 (86.0) | 591 (90.1) | 0.20 |
| Vasopressors, no. (%) | 73 (68.2) | 423 (64.5) | 0.45 |
| Sepsis, no. (%) | 28 (26.2) | 166 (25.3) | 0.85 |
| Severe sepsis, no. (%) | 26 (24.3) | 207 (31.5) | 0.13 |
| Chronic respiratory, no. (%) | 33 (30.8) | 124 (18.9) | 0.005 |
| Chronic cardiac, no. (%) | 54 (50.5) | 103 (15.7) | < 0.0001 |
| Chronic renal, no. (%) | 29 (27.1) | 74 (11.3) | < 0.0001 |
| Chronic liver, no. (%) | 4 (3.7) | 50 (7.6) | 0.15 |
| Chronic immunocompromised, no. (%) | 10 (9.4) | 56 (8.5) | 0.78 |

SD: standard deviation, APACHE II: Acute physiology and chronic health evaluation II; SOFA: Sequential organ failure assessment; INR: International normalised ratio; GCS: Glasgow coma scale.

*To convert units to mg/dl, divide by 88.4 for creatinine and 17.1 for bilirubin

**Table 2 Association between statin use and primary outcomes compared with the non-statin group using adjusted analyses**

| | Statin<br>n = 107 | Non-statin<br>n = 656 | Adjusted odds ratio (aOR)[a] | 95% confidence interval | P-value |
|---|---|---|---|---|---|
| ICU mortality, no. (%) | 19/107 (17.8) | 108/656 (16.5) | 0.84 | (0.47 - 1.51) | 0.56 |
| Dose < 40 mg | 7/47 (14.9) | 108/656 (16.5) | 0.67 | (0.28 - 1.63) | 0.43 |
| Dose ≥ 40 mg | 12/60 (20.0) | 108/656 (16.5) | 0.97 | (0.48 - 1.99) | 0.98 |
| Hospital mortality, no. (%) | 42/107 (39.3) | 200/656 (30.5) | 0.60 | (0.36 - 0.99) | 0.05 |
| Dose < 40 mg | 19/47 (40.4) | 200/656 (30.5) | 0.69 | (0.35 - 1.40) | 0.30 |
| Dose ≥ 40 mg | 23/60 (38.3) | 200/656 (30.5) | 0.53 | (0.28 - 1.00) | 0.05 |

Variables entered initially in the stepwise regression model including age, gender, admission category, APACHE II score, history of diabetes, creatinine, platelets, GCS, $PaO_2/FiO_2$, and chronic cardiac, renal, and respiratory diseases.

demonstrated a significant reduction in mortality with statin therapy in critically ill patients and patients with sepsis, severe sepsis and septic shock. The effect was primarily observed with higher doses of statins.

In contrast, some investigators have not found statin therapy to be beneficial. Fernandez et al. analysed data from 438 patients receiving mechanical ventilation for more than 96 hr and found that hospital mortality was significantly higher with statin therapy (61% vs. 42%), even after adjusting for APACHE II predicted risk (observed/expected ratio 1.53 vs. 1.17). In a population-based study of community-acquired pneumonia, Majumdar et al. found that statin users were less likely to die or to be admitted to the ICU than non-users (50/325 [15%] vs. 574/3090 [19%], respectively; OR 0.80, p = 0.15). However, after a more complete adjustment for confounding factors, the OR changed from potential benefit (0.78, adjusted for age and sex) to potential harm (1.10, fully adjusted, including propensity scores, 95% CI 0.76-1.60). This disagreement with the findings of our study may be explained by differences in illness severity. As subjects of a population-based study, the patients of Majumdar et al. were relatively healthy users [15] compared with our population. Additionally, it remains unclear whether these findings, which were observed in patients with community-acquired pneumonia, are applicable to all critically ill patients. Yang et al. conducted a retrospective study and found no difference in mortality between the two groups, despite the presence in patients in the statin group of less organ dysfunction, lower APACHE II scores, less inotropic support, and less shock [16]. The lack of benefit observed in these studies might be related to differences in the patient disease mix, severity of illness, or statin type/dose.

Our study demonstrated a mortality reduction in older patients and those with more severity of illness. This result confirms what other previous studies have shown. Dobesh et al. evaluated patients over the age of 40 with severe sepsis who were exposed to statins before and/or during hospitalisation. The mean APACHE II score in

the statin group was 26. Patients in the statin group showed a lower mortality compared with the no statin group (31.7% vs. 48.4%; p = 0.04), and this effect was more evident in older patients and those with higher APACHE II score [18]. Schmidt et al. evaluated statin therapy in patients with multi-organ dysfunction and a mean APACHE II score ≥ 30. The study demonstrated that 28-day mortality was significantly lower in the statin group compared with the no statin group (33% vs. 53%; p = 0.03).

We observed a mortality reduction with simvastatin but not atorvastatin. A similar finding was noted by Christensen et al. [19]. This result might be related to the higher lipophilicity of simvastatin, which enables it to better penetrate cells [29]. However, large sample size is required to confirm these findings.

The observed beneficial effects of statins on diabetic patients, patients with chronic cardiovascular disease and those with low GCS (a surrogate for neurologic disease) are consistent with its reported benefits in acute myocardial infarction and acute stroke [30,31]. Our results are also consistent with the findings of a population-based study by Hackam et al., who found that statin use in patients with atherosclerosis was associated with a reduced risk of subsequent sepsis [32].

Our findings confirm the need for randomised, controlled trials to verify the relationship between statin therapy and the observed outcomes. Other issues still require resolution, including the dose-effect relationship, whether the mechanism of action is related to the pleiotropic or lipid-lowering effect of statins, and whether the observed effect is a class effect or an individual statin effect [33]. We hope that the ongoing clinical trials in patients with sepsis, septic shock, ventilator-associated pneumonia, and influenza, as well as the trials investigating the prevention of acute lung injury and adult respiratory distress syndrome will help address these questions [34-38].

The findings of our study must be interpreted in the light of its strengths and weaknesses. The strengths include being a nested cohort within randomised

**Table 3 Association between statin therapy and hospital mortality, stratified by different relevant characteristics**

| | Statin n = 107 | Non-statin n = 656 | Adjusted odds ratio (aOR)[a] | 95% confidence interval | P-value |
|---|---|---|---|---|---|
| Hospital mortality, no. (%) | 42/107 (39.3) | 200/656 (30.5) | 0.60 | (0.36 - 0.99) | 0.05 |
| Stratified by age, no. (%) | | | | | |
| ≤ 58 yrs | 6/14 (42.9) | 62/374 (16.6) | 0.73 | (0.19 - 2.81) | 0.64 |
| > 58 yrs | 36/93 (38.7) | 138/282 (49.0) | 0.58 | (0.35 - 0.97) | 0.04 |
| Gender, no. (%) | | | | | |
| Male | 21/63 (33.3) | 126/492 (25.6) | 0.56 | (0.29 - 1.08) | 0.08 |
| Female | 21/44 (47.7) | 74/164 (45.0) | 0.74 | (0.35 - 1.58) | 0.43 |
| Admission category, no. (%) | | | | | |
| Postoperative | 1/4 (25.0) | 19/119 (16.0) | 0.75 | (0.04 - 14.82) | 0.85 |
| Nonoperative | 41/103 (40.0) | 181/537 (34.0) | 0.62 | (0.34 - 1.03) | 0.06 |
| APACHE II, no. (%) | | | | | |
| APACHE≤ 22 | 8/33 (24.2) | 53/370 (14.3) | 0.77 | (0.27 - 2.21) | 0.63 |
| APACHE>22 | 34/74 (46.0) | 147/286 (51.4) | 0.54 | (0.31 - 0.96) | 0.03 |
| SOFA, no. (%) | | | | | |
| ≤ 9 | 13/58 (22.4) | 63/346 (18.2) | 0.55 | (0.26 - 1.17) | 0.12 |
| > 9 | 29/49 (59.1) | 137/310 (44.2) | 0.73 | (0.36 - 1.48) | 0.38 |
| History of diabetes, no. (%) | | | | | |
| Yes | 31/84 (37.0) | 106/209 (48.4) | 0.52 | (0.30 - 0.90) | 0.02 |
| No | 11/23 (47.8) | 94/437 (21.5) | 1.31 | (0.49 - 3.54) | 0.59 |
| History of cardiovascular, no. (%) | | | | | |
| Yes | 23/54 (42.6) | 58/103 (56.3) | 0.59 | (0.3 - 1.2) | 0.13 |
| No | 19/53 (35.9) | 142/553 (25.7) | 0.52 | (0.27 - 1) | 0.06 |
| Vasopressor therapy, no. (%) | | | | | |
| Yes | 31/73 (42.5) | 151/423 (35.7) | 0.53 | (0.29 - 0.97) | 0.04 |
| No | 23/34 (67.7) | 184/233 (79.0) | 0.92 | (0.37 - 2.25) | 0.84 |
| Sepsis, no. (%) | | | | | |
| Yes | 12/28 (43.0) | 88/166 (53.0) | 0.64 | (0.26 - 1.58) | 0.33 |
| No | 30/79 (38.0) | 112/490 (23.0) | 0.72 | (0.41 - 1.28) | 0.26 |
| Severe sepsis and septic shock no. (%) | | | | | |
| Yes | 14/26 (53.9) | 84/207 (40.6) | 0.22 | (0.07 - 0.66) | 0.007 |
| No | 28/81 (34.6) | 116/449 (25.7) | 0.78 | (0.45 - 1.37) | 0.38 |
| Creatinine, no. (%) | | | | | |
| ≤ 100 µmol/L | 4/26 (15.4) | 70/351 (20.0) | 0.14 | (0.04 - 0.51) | 0.002 |
| > 100 µmol/L | 38/81 (47.0) | 130/305 (43.0) | 1.01 | (0.58 - 1.77) | 0.96 |
| Platelets, no. (%) | | | | | |
| ≤ 180 | 12/25 (48.0) | 125/358 (35.0) | 0.62 | (0.24 - 1.62) | 0.33 |
| > 180 | 30/82 (36.6) | 75/298 (25.2) | 0.78 | (0.43 - 1.42) | 0.42 |
| Bilirubin, no. (%) | | | | | |
| ≤ 16 µmol/L | 10/38 (26.3) | 54/212 (25.5) | 0.49 | (0.21 - 1.20) | 0.11 |
| > 16 µmol/L | 10/22 (45.5) | 73/223 (32.7) | 0.67 | (0.23 - 1.97) | 0.47 |
| INR, no. (%) | | | | | |
| ≤1.2 | 20/59 (34.0) | 68/312 (21.8) | 0.79 | (0.40 - 1.58) | 0.51 |
| >1.2 | 22/48 (45.8) | 132/344 (38.4) | 0.53 | (0.26 - 1.09) | 0.09 |
| GCS, no. (%) | | | | | |
| ≤ 9 | 19/50 (38.0) | 114/364 (31.3) | 0.34 | (0.17 - 0.71) | 0.004 |
| > 9 | 23/57 (40.4) | 86/292 (29.5) | 092 | (0.46 - 1.85) | 0.81 |
| Length of stay, no. (%) | | | | | |
| ≤ 5 days | 4/39 (10.3) | 32/192 (16.7) | 0.40 | (0.13 - 1.28) | 0.12 |
| > 5 days | 38/68 (55.9) | 168/464 (36.2) | 0.63 | (0.34 - 1.19) | 0.16 |
| Mechanical ventilation, no. (%) | | | | | |
| Yes | 40/92 (43.5) | 183/591 (31.0) | 0.66 | (0.34 - 1.10) | 0.11 |

**Table 3 Association between statin therapy and hospital mortality, stratified by different relevant characteristics** *(Continued)*

| No | 2/15 (13.3) | 17/65 (26.2) | 0.75 | (0.09 - 6.43) | 0.79 |
| Simvastatin, no. (%) | 12/44 (27.3) | 200/656 (30.5) | 0.37 | (0.17 - 0.81) | 0.01 |
| Atorvastatin, no. (%) | 30/63 (47.6) | 200/656 (30.5) | 0.80 | (0.84 - 1.46) | 0.47 |

APACHE II: Acute physiology and chronic health evaluation II; SOFA: Sequential organ failure assessment; INR: International normalised ratio; GCS: Glasgow coma scale.
*To convert units to mg/dl, divide by 88.4 for creatinine and 17.1 for bilirubin

**Table 4 Association between statin use and outcomes stratified by statin dose**

| | Statin therapy n = 107 | Non-statin therapy n = 656 | Adjusted odds ratio (aOR)[a] | 95% confidence interval | P-value |
| --- | --- | --- | --- | --- | --- |
| Sepsis, no.% | 32/107 (29.9) | 280/656 (42.7) | 0.84 | (0.51 - 1.37) | 0.49 |
| Dose < 40 mg | 16/47 (34.0) | 280/656 (42.7) | 1.11 | (0.57 - 2.20) | 0.74 |
| Dose ≥ 40 mg | 16/60 (25.7) | 280/656 (42.7) | 0.67 | (0.36 - 1.30) | 0.22 |
| Severe sepsis, no. % | 26/107 (24.3) | 207/656 (31.6) | 0.87 | (0.51 - 1.50) | 0.60 |
| Dose < 40 mg | 11/47 (23.4) | 207/656 (31.6) | 0.88 | (0.42 - 1.90) | 0.74 |
| Dose ≥ 40 mg | 15/60 (25.0) | 207/656 (31.6) | 0.85 | (0.44 - 1.65) | 0.64 |
| ICU LOS, mean ± SD, days | 10.2 ± 12.7 | 11.3 ± 10.6 | * | * | 0.33 |
| Hospital LOS, mean ± SD, days | 67.6 ± 118.1 | 58.6 ± 81.4 | * | * | 0.37 |
| MVD, mean ± SD, days | 9.0 ± 11.9 | 10.1 ± 10.3 | * | * | 0.33 |

Variables entered initially in the stepwise regression model including age, gender, admission category, APACHE II, history of diabetes, creatinine, platelets, GCS, and chronic cardiac, renal, and respiratory diseases.

controlled trials with prospective data collection. Among the limitations of our study are its monocenter nature, its post-hoc design, and the lack of data on the duration of statin therapy prior to ICU admission, lipid profile, and statin side effects. Because of the observational nature of the study, there were imbalances at baseline between the statin and non-statin groups. However, we have adjusted for these imbalances using multivariate analysis.

## Conclusion
Our study demonstrated that statin therapy during ICU admission was associated with lower hospital mortality, particularly among elderly patients, diabetics, patients with high APACHE II and low GCS, those on vasopressors, and those on simvastatin. In addition, using doses greater than 40 mg per day was associated with lower hospital mortality. Further randomised, controlled trials are needed to confirm these findings.

## Acknowledgements
None

## Author details
[1]Intensive Care Department, King Abdulaziz Medical City, Riyadh, Saudi Arabia. [2]Epidemiology and Biostatistics, College of Medicine, King Saud bin Abdulaziz University for Health Sciences, King Abdulaziz Medical City, Riyadh, Saudi Arabia. [3]Intensive Care Department, Medical Director, Respiratory Services, and Associate Professor, College of Medicine, King Saud bin Abdulaziz University for Health Sciences, King Abdulaziz Medical City, Riyadh, Saudi Arabia.

**Authors' contributions**
SAA: Had full access to all data in the study and takes full responsibility for the data, conception and design, participated in the data acquisition, analysis and interpretation, and drafted the manuscript; HMT: Conception and design, data analysis and interpretation and critical revision of the manuscript; YMA: Conception and design, statistical analysis, critical revision of the manuscript and overall supervision.
All authors have read and approved the final manuscript for publication.

**Competing interests**
The authors declare that they have no competing interests.

**References**
1. Weitz-Schmidt G: Statins as anti-inflammatory agents. *Trends Pharmacol Sci* 2002, **23**:482-486.
2. Blanco-Colio LM, Tunon J, Martin-Ventura JL, Egido J: **Anti-inflammatory and immunomodulatory effects of statins.** *Kidney Int* 2003, **63**:12-23.
3. Terblanche M, Almog Y, Rosenson RS, Smith TS, Hackman DG: **Statins and sepsis: multiple modifications at multiple levels.** *Lancet Infect Dis* 2007, **7**:358-368.
4. Martin CP, Talbert RL, Burgess DS, Peters JI: **Effectiveness of statins in reducing the rate of severe sepsis: a retrospective evaluation.** *Pharmacotherapy* 2007, **27**:20-26.
5. Weitz-Schmidt G, Welzenbach K, Brinkmann V, Kamata T, Kallen J, Bruns C, Cottens S, Takada Y, Hommel U: **Statins selectively inhibit leukocyte function antigen-1 by binding to a novel regulatory integrin site.** *Nat Med* 2001, **7**:687-692.
6. Weitz-Schmidt G: **Lymphocyte function-associated antigen-1 blockade by statins: molecular basis and biological relevance.** *Endothelium* 2003, **10**:43-47.
7. Zingarelli B: **Nuclear factor-kappaB.** *Crit Care Med* 2005, **33**:S414-416.
8. Falagas ME, Makris GC, Matthaiou DK, Rafailidis PI: **Statins for infection and sepsis: a systematic review of the clinical evidence.** *J Antimicrobial Chemotherapy* 2008, **61**:774-785.

9.  Kronmann L, Hatfield C, Kronmann K: **Statin therapy: not just used to lower cholesterol?** *Crit Care Nurs, Q* 2007, **30**:154-160.

10. Iijima K, Ouchi Y: **Can statins slow the process of vascular calcification? Possibilities of lipid-lowering therapy and pleiotropic effect by statin treatment.** *Clin Calcium* 2010, **20**:1719-28.

11. Liappis AP, Kan VL, Rochester CG, Simon GL: **The effect of statins on mortality in patients with bacteremia.** *Clin Infect Dis* 2001, **33**:1352-1357.

12. Almog Y, Shefer A, Novack V, Maimon N, Barski L, Eizinger M, Friger M, Zeller L, Danon A: **Prior statin therapy is associated with a decreased rate of severe sepsis.** *Circulation* 2004, **110**:880-885.

13. Kruger P, Fitzsimmons K, Cook D, Jones M, Nimmo G: **Statin therapy is associated with fewer deaths in patients with bacteraemia.** *Intensive Care Med* 2006, **32**:75-79.

14. Fernandez R, De Pedro VJ, Artigas A: **Statin therapy prior to ICU admission: protection against infection or a severity marker?** *Intensive Care Med* 2006, **32**:160-164.

15. Majumdar SR, McAlister FA, Eurich DT, Padwal RS, Marrie TJ: **Statins and outcomes in patients admitted to hospital with community acquired pneumonia: population based prospective cohort study.** *BMJ* 2006, **333**:999-1001.

16. Yang KC, Chien JY, Tseng WK, Hsueh PR, Yu CJ, Wu CC: **Statins do not improve short-term survival in an oriental population with sepsis.** *Am J Emerg Med* 2007, **25**:494-501.

17. Thomsen RW, Hundborg HH, Johnsen SP, Pedersen L, Sorensen HT, Schonherder HC, Lervang hh: **Statin use and mortality within 180 days after bacteremia: a population-based cohort study.** *Crit Care Med* 2006, **34**:1080-1086.

18. Dobesh PP, Klepser DG, McGuire TR, Morgan CW, Olsen KM: **Reduction in mortality associated with statin therapy in patients with severe sepsis.** *Pharmacotherapy* 2009, **29**:621-630.

19. Christensen S, Thomsen RW, Johansen MB, Pedersen L, Jensen R, Larsen KM, Larsson A, Tonnesen E, Sorensen HR: **Preadmission statin use and one-year mortality among patients in intensive care - a cohort study.** *Crit Care* 2010, **14**:R29.

20. Mortensen EM, Restrepo MI, Anzueto A, Pugh J: **The effect of prior statin use on 30-day mortality for patients hospitalized with community-acquired pneumonia.** *Respir Res* 2005, **6**:82.

21. Arabi Y, Alshimemeri A, Taher S: **Weekend and weeknight admissions have the same outcome of weekday admissions to an intensive care unit with onsite intensivist coverage.** *Crit Care Med* 2006, **34**:605-611.

22. Arabi YM, Dabbagh OC, Tamim HM, Al-Shimemeri AA, Memish ZA, Haddad SH, Syed SJ, Giridhar HR, Rishu AH, Al-Daker MO, Kaahoul Sh, Rritts RK, Sakkijha MH: **Intensive versus conventional insulin therapy: a randomized controlled trial in medical and surgical critically ill patients.** *Crit Care Med* 2008, **36**:3190-3197.

23. Arabi Y, Tamim H, Shifaat G, Sakkijha M, Al-Dawood A, Al-Sultan M: **Permissive Underfeeding Versus Target Feeding in Critically Ill Patients: Randomized Controlled Trial.** *Am J Respir Crit Care Med* 2009, **179**:A2167.

24. Knaus WA, Draper EA, Wagner DP, Zimmerman JE: **APACHE II: a severity of disease classification system.** *Crit Care Med* 1985, **13**:818-829.

25. Ferreira FL, Bota DP, Bross A, Melot C, Vincent JL: **Serial evaluation of the SOFA score to predict outcome in critically ill patients.** *JAMA* 2001, **286**:1754-1758.

26. Livingston BM, Mackenzie SJ, MacKirdy FN, Howie JC: **Should the pre-sedation Glasgow Coma Scale value be used when calculating Acute Physiology and Chronic Health Evaluation scores for sedated patients?.** Scottish Intensive Care Society Audit Group. *Crit Care Med* 2000, **28**:389-394.

27. Levy MM, Fink MP, Marshall JC, Abraham E, Angus D, Cook D, Cohen J, Opal SM, Vincent JL, Ramsay G: **2001 SCCM/ESICM/ACCP/ATS/SIS International Sepsis Definitions Conference.** *Crit Care Med* 2003, **31**:1250-1256.

28. Janda S, Young A, FitzGerald J, Etminan M, Swiston J: **The effect of statins on mortality from severe infections and sepsis: A systemic review and meta-analysis.** *Journal of Critical Care* 2010, **25**:656.e7-656.e22.

29. Dobesh P, Swahn S, Peterson E: **Statins in sepsis.** *Journal of Pharmacy Practice* 2010, **1**:38-49.

30. Stenestrand U, Wallentin L: **Early statin treatment following acute myocardial infarction and 1-year survival.** *JAMA* 2001, **285**:430-6.

31. Aslanyan S, Weir CJ, McInnes GT, Reid JL, Walters MR, Lees KR: **Statin administration prior to ischemic stroke onset and survival: exploratory evidence from matched treatment-control study.** *Eur J Neurol* 2005, **12**:493-8.

32. Hackam DG, Mamdani M, Li P, Redelmeier DA: **Statins and sepsis in patients with cardiovascular disease: a population-based cohort analysis.** *Lancet* 2006, **367**:413-418.

33. Weant KA, Cook AM: **Potential roles for statins in critically ill patients.** *Pharmacotherapy* 2007, **27**:1279-1296.

34. **Statins for early treatment of sepsis.** ClinicalTrials.gov Identifier: NCT00528580. [http://clinicaltrials.gov/show/NCT00528580], Accessed October 17, 2010.

35. **Simvastatin in patients with septic shock.** ClinicalTrials.gov Identifier: NCT00450840. [http://clinicaltrials.gov/show/NCT00450840], accessed October 17, 2010.

36. **Pravastatin and ventilatory associated pneumonia.** ClinicalTrials.gov Identifier: NCT00702130. [http://clinicaltrials.gov/show/NCT00702130], Accessed October 17, 2010.

37. **Simvastatin effect on the incidence of acute lung injury/adult respiratory distress syndrome.** NCT01195428. [http://clinicaltrials.gov/show/NCT00702130], Accessed October 17, 2010.

38. **Statin trial for influenza patients.** ClinicalTrials.gov Identifier: NCT00970606. [http://clinicaltrials.gov/show/NCT00970606], accessed October 17, 2010.

# 21

# Nitric oxide and histone deacetylases modulate cocaine-induced mu-opioid receptor levels in PC12 cells

Warren Winick-Ng[1], Francesco Leri[2] and Bettina E Kalisch[1*]

## Abstract

**Background:** Cocaine exposure has been reported to alter central μ-opioid receptor (MOR) expression *in vivo*. The present study employed an *in vitro* cellular model to explore possible mechanisms that may be involved in this action of cocaine.

**Methods:** To assess the effects of cocaine on MOR levels, two treatment regimens were tested in PC12 cells: single continuous or multiple intermittent. MOR protein levels were assessed by western blot analysis and quantitative PCR was used to determine relative MOR mRNA expression levels. To evaluate the role of nitric oxide (NO) and histone acetylation in cocaine-induced MOR expression, cells were pre-treated with the NO synthase inhibitor N$^{\omega}$-nitro-L-arginine methylester (L-NAME) or the non-selective histone acetyltransferase inhibitor curcumin.

**Results:** Both cocaine treatment regimens significantly increased MOR protein levels and protein stability, but only multiple intermittent treatments increased MOR mRNA levels as well as *c-fos* mRNA levels and activator protein 1 binding activity. Both regimens increased NO production, and pre-treatment with L-NAME prevented cocaine-induced increases in MOR protein and mRNA levels. Single and multiple cocaine treatment regimens inhibited histone deacetylase activity, and pre-treatment with curcumin prevented cocaine-induced up-regulation of MOR protein expression.

**Conclusions:** In the PC12 cell model, both NO and histone deacetylase activity regulate cocaine-induced MOR expression at both the transcriptional and post-transcriptional levels. Based on these novel findings, it is hypothesized that epigenetic mechanisms are implicated in cocaine's action on MOR expression in neurons.

**Keywords:** Cocaine, PC12 cells, Histone acetylation, Nitric oxide, Mu-opioid receptor

## Background

Endogenous opioid systems are involved in several aspects of cocaine addiction [1-5], and several studies have indicated that cocaine increases μ-opioid receptor (MOR) mRNA and peptide expression [6-11] in regions of the brain known to regulate incentive motivation and stress reactivity [12-14]. In rats, cocaine-induced increases in MOR mRNA expression have been consistently observed in the ventral striatum [15,16], a region of the brain critical to drug motivated behaviors [17,18]. Furthermore, PET studies in abstinent cocaine users have established correlations between elevations in MOR binding in mesocorticolimbic areas and intensity of cocaine cravings [19-21]. These data suggest the importance of elucidating the molecular mechanisms through which cocaine alters MOR levels in the central nervous system.

The experiments reported in this manuscript were designed to investigate two possible, and related, mechanisms. First, cocaine administration elevates concentrations of nitric oxide (NO) in the rat brain [22,23], and both cocaine and NO increase levels, and binding activity, of members of the activator protein 1 (AP-1) transcription factor family [24-32]. Because the promoter region of the MOR gene contains consensus sequences for AP-1 transcription factors [33], it is possible that cocaine modulates MOR expression via alterations in NO and AP-1 activity.

* Correspondence: bkalisch@uoguelph.ca
[1]Department of Biomedical Sciences, University of Guelph, Guelph, Ontario N1G 2W1, Canada
Full list of author information is available at the end of the article

Second, NO also decreases the activity of histone deacety-lases (HDACs) [34,35], enzymes implicated in the behavioral effects of cocaine in rats [36,37], as well as in morphine-induced MOR expression [38,39]. HDACs affect chromatin structure through the removal of acetyl groups from histones [40-42], and thus contribute to gene transcription [43-47]. Therefore, it is also likely that cocaine modulates MOR expression via alterations in histone acetylation.

These experiments employed PC12 cells to investigate the role of NO and HDACs in cocaine-induced alterations of MOR expression. This *in vitro* cellular model was selected because PC12 cells express the MOR gene [48-50], their NO pathway has been fairly well characterized [51-54], and they are sensitive to changes in HDACs activity [55]. Three main results were obtained. First, cocaine increased MOR protein expression and protein stability after both single continuous and multiple intermittent treatment regimens, but only the multiple intermittent treatment regimen increased expression of MOR and c-fos mRNAs, as well as AP-1 binding activity. Second, NO was identified as an important modulator, as cocaine increased NO production, and the NO synthase (NOS) inhibitor $N^{\omega}$-nitro-L-arginine methylester (L-NAME) attenuated cocaine-induced increases in MOR protein and mRNA expression. Third, it was found that cocaine decreased HDACs activity, and inhibition of histone acetyltransferase (HAT) attenuated cocaine-induced increases in MOR protein expression following both treatment regimens.

## Methods
### Materials
Dulbecco's modified Eagle medium (DMEM), horse serum, gentamycin, DNAse I, Oligo dT, Superscript II, primers, Platinum Taq and Lipofectamine 2000 were purchased from Invitrogen (Mississauga, ON, Canada) and fetal bovine serum (FBS) was obtained from HyClone Laboratories (Logan, UT, USA). Cocaine HCl was purchased from Dumex (Toronto, ON, Canada), L-NAME, curcumin, and mouse monoclonal anti-α-tubulin were purchased from Sigma Aldrich (St. Louis, MO, USA). The complete mini tablets were purchased from Roche Diagnostics (Laval, QC, Canada), the sodium dodecyl sulfate (SDS) sample buffer, DTT, and protein standards were obtained from New England Biolabs (Ipswich, MA) and the polyclonal MOR antibody was from Abcam (Cambridge, MA, USA) or Santa Cruz Biotechnology Inc. (Santa Cruz, CA, USA). Luminol was also purchased from Santa Cruz. Hybond-C blotting membranes, sheep anti-mouse IgG and enhanced chemiluminescence (ECL) kit were obtained from Amersham/GE Health Care (Piscataway, NJ, USA), poly-D-lysine was from BD Biosciences (Mississauga, ON, Canada) and 4,5-diaminofluorescein

diacetate (DAF-2 DA) was purchased from Calbiochem (San Diego, CA, USA). Syber Green PCR master mix was obtained from Qiagen (Toronto, ON, Canada) and the HDAC Assay kit was from Active Motif (Carlsbad, CA, USA). The PathDetect pAP-luciferase reporter plasmid was obtained from Stratagene (La Jolla CA, USA) and the Luciferase Assay and Galacto-Light (Tropix) kits were from Promega (Madison, WI, USA) and Applied Biosystems (Bedford, MA, USA), respectively. All other chemicals were molecular or electrophoresis grade and obtained from Fisher Scientific (Ottawa, ON, Canada) or DiaMed Laboratories (Mississauga, ON, Canada).

### Cell culture, viability and treatments
PC12 cells were maintained in DMEM containing 5% FBS, 5% horse serum and 50 µg/mL gentamycin at 37°C in 5% $CO_2$. To evaluate the effects of cocaine, NO synthase (NOS) inhibitors, and curcumin on MOR protein and mRNA levels, cells were plated on Corning® 60 mm dishes at a density of 1.0 million cells per plate for protein, and 1.5 million cells per plate for RNA. For the AP-1 study, PC12 cells were plated on 12-well culture dishes at a concentration of $2.0 \times 10^5$ cells per well. For NO production imaging, PC12 cells were plated on 6-well culture dishes containing poly-D-lysine coated coverslips at a concentration of $2.0 \times 10^5$ cells per well. For nuclear extraction, PC12 cells were plated on 100 mm culture dishes at a concentration of $4.0 \times 10^6$ cells per plate. All plating was performed 24h prior to any treatment.

The effects of cocaine were determined by exposing PC12 cells to various concentrations of cocaine using two different treatments. The doses of cocaine selected for this study (10, 100, and 500 µM) were based on previous reports investigating the effects of cocaine on morphological changes and proto-oncogene expression in PC12 cells [56]. Two treatment regimens were chosen based on previous findings indicating that different exposure patterns can differentially affect MOR binding affinity and receptor density in several regions of the rat brain [57,58]. These treatments were: single continuous treatment (SCT) or repeated intermittent treatment (RIT) (see Table 1). The latter regimen included 3 daily treatments, each lasting 30 min, separated by 60 min exposures to cocaine-free media. Cells were harvested 72 h after the beginning of treatment, except where otherwise indicated.

PC12 cell viability was assessed in control cells and those exposed to 500 µM *SCT* or 100 µM *RIT* with cocaine for 72 h by the reduction of 3-(4,5-dimethylthiazole-2-yl)-2,5-diphenyltetrazolium bromide (MTT) as described by Cheung et al. [59]. Culture media was replaced with media containing MTT (0.5mg/mL final concentration) and the cells were incubated at 37°C for 30 min. The reduced formazan product was lysed from the cells using a 100% dimethylsulfoxide solution and the absorbance was subsequently measured at 570nm using the FLUOstar Optima plate-reader (BMG, Fisher Scientific).

The effect of NOS and HAT inhibitors was determined by pre-treating PC12 cells with inhibitor, for 1 h prior to cocaine exposure. We determined previously that NGF increases NOS activity and NO production in PC12 cells and that this increase is attenuated when cells are pre-treated with 20 mM L-NAME [53]. Therefore, cells were pretreated with this dose of L-NAME to examine the involvement of NO in the cocaine-induced expression of MOR. Cells were also pretreated with 1, 3 or 5 μM of the non-selective HAT inhibitor curcumin, based on a previous report by Siddiqui et al. [60], which explored the impact of curcumin on oxidative stress in PC12 cells. Curcumin was selected for these experiments because it inhibits HAT in both *in vitro* and *in vivo* models [61-63] and it modulates cocaine place preference in rats [36]. For *RIT*, each 30 min cocaine treatment was followed by the addition of PC12 cell culture media containing only L-NAME (20 mM) or curcumin (1, 3, 5 μM).

### Immunoblot analysis

Control and treated PC12 cells were lysed in 250 μL of radioimmunoprecipitation assay (RIPA) buffer (final concentration: 50 mM Tris, 150 mM NaCl, 1% NP-40, 0.25% sodium deoxycholate, 0.5% SDS, 1 mM each of EDTA, sodium fluoride, sodium orthovanadate and protease inhibitor (1 Complete Mini Tablet (Roche Diagnostics)/10 mL], pH 7.4). Samples were rocked on ice for 15 min, sonicated, centrifuged at 17 530 g for 15 min and the protein content of the supernatant determined by the method of Bradford [64]. Cell lysates (100 μg) were then boiled in SDS sample buffer (final concentration: 62.5 mM Tris-HCl; pH 6.8, 2% SDS, 42 μM DTT, 10% glycerol and 0.01% phenol red) and loaded onto a 10% SDS/polyacrylamide gel.

Following electrophoresis, proteins were transferred onto nitrocellulose membranes (Hybond-C) using a Trans-blot semidry transfer unit (Bio-Rad Laboratories, Mississauga, ON, Canada) with transfer buffer (final concentration: 28 mM Tris, 39 mM glycine and 20% methanol, pH 9.2). Membranes were blocked in 2.5% or 5% non-fat milk in tris-buffered saline (TBS) containing 0.1% Tween-20 (TBS-T) for 1 h. Blots were then incubated in 1:750 rabbit MOR antibody in 1% bovine serum albumin (BSA) in TBS-T for 2 h (Abcam), or in 1:200 rabbit MOR antibody in 1% non-fat milk in TBS-T (Santa Cruz) overnight. Antibody detection was achieved using 1:2500 horseradish peroxidase-conjugated donkey anti-rabbit IgG in either 1 % BSA or 5% non-fat milk in TBS-T for 1 h, followed by ECL or luminol.

Membranes were scanned using the STORM 860 (Molecular Dynamics, subsidiary of Amersham) for ECL, or

the Fluorchem 9900 imaging system (Alpha Innotech, Santa Clara, CA, USA) for luminol. Bands were analyzed densitometrically using Imagequant (Molecular Dynamics) or Fluorchem 9900 software. Blots were stripped with 62.5 mM Tris, pH 6.7, containing 2% SDS and 100 mM 2-mercaptoethanol at 50°C for 20 min. Membranes were then rinsed in TBS for at least 4 h before blocking with 5 % milk in TBS-T for 1 h and reprobing with 1:50 000 mouse monoclonal anti-α tubulin antibody overnight. Blots were then exposed to 1:2500 goat anti-mouse IgG-horse radish peroxidase conjugated secondary antibody, in 5% milk in TBS-T and the protein bands visualized as described above.

### MOR half-life analysis

Following 72 h of treatment, control and *SCT* or *RIT* PC12 cells were exposed to 10 μg/mL cycloheximide [65], a *de novo* protein translation inhibitor, for 4, 8, 12, 24 and 48 h. Cells were then lysed in 250 μL RIPA buffer, and western blot analysis for MOR and α-tubulin was performed as described above.

### Analysis of NO production

NO production was assessed using the fluorescent probe DAF-2 DA. PC12 cells were treated with cocaine (100 or 500 μM) in the presence or absence of 20 mM L-NAME for 3 days, washed once with media and loaded with 10 μM DAF-2 DA in 1 mL culture media. Following 2 h of incubation cells were washed 4 times with 2 mL media and DAF-2 fluorescence was visualized using an Olympus IX-81 fluorescence microscope (excitation at 488 nm, emission at 520 nm) with an Olympus LucPlan FL 0.40 aperture lens (at 20 x magnification) in phosphate buffered saline at room temperature. Digital images were captured using a Cascade 512F camera (Photometrics, Tucson, AZ, USA), and processed in Q-Capture and Adobe Photoshop 5.0.

### qPCR and PCR analysis

In our previous studies of gene expression in PC12 cells, changes in mRNA typically occurred 24 to 36 h prior to changes in protein expression [53]. Therefore we initially examined MOR mRNA following 48h of *SCT* and *RIT* with cocaine. Control and treated PC12 cells were lysed in 1 mL of Trizol reagent to obtain total RNA. The extracted RNA was treated with DNase I and reverse transcribed using superscript II with oligo-dT as the primer for 75 min at 43°C [53]. The resulting cDNA was then used for real time PCR (qPCR) using a LightCycler (Roche). qPCR was performed using 1 μL cDNA and 9 μL of QuantiTect SYBR Green PCR master mix. There was a 15 min incubation period at 95°C prior to the first cycle, and a melting curve was obtained for each sample following the final cycle [65]. Primer pairs and cycling conditions were: β-2-

microglobulin (Genbank Accession number NM_012512): 5' primer: 5'-TGACCGTGATCTTTCTGGTG-3' and 3' primer: 5'-ATCTGAGGTGGGTGGAACTG-3', 45 cycles of 95°C: 15 s, 55°C: 25 s, 72°C: 15 s; MOR coding region (Genbank Accession Number U02083.1): 5' primer: 5'-CTGTGTGTTACGGCCTGATG-3' and 3' primer: 5'-ATGCAGAAGTGCCAGGAAAC-3', 55 cycles of 95°C: 15 s, 52°C: 25 s, 72°C: 15 s. After each cycle, fluorescent activity was determined, and a final crossing point (threshold cycle, $C_T$) was calculated. Steady-state MOR mRNA levels relative to β-2 microglobulin were determined with RelQuant software

To qualitatively observe the effect of cocaine on *c-fos* levels, total RNA was extracted from control and treated PC12 cells as described above 0.5, 1 or 2 h after the final 30 min 100 μM cocaine treatment on the first day of *RIT*. Following reverse transcription, 5 μL cDNA was combined with 45 μL of master mix containing (final concentration): 15 mM MgCl$_2$, 10 mM dNTPs, 5 μM of forward and reverse primers, 10 x PCR buffer, 0.2 μL of Platinum Taq and water [53,65]. Each PCR was performed with an initial 2 min, 95°C strand separation and a final 2 min, 72°C elongation. Primer pairs and cycling conditions were: β-actin (Genbank Accession number NM_031144): 5' primer 5'-TCATGAAGTGT-GACGGTTGACATCCGT-3' and 3' primer 5'-CCTA-GAAGATTTGCGGTGCACGATG-3', 30 cycles of 95°C: 30 s, 55°C: 30 s, 72°C: 45 s; *c-fos* coding region (Genbank Accession number NM_022197 XM_234422): 5' primer: 5'-ACGCGGACTACGAGGCGTCA-3' and 3' primer: 5'-GCTCTGGTCTGCGATGGGGC-3', 40 cycles of 95°C: 30 s, 55°C: 30 s, 72°C: 45 s. PCR products were separated on a 1.5% agarose gel stained with ethidium bromide. Fragments were visualized using the Pharmacia Biotech ImageMaster VDS, and images captured were processed in Microsoft Office Picture Manager. To quantify steady-state mRNA levels qPCR was performed as described above and analysis of *c-fos* levels relative to β-2 microglobulin determined using RelQuant software.

### AP-1 luciferase activity

PC12 cells were fed with antibiotic free media 30 min prior to transfection. For each well 1.0 μg luciferase reporter plasmid containing 7 AP-1 transcription factor binding elements was incubated with 0.5 μg of a pSV- β-galactosidase (β-gal) plasmid and 2 μL Lipofecta-mine2000 in 100 μL OptiMEM for 30 min at room temperature [51]. The mixture was added to PC12 cells and the plates returned to the cell culture incubator for 5 h. The transfection medium was replaced with regular PC12 culture medium and the cells returned to the incubator overnight. Following 6 h of *SCT* or *RIT* with cocaine or 50 ng/mL NGF (used as a positive control for AP-1 activation [51]) treatment, PC12 cells were lysed

with 200 μL 1X passive lysis buffer (Promega). Lysates were incubated for 30 min at 4°C, followed by centrifugation at 12 000 x *g* for 2 min. Duplicate 20 μL samples of the supernatant were then transferred to a 96 well plate. To measure luciferase activity, 50μL of Luciferase Assay Reagent was added to each well, and after a 2 s delay, luciferase activity was read for 10 s. Luciferase activity was an indicator for AP-1 plasmid activation. Duplicate samples from the same lysate were used to measure β-gal activity with the Galacto-Light kit. First, 25 μL of galacton (1:100 with reaction buffer diluent) was added to each well and the samples were incubated for 30 to 60 min. This was then followed by the addition of 50μL of accelerator (provided in the Galacto-Light kit) to each well, and after a 2 s delay, β-gal activity was read for 1 s. Luciferase and β-gal activity was measured using the FLUOstar Optima plate-reader luminometer (BMG, Fisher Scientific).

### Nuclear extraction and HDAC enzyme activity assay

Since *c-fos* expression and AP-1 activity were altered within 24 h of treatment, it was hypothesized that cocaine would alter HDAC activity within a similar time frame. Following 24 and 36h of *SCT* and *RIT* with cocaine, PC12 cells were harvested in nuclear extraction buffer A (final concentration: 10 mM HEPES; pH 7.9, 1.5 mM MgCl$_2$, 10 mM KCl, 0.5 μM DTT and protease inhibitor (1 complete MINI tablet/10 mL)) containing phosphatase inhibitors (1mM each of sodium fluoride, sodium orthovanadate). Cells were lysed using a 27.5 gauge needle, and the nuclei were pelleted by centrifugation at 14 000 x *g* for 5 min at 4°C. The supernatant was discarded and the pellet was rinsed in buffer A. Cells were again centrifuged at 14 000 x *g* for 5 min at 4°C, the supernatant discarded and the pellet re-suspended in nuclear extraction buffer B (final concentration: 20 mM HEPES; pH 7.9, 1.5 mM MgCl$_2$, 420 mM KCl, 0.5 μM DTT, 25% glycerol, 2 mM EDTA, 1mM each of sodium fluoride, sodium orthovanadate, and protease inhibitor (1 complete MINI tablet/10 mL)) and kept on ice for 15 min. Following the addition of nuclear extraction buffer C (final concentration: 20 mM HEPES; pH 7.9, 0.5 μM DTT, 25% glycerol, 0.2 mM EDTA, 1mM each of sodium fluoride, sodium orthovanadate, and protease inhibitor (1 complete MINI tablet/10 mL)), samples were centrifuged at 10 000 x *g* for 5 min. The nuclear fraction in the supernatant was quantified using the method of Bradford [64].

Samples were used to detect HDAC enzyme activity using an HDAC assay kit according to the manufacturer's recommendations. Briefly, nuclear extracts (7 μg) were added to a 96-well half-volume black plate, mixed with HDAC assay buffer and HDAC substrate (final concentration: 100 μM), and incubated at 37°C for 50 min.

Following incubation, HDAC reactions were halted using HDAC developer (containing 2 μM Trichostatin A, final concentration: 1 μM) and incubated at room temperature for 12 to15 min. Fluorescence was detected using the FLUOstar Optima plate reader with an excitation wavelength at 350 nm and an emission wavelength at 460 nm.

### Data Analysis & Statistics

For western blot analysis, each band was analyzed densitometrically as described previously [52,65]. To account for variability between blots, the densitometric value for each individual MOR band was expressed as a fraction of the total amount of MOR protein present on the entire blot (ie. sample MOR density/sum of density of all MOR bands on blot). The same analysis was carried out for α-tubulin and then MOR protein values were normalized to α-tubulin values from the same sample.

For qPCR analysis, relative mRNA levels were determined using the delta-deltaCt method of analysis. A threshold cycle ($C_T$) was determined for each data point. A ratio was then determined for each sample using by the following formula:

$$Ratio = 2^{-[CT(GENE)-CT(\beta 2M)]} \qquad (1)$$

where $C_{T(GENE)}$ was the gene of interest, and $C_{T(\beta 2M)}$ was the $C_T$ for β-2-microglobulin. Each data point was then expressed relative to the control sample.

In order to determine HDAC enzyme activity, a standard curve was prepared using known HDAC assay standard dilutions. The amount of fluorescence recorded was then extrapolated to the pM amount of product formed (PF) from the standard curve. The specific activity (SpA) in pM/min/mg was then determined using the PF, incubation time in min (IT), and mass of nuclear extract in mg (mnx), by using the following formula:

$$SpA = (PF/IT)/mnx \qquad (2)$$

To determine relative luciferase activity, each sample was expressed as a percentage of the total amount of luciferase activity detected for each sample set. Luciferase activity was then normalized to β-gal activity within the same sample.

Data are representative of 5 independent experiments (except where otherwise indicated) and are presented as the mean ± standard error of the mean (SEM). Data were assessed for normality and homogeneity of variance and statistical analysis was carried out using a one or two-way analysis of variance (ANOVA). In the case of a one-way ANOVA, analysis was followed by Dunnett's test or the Tukey-Kramer Multiple Comparisons test to determine which groups were significantly different. One-way ANOVA analysis was carried out for protein

and RNA analysis of MOR levels following cocaine treatment, or for experiments with L-NAME pretreatment. For RNA analysis with cocaine and L-NAME, the data did not pass the Bartlett test for homogeneity of variance, therefore a Kruskal-Wallis non-parametric ANOVA was performed. For two-way ANOVA with interaction, analysis was followed by Bonferroni's multiple comparisons t-test to determine which groups were significantly different. This analysis was used to determine significant changes in MOR protein expression following cocaine and curcumin treatments, and used to determine significant changes in c-fos mRNA expression following cocaine treatments over time. For two-way ANOVA without interaction, analysis was followed by contrast analysis to determine which groups were significantly different, and was used to determine significant changes in histone deacetylase activity following cocaine administration. Mean values were considered different if p<0.05.

For the protein half-life and AP-1 experiments, following western blot and luciferase analysis as described above, data were assessed for normality and homogeneity of variance. Due to a large disparity between variances, the natural log was taken for each data point. For the AP-1 luciferase analysis experiment, statistical analysis was carried out using a one-way ANOVA. Following transformation in the protein half-life experiment, data were analyzed using an analysis of co-variance (ANCOVA) to determine the effect of each treatment, as well as significant differences that may exist between the slopes of the resulting regression lines. The original raw data was also used to perform an ANCOVA, and, where possible, the resulting regression line was used to determine an approximate MOR half-life for each treatment. Mean values were considered different if p<0.05.

Data analysis was carried out using GraphPad InStat for one way ANOVA analysis, GraphPad Prism 4.0 or SAS 9.2 (SAS Institute, Cary, NC) for two-way ANOVA analysis with interaction, and SAS 9.2 for two-way ANOVA analysis without interaction, as well as ANCOVA analysis.

## Results

### Cocaine modulates MOR protein and mRNA levels, and protein half-life

The effect of cocaine on MOR protein levels was evaluated in extracts of control and treated (see Table 1 for treatment details) PC12 cells using western blot analysis. Figure 1A displays a representative immunoblot of MOR levels (upper panel) and corresponding α-tubulin levels (lower panel) obtained from cells treated with SCT or RIT with 10, 100 or 500 μM cocaine for 72 h. Densitometric analysis (Figure 1B) revealed a significant increase in MOR protein levels [F(6,33)= 5.75] relative to control in cells exposed to 500 μM SCT (p<0.05) or 100 μM RIT

**Table 1** *Cocaine treatment regimens*

| Regimen | Description |
| --- | --- |
| *SCT* | A single dose of cocaine added to the cell culture media and not removed over the entire time-course |
| *RIT* | Three daily intermittent 30 min treatments applied to the cells separated by 1 h of regular cell culture media. |

PC12 cells were either given a single continuous treatment (SCT) or a repeated intermittent treatment (RIT) of cocaine.

($p<0.01$) cocaine. These treatments did not compromise PC12 cell viability: metabolic activity assessed with the MTT reduction assay indicated that, relative to control, there was only a modest decrease in activity in cocaine-treated cells (100 μM RIT: 90.1 ± 4.2 % of control, n=4; 500 μM SCT: 93.4 ± 2.9 % of control, n=4), which was not statistically significant. On the basis of these data,

500 μM *SCT* and 100 μM *RIT* cocaine were used in subsequent experiments.

To determine whether the cocaine-induced increase in MOR protein level was due to an increase in protein stability, protein extracts were obtained from cells treated for 72 h with 500 μM *SCT* or 100 μM *RIT* cocaine followed by 10 μg/mL cycloheximide for 4, 8, 12, 24 or 48 h. Densitometric analysis of MOR protein levels relative to α-tubulin revealed an estimated MOR half-life of 36.3 h in control (untreated) cells (Figure 1C), and a statistically significant effect of cocaine [$F_{(2, 103)}= 13.94$, $p<0.0001$] and time (h) [$F_{(1, 103)} = 17.11$, $p<0.0001$]. Both treatment regimens significantly changed the slope of protein decay compared to control, indicating that cocaine increased MOR half-life. Although it was not possible to calculate a predicted half-life for the cells treated

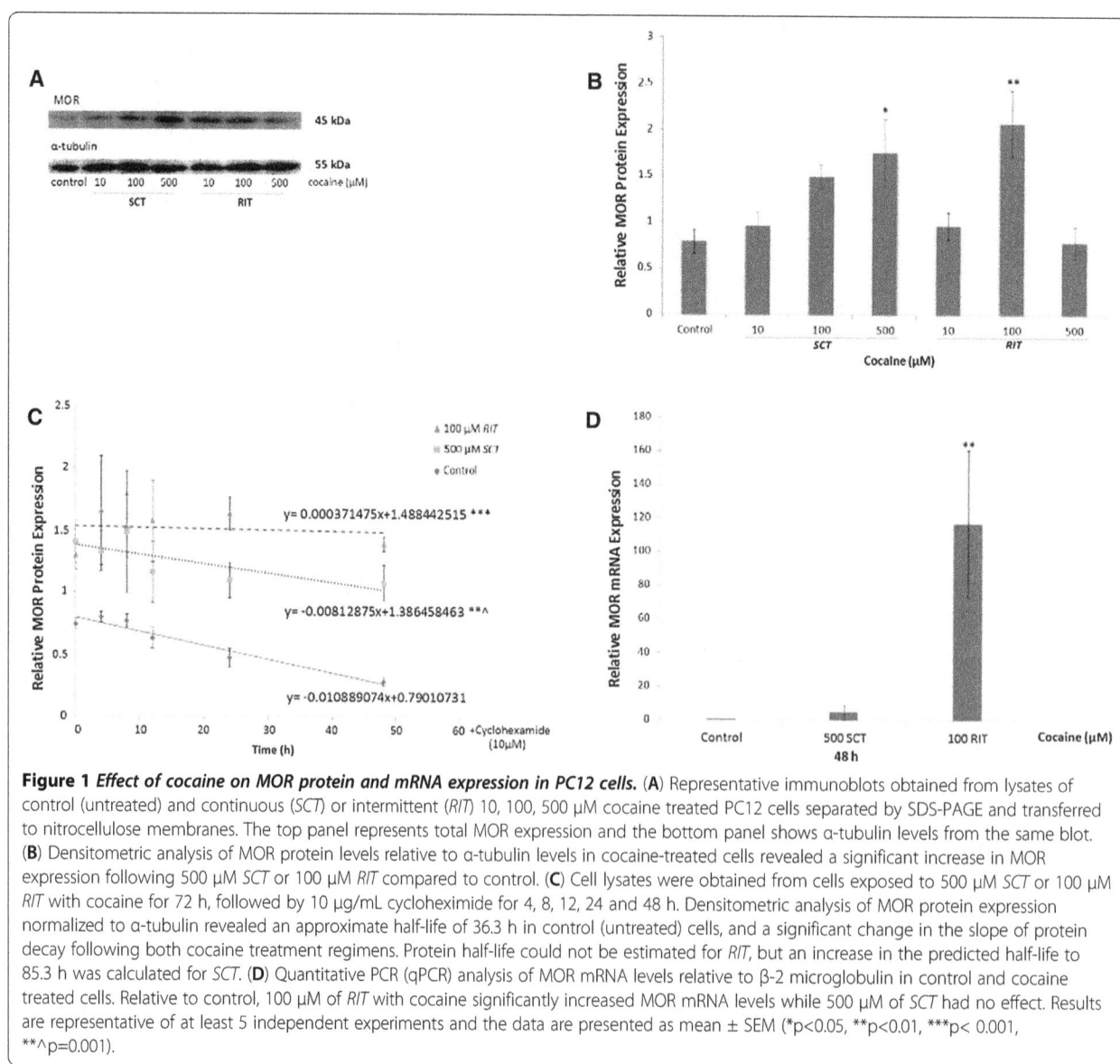

**Figure 1** *Effect of cocaine on MOR protein and mRNA expression in PC12 cells.* (**A**) Representative immunoblots obtained from lysates of control (untreated) and continuous (*SCT*) or intermittent (*RIT*) 10, 100, 500 μM cocaine treated PC12 cells separated by SDS-PAGE and transferred to nitrocellulose membranes. The top panel represents total MOR expression and the bottom panel shows α-tubulin levels from the same blot. (**B**) Densitometric analysis of MOR protein levels relative to α-tubulin levels in cocaine-treated cells revealed a significant increase in MOR expression following 500 μM *SCT* or 100 μM *RIT* compared to control. (**C**) Cell lysates were obtained from cells exposed to 500 μM *SCT* or 100 μM *RIT* with cocaine for 72 h, followed by 10 μg/mL cycloheximide for 4, 8, 12, 24 and 48 h. Densitometric analysis of MOR protein expression normalized to α-tubulin revealed an approximate half-life of 36.3 h in control (untreated) cells, and a significant change in the slope of protein decay following both cocaine treatment regimens. Protein half-life could not be estimated for *RIT*, but an increase in the predicted half-life to 85.3 h was calculated for *SCT*. (**D**) Quantitative PCR (qPCR) analysis of MOR mRNA levels relative to β-2 microglobulin in control and cocaine treated cells. Relative to control, 100 μM of *RIT* with cocaine significantly increased MOR mRNA levels while 500 μM of *SCT* had no effect. Results are representative of at least 5 independent experiments and the data are presented as mean ± SEM (*$p<0.05$, **$p<0.01$, ***$p< 0.001$, **^$p=0.001$).

with 100 µM *RIT* cocaine, MOR protein half-life following exposure to 500 µM *SCT* was estimated to be 85.3 h.

The effect of cocaine on MOR mRNA levels was also examined (Figure 1D). RNA was isolated from cells treated for 48 h with either 500 µM *SCT* or 100 µM *RIT* cocaine and levels of MOR mRNA relative to β2-microglobulin were assessed by reverse transcriptase (RT)-real time PCR (qPCR) analysis. Compared to control, a statistically significant increase in relative MOR mRNA levels was detected in cocaine-treated cells following *RIT* [F(2,15)= 6.80, p<0.01], but not *SCT*.

### Effect of cocaine on nitric oxide, and its role in MOR protein and mRNA expression

To examine the effect of cocaine on NO production, PC12 cells were treated with 500 µM *SCT* or 100 µM *RIT* for 72 h and diaminofluorescein-2 (DAF-2) fluorescence was examined. A low level of DAF-2 fluorescence, indicative of NO production, was observed in untreated PC12 cells (Figure 2A). DAF-2 fluorescence was increased in cocaine-treated cells with both treatments, and this increase was prevented when cells were pretreated with the non-selective NOS inhibitor L-NAME (20 mM).

In the subsequent experiment, PC12 cells were treated with 20 mM of L-NAME prior to 500 µM *SCT* or 100 µM *RIT* cocaine. Representative western blots depicting MOR and α-tubulin levels in extracts obtained from cells treated with cocaine in the presence or absence of L-NAME are presented in Figure 2B, and densitometric analysis of MOR expression relative to α-tubulin is depicted in Figure 2C. Relative to control, a significant increase in MOR protein levels was observed in cells treated for 72 h with either 500 µM *SCT* or 100 µM *RIT* cocaine [F(5,26)= 3.43, p<0.05 for both treatments]. This increase was not observed in cells pretreated with L-NAME.

The final experiment assessed the effect of 20 mM L-NAME pretreatment on MOR mRNA levels increased following 100 µM *RIT* cocaine. Compared to control, qPCR analysis (Figure 2D) revealed that cocaine significantly increased relative MOR mRNA levels (Kruskal-Wallis statistic= 15.36, p<0.001), and that this was prevented by pretreatment with L-NAME.

### Effect of cocaine on c-fos mRNA levels and AP-1 binding

Qualitative assessment of *c-fos* levels in PC12 cells treated with 100 µM *RIT* cocaine for 0.5, 1 or 2 h, revealed increases in steady-state *c-fos* mRNA (Figure 3A) relative to control. This was confirmed by qPCR analysis (Figure 3B) which revealed cocaine significantly increased relative *c-fos* mRNA levels [F(1,21)=11.41, p<0.01]. No increase in *c-fos* was detected following *SCT* cocaine. To investigate the effect of cocaine on AP-1 activity, PC12 cells were transiently transfected with a plasmid containing 7 AP-1 binding elements upstream from a luciferase

reporter gene. The day after transfection, cells were exposed to 10, 100 or 500 µM *SCT* or *RIT* cocaine and harvested 6 h after the start of treatment (Figure 3C). As a positive control, other cells were treated with 50 ng/mL nerve growth factor (NGF) for 6 h [51]. Although modest compared to the NGF-mediated increase in AP-1 activity, both 10 and 100 µM *RIT* cocaine significantly increased AP-1 activity compared to control [F(7,33)= 10.181, p<0.01 for NGF, p<0.05 for cocaine]. No increase in luciferase activity was detected following *SCT* at all of the doses tested.

### Effect of cocaine on HDACs, and the role of histone acetylation in MOR protein expression

PC12 cells were treated with 500 µM *SCT* or 100 µM *RIT* cocaine, and HDACs activity in nuclear extracts was evaluated 24 or 36 h after treatment (Figure 4A). Following both time points and treatments, HDACs activity was significantly inhibited in comparison to control [F(2, 29)= 3.43, p<0.05]. There was no difference in the level of HDAC inhibition between either treatment conditions or treatment times.

In a subsequent experiment, PC12 cells were treated with 1, 3 or 5 µM curcumin, a non-selective HAT inhibitor, for 1h prior to exposure to either 500 µM *SCT* or 100 µM *RIT* cocaine for 72h. Relative levels of MOR protein from these cell extracts was compared to those obtained from untreated cells, and those treated with the inhibitor or cocaine alone. Statistical analysis revealed an overall significant interaction between the effects of curcumin and cocaine on MOR protein expression [F(6, 52)= 15.25, p<0.0001], a significant effect of curcumin alone [F(3, 52)= 20.62, p<0.0001], and a significant effect of cocaine alone [F(2, 52)= 15.87, p<0.0001]. Pre-treatment with 3 µM curcumin significantly decreased MOR expression in cells treated with 500 µM *SCT* cocaine compared to cocaine alone (p<0.0001). Additionally, MOR levels in cells pre-treated with 1, 3, and 5 µM curcumin followed by 100 µM *RIT* cocaine were significantly lower than those receiving *RIT* cocaine alone (p<0.05 for 1 µM, p<0.0001 for 3 and 5 µM curcumin).

### Discussion

The present study identified a number of cellular mechanisms by which cocaine alters MOR expression. Treatment of PC12 cells with either a single dose or repeated doses of cocaine increased MOR protein levels. The mechanisms regulating this increase were dependent on the treatment regimen used. Both *SCT* and *RIT* increased MOR protein stability, indicating that both regimens increased MOR protein levels post-transcriptionally. *RIT* elevated MOR and *c-fos* mRNA levels and AP-1 activity, but a single dose of cocaine did not, indicating that multiple

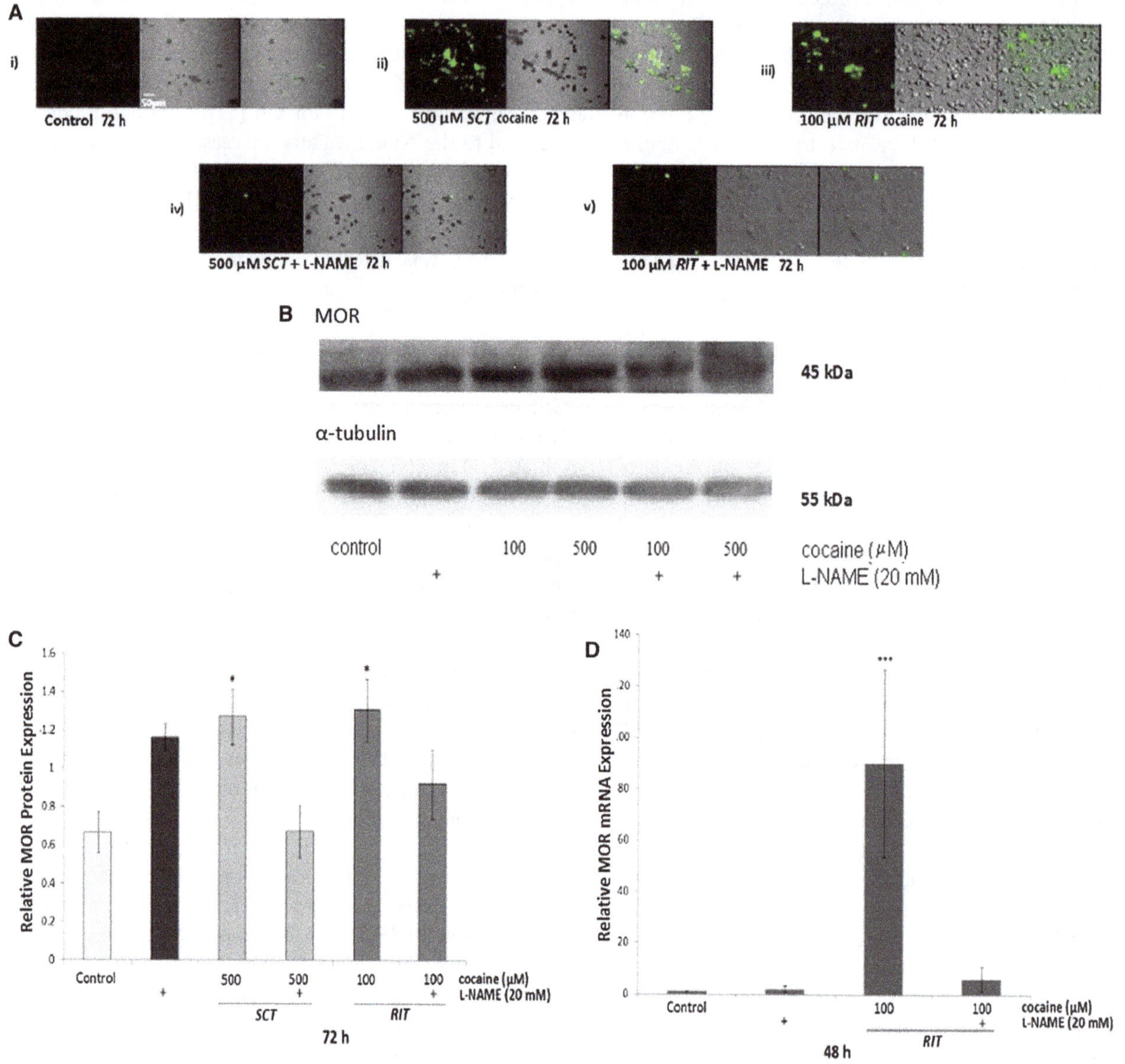

**Figure 2** *Effect of cocaine on NO levels, and NOS inhibition on MOR protein and mRNA levels.* (**A**) Representative images depicting DAF-2 fluorescence in (i) control (untreated) cells and cells treated with (ii) 500 µM *SCT*, or (iii) 100 µM *RIT* with cocaine for 72 h. The left column depicts fluorescence, the middle column is the corresponding Nomarski differential interference contrast image, and the right column is the overlay of these two images. Basal fluorescence was detected in control treated PC12 cells. Following exposure of cells to 500 µM *SCT* and 100 µM *RIT*, fluorescence intensity increased. The cocaine-induced increase in DAF-2 fluorescence was prevented when cells were pretreated with 20 mM L-NAME in both treatment regimens (iv and v). (**B**) Representative immunoblot of MOR protein (upper panel) and α-tubulin (lower panel) levels obtained from lysates of control (untreated) and cocaine-treated PC12 cells grown in the presence or absence of 20 mM L-NAME. Cells were exposed to 500 µM *SCT* or 100 µM *RIT* with cocaine for 72 h. (**C**) Densitometric analysis of MOR protein expression relative to α-tubulin in control, cocaine and L-NAME treated cells. Relative to control, cocaine (*SCT* and *RIT*) significantly increased relative MOR protein levels and this increase was prevented in cells pretreated with L-NAME. (**D**) qPCR analysis of MOR mRNA expression relative to β-2 microglobulin in control, cocaine (100 µM *RIT*) and L-NAME (alone or in combination with 100 µM *RIT* cocaine) treated PC12 cells. Relative to control, 100 µM *RIT* of cocaine significantly increased MOR mRNA, and this increase was prevented by pre-treatement with 20 mM L-NAME. Results are representative of at least 5 independent experiments and the data are shown as mean ± SEM (*p<0.05, ***p<0.001).

cocaine doses were required for transcriptional regulation of MOR. Both dosing regimens also increased NO production and inhibited HDACs activity. Finally, cocaine-induced increases in MOR expression were attenuated by pretreatment with the NOS inhibitor L-NAME, and by the non-selective HAT inhibitor curcumin. Therefore, in PC12 cells, both NO and histone acetylation play an important role in the transcriptional and post-transcriptional regulation of MOR levels by cocaine.

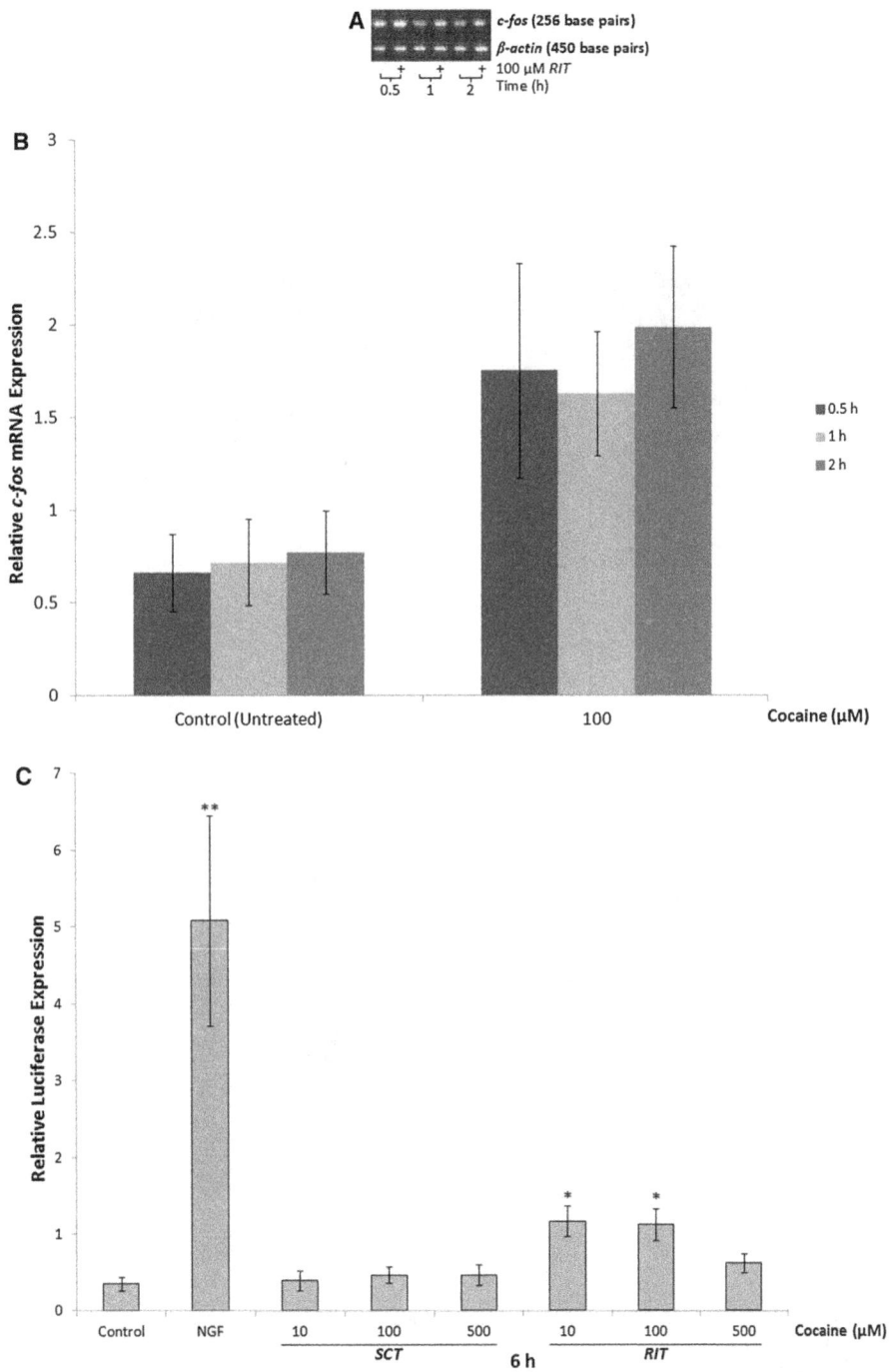

**Figure 3** *Effect of cocaine on c-fos mRNA levels and AP-1 activity.* (**A**) Representative ethidium bromide-stained gel showing amplification of *c-fos* (upper band) and β-actin (lower band) transcripts obtained from RNA extracted from control and cocaine-treated (100 μM *RIT*) PC12 cells, and harvested 0.5, 1, or 2 h after the last of three intermittent cocaine treatments. Qualitative assessment indicated that compared to control, cocaine exposure increased levels of *c-fos* mRNA at all of the time-points examined. (**B**) Quantitative PCR (qPCR) analysis of *c-fos* mRNA levels relative to β-2 microglobulin in control and cocaine treated cells. Relative to control, 100 μM of *RIT* with cocaine significantly increased *c-fos* mRNA levels [F(1,21)=11.41, p<0.01]. (**C**) PC12 cells were transiently transfected with a luciferase-reporter plasmid containing 7 AP-1 transcription factor binding sites prior to treatment with 50 ng/mL NGF or cocaine (10, 100, or 500 μM *SCT* or *RIT*) for 6 h. Luciferase activity in each sample was normalized to its corresponding β-gal activity. Relative to control, there was a significant increase in luciferase activity in PC12 cells treated with NGF, or 10 or 100 μM *RIT* with cocaine. Results are representative of at least 5 independent experiments and data are presented as the mean ± SEM (*p<0.05, **p<0.01).

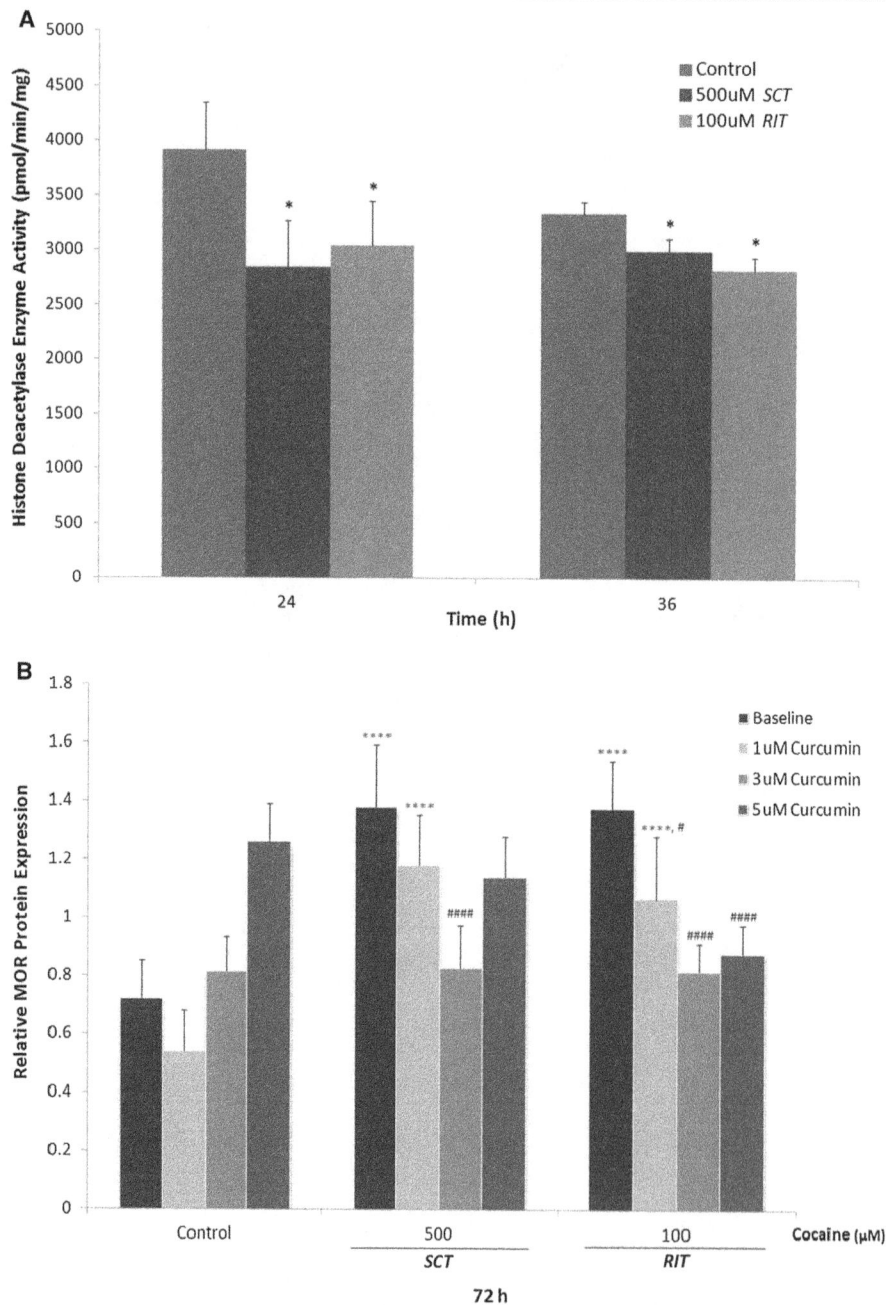

**Figure 4** *Effect of cocaine on HDAC activity, and inhibition of HAT on cocaine-induced MOR protein levels.* (**A**) Nuclear extracts were obtained from lysates of PC12 cells treated with cocaine (500 µM *SCT* or 100 µM *RIT*) for 24 or 36 hours. HDAC enzyme activity was determined using a fluorescent microplate reader and expressed as specific activity, in pM/min/mg. Statistical analysis revealed a significant decrease in HDAC activity following both cocaine treatment regimens at both 24 and 36 h. (**B**) Densitometric analysis of MOR protein levels relative to α-tubulin in control and 72 h cocaine (100 µM *SCT* and 500 µM *RIT*) treated cells grown in the presence and absence of 1, 3 or 5 µM curcumin. Compared to control, both *SCT* and *RIT* with cocaine increased MOR protein levels. For *SCT*, there was a significant decrease in MOR expression after pre-treatment with 3 µM curcumin compared to cells treated with cocaine alone. Pre-treatment with 1, 3 and 5 µM curcumin also prevented the increase in relative MOR protein levels resulting from 100 µM *RIT*. Results are representative of at least 5 independent experiments and data are presented as mean ± SEM (*p<0.05, ****p<0.0001 compared to control, #p<0.05, ####p<0.0001 compared to cocaine alone).

Cocaine has been reported to increase MOR mRNA levels and receptor density in several regions of the rat brain [6,7,66]. In the PC12 cellular model, both repeated doses and a single dose of cocaine increased MOR protein levels, but only repeated doses elevated MOR mRNA levels. This suggests that different treatment regimens regulate MOR expression through different mechanisms, and that multiple doses of cocaine are necessary for transcriptional regulation of the MOR. To investigate this possibility further, the effect of *RIT* and *SCT* cocaine on potential transcriptional regulators of MOR expression, *c-fos* expression and AP-1 activity, was also assessed.

Several studies have demonstrated increases in c-Fos levels following cocaine administration [27,30,31,40,67]. c-Fos binds to members of the Jun immediate early gene family to form the AP-1 transcription factor [68,69]. Since the promoter of the MOR gene contains consensus sequences for binding AP-1 transcription factors [33], AP-1 activity was assessed in PC12 cells treated with cocaine. It was found that the effect of cocaine on AP-1 activity was dependent on the treatment regimen. In fact, only exposure to multiple cocaine doses increased *c-fos* mRNA levels and AP-1 activity, suggesting that increased MOP-r mRNA levels induced by 100 uM *RIT* in PC12 cells could be mediated by AP-1. Increased *c-fos* expression following repeated *in vivo* cocaine administration has been linked to cocaine-induced phosphorylation of CREB [70]. Since CREB is an important regulator of *c-fos* transcription (reviewed in [71]), it is possible the increased *c-fos* mRNA levels observed following RIT in the present study are the result of cocaine-induced CREB phosphorylation. Although we only focused on one potential candidate, other transcription factors, such as SP-1 and NF-κB are also increased in PC12 cells following cocaine administration. [72,73] and activation of these transcription factors has been linked to increases in MOR transcription and mRNA expression [74-76]).

The present study also investigated the role of NO in regulating cocaine-induced changes in MOR protein levels. NO has been found to contribute to the behavioral effects of cocaine, including conditioned place preference and sensitization [77-83]. In addition, NO has been reported to modulate CREB phosphorylation and DNA binding [84,85], increase the expression of immediate early genes such as c-Fos and Jun-B [25,28,29] and increase transcription from AP-1 responsive promoters [25,29], suggesting that NO could also be involved in regulating MOR transcription. In PC12 cells, pre-treatment with the NOS inhibitor L-NAME prevented cocaine-induced up-regulation of MOR mRNA and protein. Additionally, NO production was assessed visually by loading the cells with DAF-2DA as described previously [53]. Both 100 μM *RIT* and 500 μM *SCT* cocaine substantially enhanced DAF-2 fluorescence relative to control (untreated) cells indicating both dosing regimens result in increased NO production. This cocaine-mediated increase in DAF-2 fluorescence was blocked by pre-treated with 20 mM L-NAME, the dose of L-NAME that also prevented cocaine-induced increases in MOR protein and mRNA levels. Taken together, these findings indicate that NO

modulates cocaine-induced changes in MOR protein levels. Interestingly, in *in vivo* neuronal models, cocaine increases NO production by increasing neuronal NOS (nNOS) protein levels and activation [22,23,78,79] via dopamine-, glutamate- and MOR-dependent mechanisms [22,23,79]. Because the PC12 cell culture model does not contain these pre- and post-synaptic systems, the current findings support the intriguing possibility that cocaine can alter NO levels and/or activity by direct intracellular actions. The specific target of these direct actions, and its biological significance, will require further investigation.

These experiments in PC12 cells identified another possible mechanism through which cocaine could increase MOR expression. NO has been reported to decrease HDACs activity [34,35], enzymes that are linked to the behavioral effects of cocaine in rats [36,37], and inhibition of these enzymes prolongs histone acetylation and contributes to enhanced transcription [43-47]. In the present study, both *RIT* and *SCT* cocaine decreased HDACs activity indicating that *in vitro* cocaine exposure enhances histone acetylation. In addition, pre-treatment with the non-selective HAT inhibitor curcumin prevented the cocaine-induced up-regulation of MOR protein levels for both dosing regimens. *In vivo* studies in rats have demonstrated that cocaine increases histone acetylation [36,86,87]. Our findings complement and extend these findings, and suggest that cocaine-mediated alterations in histone acetylation could be an important regulator of MOR protein levels. However, additional actions of curcumin could also contribute to these effects. In fact, cocaine induces the expression of cytokines, such as interleukin-1β [88] which can also regulate MOR transcription [89]. Curcumin inhibits interleukin-1β-induced NF-κB activation [90], suggesting the possibility that the anti-inflammatory properties of curcumin could contribute to its ability to inhibit MOR transcription.

The relationship between NO and HDACs is also complex. Although the cocaine-induced increase in NO observed in the present study could be responsible for decreasing HDACs activity, inhibition of HDACs has also been associated with increases in eNOS mRNA [91]. Increased constitutive NOS levels and increases in NO production resulting in S-nitrosylation have been reported to regulate protein stability [43,44,47]. Thus, in the PC12 cell model, NO and HDACs could modulate MOR expression independently, or may regulate each other to affect MOR transcription and protein stability. As well, the cocaine-induced increase in c-fos expression and AP-1 activity, only observed after RIT, together with increased histone acetylation could be involved in the transcriptional regulation of MOR. Interestingly, both cocaine and NO were reported to increase *c-fos* expression *in vivo* [92], and increases in *c-fos* are correlated with hyperacetylation of H3 histones during chronic co-caine administration and H4 histones after a single acute dose [93], suggesting that similar cellular mechanisms could be regulating the effects of cocaine *in vitro* and *in vivo*.

Although we identified NO and histone acetylation as important regulators of cocaine-induced MOR protein expression, how cocaine initiated the observed effects remains unclear. Blockade of sodium channels following passive entry of cocaine into PC12 cells is one possibility. However, this may not be the only mechanism because, in PC12 cells, NO activity is associated with extracellular signal-regulated kinase (ERK) pathway activation [94-97], and Tan et al. [98] found that the selective sodium channel inhibitor tetrodotoxin had no effect on this pathway. We determined previously that NO modulates ERK activity in PC12 cells [54], and since blockade of ERK phosphorylation in the nucleus accumbens of rats inhibits cocaine-induced behavioural sensitization [99], it is possible that in our system NO-mediated activation of ERK contributes to cocaine-induced MOR expression. *In vivo* cocaine exposure increases dopamine accumulation, through inhibition of dopamine reuptake by the dopamine transporter (for reviews, see: [14,100]), and the dopamine transporter inhibitor sydnocarb has been shown to increase NO generation [101]. Interestingly, Imam et al. [56] reported that cocaine, increased NFκB expression, and dose-dependently decreased both dopamine transporter expression and intracellular dopamine concentrations in differentiated PC12 cells. Elevations in extracellular dopamine could result in dopamine receptor activation, and inhibition of the D1 sub-type of dopamine receptor was reported to partially inhibit cocaine-induced increase in NF-κB [73]. Because NF-κB has also been implicated in regulating NOS expression and NO production [102,103], indirect activation of the D1 receptor by cocaine could enhance NO production. Whether the increases in NO observed in the current study resulted from cocaine-induced dopamine accumulation and dopamine receptor activation requires further investigation. Finally, cocaine has also been reported to diffuse through the membrane of cells [104], suggesting that it may exert direct effects on gene or protein expression.

There are several advantages to identify cellular mechanisms in cell lines, however some limitations of this system need to be considered. In contrast to neurons, PC12 cells continue to divide, and this could make

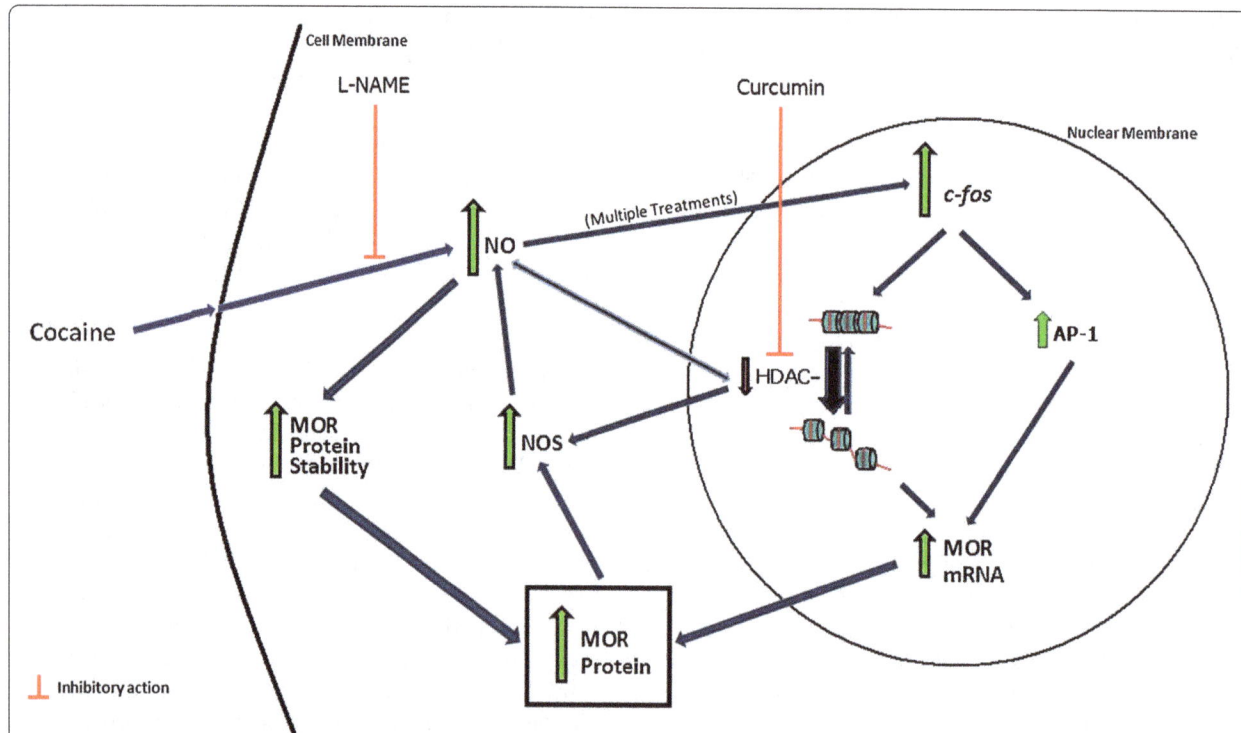

**Figure 5** *Schematic representation of the proposed mechanisms for the in vitro action of cocaine on MOR expression.* Cocaine increases NO production and decreases HDAC activity, which could lead to further increases in NO production as well as enhanced MOR protein stability. Multiple repeated treatments with cocaine also lead to increases in the levels of *c-fos* mRNA. c-Fos can bind to Jun transcription family members to stimulate AP-1 activity, which, in combination with HDAC inhibition, may contribute to an up-regulation in MOR mRNA levels through enhanced transcription. Sites of inhibition (⊥) by curcumin and L-NAME are indicated.

them less vulnerable to neurotoxic compounds. Although we have identified many similarities between our findings and previous *in vivo* studies, differences in the biology of cocaine in the intact organisms compared to the effects observed *in vitro* are likely to exist. The physiological relevance of the doses and regimens employed in these *in vitro* studies is also not known. The doses selected for the present study were based on a previous study that characterized changes in proto-oncogene expression in differentiated PC12 cells [56]. It is not known whether similar treatment regimens, or doses of cocaine, would exert similar effects in an *in vitro* neuronal model or *in vivo*. Further the authors are not aware of any study that has established concentrations of cocaine in the extracellular fluid required to initiate changes in NO production or epigenetic modifications in neurons, or whether cocaine can act on these mechanisms by pathways that do not involve the transporters of catecholamines. Therefore, the current results in the PC12 cell model are important as they propose testable hypotheses about cellular and molecular mechanisms through which cocaine modulates MOR protein and gene expression in neurons.

## Conclusions

The data presented in this study support a model in which cocaine enhances MOR protein expression by increasing cellular NO levels and by decreasing HDAC activity (Figure 5). In addition to cocaine activating these effects independently, elevations in NO could also alter HDAC activity. Inhibition of HDACs could further enhance NO production, resulting in increased MOR expression and protein stability. Additionally, increases in *c-fos* (following multiple treatments) may lead to a modest increase in AP-1 activity that, in combination with enhanced histone acetylation, could contribute to the up-regulation of MOR transcription. Whether these mechanisms occur in neurons, and whether they have implications for the behavioral effects of cocaine, should be the focus of additional investigations.

### Abbreviations
ANOVA: analysis of variance; ANCOVA: analysis of co-variance; AP-1: activator protein 1; DAF-2 DA: 4,5-diaminofluorescein diacetate; HAT: histone acetyltransferase; HDAC: histone deacetylase; L-NAME: N$^\omega$-nitro-L-arginine methyl ester; MOR: μ-opioid receptor; nNOS: neuronal nitric oxide synthase; RIPA: radioimmunoprecipitation assay; SEM: standard error of the mean; TBS-T: TBS containing 0.1 % tween 20.

### Competing interests
The authors declare that they have no competing interests.

### Authors' contributions
WW carried out all of the above experiments, performed the statistical analysis and contributed to the preparation of the manuscript. FL participated in the experimental design of the study, provided some of the materials used, and edited the manuscript. BK supervised the experiments, provided the laboratory facilities and the majority of the reagents used in

the study, and contributed to the preparation of the manuscript. All authors participated equally in the conception of the study, the interpretation of the data and have read and approved the final manuscript.

### Acknowledgements
We wish to thank Mrs. Jennifer Winick-Ng for her help and expertise in the statistical analysis of this study, as well as Dr. Neil MacLusky for his careful review and editing of the manuscript. This work was supported by operating grants from the Natural Sciences and Engineering Research Council of Canada (NSERC) to BK and FL.

### Author details
[1]Department of Biomedical Sciences, University of Guelph, Guelph, Ontario N1G 2W1, Canada. [2]Department of Psychology, University of Guelph, Guelph, Ontario N1G 2W1, Canada.

### References
1. Cummins E, Leri F: Animal studies trigger new insights on the use of methadone maintenance. *Exp Opin Drug Disc* 2009, 4:577.
2. Kreek MJ, Zhou Y, Butelman ER, Levran O: Opiate and cocaine addiction: from bench to clinic and back to the bench. *Curr Opin Pharmacol* 2009, 9:74–80.
3. Roth-Deri I, Green-Sadan T, Yadid G: Beta-endorphin and drug-induced reward and reinforcement. *Prog Neurobiol* 2008, 86:1–21.
4. Shippenberg TS, Zapata A, Chefer VI: Dynorphin and the pathophysiology of drug addiction. *Pharmacol* 2007, 116:306–321.
5. Wee S, Koob GF: The role of the dynorphin-kappa opioid system in the reinforcing effects of drugs of abuse. *Psychopharmacology (Berl)* 2010, 210:121–135.
6. Azaryan AV, Clock BJ, Cox BM: Mu opioid receptor mRNA in nucleus accumbens is elevated following dopamine receptor activation. *Neurochem Res* 1996, 21:1411–1415.
7. Bailey A, Yuferov V, Bendor J, Schlussman SD, Zhou Y, Ho A, Kreek MJ: Immediate withdrawal from chronic "binge" cocaine administration increases mu-opioid receptor mRNA levels in rat frontal cortex. *Brain Res Mol Brain Res* 2005, 137:258–262.
8. Cohen BM, Nguyen TV, Hyman SE: Cocaine-induced changes in gene expression in rat brain. *NIDA Res Monogr* 1991, 105:175–181.
9. Unterwald EM: Regulation of opioid receptors by cocaine. *Ann N Y Acad Sci* 2001, 937:74–92.
10. Zhou Y, Spangler R, Schlussman SD, Yuferov VP, Sora I, Ho A, Uhl GR, Kreek MJ: Effects of acute "binge" cocaine on preprodynorphin, preproenkephalin, proopiomelanocortin, and corticotropin-releasing hormone receptor mRNA levels in the striatum and hypothalamic-pituitary-adrenal axis of mu-opioid receptor knockout mice. *Synapse* 2002, 45:220–229.
11. Zhou Y, Proudnikov D, Yuferov V, Kreek MJ: Drug-induced and genetic alterations in stress-responsive systems: Implications for specific addictive diseases. *Brain Res* 2010, 1314:235–252.
12. Di Chiara G: The role of dopamine in drug abuse viewed from the perspective of its role in motivation. *Drug Alcohol Depend* 1995, 38:95–137.
13. Koob G, Kreek MJ: Stress, dysregulation of drug reward pathways, and the transition to drug dependence. *Am J Psychiatry* 2007, 164:1149–1159.
14. Wise RA: Neurobiology of addiction. *Curr Opin Neurobiol* 1996, 6:243–251.
15. Leri F, Zhou Y, Goddard B, Cummins E, Kreek MJ: Effects of high-dose methadone maintenance on cocaine place conditioning, cocaine self-administration, and mu-opioid receptor mRNA expression in the rat brain. *Neuropsychopharmacology* 2006, 31:1462–1474.
16. Leri F, Zhou Y, Goddard B, Levy A, Jacklin D, Kreek MJ: Steady-state methadone blocks cocaine seeking and cocaine-induced gene expression alterations in the rat brain. *Eur Neuropsychopharmacol* 2009, 19:238–249.
17. Mogenson GJ, Yim CC, Willner P, Scheel-Kruger J: Neuromodulatory functions of the mesolimbic dopamine system: electrophysiological and behavioural studies. In *The mesolimbic dopamine system: from motivation to action*. Edited by Wilner P, Scheel-Kruger J. West Sussex: John Wiley & Sons; 1991:106–130.

18. Stewart J: **Pathways to relapse: the neurobiology of drug- and stress-induced relapse to drug-taking.** *J Psychiatry Neurosci* 2000, **25**:125–136.

19. Ghitza UE, Preston KL, Epstein DH, Kuwabara H, Endres CJ, Bencherif B, Boyd SJ, Copersino ML, Frost JJ, Gorelick DA: **Brain mu-opioid receptor binding predicts treatment outcome in cocaine-abusing outpatients.** *Biol Psychiatry* 2010, **68**:697–703.

20. Gorelick DA, Kim YK, Bencherif B, Boyd SJ, Nelson R, Copersino M, Endres CJ, Dannals RF, Frost JJ: **Imaging brain mu-opioid receptors in abstinent cocaine users: time course and relation to cocaine craving.** *Biol Psychiatry* 2005, **57**:1573–1582.

21. Zubieta JK, Gorelick DA, Stauffer R, Ravert HT, Dannals RF, Frost JJ: **Increased mu opioid receptor binding detected by PET in cocaine-dependent men is associated with cocaine craving.** *Nat Med* 1996, **2**:1225–1229.

22. Lee DK, Koh WC, Shim YB, Shim I, Choe ES: **Repeated cocaine administration increases nitric oxide efflux in the rat dorsal striatum.** *Psychopharmacology* 2010, **208**:245–256.

23. Sammut S, West AR: **Acute cocaine administration increases NO efflux in the rat prefrontal cortex via a neuronal NOS-dependent mechanism.** *Synapse* 2008, **62**:710–713.

24. Chan SH, Chang KF, Ou CC, Chan JY: **Nitric oxide regulates c-fos expression in nucleus tractus soliarii induced by baroreceptor activation via cGMP-dependent protein kinase and cAMP response element-binding protein phosphorylation.** *Mol Pharmacol* 2004, **65**:19–325.

25. Haby C, Lisovoski F, Aunis D, Zwiller J: **Stimulation of the cyclic GMP pathway by NO induces expression of the immediate early genes c-fos and junB in PC12 cells.** *J Neurochem* 1994, **62**:496–501.

26. Imam SZ, Jankovic J, Ali SF, Skinner JT, Xie W, Conneely OM, Le WD: **Nitric oxide mediates increased susceptibility to dopaminergic damage in Nurr1 heterozygous mice.** *FASEB J* 2005, **19**:1441–1450.

27. Kreuter JD, Mattson BJ, Wang B, You ZB, Hope BT: **Cocaine-induced Fos expression in rat striatum is blocked by chloral hydrate or urethane.** *Neuroscience* 2004, **127**:233–242.

28. Morris BJ: **Stimulation of immediate early gene expression in striatal neurons by nitric oxide.** *J Biol Chem* 1995, **270**:24740–24744.

29. Pilz RB, Suhasini M, Idriss S, Meinkoth JL, Boss GR: **Nitric oxide and cGMP analogs activate transcription from AP-1 responsive promoters in mammalian cells.** *FASEB J* 1995, **9**:552–558.

30. Radwanska K, Caboche J, Kaczmarek L: **Extracellular signal-regulated kinases (ERKs) modulated cocaine-induced gene expression in the mouse amygdala.** *Eur J Neurosci* 2005, **22**:939–948.

31. Zahm DS, Becker ML, Freiman AJ, Strauch S, Degarmo B, Geisler S, Meredith GE, Marinelli M: **Fos after single and repeated self-administration of cocaine and saline in the rat: emphasis on the Basal forebrain and recalibration of expression.** *Neuropsychopharmacology* 2010, **35**:445–463.

32. Zhuravliova E, Barbakadze T, Narmania N, Ramsden J, Mikeladze D: **Inhibition of nitric oxide synthase and farnesyltransferase change the activities of several transcription factors.** *J Mol Neurosci* 2007, **31**:281–287.

33. Börner C, Höllt V, Kraus J: **Involvement of activator protein-1 in transcriptional regulation of the human mu-opioid receptor gene.** *Mol Pharmacol* 2002, **61**:800–805.

34. Feng J, Jing F, Fang H, Gu L, Xu W: **Expression, purification, and S-nitrosylation of recombinant histone deacetylase 8 in Escherichia coli.** *Biosci Trends* 2011, **5**:17–22.

35. Sha Y, Marshall HE: **S-nitrosylation in the regulation of gene transcription.** *Biochim Biophys Acta*, in press [Epub ahead of print].

36. Hui B, Wang W, Li J: **Biphasic modulation of cocaine-induced conditioned place preference through inhibition of histone acetyltransferase and histone deacetylase.** *Saudi Med J* 2010, **31**:389–393.

37. Sun J, Wang L, Jiang B, Hui B, Lv Z, Ma L: **The effects of sodium butyrate, an inhibitor of histone deacetylase, on the cocaine- and sucrose-maintained self-administration in rats.** *Neurosci Letters* 2008, **441**:72–76.

38. Hwang CH, Song KY, Kim CS, Choi HS, Guo X, Law P, Wei L, Loh HH: **Epigenetic programming of μ-opioid receptor gene in mouse brain is regulated by MeCP2 and brg1 chromatin remodelling factor.** *J Cell Mol Med* 2008, **13**:3591–3615.

39. Hwang CK, Kim CS, do K K, Law PY, Wei LN, Loh HH: **Up-regulation of the mu-opioid receptor gene is mediated through chromatin remodeling and transcriptional factors in differentiated neuronal cells.** *Mol Pharmacol* 2010, **78**:58–68.

40. Guan X, Tao J, Li S: **Dopamine D1 receptor, but not dopamine D2 receptor, is a critical regulator for acute cocaine-enhanced gene expression.** *Neurol Res* 2009, **31**:17–22.

41. Jablonka E, Lachman M, Lamb MJ: **Evidence, mechanisms and models for the inheritance of acquired characters.** *J Theor Biol* 1992, **158**:245–268.

42. Liu Y, Lu C, Yang Y, Fan Y, Yang R, Liu CF, Korolev N, Nordenskiöld L: **Influence of Histone Tails and H4 Tail Acetylations on Nucleosome-Nucleosome Interactions.** *J Mol Biol* 2011, **414**:749–764.

43. Kwak Y, Ma T, Diao S, Zhang X, Chen Y, Hsu J, Lipton S, Masliah E, Xu H, Liao F: **NO signaling and S-nitrosylation regulate PTEN inhibition in neurodegeneration.** *Mol Neurodegener* 2010, **5**:49–61.

44. Palmer LA, Gaston B, Johns RA: **Normoxic stabilization of hypoxia-inducible factor-1 expression and activity: redox-dependent effect of nitrogen oxides.** *Mol Pharmacol* 2000, **58**:1197–1203.

45. Schlake T, Klehr-Wirth D, Yoshida M, Beppu T, Bode J: **Gene expression within a chromatin domain: the role of core histone hyperacetylation.** *Biochemistry* 1994, **33**:4197–4206.

46. Ura K, Kurumizaka H, Dimitrov S, Almouzni G, Wolffe AP: **Histone acetylation: influence on transcription, nucleosome mobility and positioning, and linker histone-dependent transcriptional repression.** *EMBO J* 1997, **16**:2096–2107.

47. Zhou J, Fandrev J, Schiiman J, Tiegs G, Brüne B: **NO and TNF- released from activated macrophages stabilize HIF-1 in resting tubular LLC-PK1 cells.** *Am J Physiol* 2003, **284**:C439–C446.

48. Borowitz JL, Gunasekar PG, Isom GE: **Hydrogen cyanide generation by mu-opiate receptor activation: possible neuromodulatory role of endogenous cyanide.** *Brain Res* 1997, **768**:294–300.

49. Niu S, Kuo CH, Gan Y, Nisikawa E, Sadakata T, Ichikawa H, Miki N: **Increase of calmodulin III gene expression by mu-opioid receptor stimulation in PC12 cells.** *Jpn J Pharmacol* 2000, **84**:412–417.

50. Yoshikawa M, Ueno S, Hirano M, Nakayama H, Furuya H: **Effects of fentanyl on survival of serum-deprived rat pehochromocytoma cells.** *Pharm Pharmacol Commun* 1999, **5**:603–607.

51. Baskey JC, Kalisch BE, Davis WL, Meakin SO, Rylett RJ: **PC12^nnr5 cells expressing TrkA receptors undergo morphological but not cholinergic phenotypic differentiation in response to NGF.** *J Neurochem* 2002, **80**:501–511.

52. Binnington JC, Kalisch BE: **Nitric oxide synthase inhibitors modulate nerve growth factor-mediated regulation of amyloid precursor protein expression in PC12 cells.** *J Neurochem* 2007, **101**:422–433.

53. Kalisch BE, Bock NA, Davis W, Rylett RJ: **Inhibitors of nitric oxide synthase attenuate nerve growth factor-mediated increases in choline acetyltransferase gene expression in PC12 cells.** *J Neurochem* 2002, **81**:624–635.

54. Kalisch BE, Demeris CS, Ishak M, Rylett RJ: **Modulation of nerve growth factor-induced activation of MAP kinase in PC12 cells by inhibitors of nitric oxide synthase.** *J Neurochem* 2003, **87**:1321–1332.

55. Gotfryd K, Skladchikova G, Lepekhin EA, Berezin V, Bock E, Walmod PS: **Cell type-specific anti-cancer properties of valproic acid: independent effects on HDAC activity and Erk1/2 phosphorylation.** *BMC Cancer* 2010, **10**:383.

56. Imam SZ, Duhart HM, Skinner JT, Ali SF: **Cocaine induces a differential dose-dependent alteration in the expression profile of immediate early genes, transcription factors, and caspases in PC12 cells: a possible mechanism of neurotoxic damage in cocaine addiction.** *Ann NY Acad Sci* 2005, **1053**:482–490.

57. Unterwald EM, Cox BM, Kreek MJ, Cote TE, Izenwasser S: **Chronic repeated cocaine administration alters basal and opioid-regulated adenylyl cyclase activity.** *Synapse* 1993, **15**:33–38.

58. Izenwasser S, Heller B, Cox BM: **Continuous cocaine administration enhances mu- but not delta-opioid receptor-mediated inhibition of adenylyl cyclase activity in nucleus accumbens.** *Eur J Pharmacol* 1996, **297**:187–191.

59. Cheung NS, Pascoe CJ, Giardina SF, John CA, Beart PM: **Micromolar L-glutamate induces extensive apoptosis in an apoptotic-necrotic continuum of insult-dependent, excitotoxic injury in cultured cortical neurones.** *Neuropharmacol* 1998, **37**:1419–1429.

60. Siddiqui MA, Kashyap MP, Kumar V, Tripathi VK, Khanna VK, Yadav S, Pant AB: **Differential protection of pre-, co- and post-treatment of curcumin against hydrogen peroxide in PC12 cells.** *Hum Exp Toxicol* 2011, **30**:192–198.

61. Chen W, Bacanamwo M, Harrison DG: **Activation of p300 histone acetyltransferase activity is an early endothelial response to laminar

shear stress and is essential for stimulation of endothelial nitric-oxide synthase mRNA transcription. *J Biol Chem* 2008, **283**:16293-16298.

62. Kang SK, Cha SH, Jeon HG: Curcumin-induced histone hypoacetylation enhances caspase-3-dependent glioma cell death and neurogenesis of neural progenitor cells. *Stem Cells Dev* 2006, **15**:165-174.

63. Sun H, Yang X, Zhu J, Lv T, Chen Y, Chen G, Zhong L, Li Y, Huang X, Huang G, Tian J: Inhibition of p300-HAT results in a reduced histone acetylation and down-regulation of gene expression in cardiac myocytes. *Life Sci* 2010, **87**:707-714.

64. Bradford M: A rapid and sensitive method for the quantitation of microgram quantities of protein utilizing the principle of protein-dye binding. *Anal Biochem* 1976, **72**:248-254.

65. MacKinnon JC, Huether P, Kalisch BE: Effects of nerve growth factor and nitric oxide synthase inhibitors on amyloid precursor protein mRNA levels and protein stability. *Open Biochem J* 2012, **6**:31-39.

66. Unterwald EM, Kreek MJ, Cuntapay M: The frequency of cocaine administration impacts cocaine-induced receptor alterations. *Brain Res* 2001, **900**:103-109.

67. Larson EB, Akkentli F, Edwards S, Graham DL, Simmons DL, Alibhai IN, Nestler EJ, Self DW: Striatal regulation of ΔFosB, FosB, and cFos during cocaine self-administration and withdrawal. *J Neurochem* 2010, **115**:112-122.

68. Bossis G, Malnou CE, Farras R, Andermarcher E, Hipskind R, Rodriguez M, Schmidt D, Muller S, Jariel-Encontre I, Piechaczyk M: Down-regulation of c-Fos/c-Jun AP-1 dimer activity by sumoylation. *Mol Cell Biol* 2005, **25**:6964-6979.

69. Chinenov Y, Kerppola TK: Close encounters of many kinds: Fos-Jun interactions that mediate transcription regulatory specificity. *Oncogene* 2001, **20**:2438-2452.

70. Mattson BJ, Bossert JM, Simmons DE, Nozaki N, Nagarkar D, Kreuter JD, Hope BT: Cocaine-induced CREB phosphorylation in nucleus accumbens of cocaine-sensitized rats is enabled by enhanced activation of extracellular signal-related kinase, but not protein kinase A. *J Neurochem* 2005, **95**:1481-1494.

71. Mayr B, Montminy M: Transcriptional regulation by the phosphorylation-dependent factor CREB. *Nat Rev Mol Cell Biol* 2001, **2**:599-609.

72. Imam SZ, Duhart HM, Skinner JT, Ali SF: Cocaine induces a dose-dependent alteration in the expression of immediate early genes c-fos and SP-1 and in nuclear factor NF-kappabeta in PC12 cells. *Ann NY Acad Sci* 2003, **993**:362.

73. Lepsch LB, Munhoz CD, Kawamoto EM, Yshii LM, Lima LS, Curi-Boaventura MF, Salgado TM, Curi R, Planeta CS, Scavone C: Cocaine induces cell death and activates the transcription nuclear factor kappa-B in PC12 cells. *Mol Brain* 2009, **2**:3.

74. Beltran JA, Peek J, Chang SL: Expression and regulation of the mu opioid peptide receptor in TPA-differentiated HL-60 promyelocytic leukemia cells. *Int Immunopharmacol* 2006, **6**:1331-1340.

75. Gach K, Piestrzeniewicz M, Fichna J, Stefanska B, Szemraj J, Janecka A: Opioid-induced regulation of mu-opioid receptor gene expression in the MCF-7 breast cancer cell line. *Biochem Cell Biol* 2008, **86**:217-226.

76. Lin YC, Flock KE, Cook RJ, Hunkele AJ, Loh HH, Ko JL: Effects of trichostatin A on neuronal mu-opioid receptor gene expression. *Brain Res* 2008, **1246**:1-10.

77. Pudiak CM, Bozarth MA: The effect of nitric oxide synthesis inhibition on intravenous cocaine self-administration. *Prog Neuropsychopharmacol Biol Psychiatry* 2002, **26**:189-196.

78. Bhargava HN, Kumar S: Sensitization to the locomotor stimulant activity of cocaine is associated with increases in nitric oxide synthase activity in brain regions and spinal cord of mice. *Pharmacol* 1997, **55**:292-298.

79. Yoo JH, Cho JH, Lee SY, Lee S, Loh HH, Ho IK, Jang CG: Differential effects of morphine- and cocaine-induced nNOS immunoreactivity in the dentate gyrus of hippocampus of mice lacking mu-opioid receptors. *Neurosci Lett* 2006, **395**:98-102.

80. Collins SL, Kantak KM: Neuronal nitric oxide synthase inhibition decreases cocaine self-administration behavior in rats. *Psychopharmacology (Berl)* 2002, **159**:361-369.

81. Itzhak Y, Martin JL, Black MD, Huang PL: The role of neuronal nitric oxide synthase in cocaine-induced conditioned place preference. *Neuroreport* 1998, **9**:2485-2488.

82. Itzhak Y: Role of the NMDA receptor and nitric oxide in memory reconsolidation of cocaine-induced conditioned place preference in mice. *Ann N Y Acad Sci* 2008, **1139**:350-357.

83. Martin JL, Itzhak Y: 7-Nitroindazole blocks nicotine-induced conditioned place preference but not LiCl-induced conditioned place aversion. *Neuroreport* 2000, **11**:947-949.

84. Ohki K, Yoshida K, Hagiwara M, Harada T, Takamura M, Ohashi T, Matsuda H, Imaki J: Nitric oxide induces c-fos gene expression via cyclic AMP response element binding protein (CREB) phosphorylation in rat retinal pigment epithelium. *Brain Res* 1995, **696**:140-144.

85. Riccio A, Alvania RS, Lonze BE, Ramanan N, Kim T, Huang Y, Dawson TM, Snyder SH, Ginty DD: A nitric oxide signaling pathway controls CREB-mediated gene expression in neurons. *Mol Cell* 2006, **21**:283-294.

86. Sanchis-Segura C, Lopez-Atalaya JP, Barco A: Selective boosting of transcriptional and behavioral responses to drugs of abuse by histone deacetylase inhibition. *Neuropsychopharmacol* 2009, **34**:2642-2654.

87. Wang L, Lv Z, Hu Z, Sheng J, Hui B, Sun J, Ma L: Chronic cocaine-induced H3 acetylation and transcriptional activation of CaMKII alpha in the nucleus accumbens is critical for motivation for drug reinforcement. *Neuropsychopharmacol* 2010, **35**:913-928.

88. Cearley CN, Blindheim K, Sorg BA, Krueger JM, Churchill L: Acute cocaine increases interleukin-1β mRNA and immunoreactive cells in the cortex and nucleus accumbens. *Neurochem Res* 2011, **36**:686-692.

89. Zhang L, Belkowski JS, Briscoe T, Rogers TJ: Regulation of Mu Opioid Receptor Expression in Developing T Cells. *J Neuroimmune Pharmacol* 2012, [Epub ahead of print].

90. Buhrmann C, Mobasheri A, Busch F, Aldinger C, Stahlmann R, Montaseri A, Shakibaei M: Curcumin modulates nuclear factor kappaB (NF-kappaB)-mediated inflammation in human tenocytes in vitro: role of the phosphatidylinositol 3-kinase/Akt pathway. *J Biol Chem* 2011, **286**:28556-28566.

91. Gan Y, Shen YH, Utama B, Wang J, Coselli J, Wang XL: Dual effects of histone deacetylase inhibition by trichostatin A on endothelial nitric oxide synthase expression in endothelial cells. *Biochem Biophys Res Commun* 2006, **340**:29-34.

92. Thiriet N, Aunis D, Zwiller J: The nitric oxide releasing agent sodium nitroprusside modulates cocaine-induced immediate early gene expression in rat brain. *Ann NY Acad Sci* 2002, **965**:47-54.

93. Kumar A, Choi KH, Renthal W, Tsankova NM, Theobald DE, Truong HT, Russo SJ, Laplant Q, Sasaki TS, Whistler KN, Neve RL, Self DW, Nestler EJ: Chromatin remodeling is a key mechanism underlying cocaine-induced plasticity in striatum. *Neuron* 2005, **48**:303-314.

94. Miyamoto Y, Sakai R, Maeda C, Takata T, Ihara H, Tsuchiya Y, Watanabe Y: Nitric oxide promotes nicotine-triggered ERK signaling via redox reactions in PC12 cells. *Nitric Oxide* 2011, **25**:344-349.

95. Yasui H, Ito N, Yamamori T, Nakamura H, Okano J, Asanuma T, Nakajima T, Kuwabara M, Inanami O: Induction of neurite outgrowth by alpha-phenyl-N-tert-butylnitrone through nitric oxide release and Ras-ERK pathway in PC12 cells. *Free Radic Res* 2010, **44**:645-654.

96. Jang JH, Surh YJ: AP-1 mediates beta-amyloid-induced iNOS expression in PC12 cells via the ERK2 and p38 MAPK signaling pathways. *Biochem Biophys Res Commun* 2005, **331**:1421-1428.

97. Kim TW, Lee CH, Choi CY, Kwon NS, Baek KJ, Kim YG, Yun HY: Nitric oxide mediates membrane depolarization-promoted survival of rat neuronal PC12 cells. *Neurosci Lett* 2003, **344**:209-211.

98. Tan Z, Dohi S, Ohguchi K, Nakashima S, Nozawa Y: Local anesthetics inhibit muscarinic receptor-mediated activation of extracellular signal-regulated kinases in rat pheochromocytoma PC12 cells. *Anesthesiology* 1999, **91**:1014-1024.

99. Kim S, Shin JK, Yoon HS, Kim JH: Blockade of ERK Phosphorylation in the Nucleus Accumbens Inhibits the Expression of Cocaine-induced Behavioral Sensitization in Rats. *Korean J Physiol Pharmacol* 2011, **15**:389-395.

100. Self DW, Nestler EJ: Molecular mechanisms of drug reinforcement and addiction. *Annu Rev Neurosci* 1995, **18**:463-495.

101. Bashkatova V, Mathieu-Kia AM, Durand C, Penit-Soria J: Neurochemical changes and neurotoxic effects of an acute treatment with sydnocarb, a novel psychostimulant: comparison with D-amphetamine. *Ann NY Acad Sci* 2002, **965**:180-192.

102. Broadbelt NV, Chen J, Silver RB, Poppas DP, Felsen D: Pressure activates epidermal growth factor receptor leading to the induction of iNOS via NFkappaB and STAT3 in human proximal tubule cells. *Am J Physiol Renal Physiol* 2009, **297**:F114-F124.

103. Hwang MH, Damte D, Lee JS, Gebru E, Chang ZQ, Cheng H, Jung BY, Rhee MH, Park SC: **Mycoplasma hyopneumoniae induces pro-inflammatory cytokine and nitric oxide production through NFκB and MAPK pathways in RAW264.7 cells.** *Vet Res Commun* 2011, **35:**21–34.

104. Rang HP, Dale MM, Ritter JM: **Local anaesthetics and other drugs that affect ion channels.** In *Pharmacology.* 4th edition. Edinburgh: Harcourt Publishers Ltd; 2001:634–645.

# 22

# Decreased cervical epithelial sensitivity to nonoxynol-9 (N-9) after four daily applications in a murine model of topical vaginal microbicide safety

Karissa Lozenski[1], Robert Ownbey[2], Brian Wigdahl[1], Tina Kish-Catalone[1] and Fred C Krebs[1*]

## Abstract

**Background:** The disappointing clinical failures of five topical vaginal microbicides have provided new insights into factors that impact microbicide safety and efficacy. Specifically, the greater risk for human immunodeficiency virus type 1 (HIV-1) acquisition associated with multiple uses of a nonoxynol-9 (N-9)-containing product has highlighted the importance of application frequency as a variable during pre-clinical microbicide development, particularly in animal model studies.

**Methods:** To evaluate an association between application frequency and N-9 toxicity, experiments were performed using a mouse model of cervicovaginal microbicide safety. In this model system, changes in cervical and vaginal epithelial integrity, cytokine release, and immune cell infiltration were assessed after single and multiple exposures to N-9.

**Results:** After the initial application of N-9 (aqueous, 1%), considerable damage to the cervical epithelium (but not the vaginal epithelium) was observed as early as 10 min post-exposure and up to 8 h post-exposure. Subsequent daily exposures (up to 4 days) were characterized by diminished cervical toxicity relative to single exposures of like duration. Levels of pro-inflammatory cytokines released into the cervicovaginal lumen and the degree of CD14-positive immune cell infiltration proximal to the cervical epithelium were also dependent on the number of N-9 exposures.

**Conclusions:** Rather than causing cumulative cervical epithelial damage, repeated applications of N-9 were characterized by decreased sensitivity to N-9-associated toxicity and lower levels of immune cell recruitment. These results provide new insights into the failure of N-9-based microbicides and illustrate the importance of considering multiple exposure protocols in pre-clinical microbicide development strategies.

**Keywords:** Microbicide, N-9, Cervix, Mouse, Toxicity

## Background

The global human immunodeficiency virus type 1 (HIV-1) epidemic currently includes approximately 33 million HIV-1-infected people worldwide, with a particularly high incidence of infection (~23 million individuals) in Sub-Saharan Africa [1]. Since the discovery of HIV-1 over 30 years ago, the face of this global epidemic has changed dramatically, with heterosexual intercourse now considered the predominant route for the spread of the virus [1]. As a result, women are at much greater risk for acquiring HIV-1 and have a much greater need for methods that effectively reduce or eliminate the risk of infection during sexual intercourse. Although condoms (male and female) are highly effective barrier methods, they are not female-controlled and are unlikely to be used with great adherence in developing countries. To answer the critical need for effective female-controlled methods of protection, continued efforts are being directed toward the development of microbicides. A microbicide is a chemical

---

* Correspondence: fred.krebs@drexelmed.edu
[1]Department of Microbiology and Immunology, and Center for Molecular Therapeutics and Resistance, Center for Sexually Transmitted Disease, Institute for Molecular Medicine and Infectious Disease, Drexel University College of Medicine, 245 N. 15th Street, Philadelphia, PA 19102, USA
Full list of author information is available at the end of the article

entity that can be applied vaginally or rectally to eliminate or reduce the risk of HIV-1 transmission. Efforts to develop topical vaginal microbicides have resulted in the advancement of many candidate microbicide compounds through pre-clinical studies and clinical trials of both safety and efficacy [2-4].

Unfortunately, clinical trials involving the microbicides COL-1492 (nonoxynol-9 or N-9), Savvy (C31G), Ushercell (cellulose sulfate), Carraguard (carrageenan), and PRO 2000 [5-7] failed to demonstrate any product efficacy despite promising activities in pre-clinical studies and apparently acceptable levels of safety in early clinical studies. The results of these failed trials emphasized the urgent need for more stringent pre-clinical protocols, with emphasis on microbicide safety and the use of non-human primate models to evaluate the efficacy and safety of potential microbicides [8].

The clear need for more thorough pre-clinical evaluations is particularly apparent in retrospective analyses of the development of N-9 as a microbicide [9]. Pre-clinical assessments of N-9 failed to predict the inability of N-9 to inhibit HIV-1 transmission and the adverse effects of N-9 exposure on the risk of infection. Early in vitro studies of N-9, which has been widely used as a spermicidal agent for more than 40 years [9], yielded promising results, demonstrating that N-9 possessed broad-spectrum activity against several sexually transmitted disease (STD) pathogens, including *Chlamydia trachomatis*, *Neisseria gonorrhoeae*, herpes simplex virus type 2 (HSV-2), and HIV-1 [10-18]. The widespread and apparently safe use of N-9 as a human contraceptive agent further supported the development of this compound as a topical microbicide. As a consequence, N-9 was advanced into human clinical trials. However, the final phase 2/3 clinical trial of N-9 (formulated as COL-1492 with 52.5 mg N-9 per treatment dose) demonstrated that high frequency use of this product was associated with an almost 2-fold greater risk of HIV-1 acquisition [5]. Increased HIV-1 infection after N-9 application, in hindsight, has been attributed to the disruption of the cervicovaginal epithelial barrier as well as inflammation and irritation associated with N-9 application [9,19-22]. While these findings ended the further development of N-9 as a microbicide, they also raised new questions about mechanisms by which potential topical microbicides can fail.

The apparent association between N-9 application frequency and increased risk of HIV-1 infection prompted an expansion of our previous N-9 toxicity studies involving a Swiss Webster mouse model of cervicovaginal toxicity. The value of this model system was demonstrated in investigations that reiterated the clinical toxicity of N-9 (after a single application) and paralleled indications of irritation associated with topical application of 1.7% C31G [19,23,24]. Furthermore, mouse model experiments involving topical vaginal application of N-9 clearly demonstrated that (i) N-9-associated tissue damage was greatest approximately two to four hours post-application, (ii) epithelial damage was limited to the cervix, and (iii) repair and regeneration of cervical epithelial tissues was essentially complete 24 h after a single application of N-9 [19].

The present studies were conducted using the mouse model of microbicide toxicity to examine the effects of multiple daily exposures to N-9. These experiments were designed to provide a comprehensive assessment of changes in cervicovaginal integrity with respect to post-application exposure duration and the number of topical applications of N-9. The results of these investigations indicated that (i) multiple exposures to N-9 resulted in diminished cervical sensitivity to N-9 application relative to the initial exposure and (ii) cytokine release and CD14-positive cell infiltration subsequent to N-9 exposure varied with the number of exposures. These studies provide new insights into the mechanisms underlying the failure of N-9 as a microbicide and suggest a new parameter for assessing future microbicide candidate molecules.

## Methods
### Animals
Five- to six-week-old female outbred Swiss-Webster mice (CFW®) were utilized for all experiments (Charles River Laboratories International, Inc., Wilmington, MA). Mice were synchronized 7 and 3 days prior to the start of each experiment with a 0.2 mL subcutaneous injection of Depo-Provera® (Pharmacia and Upjohn Company) diluted in Lactated Ringer's Solution (Baxter) for a final dose of 3 mg/animal. Prior to intravaginal application, mice were anesthetized with a formulation of ketamine/xylazine (100–200 mg/kg and 5–10 ng/kg, respectively). Anesthetized animals then received a single intravaginal inoculation (60 µL) of saline or N-9 diluted in saline. Mice treated with saline alone were included as controls at all time points to evaluate the normal tissue morphology in the cervicovaginal mucosa. After treatment, mice were humanely sacrificed and the cervicovaginal tracts were surgically excised and prepared for histological examination. Each experiment evaluated three animals at each time point within each test group. All animal studies conformed to the "Guiding Principle in the Care and Use of Animals" approved by the American Physiological Society, and were approved by The Drexel University College of Medicine Institutional Animal Care and Use Committee (IACUC).

### Multiple exposure experiments
The previously described single application protocol [23,25] was adapted to investigate the effects of multiple N-9 exposures. In the first set of experiments, four

consecutive daily applications of N-9 were administered to the mice. This protocol parallels the FDA standardized rabbit vaginal irritation (RVI) study design, which utilizes 10 consecutive daily applications. Unlike the RVI protocol, however, the present experimental design also included intermediate assessments of tissue damage at acute post-application time points. Specifically, animals were sacrificed at acute exposure durations of 10 min, 2 h, and 4 h, and at longer exposure times of 8 h and 24 h following each application for additional and more stringent assessments of cervicovaginal toxicity (Figure 1A). These acute exposure durations were previously used to characterize the onset and development of epithelial damage following single microbicide application [23,25]. In addition, these exposure durations are presumed to be within a likely window of STD pathogen exposure and infection. The longer exposure durations have been shown to be

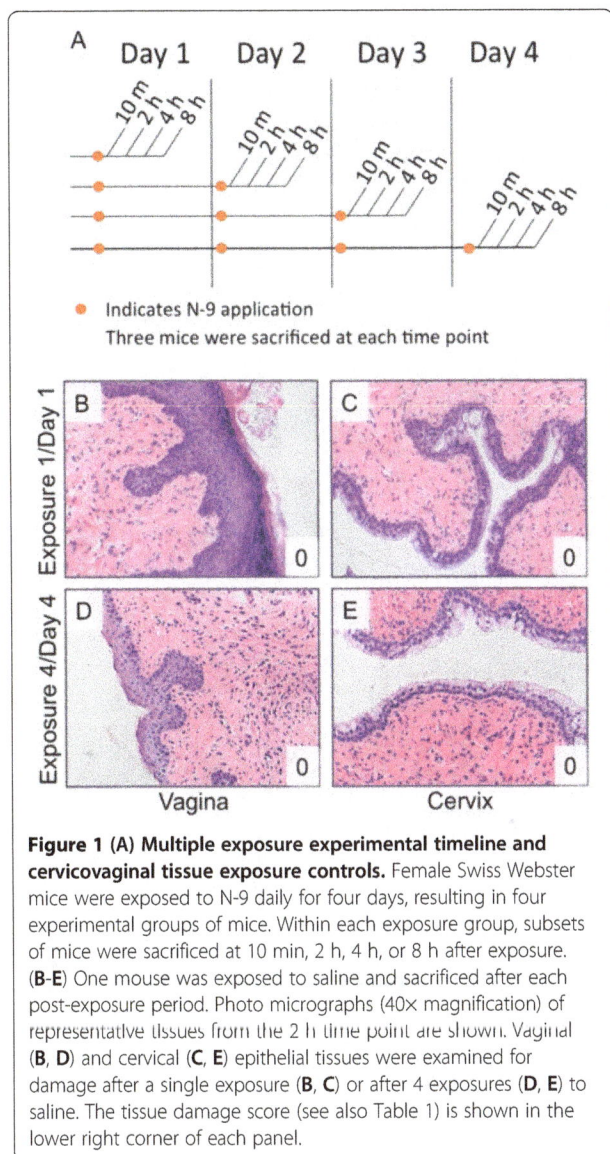

Figure 1 (A) Multiple exposure experimental timeline and cervicovaginal tissue exposure controls. Female Swiss Webster mice were exposed to N-9 daily for four days, resulting in four experimental groups of mice. Within each exposure group, subsets of mice were sacrificed at 10 min, 2 h, 4 h, or 8 h after exposure. (B-E) One mouse was exposed to saline and sacrificed after each post-exposure period. Photo micrographs (40× magnification) of representative tissues from the 2 h time point are shown. Vaginal (B, D) and cervical (C, E) epithelial tissues were examined for damage after a single exposure (B, C) or after 4 exposures (D, E) to saline. The tissue damage score (see also Table 1) is shown in the lower right corner of each panel.

important for characterizing the time course of epithelial repair and subsequent tissue inflammation.

Prior to excision of the reproductive tracts, animals were vaginally lavaged using 150 µl Lactated Ringer's Solution (Baxter) by reverse pipetting. Lavage fluids were collected and stored at –80°C prior to analyses of cytokine content. The cervicovaginal tract was then excised, formalin-fixed, and embedded in paraffin using standard procedures. Tissue sections set aside for further processing were chosen to show epithelial tissues from the lower vaginal tract and the cervix. Sections were stained with hematoxylin and eosin (H&E) for assessment of tissue damage; representative fields from each treatment group were imaged and documented using deconvolution microscopy.

### Measurement of cytokine levels in vaginal lavage fluids

Cytokine levels in collected vaginal lavages were measured using a Luminex 100/200 instrument (Luminex Corporation, Austin, TX). Two murine pro-inflammatory cytokines – interleukin-1β (IL-1β) and interleukin-6 (IL-6) – were measured using commercially available plates (Millipore). Lavage samples were thawed on ice and then centrifuged for 5 minutes at a high speed to pellet any debris or mucus and to prevent plate filter clogging. Samples (25 µL per well) were added to the plate in duplicate and processed as described by the manufacturer. Results were analyzed using Xponent 3.1 software (Luminex) and graphed using Microsoft Excel to visualize changes in cytokine levels.

### Immunohistochemical staining for immune cell localization

Paraffin-embedded tissue sections were deparaffinized and rehydrated using xylene, an ethanol gradient, and deionized water as per standard protocol. Antigen retrieval was performed using trypsin in a humidified chamber followed by steaming while treating tissue with target retrieval solution (Dako S1700) for 30 min. Following this incubation, the tissue sections were treated with hydrogen peroxide and then blocked with R.T.U. normal horse serum (Vector). Primary anti-CD14 antibody (Abcam) was applied at a 1:500 dilution followed by the secondary antibody (ImmPRESS Reagent Kit peroxidase, Vector MP-7401). After the incubation with the secondary antibody, visualization of the cells was performed using the DAB: Peroxidase Substrate Kit (Vector SK-4100). The tissue was then counterstained using hematoxylin (Vector H3401) and was processed through an alcohol gradient and xylene before application of a coverslip mounted using cytoseal XYL mounting media (Richard Allan Scientific 8312–4). Staining was performed by Paragon Bioservices. Levels of staining were assessed qualitatively in sections prepared from three mice at each time point.

**Table 1 Scoring system used for the assessment of cervicovaginal epithelial tissue damage subsequent to N-9 exposure**

| Score | Description of epithelial damage |
|---|---|
| 0 | No epithelial disturbances or sloughing of epithelial cells |
| 1 | Light epithelial damage and disruption – localized loss of tissue integrity and epithelial sloughing over less than 5% of the epithelial surface, which is otherwise contiguous and intact |
| 2 | Moderate epithelial damage and disruption – Multiple areas of epithelial disturbance representing 5-25% of the total epithelial surface and small regions of sloughing that expose the basal cell layer |
| 3 | Severe epithelial damage and disruption – Sloughing over large sections of the epithelial surface (> 25%) that exposes the basal cell layer |

## Results

### Toxicity after a single N-9 exposure is localized to the cervix

The importance of assessing the impact of multiple exposures of N-9 on epithelial integrity and inflammation was illustrated by the negative consequences of frequent N-9 exposures reported in clinical trials [20,26]. To determine if multiple applications of N-9 affected cervicovaginal tissue sensitivity and subsequent recovery rates of the damaged epithelium, Swiss Webster mice were treated with 1% unformulated N-9 once daily for 4 consecutive days. Following each application, a subset of mice was sacrificed and cervicovaginal tissues were harvested 10 min, 2 h, 4 h, and 8 h after each application and assessed for morphological damage (Figure 1A). The tissues were scored visually according to a four-point tissue scoring system (Table 1).

In control animals, saline application caused no damage to the cervicovaginal epithelium. At 2 h post-exposure, the vaginal (Figure 1B) and cervical (Figure 1C) epithelia were unaffected by a single exposure to saline. Similarly, no damage to the vaginal (Figure 1D) or cervical (Figure 1E) epithelia was apparent after four daily exposures to saline. Similar results were obtained at days 2 and 3, and after post-exposure durations shorter (10 min) or longer (4 h and 8 h) than 2 h (data not shown). Saline controls were considered representative of healthy tissue, since mock-exposed tissues and saline-exposed tissues were indistinguishable (data not shown).

A single exposure to N-9 also had a minimal effect on vaginal epithelial integrity. There was little to no damage to the vaginal epithelium detectable 10 min after a single exposure to 1% N-9 (Figure 2A), despite the concurrent appearance of moderate to severe damage in the cervix (Figure 2B). Although some indications of toxicity were apparent in the upper layers of the vaginal epithelium at 2 h post-exposure, this damage was very limited; the majority of the lower vaginal epithelium appeared to be intact (Figure 2C). At 4 h post-application, the vaginal

epithelium appeared to be unaffected by N-9 exposure (Figure 2E). At 8 h following the single application of N-9, light tissue sloughing was observed in the vagina (Figure 2G).

In sharp contrast, damage to the cervix was readily apparent by 10 min after a single application of N-9 (Figure 2B), with swelling of cells in the columnar epithelium, sloughing of the superficial layers of the epithelium, and presumed apoptosis. Severe sloughing across most of the superficial epithelium (leaving the basal layer intact) was consistently observed in the cervix 2 h post-application (Figure 2D). By 4 h post-exposure, there was scant superficial epithelium remaining with some foci showing complete epithelial denudation (Figure 2F). At 8 h post-exposure, very little of the superficial columnar cell layer of the cervical epithelium remained, leaving large areas of the deeper basal cell layer almost

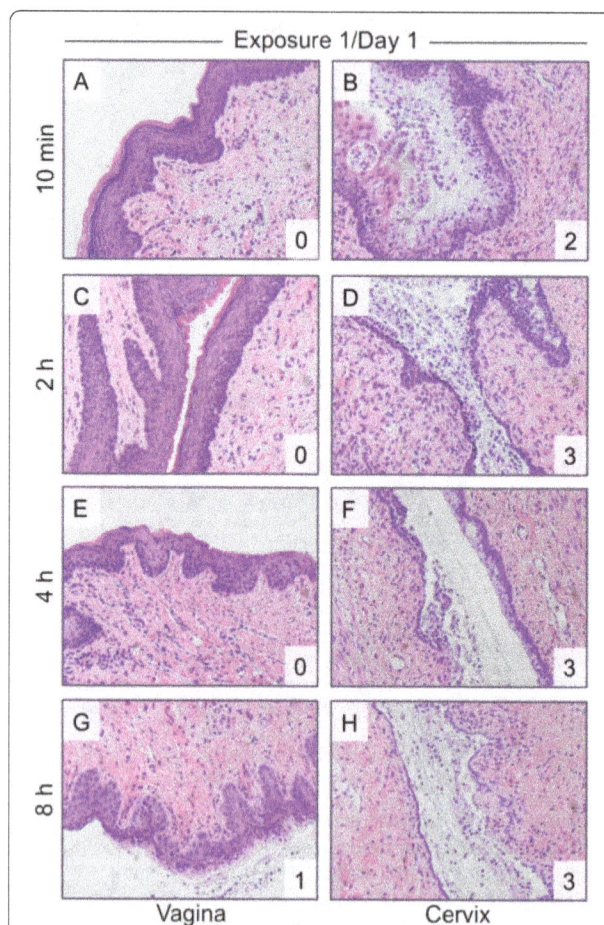

**Figure 2 After a single exposure to N-9, severe toxicity was observed in the cervix.** Mice were exposed once to unformulated N-9 at a concentration of 1% for the indicated durations. H&E-stained tissue sections (shown at 40× magnification) were assessed for vaginal (**A**, **C**, **E**, **G**) and cervical (**B**, **D**, **F**, **H**) epithelial toxicity and scored. The tissue damage score (see also Table 1) is shown in the lower right corner of each panel.

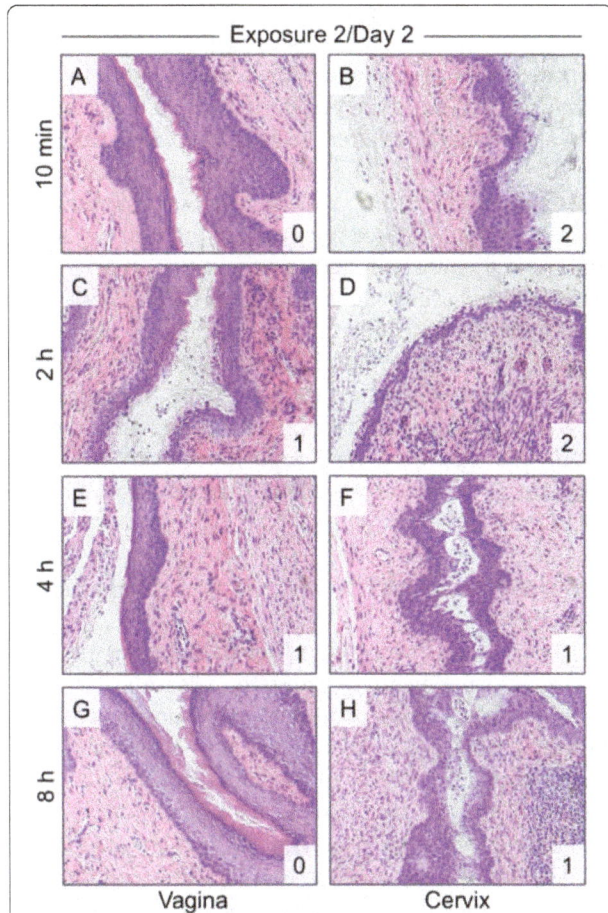

**Figure 3 Cervical epithelial damage is still apparent after two daily exposures to N-9.** Mice were exposed twice to unformulated 1% N-9 and sacrificed after the indicated post-exposure intervals following the second exposure. H&E-stained tissue sections (shown at 40x magnification) were assessed for vaginal (**A, C, E, G**) and cervical (**B, D, F, H**) epithelial toxicity and scored. The tissue damage score (see also Table 1) is shown in the lower right corner of each panel.

completely exposed. The majority of the mucosa contained only one or two layers of basal cells with larger areas of complete epithelial denudation (Figure 2H). By 24 h after N-9 application, however, the cervical epithelium more closely resembled saline-exposed tissue, suggesting a process of tissue repair during the preceding 16 hours (data not shown).

## Cervical sensitivity to N-9 exposure decreases with increasing exposure number

Assessments of tissue damage after the second exposure to N-9 continued to reveal minimal damage to the vaginal tissue and considerable toxicity in the cervix (Figure 3). Damage to the vagina after the second exposure was limited and isolated to the upper layers of the vaginal epithelium at 2 h post-exposure (Figure 3C). At 4 h after the second application, however, the majority of the vaginal

epithelium appeared to have a more compact histological presentation (Figure 3E). Although the integrity of the continuous epithelial barrier remained intact, the cell morphology appeared denser and more tightly connected. Damage to the cervix at 10 min and 2 h post-exposure was moderate, but less severe than after the first exposure (Figure 3B and D). However, moderate shedding of the epithelial layer was evident and occasional breaks in the epithelial lining, which exposed the lamina propria, were observed. Cervical epithelial repair was again evident by 24 h post-application (data not shown).

After the third N-9 exposure (Figure 4), the vaginal epithelium again appeared more compact and thinner (relative to saline-exposed tissue), especially on the lower layers of the stratified squamous epithelium. The cellular structure of the upper stratified layers appeared to have a

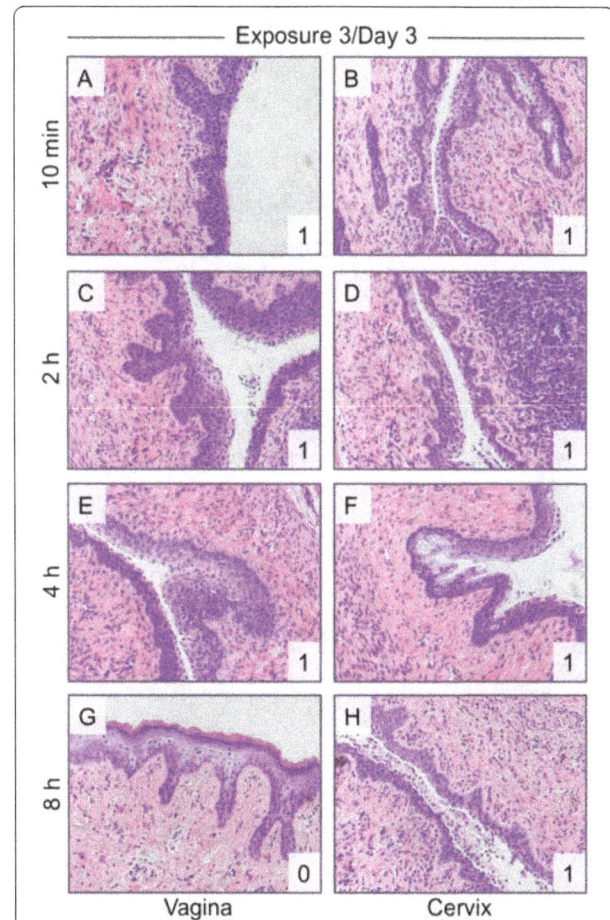

**Figure 4 Cervical epithelial damage is still apparent after three daily exposures to N-9.** Mice were exposed once daily over three days to unformulated 1% N-9 and sacrificed after the indicated post-exposure intervals following the third exposure. H&E-stained tissue sections (shown at 40x magnification) were assessed for vaginal (**A, C, E, G**) and cervical (**B, D, F, H**) epithelial toxicity and scored. The tissue damage score (see also Table 1) is shown in the lower right corner of each panel.

looser configuration, indicating that cells may have been in the process of being shed. However, the vaginal tissues were still continuous and intact, with no breaks in the tissue. Damage to the cervix after the third exposure was less at 10 min (Figure 4B) and 2 h post-exposure (Figure 4D) relative to the damage observed after like durations on day 2.

Following the fourth exposure, N-9 toxicity was evident again predominantly in the cervix (Figure 5). The vaginal epithelium was generally intact, with minimal cellular shedding in the upper layers of the mucosa at 10 min and 2 h post-application (Figure 5A and C). The lower layers of stratified squamous epithelium still exhibited a more compact appearance. However, tissues analyzed at 4 h and 8 h post-exposure were more similar to the control tissues (Figure 5E and G). As was observed on day 3, the cervical epithelium appeared to be more tolerant to N-9 exposure

after the fourth application relative to cervical epithelial tissues exposed once (day 1) or twice (day 2). With each daily exposure, the morphology of the cervix changed to a more compact structure, and appeared as a multi-layered structure at all time points after the fourth N-9 application (Figure 5B, D, F, and H). After the fourth application of 1% N-9, mucous-producing cells were absent in more than 50% of the N-9-exposed mice despite the recovery of the endocervical epithelium and reconstruction of an intact epithelial barrier over the lamina propria. This observation suggests the absence of normal mucous secretion. When tissue sections from the cervix were scored with respect to the degree of epithelial damage (Table 1), cervical epithelial damage scores at all four time points after the fourth daily exposure were significantly lower than corresponding damage scores recorded after the initial exposure on Day 1 (Table 2).

## Pro-inflammatory cytokine release varies after multiple N-9 exposures

Cervicovaginal lavages were also collected during the multiple exposure experiments to assess the release of cytokines subsequent to single or multiple exposures to N-9. We hypothesized that comparisons of pro-inflammatory cytokines released on days 1 and 4 would reveal notable differences, given the considerable and significant histological differences between cervical tissues subjected to one or four daily exposures to N-9. Because previous in vitro, rabbit, and human studies identified IL-1β and IL-6 as significant predictors of cervicovaginal toxicity following single or multiple exposures to N-9 [27,28], the present studies were focused on these factors.

Analyses of IL-1β release demonstrated that the first exposure to N-9 caused a small but steady increase in IL-1β protein release into the cervicovaginal lumen, with concentrations peaking at approximately ~10 pg/ml at 24 h post-exposure (Figure 6A). In contrast, IL-1β concentrations after the fourth N-9 exposure (Figure 6B) rapidly increased from baseline to ~115 pg/ml at 10 min post-exposure but returned to pre-exposure levels by 2 h.

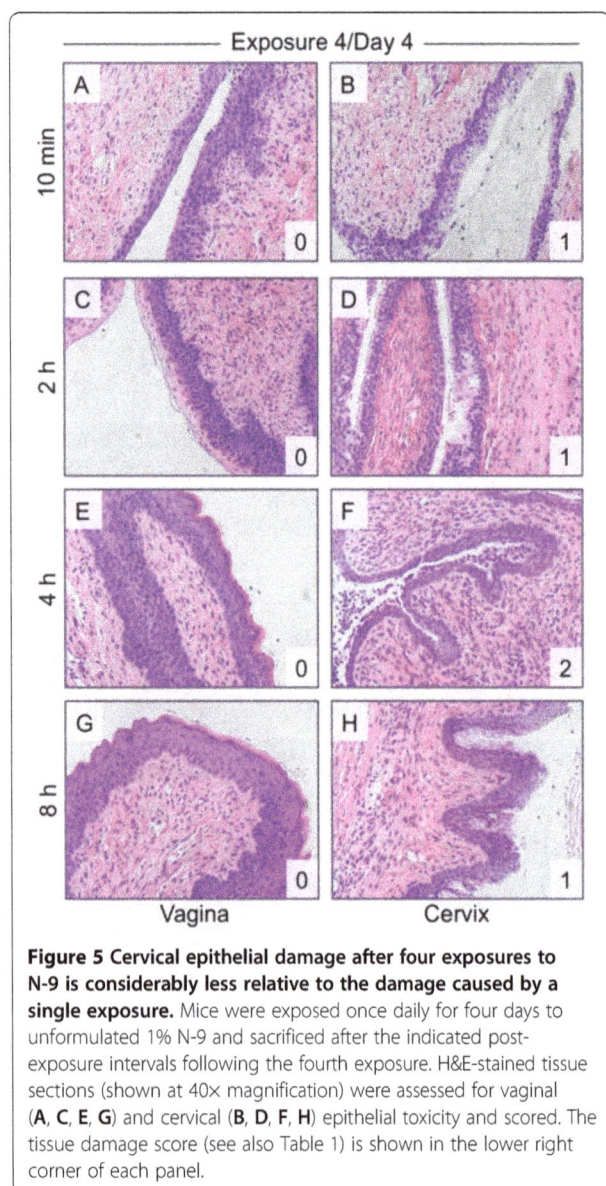

**Figure 5 Cervical epithelial damage after four exposures to N-9 is considerably less relative to the damage caused by a single exposure.** Mice were exposed once daily for four days to unformulated 1% N-9 and sacrificed after the indicated post-exposure intervals following the fourth exposure. H&E-stained tissue sections (shown at 40× magnification) were assessed for vaginal (**A**, **C**, **E**, **G**) and cervical (**B**, **D**, **F**, **H**) epithelial toxicity and scored. The tissue damage score (see also Table 1) is shown in the lower right corner of each panel.

**Table 2 Average damage scores for cervical epithelial tissues exposed to N-9**

|                        | N-9 exposure duration | | | |
|------------------------|-------------|-------------|-------------|-------------|
|                        | 10 min      | 2 h         | 4 h         | 8 h         |
| Exposure 1/Day 1       | 1.3 ± 0.3   | 3.0 ± 0.0   | 3.0 ± 0.0   | 3.0 ± 0.0   |
| Exposure 4/Day 4       | 0.0 ± 0.0   | 1.0 ± 0.0   | 1.7 ± 0.3   | 0.7 ± 0.3   |
| P value, Day 1 vs. Day 4 | 0.016     | <0.0001     | 0.016       | 0.002       |

After the first or the fourth daily exposure to N-9, mice were sacrificed following the indicated post-exposure intervals. Scores (as described in Table 1) were assigned to cervical tissue sections after multiple fields from three replicate mice at each time point within each exposure group were examined microscopically. Each value is expressed as an average score ± standard error. Significant differences between scores on Days 1 and 4 are indicated by p values less than 0.05 (as calculated by an unpaired Student's t-test).

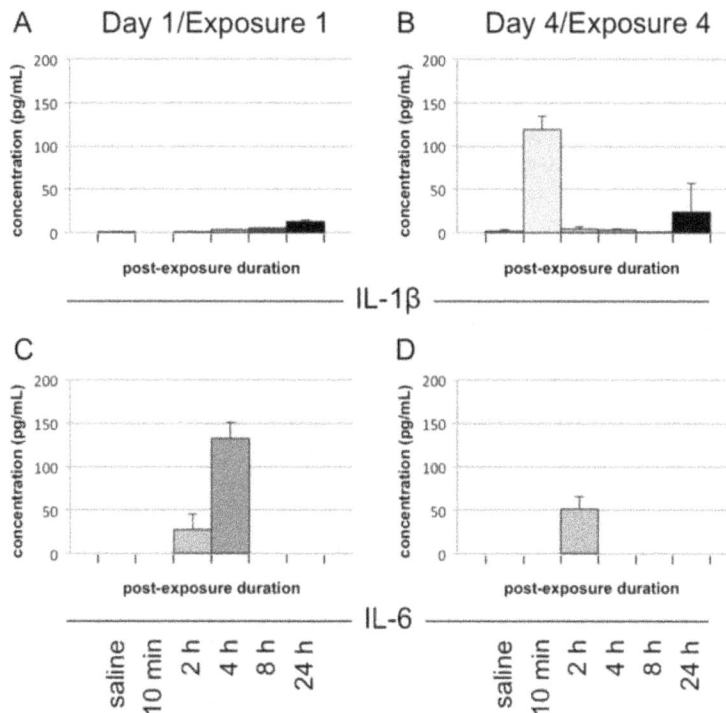

**Figure 6 IL-1β and IL-6 are differentially released following single and multiple exposures to N-9.** Female Swiss Webster mice were exposed once or once daily over 4 days to unformulated 1% N-9 and sacrificed after the indicated post-exposure intervals following the last exposure. Prior to sacrifice, saline cervicovaginal lavages were collected from the mice and analyzed for the presence of IL-1β (**A, B**) or IL-6 (**C, D**) using Luminex technology. The absence of a bar indicates no detectable cytokine release over background levels. Error bars indicate standard deviations on replicate data points.

A second but smaller release (~20 pg/ml) was detected at 24 h post-exposure. Interestingly, the levels of IL-1β release did not appear to correspond with the severity of cervical epithelial damage. Despite the appearance of moderate to severe damage between 10 min and 8 h post-exposure on day 1, increases in IL-1β were minimal. Conversely, the minimal cervical epithelial damage following the fourth exposure was accompanied by a large but transient increase in IL-1β release.

In contrast, IL-6 levels were consistent with the degree of cervical epithelial damage. On day 1 (Figure 6C), IL-6 release was first detected at 2 h post-exposure and peaked at 4 h (~130 pg/ml) before returning to baseline levels. After four daily N-9 applications (Figure 6D), IL-6 release was detected only at 2 h post-exposure at a considerably lower concentration (~50 pg/ml) relative to day 1. Both IL-6 release patterns paralleled the time course and severity of N-9-associated cervical epithelial damage. On day 1, the peak of IL-6 release corresponded with the severe damage to the cervical epithelia noted at 2–4 h post-exposure. On day 4, the comparatively lower level of IL-6 release was consistent with the reduced severity of epithelial damage and apparent tolerance to N-9 exposure, and coincided with the modest increase in epithelial damage observed at 4 h post-exposure.

## CD14+ cell infiltration in the cervix increases following a single N-9 exposure but declines after repeated daily exposures

Previous studies of N-9 toxicity in the mouse revealed intense infiltration of CD45-positive immune cells and Ly6-positive neutrophils subsequent to a 2 h exposure to unformulated N-9 [19,25]. In preliminary experiments designed to expand these findings, mice were given a single application of unformulated 1% N-9 and sacrificed at 2, 4, or 24 h post-exposure. Cells isolated from excised cervicovaginal tissues before or after N-9 exposure were analyzed by flow cytometry to identify the following immune cell populations: CD4+/CD3+ T lymphocytes, CD8+/CD3+ T lymphocytes, Ly6G + neutrophils, and CD14+/CD11C- monocytes/macrophages. In addition to the abundance of infiltrating neutrophils following N-9 exposure, these experiments indicated a 50% increase in the number of CD14+/CD11c- cells at 2 h post-exposure (data not shown). In addition, monocyte/macrophage infiltration appeared to decrease by 4 h post-exposure and returned to control levels by 24 h post-exposure (data not shown).

To localize macrophage/monocyte infiltration following single or multiple exposures to N-9 within the cervicovaginal epithelium and to confirm the preliminary findings,

CD14+ cells were visualized immunohistochemically in exposed tissues in conjunction with a CD14-specific antibody. Analyses of control tissues exposed once to saline revealed little infiltration by CD14+ cell populations into the vaginal (Figure 7A) or cervical (Figure 7B) epithelium. In contrast, tissues excised at 2 h post-exposure following a single N-9 exposure (day 1) were characterized by light infiltration into the vaginal epithelium (Figure 7C) and intense CD14 staining under the epithelial surface in the cervix (Figure 7D). Levels of CD14+ cell infiltration in the cervix were less at 4 h post-exposure and declined considerably at 24 h post-exposure (data not shown). These results indicated that CD14+ cell infiltration was concurrent with peak N-9-associated physical damage within the cervical epithelium after a single exposure.

Because peak cervical epithelial damage after four daily N-9 exposures was observed at 4 h post-exposure (Figure 5 and Table 2), similar analyses were performed on cervicovaginal tissues collected at 4 h post-exposure from mice after four daily N-9 applications. As was observed after a single N-9 exposure, few CD14+ cells were

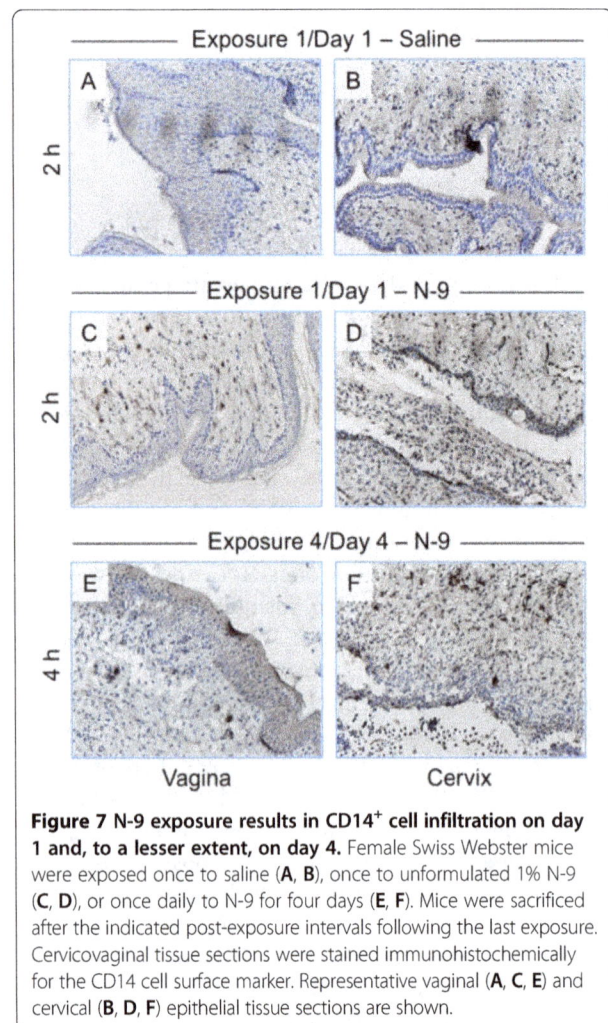

**Figure 7 N-9 exposure results in CD14+ cell infiltration on day 1 and, to a lesser extent, on day 4.** Female Swiss Webster mice were exposed once to saline (**A, B**), once to unformulated 1% N-9 (**C, D**), or once daily to N-9 for four days (**E, F**). Mice were sacrificed after the indicated post-exposure intervals following the last exposure. Cervicovaginal tissue sections were stained immunohistochemically for the CD14 cell surface marker. Representative vaginal (**A, C, E**) and cervical (**B, D, F**) epithelial tissue sections are shown.

observed in the day 4 vaginal epithelium (Figure 7E). In the cervical epithelium (Figure 7F), CD14+ cells were present in greater numbers relative to cell numbers in the corresponding vaginal tissues. However, cell infiltration was clearly not as intense as was noted at 2 h on day 1. Furthermore, the intense cervical sub-surface staining seen on day 1 was not apparent on day 4; infiltrating CD14+ cells were only present deeper in the lamina propria. CD14+ cell staining in the cervix at 4 h and 24 h post-exposure was also reduced relative to levels noted in cervical tissues on day 1 (data not shown). These results again indicate a parallel between physical epithelial damage and CD14+ cell infiltration within the cervix; apparent tolerance to N-9 exposure was accompanied by considerably lower levels of monocyte/macrophage infiltration.

## Discussion

Early efforts to develop a safe and effective microbicide ended with the observation that N-9, which had been used safely as a spermicidal agent for over four decades [9], was not only clinically ineffective against HIV-1 transmission, but was also capable of significantly increasing the risk of HIV-1 acquisition after repeated use [5]. These clinical trial results prompted a reassessment of mechanisms of N-9 toxicity and a general realization that a greater emphasis on pre-clinical microbicide safety was necessary.

One conclusion from post-failure analyses of N-9 microbicide development was that toxicity studies using the standard rabbit vaginal irritation (RVI) model provided an incomplete picture of the adverse effects of N-9 on the cervicovaginal epithelial tissues and the relevance of those effects to the risk of HIV-1 transmission. While the RVI model has provided important information regarding the safety of N-9 and other topical vaginal microbicides, there are limitations to the standard protocol. First, despite its demonstrated sensitivity to toxic topical agents, the RVI model does not assess product safety during the window of likely HIV-1 transmission. The standard RVI test protocol includes only one assessment of toxicity at 24 h after the final product application and does not provide for measures of toxicity at more acute post-exposure intervals, particularly the first hours after topical application when sexual intercourse and HIV-1 transmission are likely to occur. Our previous studies using the mouse model of cervicovaginal toxicity demonstrated that N-9- and C31G-mediated damage was greatest at 2 to 4 h post-exposure and was minimal or undetectable by 24 h post-application [19,24,25], presumably because epithelial repair mechanisms had restored the epithelium to its pre-exposure state. The standard RVI model would not reveal these important milestones in the time course of N-9 topical toxicity. Second, this model also differs from the human female reproductive tract

(FRT) in that the rabbit FRT (i) does not undergo cyclic reproductive stages, (ii) is not colonized by lactobacillus (resulting in a lack of acidity within the vaginal tract), (iii) lacks the production of cervicovaginal mucus, and (iv) is characterized by a columnar epithelium in the upper vagina (cervicovagina) and a stratified squamous epithelium in the lower vagina (urovagina) [29-32].

We developed a Swiss Webster murine model [19] to assess cervicovaginal tissue integrity and inflammation following exposure to candidate vaginal microbicides and to specifically address the need for an *in vivo* model system that can be used to provide pre-clinical results predictive of clinical trial outcomes. The Swiss Webster mouse is a readily accessible, outbred stock strain that has previously been used as a model for studies of various infectious cervicovaginal tract pathogens, including *Chlamydia trachomatis*, herpes simplex virus, and group B streptococci (GBS). These mice have also been used in various pre-clinical microbicide studies [33-37]. The Swiss Webster mouse model offers several distinct advantages over the RVI model and other approaches used for the evaluation of cervicovaginal toxicity and inflammation associated with exposure to topical microbicides. First, the Swiss Webster mouse is a relatively inexpensive animal model, permitting large, pre-clinical toxicity screens of candidate compounds under a variety of experimental conditions (including multiple exposure protocols) that can be used to evaluate cervicovaginal toxicity and inflammation at the cellular and tissue level prior to Phase I safety trials. Second, previously published observations from experiments involving this model [19,25] have indicated close parallels to clinical findings, demonstrating the value of this model as a prescreening tool to prevent costly and time-consuming clinical trials on compounds with unacceptable safety profiles. Third, the mouse model, unlike the RVI model system, can be used to assess regional differences in cervicovaginal toxicity. This is an important feature of this animal model system, since topical toxicity can be tissue-specific, as we have demonstrated in past studies [19,25,38]. Consideration of regional differences in FRT toxicity may be relevant to understanding mechanisms of HIV-1 transmission, since non-human primate studies of SIV cervicovaginal infection suggest that HIV-1 transmission within the FRT may be regionally constrained [39,40], perhaps by the nature of the epithelial barrier or by regional differences in the distribution of HIV-1-susceptible immune cell populations [41]. The model, however, is not without its limitations: the lack of colonizing lactobacillus (addressed only in the non-human primate model); a higher cervicovaginal pH relative to the human FRT; and the use of Depo-Provera to pretreat the animals prior to experimentation.

The present studies, through the single N-9 exposure aspect of these experiments, have confirmed observations reported in previously published studies [19,25]. First, the cervical epithelium is severely damaged by a single exposure to N-9, while the vaginal epithelium remains relatively intact. The damage to the cervical epithelium is characterized by breaks in the columnar tissue architecture and severe tissue sloughing. Second, N-9-associated cervical epithelial damage occurs relatively rapidly. After a single exposure to 1% N-9, the damage to the cervical epithelium was greatest at 2 to 4 h post-exposure. Third, physical damage can be accompanied by intense immune cell infiltration. Unlike the present studies, past experiments identified the infiltrating cells as positive for CD45, which is a pan-leukocyte cell surface marker. Finally, the damage caused by a single N-9 exposure is transient and resolved over a period of approximately 24 h post-exposure.

The single exposure results also suggest that tissue damage may not be strictly associated with the anatomy of the cervicovaginal tract. We consistently observed severe N-9-associated damage to the columnar epithelium of the cervix and minimal damage to the stratified squamous epithelium of the lower vagina. However, one of the vaginal sections (Figure 3C, Day 2/Exposure 2, 2 h) shows intact stratified squamous epithelium adjacent to damaged columnar epithelium (roughly the lower half of the field), which is presumed to be part of the upper vaginal tract. Under Depo-Provera pre-treatment, the upper vaginal tract assumes a morphology typified by a single layer of columnar cells overlying 1–2 layers of basal cells. These observations indicate that epithelial damage subsequent to N-9 application is dependent on the architecture of the epithelial tissue rather than its anatomical location, and that a columnar epithelium, regardless of its location, is more susceptible to N-9 toxicity than a stratified squamous epithelium.

The present studies also provide new information regarding N-9 toxicity that is relevant to increases in HIV-1 transmission after repeated exposure to N-9. During repeated daily exposures to unformulated 1% N-9, the cervical epithelium appeared to become less sensitive to the degradative effects of N-9 application. By the fourth application, the damage caused by N-9 application was less and the peak damage was observed at 4 h post-exposure rather than at 2 h post-exposure as seen following the first application of N-9. This observation suggests the possibility that changes in the epithelial architecture after the initial exposure, insult, inflammation, and repair provide a protective mechanism against the effects of subsequent N-9 exposure.

This apparent tolerance to N-9 exposure after multiple applications may likely be related to changes in cervical tissue morphology observed during these studies. After multiple N-9 exposures, the tissue appeared to be metaplastic, forming multiple layers of stratified squamous epithelium instead of the usual single layer of columnar epithelium overlying one or two layers of basal epithelium. This effect has been observed subsequent to stress applied to tissue over time [42]. The increased tolerance of this metaplastic tissue is consistent with the above conclusion that susceptibility to N-9-associated damage is dependent on tissue architecture rather than anatomical location, since the stratified cervical tissue observed in day 4 mice was more tolerant of N-9 exposure compared to the columnar cervical epithelial tissue found in day 1 mice. One focus of future studies will be to determine the amount of time required for repaired and tolerant tissues to return to their baseline structures and levels of susceptibility to damage.

The present studies also revealed new information about relationships between repeated N-9-associated damage and induced tissue inflammation. Following N-9 exposure, the release of the pro-inflammatory cytokines IL-1$\beta$ and IL-6 was detected in vaginal lavages, reinforcing the roles for these cytokines as important mediators of the inflammatory response in the vaginal tract in response to microbicide application [27,28]. However, only IL-6 release coincided with cervical epithelial damage (2–4 h postexposure) after the initial N-9 application. In contrast, minimal amounts of IL-1$\beta$ were detected on day 1. Conversely, IL-1$\beta$ was released quickly (10 min post-exposure) and in relatively large amounts on day 4 relative to day 1. While IL-6 release was also detected on day 4, the magnitude of release was considerably less. In all cases, cytokine increases were transient and returned to control levels by 8 to 24 h post-exposure as tissue regeneration was in progress. Although the significance of these observations has not yet been determined, the pattern of cytokine release suggests an association with tissue regeneration following multiple N-9 exposures and the development of tolerance to N-9 application.

Subsequent to N-9 exposure, CD14+ monocytes/macrophages were also detected as part of the immune cell infiltrate. The intense, sub-surface presence of CD14+ immune cells after the first exposure to N-9 coincided with the cervical localization of epithelial damage, the peak severity of damage at 2 to 4 h post-exposure, and the detection of IL-6 in the vaginal lavage. The association between IL-6 release and the presence of CD14+ immune cells suggests that the source of the IL-6 may be the monocyte/macrophage population within the infiltrate [43,44]. This hypothesis is also consistent with the concomitant decrease in CD14+ cells and reduction in released IL-6 at 8 and 24 h post-exposure, and with the association between the reduced levels of IL-6 and lower numbers of infiltrating CD14+ cells on day 4.

## Conclusions

These studies provide new insights and raise new questions about cervicovaginal damage associated with multiple exposures to topical agents with epithelial toxicity. Future studies will need to explore several aspects of these results, including the underlying mechanisms of cervicovaginal epithelial regeneration and tolerance to toxic agents, and the involvement of the inflammatory response in the process of tissue recovery. Additional experiments will need to examine the effects of multiple exposures to toxic agents such as N-9 during a single day, since increases in the risk of HIV-1 acquisition were attributed to multiple uses of N-9 within a single 24 h period [5]. Finally and most importantly, these studies suggest the need for multiple exposure protocols in future safety and efficacy assessments during the pre-clinical development of topical vaginal (and rectal) microbicides effective against HIV-1 transmission.

**Competing interests**

The authors declare that they have no competing interests.

**Authors' contributions**

KL established the study design, performed all experimental procedures, collected the data, analyzed the results, and prepared the manuscript. RO and BW participated in data analyses and the preparation of the manuscript. TKC contributed expertise in animal model studies and participated in data analyses. FCK participated in study planning, data analyses, and the preparation of the manuscript. All authors read and approved the final manuscript.

**Acknowledgements**

These studies were supported by a grant through the National Institute of Allergy and Infectious Diseases, National Institutes of Health (1 U19 AI076965). Dr. Krebs was also supported by faculty development funds provided by the Department of Microbiology and Immunology and the Institute for Molecular Medicine and Infectious Disease at the Drexel University College of Medicine.

**Author details**

[1]Department of Microbiology and Immunology, and Center for Molecular Therapeutics and Resistance, Center for Sexually Transmitted Disease, Institute for Molecular Medicine and Infectious Disease, Drexel University College of Medicine, 245 N. 15th Street, Philadelphia, PA 19102, USA. [2]Department of Pathology & Laboratory Medicine, Drexel University College of Medicine, 245 N. 15th Street, Philadelphia, PA 19102, USA.

**References**

1.  Global Report: UNAIDS report on the global AIDS epidemic 2010. http://www.unaids.org/globalreport/Global_report.htm.
2.  Ramjee G: **Microbicide research: current and future directions.** *Curr Opin HIV AIDS* 2010, 5(4):316–321.
3.  Nuttall J: **Microbicides in the prevention of HIV infection: current status and future directions.** *Drugs* 2010, 70(10):1231–1243.
4.  Minces LR, McGowan I: **Advances in the Development of Microbicides for the Prevention of HIV Infection.** *Curr Infect Dis Rep* 2010, 12(1):56–62.
5.  Van Damme L, Ramjee G, Alary M, Vuylsteke B, Chandeying V, Rees H, Sirivongrangson P, Mukenge-Tshibaka L, Ettiegne-Traore V, Uaheowitchai C, et al: **Effectiveness of COL-1492, a nonoxynol-9 vaginal gel, on HIV-1 transmission in female sex workers: a randomised controlled trial.** *Lancet* 2002, 360(9338):971–977.
6.  Peterson L, Nanda K, Opoku BK, Ampofo WK, Owusu-Amoako M, Boakye AY, Rountree W, Troxler A, Dominik R, Roddy R, et al: **SAVVY (C31G) gel for prevention of HIV infection in women: a Phase 3, double-blind, randomized, placebo-controlled trial in Ghana.** *PLoS One* 2007, 2(12):e1312.

7. Pirrone V, Wigdahl B, Krebs FC: The rise and fall of polyanionic inhibitors of the human immunodeficiency virus type 1. Antiviral Res 2011, 90(3):168–182.

8. Veazey RS: Microbicide safety/efficacy studies in animals: macaques and small animal models. Curr Opin HIV AIDS 2008, 3(5):567–573.

9. Hillier SL, Moench T, Shattock R, Black R, Reichelderfer P, Veronese F: In vitro and in vivo: the story of nonoxynol 9. J Acquir Immune Defic Syndr 2005, 39(1):1–8.

10. Benes S, McCormack WM: Inhibition of growth of Chlamydia trachomatis by nonoxynol-9 in vitro. Antimicrob Agents Chemother 1985, 27(5):724–726.

11. Kelly JP, Reynolds RB, Stagno S, Louv WC, Alexander WJ: In vitro activity of the spermicide nonoxynol-9 against Chlamydia trachomatis. Antimicrob Agents Chemother 1985, 27(5):760–762.

12. Asculai SS, Weis MT, Rancourt MW, Kupferberg AB: Inactivation of herpes simplex viruses by nonionic surfactants. Antimicrob Agents Chemother 1978, 13(4):686–690.

13. Jennings R, Clegg A: The inhibitory effect of spermicidal agents on replication of HSV-2 and HIV-1 in-vitro. J Antimicrob Chemother 1993, 32(1):71–82.

14. Malkovsky M, Newell A, Dalgleish AG: Inactivation of HIV by nonoxynol-9. Lancet 1988, 1(8586):645.

15. Krebs FC, Miller SR, Malamud D, Howett MK, Wigdahl B: Inactivation of human immunodeficiency virus type 1 by nonoxynol-9, C31G, or an alkyl sulfate, sodium dodecyl sulfate. Antiviral Res 1999, 43(3):157–173.

16. Polsky B, Baron PA, Gold JW, Smith JL, Jensen RH, Armstrong D: In vitro inactivation of HIV-1 by contraceptive sponge containing nonoxynol-9. Lancet 1988, 1(8600):1456.

17. Singh B, Cutler JC, Utidjian HM: Studies on development of a vaginal preparation providing both prophylaxis against venereal disease, other genital infections and contraception. 3. In vitro effect of vaginal contraceptive and selected vaginal preparations of Candida albicans and Trichomonas vaginalis. Contraception 1972, 5(5):401–411.

18. Cook RL, Rosenberg MJ: Do spermicides containing nonoxynol-9 prevent sexually transmitted infections? A meta-analysis. Sex Transm Dis 1998, 25(3):144–150.

19. Catalone BJ, Kish-Catalone TM, Budgeon LR, Neely EB, Ferguson M, Krebs FC, Howett MK, Labib M, Rando R, Wigdahl B: Mouse model of cervicovaginal toxicity and inflammation for preclinical evaluation of topical vaginal microbicides. Antimicrob Agents Chemother 2004, 48(5):1837–1847.

20. Roddy RE, Cordero M, Cordero C, Fortney JA: A dosing study of nonoxynol-9 and genital irritation. Int J STD AIDS 1993, 4(3):165–170.

21. Chvapil M, Droegemueller W, Owen JA, Eskelson CD, Betts K: tudies of nonoxynol-9. I. The effect on the vaginas of rabbits and rats. Fertil Steril 1980, 33(4):445–450.

22. Kaminsky M, Szivos MM, Brown KR, Willigan DA: Comparison of the sensitivity of the vaginal mucous membranes of the albino rabbit and laboratory rat to nonoxynol-9. Food Chem Toxicol 1985, 23(7):705–708.

23. Catalone BJ, Ferguson ML, Miller SR, Malamud D, Kish-Catalone T, Thakkar NJ, Krebs FC, Howett MK, Wigdahl B: Prolonged exposure to the candidate microbicide C31G differentially reduces cellular sensitivity to agent re-exposure. Biomed Pharmacother 2005, 59(8):460–468.

24. Catalone BJ, Miller SR, Ferguson ML, Malamud D, Kish-Catalone T, Thakkar NJ, Krebs FC, Howett MK, Wigdahl B: Toxicity, inflammation, and anti-human immunodeficiency virus type 1 activity following exposure to chemical moieties of C31G. Biomed Pharmacother 2005, 59(8):430–437.

25. Catalone BJ, Kish-Catalone TM, Neely EB, Budgeon LR, Ferguson ML, Stiller C, Miller SR, Malamud D, Krebs FC, Howett MK, et al: Comparative safety evaluation of the candidate vaginal microbicide C31G. Antimicrob Agents Chemother 2005, 49(4):1509–1520.

26. Roddy RE, Cordero M, Ryan KA, Figueroa J: A randomized controlled trial comparing nonoxynol-9 lubricated condoms with silicone lubricated condoms for prophylaxis. Sex Transm Infect 1998, 74(2):116–119.

27. Fichorova RN, Bajpai M, Chandra N, Hsiu JG, Spangler M, Ratnam V, Doncel GF: Interleukin (IL)-1, IL-6, and IL-8 predict mucosal toxicity of vaginal microbicidal contraceptives. Biol Reprod 2004, 71(3):761–769.

28. Fichorova RN, Tucker LD, Anderson DJ: The molecular basis of nonoxynol-9-induced vaginal inflammation and its possible relevance to human immunodeficiency virus type 1 transmission. J Infect Dis 2001, 184(4):418–428.

29. Noguchi K, Tsukumi K, Urano T: Qualitative and quantitative differences in normal vaginal flora of conventionally reared mice, rats, hamsters, rabbits, and dogs. Comparative medicine 2003, 53(4):404–412.

30. Costin GE, Raabe HA, Priston R, Evans E, Curren RD: Vaginal irritation models: the current status of available alternative and in vitro tests. Alternatives to laboratory animals: ATLA 2011, 39(4):317–337.

31. Eckstein P, Jackson MC, Millman N, Sobrero AJ: Comparison of vaginal tolerance tests of spermicidal preparations in rabbits and monkeys. Journal of reproduction and fertility 1969, 20(1):85–93.

32. Castle PE, Hoen TE, Whaley KJ, Cone RA: Contraceptive testing of vaginal agents in rabbits. Contraception 1998, 58(1):51–60.

33. Pal S, Fielder TJ, Peterson EM, de la Maza LM: Analysis of the immune response in mice following intrauterine infection with the Chlamydia trachomatis mouse pneumonitis biovar. Infect Immun 1993, 61(2):772–776.

34. Cox F: Prevention of group B streptococcal colonization with topically applied lipoteichoic acid in a maternal-newborn mouse model. Pediatr Res 1982, 16(10):816–819.

35. Bourne N, Stegall R, Montano R, Meador M, Stanberry LR, Milligan GN: Efficacy and toxicity of zinc salts as candidate topical microbicides against vaginal herpes simplex virus type 2 infection. Antimicrob Agents Chemother 2005, 49(3):1181–1183.

36. Milligan GN, Bernstein DI: Interferon-gamma enhances resolution of herpes simplex virus type 2 infection of the murine genital tract. Virology 1997, 229(1):259–268.

37. Milligan GN, Chu CF, Young CG, Stanberry LR: Effect of candidate vaginally-applied microbicide compounds on recognition of antigen by CD4+ and CD8+ T lymphocytes. Biol Reprod 2004, 71(5):1638–1645.

38. Lozenski K, Kish-Catalone T, Pirrone V, Rando RF, Labib M, Wigdahl B, Krebs FC: Cervicovaginal safety of the formulated, biguanide-based human immunodeficiency virus type 1 (HIV-1) inhibitor NB325 in a murine model. Journal of biomedicine & biotechnology 2011, 2011:941061.

39. Haase AT: Targeting early infection to prevent HIV-1 mucosal transmission. Nature 2010, 464(7286):217–223.

40. Li Q, Estes JD, Schlievert PM, Duan L, Brosnahan AJ, Southern PJ, Reilly CS, Peterson ML, Schultz-Darken N, Brunner KG, et al: Glycerol monolaurate prevents mucosal SIV transmission. Nature 2009, 458(7241):1034–1038.

41. Pudney J, Quayle AJ, Anderson DJ: Immunological microenvironments in the human vagina and cervix: mediators of cellular immunity are concentrated in the cervical transformation zone. Biol Reprod 2005, 73(6):1253–1263.

42. Cone RA, Hoen T, Wong X, Abusuwwa R, Anderson DJ, Moench TR: Vaginal microbicides: detecting toxicities in vivo that paradoxically increase pathogen transmission. BMC Infect Dis 2006, 6:90.

43. Grimm MC, Pavli P, Van de Pol E, Doe WF: Evidence for a CD14+ population of monocytes in inflammatory bowel disease mucosa–implications for pathogenesis. Clin Exp Immunol 1995, 100(2):291–297.

44. Clahsen T, Schaper F: Interleukin-6 acts in the fashion of a classical chemokine on monocytic cells by inducing integrin activation, cell adhesion, actin polymerization, chemotaxis, and transmigration. J Leukoc Biol 2008, 84(6):1521–1529.

# Permissions

The contributors of this book come from diverse backgrounds, making this book a truly international effort. This book will bring forth new frontiers with its revolutionizing research information and detailed analysis of the nascent developments around the world.

We would like to thank all the contributing authors for lending their expertise to make the book truly unique. They have played a crucial role in the development of this book. Without their invaluable contributions this book wouldn't have been possible. They have made vital efforts to compile up to date information on the varied aspects of this subject to make this book a valuable addition to the collection of many professionals and students.

This book was conceptualized with the vision of imparting up-to-date information and advanced data in this field. To ensure the same, a matchless editorial board was set up. Every individual on the board went through rigorous rounds of assessment to prove their worth. After which they invested a large part of their time researching and compiling the most relevant data for our readers.

The editorial board has been involved in producing this book since its inception. They have spent rigorous hours researching and exploring the diverse topics which have resulted in the successful publishing of this book. They have passed on their knowledge of decades through this book. To expedite this challenging task, the publisher supported the team at every step. A small team of assistant editors was also appointed to further simplify the editing procedure and attain best results for the readers.

Apart from the editorial board, the designing team has also invested a significant amount of their time in understanding the subject and creating the most relevant covers. They scrutinized every image to scout for the most suitable representation of the subject and create an appropriate cover for the book.

The publishing team has been an ardent support to the editorial, designing and production team. Their endless efforts to recruit the best for this project, has resulted in the accomplishment of this book. They are a veteran in the field of academics and their pool of knowledge is as vast as their experience in printing. Their expertise and guidance has proved useful at every step. Their uncompromising quality standards have made this book an exceptional effort. Their encouragement from time to time has been an inspiration for everyone.

The publisher and the editorial board hope that this book will prove to be a valuable piece of knowledge for researchers, students, practitioners and scholars across the globe.

# List of Contributors

**Helen Tomkinson**
AstraZeneca, Alderley Park, Macclesfield, UK

**John Kemp**
AstraZeneca, Alderley Park, Macclesfield, UK

**Stuart Oliver**
AstraZeneca, Alderley Park, Macclesfield, UK

**Helen Swaisland**
AstraZeneca, Alderley Park, Macclesfield, UK

**Maria Taboada**
AstraZeneca, Alderley Park, Macclesfield, UK

**Thomas Morris**
AstraZeneca, Alderley Park, Macclesfield, UK

**Almath M Spooner**
School of Pharmacy and Pharmaceutical Sciences, Trinity College Dublin, Dublin 2, Ireland

**Catherine Deegan**
Intensive Care Medicine, Adelaide and Meath Hospital, Dublin, Incorporating the National Children's Hospital, Tallaght, Dublin 24, Ireland

**Deirdre M D'Arcy**
School of Pharmacy and Pharmaceutical Sciences, Trinity College Dublin, Dublin 2, Ireland

**Caitriona M Gowing**
Intensive Care Medicine, Adelaide and Meath Hospital, Dublin, Incorporating the National Children's Hospital, Tallaght, Dublin 24, Ireland

**Maria B Donnelly**
Intensive Care Medicine, Adelaide and Meath Hospital, Dublin, Incorporating the National Children's Hospital, Tallaght, Dublin 24, Ireland

**Owen I Corrigan**
School of Pharmacy and Pharmaceutical Sciences, Trinity College Dublin, Dublin 2, Ireland

**Lawrence K Leung**
Centre of Studies in Primary Care, Queen's University, 220 Bagot Street, Kingston Ontario, Canada K7L 5E9
Department of Family Medicine, Queen's University, 220 Bagot Street, Kingston Ontario, Canada K7L 5E9
School of Medicine, Queen's University, Kingston General Hospital, 18 Stuart Street, Kingston Ontario, Canada K7L 3N6

**Francis M Patafio**
School of Medicine, Queen's University, Kingston General Hospital, 18 Stuart Street, Kingston Ontario, Canada K7L 3N6

**Walter W Rosser**
Centre of Studies in Primary Care, Queen's University, 220 Bagot Street, Kingston Ontario, Canada K7L 5E9.
Department of Family Medicine, Queen's University, 220 Bagot Street, Kingston Ontario, Canada K7L 5E9.
School of Medicine, Queen's University, Kingston General Hospital, 18 Stuart Street, Kingston Ontario, Canada K7L 3N6

**Jorge A Diaz**
Universidad Nacional de Colombia, Facultad de Ciencias, Departamento de Farmacia, Laboratorio de Asesorías e Investigaciones en Microbiología, 472. Ciudad Universitaria. Carrera 30 Calle 45. A.A.14490. Bogotá D. C. Colombia

**Edelberto Silva**
Universidad Nacional de Colombia, Facultad de Ciencias, Departamento de Farmacia, Laboratorio de Asesorías e Investigaciones en Microbiología, 472. Ciudad Universitaria. Carrera 30 Calle 45. A.A.14490. Bogotá D. C. Colombia

**Maria J Arias**
Vitalis Pharmaceutical, Proyectos Especiales, Carrera 7 No 156-80. Oficina No 1104. Bogotá D. C. Colombia

**María Garzón**
Universidad Nacional de Colombia, Facultad de Ciencias, Departamento de Farmacia, Laboratorio de Asesorías e Investigaciones en Microbiología, 472. Ciudad Universitaria. Carrera 30 Calle 45. A.A.14490. Bogotá D. C. Colombia

**Jessica Stahl**
Department of Pharmacology, Toxicology and Pharmacy, University of Veterinary Medicine Hannover, Foundation, Buenteweg 17, Hannover 30559, Germany

**Mareike Wohlert**
Department of Pharmacology, Toxicology and Pharmacy, University of Veterinary Medicine Hannover, Foundation, Buenteweg 17, Hannover 30559, Germany

**Manfred Kietzmann**
Department of Pharmacology, Toxicology and Pharmacy, University of Veterinary Medicine Hannover, Foundation, Buenteweg 17, Hannover 30559, Germany

**George I Eluwa**
Department of Operations Research, HIV/AIDS Program.
Population Council, Nigeria. Plot 759, Cadastral Zone
AO, Off Constitution Avenue, Central Business District,
Abuja, Nigeria
Department of Health Policy and Management, Diadem
Consults Ltd, Abuja, Nigeria

**Titilope Badru**
Department of Health Policy and Management, Diadem
Consults Ltd, Abuja, Nigeria

**Kesiena J Akpoigbe**
Society for Family Health, Abuja, Nigeria

**Howard A Smithline**
Department of Emergency Medicine, Tufts University
School of Medicine and Baystate Medical Center,
Springfield, MA, USA
Baystate Medical Center, 759 Chestnut Street, Springfield,
MA 01199, USA

**Michael Donnino**
Department of Emergency Medicine, Harvard University
School of Medicine and Beth Israel Deaconess Medical
Center, Boston, MA, USA

**David J Greenblatt**
Program in Pharmacology and Experimental Therapeutics,
Tufts University School of Medicine and Tufts Medical
Center, Boston, MA, USA

**Andreas Vilhelmsson**
Nordic School of Public Health (NHV), Box 121 33, SE-
402 42 Gothenburg, Sweden

**Tommy Svensson**
Department of Behavioural Sciences and Learning,
Linkoping University, Linkoping, Sweden

**Anna Meeuwisse**
School of Social Work, Lund University, Lund, Sweden

**Anders Carlsten**
Medical Products Agency, Uppsala, Sweden

**Abd-Rahman Marzilawati**
Division of Gastroenterology, Department of Medicine,
University of Malaya, Kuala Lumpur, Malaysia
Department of Medicine, Hospital Kuala Lumpur, Kuala
Lumpur, Malaysia

**Yen-Yew Ngau**
Department of Medicine, Hospital Kuala Lumpur, Kuala
Lumpur, Malaysia

**Sanjiv Mahadeva**
Division of Gastroenterology, Department of Medicine,
University of Malaya, Kuala Lumpur, Malaysia

**Prajakti A Kothare**
Eli Lilly and Company, Lilly Corporate Center,
Indianapolis, IN, USA

**Mary E Seger**
Eli Lilly and Company, Lilly Corporate Center,
Indianapolis, IN, USA

**Justin Northrup**
Eli Lilly and Company, Lilly Corporate Center,
Indianapolis, IN, USA

**Kenneth Mace**
Eli Lilly and Company, Lilly Corporate Center,
Indianapolis, IN, USA

**Malcolm I Mitchell**
Eli Lilly and Company, Lilly Corporate Center,
Indianapolis, IN, USA

**Helle Linnebjerg**
Eli Lilly and Company, Lilly Research Center, Earl Wood
Manor, Windlesham, Surrey GU20 6PH, UK

**Marie-Louise Johansson**
Department of Clinical Pharmacology and Regional
Pharmacovigilance Centre, Sahlgrenska University
Hospital, Gothenburg, Sweden

**Staffan Hägg**
Department of Drug Research/Clinical Pharmacology,
Linköping University, Linköping, Sweden

**Susanna M Wallerstedt**
Department of Clinical Pharmacology and Regional
Pharmacovigilance Centre, Sahlgrenska University
Hospital, Gothenburg, Sweden

**Yanelda García-Vega**
Clinical Investigation Department, Center for Genetic
Engineering and Biotechnology, P.O. Box 6332, Havana,
Cuba

**Idrian García-García**
Clinical Investigation Department, Center for Genetic
Engineering and Biotechnology, P.O. Box 6332, Havana,
Cuba

**Sonia E Collazo-Caballero**
"Hermanos Ameijeiras" Hospital, Dermatology Service,
Havana, Cuba

**Egla E Santely-Pravia**
"Hermanos Ameijeiras" Hospital, Dermatology Service,
Havana, Cuba

**Alieski Cruz-Ramírez**
Clinical Investigation Department, Center for Genetic
Engineering and Biotechnology, P.O. Box 6332, Havana,
Cuba

**Ángela D Tuero-Iglesias**
Clinical Investigation Department, Center for Genetic Engineering and Biotechnology, P.O. Box 6332, Havana, Cuba

**Cristian Alfonso-Alvarado**
"Hermanos Ameijeiras" Hospital, Dermatology Service, Havana, Cuba.

**Mileidys Cabrera-Placeres**
"Hermanos Ameijeiras" Hospital, Dermatology Service, Havana, Cuba

**Nailet Castro-Basart**
"Hermanos Ameijeiras" Hospital, Dermatology Service, Havana, Cuba

**Yaquelín Duncan-Roberts**
Clinical Investigation Department, Center for Genetic Engineering and Biotechnology, P.O. Box 6332, Havana, Cuba.

**Tania I Carballo-Treto**
"Hermanos Ameijeiras" Hospital, Clinical Laboratory Service, Havana, Cuba

**Josanne Soto-Matos**
"Hermanos Ameijeiras" Hospital, Clinical Laboratory Service, Havana, Cuba

**Yoandy Izquierdo-Toledo**
Genomics Department, Center for Genetic Engineering and Biotechnology, Havana, Cuba

**Dania Vázquez-Blomquist**
Genomics Department, Center for Genetic Engineering and Biotechnology, Havana, Cuba

**Elizeth García-Iglesias**
Clinical Investigation Department, Center for Genetic Engineering and Biotechnology, P.O. Box 6332, Havana, Cuba

**Iraldo Bello-Rivero**
Clinical Investigation Department, Center for Genetic Engineering and Biotechnology, P.O. Box 6332, Havana, Cuba

**Marianne Jennifer Ratcliffe**
Personalised Healthcare and Biomarkers, AstraZeneca R&D Alderley Park, Cheshire, SK 10 4TG, UK

**Iain Gordon Dougall**
IGD Consultancy Limited, Loughborough, LE 11 3JR, UK

**Thomas Babcock**
Shire Development LLC, 725 Chesterbrook Blvd, Wayne, PA 19087, USA

**Bryan Dirks,**
Shire Development LLC, 725 Chesterbrook Blvd, Wayne, PA 19087, USA

**Ben Adeyi**
Shire Development LLC, 725 Chesterbrook Blvd, Wayne, PA 19087, USA

**Brian Scheckner**
Shire Development LLC, 725 Chesterbrook Blvd, Wayne, PA 19087, USA

**Andreas Vilhelmsson**
Nordic School of Public Health, Gothenburg, Sweden

**Tommy Svensson**
Nordic School of Public Health, Gothenburg, Sweden Department of Behavioural Sciences and Learning, Linkoping University, Linkoping, Sweden

**Anna Meeuwisse**
School of Social Work, Lund University, Lund, Sweden

**Anders Carlsten**
Medical Products Agency, Uppsala, Sweden

**Christian de Mey**
ACPS - Applied Clinical Pharmacology Services, Mainz-Kastel, Germany

**Nassr Nassr**
Nycomed GmbH, Konstanz, Germany

**Gezim Lahu**
Nycomed GmbH, Konstanz, Germany

**Deirdre M D'Arcy**
School of Pharmacy and Pharmaceutical Sciences, Trinity College Dublin, Dublin 2, Ireland

**Eoin Casey**
Intensive Care Medicine, Tallaght Hospital, Dublin 24, Ireland

**Caitriona M Gowing**
Pharmacy Department, Tallaght Hospital, Dublin 24, Ireland

**Maria B Donnelly**
Intensive Care Medicine, Tallaght Hospital, Dublin 24, Ireland

**Owen I Corrigan**
School of Pharmacy and Pharmaceutical Sciences, Trinity College Dublin, Dublin 2, Ireland

**Pekka Rapeli**
Department of Psychiatry. Helsinki University Central Hospital, Finland

Department of Mental Health and Substance Abuse Services, National Institute for Health and Welfare (THL), Finland
Institute of Behavioural Sciences, University of Helsinki, Finland

**Carola Fabritius**
Department of Mental Health and Substance Abuse Services, National Institute for Health and Welfare (THL), Finland

**Hely Kalska**
Institute of Behavioural Sciences, University of Helsinki, Finland

**Hannu Alho**
Department of Mental Health and Substance Abuse Services, National Institute for Health and Welfare (THL), Finland
Research Unit of Substance AbuseMedicine, University of Helsinki, Finland

**Tobias Dreischulte**
Tayside Medicines Unit, NHS Tayside, Mackenzie Building, Kirsty Semple Way, Dundee, Scotland, DD2 4BF, UK.

**Aileen M Grant**
Population Health Sciences, University of Dundee, Mackenzie Building, Kirsty Semple Way, Dundee, Scotland, DD2 4BF, UK

**Colin McCowan**
Population Health Sciences, University of Dundee, Mackenzie Building, Kirsty Semple Way, Dundee, Scotland, DD2 4BF, UK

**John J McAnaw**
NHS 24 East Contact Centre, 2 Ferrymuir, South Queensferry, Scotland, EH3 0 9QZ, UK

**Bruce Guthrie**
Population Health Sciences, University of Dundee, Mackenzie Building, Kirsty Semple Way, Dundee, Scotland, DD2 4BF, UK

**Shmeylan A Al Harbi**
Intensive Care Department, King Abdulaziz Medical City, Riyadh, Saudi Arabia.

**Hani M Tamim**
Epidemiology and Biostatistics, College of Medicine, King Saud bin Abdulaziz University for Health Sciences, King Abdulaziz Medical City, Riyadh, Saudi Arabia

**Yaseen M Arabi**
Intensive Care Department, Medical Director, Respiratory Services, and Associate Professor, College of Medicine, King Saud bin Abdulaziz University for Health Sciences, King Abdulaziz Medical City, Riyadh, Saudi Arabia

**Warren Winick-Ng**
Department of Biomedical Sciences, University of Guelph, Guelph, Ontario N1G 2W1, Canada

**Francesco Leri**
Department of Psychology, University of Guelph, Guelph, Ontario N1G 2W1, Canada

**Bettina E Kalisch**
Department of Biomedical Sciences, University of Guelph, Guelph, Ontario N1G 2W1, Canada

**Karissa Lozenski**
Department of Microbiology and Immunology, and Center for Molecular Therapeutics and Resistance, Center for Sexually Transmitted Disease, Institute for Molecular Medicine and Infectious Disease, Drexel University College of Medicine, 245 N. 15th Street, Philadelphia, PA 19102, USA

**Robert Ownbey**
Department of Pathology & Laboratory Medicine, Drexel University College of Medicine, 245 N. 15th Street, Philadelphia, PA 19102, USA

**Brian Wigdahl**
Department of Microbiology and Immunology, and Center for Molecular Therapeutics and Resistance, Center for Sexually Transmitted Disease, Institute for Molecular Medicine and Infectious Disease, Drexel University College of Medicine, 245 N. 15th Street, Philadelphia, PA 19102, USA

**Tina Kish-Catalone**
Department of Microbiology and Immunology, and Center for Molecular Therapeutics and Resistance, Center for Sexually Transmitted Disease, Institute for Molecular Medicine and Infectious Disease, Drexel University College of Medicine, 245 N. 15th Street, Philadelphia, PA 19102, USA

**Fred C Krebs**
Department of Microbiology and Immunology, and Center for Molecular Therapeutics and Resistance, Center for Sexually Transmitted Disease, Institute for Molecular Medicine and Infectious Disease, Drexel University College of Medicine, 245 N. 15th Street, Philadelphia, PA 19102, USA